Human Development and Performance

Throughout the Lifespan

Human Development and Performance

Throughout the Lifespan

Edited by

Anne Cronin, PhD, OTR/L, BCP
Associate Professor
West Virginia University
Morgantown, West Virginia

MaryBeth Mandich, PT, PhD
Professor and Chairperson
Division of Physical Therapy
West Virginia University
Morgantown, West Virginia

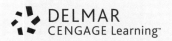

DELMAR
CENGAGE Learning

Australia • Brazil • Japan • Korea • Mexico • Singapore • Spain • United Kingdom • United States

DELMAR
CENGAGE Learning™

Human Development and Performance Throughout the Lifespan, First Edition
Anne Cronin, MaryBeth Mandich

Vice President, Health Care Business Unit:
William Brottmiller

Editorial Director: Cathy L. Esperti

Acquisitions Editor: Kalen Conerly

Developmental Editor: Juliet Byington

Editorial Assistant: James Duncan

Marketing Director: Jennifer McAvey

Marketing Coordinator: Chris Manion

Project Editor: Daniel Branagh

Art & Design Specialist: Connie
Lundberg-Watkins

Production Coordinator: Jessica McNavich

For product information and technology assistance, contact us at
Cengage Learning Customer & Sales Support, 1-800-354-9706

For permission to use material from this text or product,
submit all requests online at **www.cengage.com/permissions**
Further permissions questions can be emailed to
permissionrequest@cengage.com

Library of Congress Control Number: 2004004493

ISBN-13: 978-0-7668-4260-1

ISBN-10: 0-7668-4260-6

Delmar
Executive Woods
5 Maxwell Drive
Clifton Park, NY 12065
USA

Cengage Learning is a leading provider of customized learning solutions with office locations around the globe, including Singapore, the United Kingdom, Australia, Mexico, Brazil, and Japan. Locate your local office at **www.cengage.com/global**

Cengage Learning products are represented in Canada by Nelson Education, Ltd.

To learn more about Delmar, visit **www.cengage.com/delmar**

Purchase any of our products at your local bookstore or at our preferred online store **www.ichapters.com**

Printed in the United States of America
8 9 10   14 13 12

Dedication

We would like to express our appreciation to West Virginia University for the time and administrative support given us in order to be able to work on this project. We would also like to thank our faculty and staff colleagues, who helped us in so many ways, including writing case studies, editing, advising, and reviewing. As pediatric therapists, we would also like to thank all the children and their families who have so enriched our professional lives over the years and who have taught us so much. As academicians, we would like to thank all the students who have been in our classrooms, listened to our thoughts and information, and ultimately joined us as professional colleagues.

We would like to especially dedicate this book to the young people who are closest to us, who have provided balance and perspective to our busy professional lives, and who have been a source of joy and fulfillment:

Our children:

Bronwyn and James Cockburn (AC)

and

Heather, Sam, Scott, and Ben Harris (MBM)

Finally, a special dedication for Andrew Cockburn, husband of Anne Cronin, who has supported us in innumerable ways, from doing most of the housework in the last weeks before our publication deadline, to occupying the kids, and editing our reference pages into a consistent format. Without his support this effort would be far weaker.

Contents

PART 2   *Lifestage Characteristics*

CHAPTER 6
Prenatal Development
ELSIE R. VERGARA, SCD, OTR, FAOTA

CHAPTER 7
The Newborn
MARYBETH MANDICH, PT, PhD

CHAPTER 8
Infancy
MARYBETH MANDICH, PT, PhD

CHAPTER 9
Family and Disability Issues through Infancy
DIANNE KOONTZ-LOWMAN, EdD, OTR

CHAPTER 10
Development in the Preschool Years
ANNE CRONIN, PhD, OTR/L, BCP

CHAPTER 11
Middle Childhood and School
ANNE CRONIN, PhD, OTR/L, BCP

PART 3 *Special Topics in Human Performance*

Preface

The purpose of this text is to provide entry-level students who plan to work in rehabilitation disciplines such as occupational and physical therapy an overview of normative life tasks and roles across the lifespan. The impact of disease or disability on these normative roles is further considered in the text. Our intent has been to provide a resource that integrates information in a contemporary frame of reference—that is, the World Health Organization's International Classification of Function (ICF)—with a developmental life-task perspective. The text also serves as a resource for practicing professionals, especially those who were not educated in the conceptual framework of newer models, such as the ICF.

Since the 1960s there has been a significant change in a short period of time—one that might be considered a revolution—in the fields of disability. This revolution has significantly changed our perspectives of human function and disability, and its societal implications have had a major impact on public policy in the United States. The evidence of this impact is the passage of many pieces of legislation guaranteeing the individual with a disability the right to participate in societal functions, including the right to education and the right to employment. The sociologic models of disability, culminating in the World Health Organization models, the International Classification of Impairment, Disability & Handicap (ICIDH) model, and, most recently, the International Classification of Function (ICF) Disability and Health model, have resulted in an enduring shift in perspective that impacts all who work in the disability field.

The shift in perspective just described may be summarized as follows. First, it is impossible and erroneous to equate a medical diagnosis with function. Although such diagnoses have functional implications, they do not necessitate a definitive functional prognosis. Second, the outcome measures of success in working with individuals with a disability must be viewed at the level at which the individual is able to assume or resume those normal roles, both personal and societal, that are naturally characteristic and generally viewed as desirable. These normative roles change across the lifespan. Finally, and most recently recognized in the ICF scheme, barriers and facilitators to this optimum outcome are both intrinsic to the individual (such as motivation) and extrinsic (such as public policy allowing access to transportation, employment, and education).

NEED FOR THIS TEXT

Our experience is that there is not currently a resource available that integrates information from a number of core disciplines to permit easy understanding of the newer concepts of function and disability. Professionals such as occupational and physical therapists have always studied lifespan human development. They have also studied medical sciences, psychology, sociology, and professional roles. However, the paradigm shifts just described will demand that the rehabilitation professional of the twenty-first century be able to integrate knowledge of normative developmental life roles or tasks with other information to assist individuals with disabilities to maximize their function. The ICF model forms the conceptual foundation for the text, with a secondary developmental framework.

This text meets the needs of entry-level professionals by preparing them to look at a disability from a functional life-tasks perspective. Although lifespan development has traditionally been considered foundational knowledge, upon which to build an understanding of pathology, recent social and legislative trends have demanded an increased application of developmental information in setting goals and planning interventions. Increasingly, reimbursement for rehabilitation, especially occupational and physical therapy, is currently based on the ability to reflect and document the impact of impairment on the individual's function in interpersonal, social, and environmental contexts.

No prior knowledge of human development or disability models is required to use this text, commensurate with the entry-level target audience. However, exposure to basic anatomy and physiology will help the student understand the physical-characteristics section of each chapter. A prior course in lifespan human development, such as developmental psychology, will help the student grasp the concepts presented in the text.

ORGANIZATION OF TEXT

The text is organized into three main sections: Human Performance (an introduction to the subject), Lifestage Characteristics, and Special Topics in Human Performance. The first section, "Human Performance," introduces the reader to the newer conceptual and theoretical models in the field of disability. All health-related professionals are encouraged to develop cultural competence during their education, and the chapter on culture is designed to contribute to that knowledge. Finally, the concept of communication as an important functional concept across the lifespan is discussed. The second section of the book, "Lifestage Characteristics," follows a traditional developmental framework; however, basic physiologic content is presented in every chapter as an introduction, as well as the developmental characteristics of the particular lifestage. Few texts combine the 360-degree approach to the study of human development across body systems, as well as dimensions of performance (motor, psychologic, sociologic), as this text does. Interspersed in this section are chapters addressing the impact of disability at various life stages.

The final section of the book, "Special Topics in Human Performance," presents some contemporary topics for occupational and physical therapists, as well as others. The notion of Societal Factors from the ICF is discussed in the "Environmental Contexts" and "Public Policy and Health Care" chapters. The "Wellness and Health Promotion" chapter prepares the reader to discuss and analyze her professional role in this newest addition to the ICF paradigm. Finally, the "Assessment of Human Performance across the Lifespan" chapter introduces the reader to the concept of accountability for practice through measurement. This is an important part of documentation and outcomes research for all disciplines.

FEATURES OF TEXT

The text provides the reader with a large amount of information on lifespan development, organized around the conceptual framework of the ICF. Many chapters have case studies based on true clinical situations, which help the student apply the information in the text to the practical setting. In addition, most chapters have a section called "Speaking of . . .". These sections are informal notes from individuals—both professionals and family members of individuals with disabilities—about the application of content in the chapter. They bring to life the real challenges and experiences of individuals who have unique perspectives on the issues discussed in each chapter. These notes are intended to help the reader with the "emotional intelligence" aspect of learning.

SUPPLEMENTARY PACKAGE FOR INSTRUCTOR

An instructor's manual with three main components accompanies this text. The first component is the critical-thinking guide. For each chapter, a minimum of three questions have been selected to guide the students' thinking about the content presented. The questions are suitable for in-class discussion, small-group work, or essay questions on tests. The second component of the instructor's manual is the laboratory experiences. These are guides for activities that reinforce the chapter learning. They include such activities as Web searches and analysis of current literature. Forms are also included to allow students to analyze movement patterns of individuals across the lifespan. The final component of the instructor's manual is multiple-choice exam questions. These three components have been carefully designed to provide instructors with key tools to help facilitate student comprehension that will follow them into their professional lives.

FEEDBACK

The authors welcome comments and feedback about this text and may be contacted at the following addresses:

Anne Cronin, PhD, OTR/L, BCP
Division of Occupational Therapy
PO Box 1939
West Virginia University
Morgantown, West Virginia 26506-9139
acronin@hsc.wvu.edu

MaryBeth Mandich, PT, PhD
Division of Physical Therapy
PO Box 9226
West Virginia University
Morgantown, West Virginia 26506-9226
mmandich@hsc.wvu.edu

ACKNOWLEDGMENTS

We would like to acknowledge all those who provided us assistance in writing this text. First, to West Virginia University, which provided time and support for this endeavor. Second, our faculty colleagues who helped by taking on extra tasks so that we could be free to write deserve a special thanks. Finally, several staff, including Patti Clawges and Linda Stankos, assisted with copying and compilation of the manuscript.

We would like to thank all those who contributed to this book. First, to our chapter authors, who are all busy professionals, and who did an outstanding job in their work on this text. Second, to all the therapists who provided case studies from their practical experience—you helped to make the text applicable and relevant. Finally, to therapists and family members of individuals with disabilities who wrote "Speaking of . . ." sections and who told us "the rest of the story"—the effort would have been much less meaningful without your contribution.

Contributing Authors

Anne Cronin, PhD, OTR/L, BCP
Associate Professor
Division of Occupational Therapy
West Virginia University
Morgantown, West Virginia

Sandee Dunbar, DPA, OTR/L
Associate Professor
Nova Southeastern University
Fort Lauderdale, Florida

Bernadette Hattjar, MEd, OTR
Occupational Therapy
Florida A & M University
Tallahassee, Florida

Barbara L. Kornblau, JD, OT/L, FAOTA,
    DAAPM, CCM, CDMS
Professor, Occupational Therapy and Law
Nova Southeastern University
Fort Lauderdale, Florida

Toby Long, PhD, PT
Associate Professor, Department of
    Pediatrics
Associate Director for Training, Center for
    Child and Human Development
Director, Division of Physical Therapy, Center
    for Child and Human Development
Georgetown University
Washington, D.C.

Dianne Koontz-Lowman, EdD, OTR
Assistant Professor
Department of Occupational Therapy
Virginia Commonwealth University
Richmond, Virginia

MaryBeth Mandich, PT, PhD
Professor and Chairperson
Division of Physical Therapy
West Virginia University
Morgantown, West Virginia

Diana Middleton-Davis, OTR/L
Assistant Professor
Division of Occupational Therapy
West Virginia University
Morgantown, West Virginia

Susannah Grimm Poe, EdD
Assistant Professor
Department of Pediatrics
WVU School of Medicine
WG Klingberg Center for Child Development
Morgantown, West Virginia

Christine L. Raber, MS, OTR/L
Assistant Professor
Department of Occupational Therapy
Shawnee State University
Portsmouth, Ohio

Pamela Reynolds, PT, EdD
Associate Professor
Gannon University
Erie, Pennsylvania

Dennis M. Ruscello, PhD
Professor of Speech Pathology and Audiology
Adjunct Professor of Otolaryngology
Department of Speech Pathology and
    Audiology
West Virginia University
Morgantown, West Virginia

Winifred Schultz-Krohn, PhD, OTR, BCP, FAOTA
Associate Professor of Occupational Therapy
San Jose State University
San Jose, California

Keiba Shaw, EdD, PT
Assistant Professor
University of South Florida
Tampa, Florida

Dianne F. Simons, PhD, OTR/L
Assistant Professor
Department of Occupational Therapy
Virginia Commonwealth University
Richmond, Virginia

Ralph Utzman, PT, MPH
Assistant Professor
Division of Physical Therapy
West Virginia University
Morgantown, West Virginia

Elsie R. Vergara, ScD, OTR, FAOTA
Occupational Therapy Program
Department of Rehabilitation Sciences
Sargent College, Boston University
Boston, Massachusetts

Steven Wheeler, PhD, OTR/L
Assistant Professor
Division of Occupational Therapy
West Virginia University
Morgantown, West Virginia

Contributors:
Case Studies and
"Speaking of . . ."

Colleen Anderson
Senior Parent Network Specialist
WVU Center for Excellence in Disabilities
Robert C. Byrd Health Sciences Center
West Virginia University
Morgantown, West Virginia
"Speaking of . . ." Chapter 14

Cristina H. Bolanos, PhD, OT
Instituto de Terapia Ocupacional
General Director
Mexico City, Mexico
"Speaking of . . ." Chapter 4

Ann Chester, PhD
Assistant Vice-President for Social Justice
WVU Health Sciences Center
West Virginia University
Morgantown, West Virginia
"Speaking of . . ." Chapter 15

Carrie Cobun
Parent Resource Specialist
WVU Klingberg Center for Child Development
West Virginia University
Morgantown, West Virginia
"Speaking of . . ." Chapter 13

Anne Cronin, PhD, OTR/L, BCP
Associate Professor
Division of Occupational Therapy
West Virginia University
Morgantown, West Virginia
"Speaking of . . ." Chapters 2, 3, 5, 6, 10, and 19

Colleen Cronin
Senior citizen and retired dietician
Mooresville, North Carolina
"Speaking of . . ." Chapter 16

Scott Davis, PT, MS, OCS
Assistant Professor
Division of Physical Therapy
West Virginia University
Case 2, Chapter 12

Barbara Haase, MHS, OTR, BCN
Occupational Therapist
and
Richard Haase, MA
Rehabilitation Counselor
Huron, Ohio
"Speaking of . . ." Chapter 16

Tracy Hough, BS, AS
Staff COTA
University of Pittsburgh Medical Center
    Shadyside
Pittsburgh, Pennsylvania
"Speaking of . . ." Chapter 15

Susan Lynch, MD
Assistant Professor
Department of Pediatrics, Section of
    Neonatology
West Virginia University
Morgantown, West Virginia
"Speaking of . . ." Chapter 8

Corrie Mancinelli, PT, PhD
Associate Professor
Division of Physical Therapy
West Virginia University
Morgantown, West Virginia
"Speaking of . . ." Chapter 17

MaryBeth Mandich, PT, PhD
Professor and Chairperson
Division of Physical Therapy
West Virginia University
Morgantown, West Virginia
"Speaking of . . ." Chapters 1, 7, and 18
Case 1, Chapter 6

Hannah McMonagle
Parent
Morgantown, West Virginia
"Speaking of . . ." Chapter 11

Andrea Earle Mullins, MS, OTR/L
Occupational Therapist
Grafton School
Richmond, Virginia
"Speaking of . . ." Chapter 12

Hugh Murray, PT, DMDT
President, Huntington Physical Therapy
Huntington, West Virginia
"Speaking of . . ." Chapter 20

Jenny Patterson, MOT
Staff Occupational Therapist
Ruby Memorial Hospital
Morgantown, West Virginia
"Speaking of . . ." Chapter 21

Jane Pertko, PT, GCS
Morgantown, West Virginia
Case 1, Chapter 16

Susie Ritchie, RN, MPH, CPNP
Research Associate Professor
Department of Pediatrics
West Virginia University
Morgantown, West Virginia
"Speaking of . . ." Chapter 9

About the Editors

ANNE CRONIN, PhD, OTR/L, BCP, has been practicing pediatric occupational therapy for many years. She received her BS in occupational therapy from the University of Missouri and an MA in health services management from Webster University in St. Louis, Missouri. Her PhD was received from the University of Florida in medical sociology. Dr. Cronin has taught extensively in occupational therapy curricula, including content in human development, research, clinical practice of occupational therapy, pediatrics, and educational practice. Her own research interests include community integration of children with disabilities, feeding and swallowing, and pediatric occupational therapy practice issues. Dr. Cronin is currently an associate professor of occupational therapy at West Virginia University.

MARYBETH MANDICH, PT, PhD, has been practicing pediatric physical therapy for many years. She received BS and MS degrees in physical therapy from the Medical College of Virginia/Virginia Commonwealth University. She went on to receive a PhD in development psychology from West Virginia University, with a major area of emphasis in infancy and a minor area of emphasis in developmental neurobiology. Dr. Mandich has taught extensively in physical therapy curricula, including content in neuroanatomy and neurophysiology, embryology, human development, and pediatric and adult neurologic rehabilitation and research. Her own research interests have focused primarily on premature, high-risk infants. She has published studies on both outcome and effects of therapeutic intervention for this population. Dr. Mandich is currently a professor of physical therapy at West Virginia University.

Human Performance

Human Performance, Function, and Disablement

MaryBeth Mandich, PT, PhD
Professor and Chairperson
Division of Physical Therapy
West Virginia University
Morgantown, West Virginia

and

Anne Cronin, PhD, OTR/L, BCP
Associate Professor
Division of Occupational Therapy
West Virginia University
Morgantown, West Virginia

Objectives

Upon completion of this chapter, the reader should be able to

▓ Discuss international classification systems, including the ICF.

▓ Discuss the component domains of human performance.

▓ Define the framework dimensions of ICF: Body Structure and Function, Activity and Participation, Personal Factors, and Environmental Factors.

▓ Differentiate hierarchical models of development and dynamical systems theory as they pertain to human function.

▓ Define the following domains of human function: physical, psychological, and social.

▓ Define the concept of disablement and apply the concept to practical situations.

▓ Describe the medical and the social models of function, activity limitation, and disability.

▓ Differentiate contextual factors in the process of human activity.

Key Terms

activities of daily living (ADLs)
activity limitation
Affective Domain
agonist
antagonist
anticipatory control
autonomic nervous system (ANS)
cardiopulmonary system
central nervous system (CNS)
cognitive domain
Contextual Factors
control parameters
development
disability
disablement
disablement model
dynamical systems
effector system of motor control

emergent control
environmental constraints
Environmental Factors
frame of reference
function
growth
hierarchical model
International Classification of
    Functioning and Disability (ICF)
instrumental activities of daily living
    (IADLs)
learning
maturation
medical model
Model of Function and Disability
motor control
motor program
musculoskeletal system

occupational model
Occupational Therapy Practice
    Framework
parasympathetic nervous system
peripheral nervous system (PNS)
Personal Factors
physical function
proprioceptors
psychological function
psychomotor domain
readiness
social function
social model
societal limitation
somatosensory
special senses
sympathetic nervous
    system

INTRODUCTION

The human being is a complex creature capable of a myriad of accomplishments. Furthermore, humans are unique in that they have the ability to study, learn about, and analyze mental processes within the self. No other creature displays the curiosity, the cognition, and the drive to attempt to explain its own behavior and actions. Such areas of study as meta-cognition, which is the study of thought, represent the pinnacle of the human being's abilities.

Like all living things, the human being has a life cycle: birth, infancy, puberty, adulthood, and old age, eventually leading to death. It is now possible for the human lifespan to encompass a century or more. However, quality and quantity of life are separate issues. Quality of life may be defined as a life that promotes fulfillment both of basic and of complex needs, leading to life satisfaction. Maslow defines the human needs as a hierarchy, from the most basic need for sustenance to the need for self-actualization and love (Maslow, 1954). A good quality of life implies that all the individual's needs are being adequately met.

Throughout the human lifespan there unfolds an array of challenges or tasks that must be accomplished. Some of these tasks are normative, such as learning to walk or to read. Some of the tasks are nonnormative, such as adapting to a disease or disability. A person's capacity to meet these challenges depends on many factors, both intrinsic and extrinsic, and varies across the

lifespan. For those professions seeking to promote a high quality of life for all individuals, it is important to understand these variations in people's capacity to meet different challenges. The purpose of this chapter is to introduce the terminology and the constructs of function and disablement that enable a discussion of the subject.

INTERNATIONAL CLASSIFICATION OF FUNCTIONING AND DISABILITY (ICF)

Historically there have been several efforts to standardize the language associated with health and disability. The World Health Organization (WHO) developed the most current of these, the **International Classification of Functioning and Disability (ICF),** as a classification system of human function and abilities. This system offers the uniform language and framework that will provide the framework for this text.

SCOPE OF ICF

The ICF was developed to establish a common language for information sharing and policy planning internationally by encompassing in its descriptions all aspects of human functioning and disability. These descriptions are organized according to two

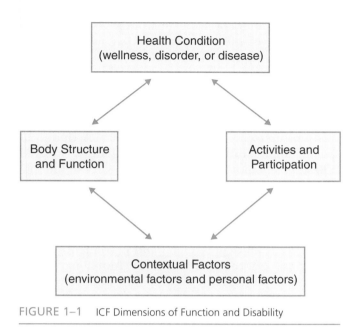

Health Condition
(wellness, disorder, or disease)

Body Structure
and Function

Activities and
Participation

Contextual Factors
(environmental factors and personal factors)

FIGURE 1–1   ICF Dimensions of Function and Disability

dimensions of functioning and disability: (1) Body Structure and Function and (2) Activities and Participation. In addition, there are two dimensions of **Contextual Factors:** Personal Factors and Environmental Factors. A schematic of the interaction of these dimensions is presented in Figure 1–1.

In the ICF and in this text, the term **function** refers to all body functions, activities, and types of participation. The ICF is unique in that it has rejected using the word *disability* as a descriptor, preferring the term **activity limitation.** Activity limitation is a less value-laden term to describe impairments and participation restrictions. However, as **disability**—defined as "something that hinders or incapacitates" (*American Heritage,* 2000)—is the term typically used to describe activity limitations in the professional literature, both terms will be used in this text interchangeably.

Body Structure and Function

The ICF dimension of Body Structure and Function comprises two sets of classifications, one for functions of the body systems and one for body structure. *Body functions* are the physiologic or psychological functions of the body systems. *Body structures* are the anatomic parts and their components. The specific aspects of interest in this dimension are changes in physiologic body function and anatomic changes in body structure.

Activities and Participation

The Activities and Participation dimension covers the complete range of tasks and actions performed by an individual. The specific focus is on the individual's capacity in executing tasks and the quality of his or her performance. This dimension classifies areas of life in

which an individual is involved, has access to, and encounters societal opportunities or barriers in regard to health conditions, body functions, activities, and contextual factors (World Health Organization, 2002). All the tasks involved in caring for oneself and others, education, work, and leisure preferences are considered in the analysis of Activities and Participation.

Personal and Environmental Factors

Personal Factors are contextual influences on function and activity limitation that are intrinsic, internal to the person. They include features like gender, age, temperament, intelligence, social background, education, past and current experiences, and personality. Personal Factors are considered in the context of their impact on a person's ability to function.

Environmental Factors are contextual influences on function that are extrinsic, or external, to the person. Tools in an individual's immediate environment, aspects of the physical environment, or social pressures on the person are examples of Environmental Factors, which, like Personal Factors, may be barriers or facilitators for both capacity and performance of actions and tasks in daily living (World Health Organization, 2002).

Conclusion

In each chapter, as it relates to the chapter content, we will present relevant aspects of the three dimensions used in the ICF categories. Contextual Factors, especially the category of Environmental Factors, are unique to the ICF model and reflect a change in thinking about activity limitation and function from earlier models of disability and disablement.

DOMAINS OF HUMAN PERFORMANCE

Traditionally, the study of human development has addressed three domains of human performance: cognitive, affective, and psychomotor. Most traditional textbooks and research on human development prior to the adoption of the ICF model have used this framework, in which the three domains are driven by innate physiologic functions that are acted upon and react to the environment (Payne & Isaacs, 1999). It is important to understand this traditional approach because the bulk of existing knowledge is based on it.

COGNITIVE DOMAIN

The **cognitive domain** involves thought. The functions commonly attributed to the cognitive domain are described in the ICF as "mental functions." Examples of this domain include (1) the ability to express one-self through written and spoken language and (2) the ability to read, think, and perform tasks from planning through completion. The "specific mental functions" domain of the ICF includes such aspects of the cognitive domain as attention, memory, and thought functions. Other traditionally described features of the cognitive domain—consciousness, orientation, and intelligence—are described in ICF as "global mental functions." Figure 1–2 illustrates areas of consistency between the ICF model and the traditional model.

The ICF concept of Body Structure and Function is largely parallel with the traditional one of psychomotor domain, although the psychomotor domain overlaps to include some specific activities. Similarly, the cognitive domains of the older model encompass aspects of all of the ICF Activities and Participation dimension, as well as having some overlap into other ICF dimensions. The affective domain from the traditional model is the most difficult to directly place within the ICF model but most closely parallels the Contextual Factors of the ICF.

AFFECTIVE DOMAIN

The **affective domain** involves feelings. Happiness, sadness, anger, and so forth are all part of the normal human experience. The ICF domain of global mental functions encompasses traditional affective thought, including intelligence, temperament, and personality. Emotional functions are a specific mental function. While much of what is traditionally the affective domain is intrinsic to the individual, the affective domain influences work, social participation, leisure, and communication, all characterized among Activities and Participation in the ICF.

PSYCHOMOTOR DOMAIN

Finally, the **psychomotor domain** involves movement. This domain includes all those activities that give the individual mastery over the environment—at the most elemental level, the ability to stand, sit, walk, and conquer gravity. At the most advanced level, this domain involves breaking records of environmental mastery including speed, accuracy, and performance (Bloom, 1956). Of the three traditional developmental domains, the psychomotor domain is the most confusing in its relationship to the ICF language. In its description of specific mental functions, the ICF includes a category called "psychomotor functions" that relates to the specific mental functions of control over motor events but is not synonymous with the developmental process of **motor control.**

An additional category of analysis offered in the ICF is "neuromusculoskeletal and movement-related functions." Subcategories include functions of the bones and joints, muscle functions, and movement functions. All of these functions have been traditionally included as part of the psychomotor domain.

HUMAN DEVELOPMENT

An individual acquires an increasing number of behaviors within these domains of performance, particularly in early life. Two processes are fundamental to acquisition of these new behaviors. The first process, development, refers to those changes in performance that are heavily influenced by maturational processes, such as learning to walk. Despite wide varieties of environmental influences, when all body systems are sufficiently mature, most infants will begin walking. The quantitative changes that occur over time in the human (changes in height, weight, and physical characteristics) are categorized as **growth.** Qualitative changes related to organizational and process change may be considered **maturation.** For example, maturation of the brain plays a key role in support of early behavioral acquisition, particularly in early childhood. Both growth and maturation underlie human development (Payne & Isaacs, 1999).

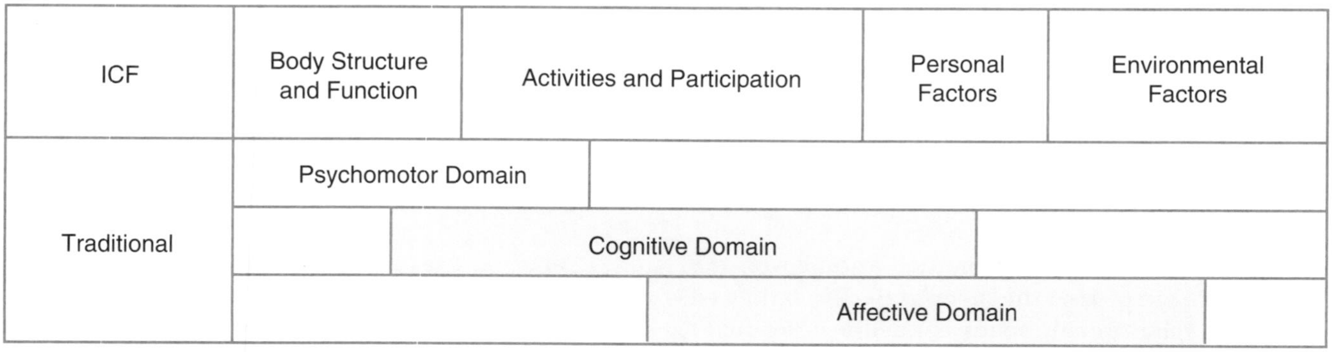

ICF	Body Structure and Function	Activities and Participation		Personal Factors	Environmental Factors
Traditional	Psychomotor Domain				
		Cognitive Domain			
			Affective Domain		

FIGURE 1–2 Comparison of ICF Model and Traditional Model

The second fundamental process, **learning,** is the acquisition of new behavior as influenced by interaction with the environment. Learning is dependent not only on environmental exposure, but also on such factors as feedback and practice. Of course, in order to be able to learn skills such as gymnastics or handwriting, certain elements of maturation and growth are necessary as well. Although maturation and growth have more influence on early developmental processes than on learning, these factors are not excluded from learning.

One of the first individuals to differentiate between skills acquired primarily by development and those acquired by learning was Myrtle McGraw. In her classic studies of the 1930s, identical twins, Johnny and Jimmy, were observed while one was given more toys and overall greater opportunities for stimulation over the first two years of life. Several key findings of these classic studies are still accepted today. For example, some skills, such as roller-skating, appear to be learned and retained better when introduced at an early age. However, skills such as walking, creeping, and so on are less affected by environmental exposure. Another finding of McGraw was the concept of **readiness:** some behaviors are not acquired until sufficient growth and maturation have occurred, irrespective of the amount of exposure. McGraw also discovered that there was a *level of fixity* for certain skills, meaning a point where the skill will not be lost even if the child stops performing it for a while. We all know that skills such as riding a bicycle, when they have obtained a sufficient level of fixity, are never forgotten (McGraw, 1935).

HIERARCHICAL MODELS OF HUMAN DEVELOPMENT

For all three domains of behavior, a key aspect of normal function is the nervous system. The human nervous system consists of a central and a peripheral component. The **central nervous system (CNS),** for the purposes of this text, is the brain and spinal cord, that is, the parts of the nervous system that are protected by the bony covering of skull and vertebral column. The **peripheral nervous system (PNS)** consists primarily of nerves and nerve roots that connect the control centers of the CNS to external sites, such as muscles, glands, or skin.

The cognitive domain of function relies nearly exclusively on the function of the brain. The affective domain of function is tied to parts of the CNS and PNS, often referred to as the **autonomic nervous system (ANS).** The ANS is directed by special parts of the brain and peripheral nervous system. The parts of the ANS that communicate with the periphery are subdivided into the **sympathetic** and **parasympathetic systems.** The sympathetic nervous system controls "fight or flight" behaviors and is associated with a high level of arousal.

Conversely, the parasympathetic nervous system mediates basic physiologic behaviors such as digestion, elimination, and sexual function.

Our understanding of the role of the CNS in psychomotor function has changed considerably over the years. The neurobiologic processes underlying human movement are called *motor control.* It used to be thought that the brain and its maturational status were determinant in prescribing the form of motor behavior. McGraw (1945) attempted to specifically tie the acquisition of developmental milestones such as rolling to the level of brain maturation. Therefore, traditional theorists tended to adopt a **hierarchical model** to explain human motor behavior, with the cerebral cortex ultimately determining the form and function of human movement.

DYNAMICAL SYSTEMS THEORY

The hierarchical concept just mentioned has been replaced by newer theoretical models, the most commonly applied being the **dynamical systems** theory. This theory has its roots in a concept of human physics that refers to self-organization of complex particles. Several key elements of dynamical systems theory as they apply to motor control should be understood. First is the idea that behavior at any given point in time is the result of variable interaction of a number of complex systems. This interaction occurs in accordance with control parameters and environmental constraints (Kamm et al., 1991).

Control parameters are the conditions in existence at the time the task is executed. A control parameter could be executed by change in any one of the subsystems. For example, pain may function as a control parameter when an attempt is made to bear weight on a sprained ankle, resulting in a change in the movement pattern executed. **Environmental constraints** are the prevailing environmental conditions that help shape the movement. For example, walking on a slippery floor would be an environmental constraint, changing the pattern of walking. As is implied by the preceding discussion, in systems theory, the CNS is no longer the prime determinant of human motor function but is rather one of the key subsystems mediating the motor behavior (Shumway-Cook & Woollacott, 2001).

A second key element of dynamical systems theory is the idea of **emergent control** of behavior, meaning that the individual will alter a task in myriad ways in order to meet the current conditions. Emergent control goes along with the idea of **anticipatory control,** meaning that the motor program is adjusted even before any interaction with the environment. Moreover, behavior from a systems perspective is believed to be self-organizing. This concept implies that there is an extremely complex interaction between systems, which act together in an infinite number of ways to produce a behavioral result (Kamm et al., 1991).

Dynamical systems theory addresses the importance of systems and subsystems other than the CNS in determining psychomotor behavior. One of the key systems in executing motor behavior is the **musculoskeletal system,** considered to be the **effector system of motor control.** The specific parameters of how the muscular system is to act are coded in a message called the **motor program,** sent from the CNS to the spinal cord and out to the muscles. The muscles act in accordance with this program. For example, the motor program may specify the amount of reciprocal versus co-contraction of agonist and antagonist muscles.

An **agonist** muscle is the prime mover, as in extension of the wrist. The **antagonist** muscles to wrist extension would be the wrist flexors. When there is a lot of reciprocal inhibition specified by the motor program, the wrist flexors would be relatively inactive during wrist extension, permitting a very pliable wrist joint as it moves into extension. An example of a task requiring a relatively pliable wrist joint is playing the piano. However, when the CNS specifies a large amount of co-contraction of antagonist muscles, the joint is relatively stiff. An example of a task requiring a relatively stiff wrist would be stabilizing the wrist to pick up a pot of boiling water. Therefore, the motor program specifies the amount and pattern of muscle contraction to control joint stiffness.

Other aspects of movement controlled through the motor program, as executed by the muscles, are the amount of force or tension, timing, and direction of the movement. Of course, the muscles are able to effect the motor program because they act over a system of bones, connected by joints. The bones and joints actually form an elaborate system of levers, with forces being applied over the levers by the contraction of muscles.

The sensory system is also a key element of motor control. The organs of **special senses,** such as vision and hearing, inform us about environmental constraints and provide important feedback about the results of the movement. The **somatosensory** system includes those sensory receptors located in the skin that provide information about touch, pressure, pain, and temperature. **Proprioceptors** are sensory receptors located in muscles, tendons, joints, and ligaments. The vestibular system of the inner ear is also functionally a proprioceptive system. The proprioceptors give us information about position and movement of the body in space. In addition to playing a key role in mediating the motor domain of function, the sensory system also plays a key role in cognitive and affective domains. The ability to receive and process sensory input is important, then, across all domains of behavior, and, conversely, deficits in this ability have implications for all three behavioral domains.

The **cardiopulmonary system** is another key physiologic system in mediating behavior, particularly motor behavior. It is from the cardiopulmonary system that oxygenated blood is supplied to all organs, permitting normal function. Characteristics of motor performance, such as endurance, are supported by this system.

These physiologic systems are all essential in promoting normal function across behavioral domains. The three traditional domains—cognitive, affective, and psychomotor—refer to the individual's behavior from an intrinsic perspective. However, the individual does not exhibit behavior in isolation. Behaviors typically occur in an environmental context and frequently involve acting on or modifying the environment. An extrinsic view of human performance can be considered a study of human factors.

DOMAINS OF HUMAN FUNCTION

Function is defined in *Merriam-Webster's Dictionary* as "the action for which a person or thing is specially fitted, used or responsible, or for which a thing exists: the activity appropriate to the nature or position of a person or thing" (2003). Human function may be generally defined as the ability to set and successfully attain goals. Frequently these goals involve some form of mastery of tasks from simple to complex. A simple task might be moving from a sitting position to a standing one. A complex task might be running a marathon. Function is the ability to meet these goals, and, conversely, dysfunction is an inability to meet either internally or externally established goals.

The domains of human function differ slightly from the traditional classifications of psychomotor, cognitive, and affective. Human function relies on the behaviors but places them in an environmental, behavior, and task-specific context. To that end, the domains of human function widely used in the rehabilitation professions have been categorized as physical, psychological, and social functions. Figure 1–3 builds on the earlier figure to show how this rehabilitation-based classification system compares with the other two systems.

Note the great consistency among the constructs of Body Functions and Structure from the ICF, the psychomotor domain from the traditional model, and physical function in the domains of human function. Strong parallels exist between the traditional cognitive domains and psychological functions, and between the affective domain and social function.

PHYSICAL FUNCTION

Physical function is the ability to react to and act upon the environment using the existing behavioral repertoire. As identified previously, the behavioral repertoires are acquired through different processes,

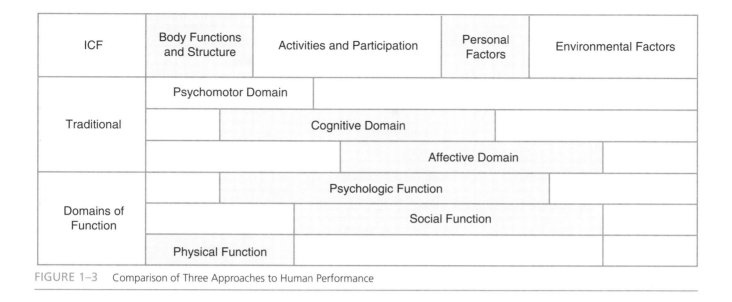

ICF	Body Functions and Structure	Activities and Participation	Personal Factors	Environmental Factors
Traditional	Psychomotor Domain			
		Cognitive Domain		
		Affective Domain		
Domains of Function		Psychologic Function		
		Social Function		
	Physical Function			

FIGURE 1–3   Comparison of Three Approaches to Human Performance

including development and learning. Physical function involves all areas of human performance, including the simplest tasks of self-care, known as **activities of daily living (ADLs).** Examples of ADLs are personal hygiene (toileting, bathing), feeding, dressing, and grooming. A more complex set of functional behaviors is the **instrumental activities of daily living (IADLs).** These are the activities of daily living that typically involve cognitive sequencing as well as chains of behaviors. Examples are grocery shopping, managing money, planning and preparing meals, and using transportation. Physical function also includes the ability to maneuver in the environment through some means of locomotion. Physical function abilities underlie the execution of work, productive activities, and leisure.

The domain of physical function implies mastery of certain aspects of all three behavioral domains. In the cognitive domain, the individual must be capable of planning and executing the tasks of ADLs, IADLs, and other more complex challenges. In the affective domain, the individual must be motivated to perform these tasks. In the psychomotor domain, the individual must be physically capable of carrying out these behaviors.

PSYCHOLOGICAL FUNCTION

The domain of **psychological function** encompasses both cognitive and affective behavioral domains. In this functional arena, cognitive ability, motivation, and affect all play a part. Psychological function is exemplified by the individual's ability to complete tasks associated with life roles, such as success in academic endeavors. Psychological function also encompasses the

affective behaviors necessary to effectively master the environment. We are all aware of the devastating impact of psychologic dysfunction, such as mental illness, on the attempt to master environmental challenges. This domain also includes aspects of motivation, mood, temperament, and other intrinsic qualities as they affect activities and participation.

SOCIAL FUNCTION

Finally, the domain of **social function** encompasses all three behavioral domains: motor, cognitive, and affective, placing them in the larger social context. Social function is the ability to participate in a social environment, filling social roles and expectations. Included are the ability to earn a living through meaningful work, the ability to participate in family and community life, and the ability to participate in leisure activities. As in the other functional domains, all three behavioral domains mediate social function. Motor behaviors are necessary to fully participate in social roles and experiences. Cognitive and affective behaviors are necessary to understand and relate to the social environment (Cech & Martin, 1995).

MODELS OF FUNCTION AND DISABILITY

An understanding of normative human performance is necessary to grasp the implications and consequences of disease or activity limitation on the ability

ICF	Function and Disability		Contextual Factors	
	Body Functions and Structure	Activities and Participation	Personal Factors	Environmental Factors
Positive aspects	Physical Integrity	Competency	Facilitators	
Negative aspects	Impairments	Limitations and restrictions	Barriers	

FIGURE 1–4   ICF Model of Function and Disability

of an individual to function in any or all of the aforementioned domains. This understanding is what the ICF attempts to impart in its **Model of Function and Disability.** Figure 1–4 is intended to help the reader visualize the current understanding of the interactions between various components of the classification system in the ICF model. The model presents the "health condition as a factor that influences the three major dimensions of the model, body functions and structure, activity, and participation. The outcome of this process is the ability of the individual to maintain current and future life roles" (World Health Organization, 2002, p. 24).

In rehabilitation, differing professional groups have approached this interaction in slightly different ways. For example, the *Guide to Physical Therapy Practice* refers to function as "those activities identified by an individual as essential to support physical, social, and psychologic well-being and to create a personal sense of meaningful living" (APTA, 1997, p. 1173). Occupational therapists use the term *occupation* to encompass "all of the activities that occupy people's time and give meaning to their lives" (Neistadt & Crepeau, 1998, p. 5). Both groups are, in the end, considering the ability of the individual to live a meaningful life.

DISABLEMENT

A sociologic concept known as **disablement** is commonly used to put into concrete terms the impact of a disease or activity limitation on human function. The disablement concept recognizes that functional states associated with health conditions are not identical to the conditions themselves. For example, two people might have the health condition known as chronic low back pain. One of these persons may have been accommodated to the workplace and life activities and may continue to participate in the accommodated

environment. Another person may become quite sedentary, removed from normal roles such as vocation, and hence may be very depressed. Therefore, the functional status of these individuals should not rest in the medical condition itself.

Models of Disablement

A **disablement model** is a theoretical attempt to categorize activity limitation in terms of the person's social and cultural environment. One of the first individuals to write about the disablement concept as distinct from diagnosis was a sociologist, Saad Nagi. Nagi's original disablement model was published in 1965. This model involved the following four classifications. First, *active pathology* was defined as interruption of normal physiologic processes, as by disease. Second, *impairment* included the anatomic, physiological, mental, or emotional abnormalities brought about by the pathology. Third, *functional limitation* was the limitation in performance as it related to the individual. Finally, *disability* was the limitation in performance of socially defined roles and tasks.

Some years later, the World Health Organization (WHO) presented its own classification system, known as the International Classification of Impairments, Disabilities, and Handicaps (ICIDH) model. The reader may be able to relate this to another classification system set forth by WHO, the International Classification of Disease (ICD), which forms the basis today for medical diagnostic codes (ICD-9). The purpose of these classification systems as established by WHO is to permit international communication for acquiring data banks used for epidemiology and outcome studies on a large scale.

The ICIDH classification system of 1980 was a significant step forward in recognizing the concept of disablement. The first ICIDH classification system was similar to the Nagi model, with some differences in terminology. The term *disease* was used to define the intrinsic pathology. The term *impairment* was used to define the loss or abnormality of structure or function at the organ level. The original ICIDH classification system differed from the Nagi model in the last two classification categories. In the ICIDH system, *disability* referred to the restriction or lack of ability to perform an activity in the normal manner, and the term *handicap* referred to the societal implication of this activity limitation.

In 1991 the National Center for Medical Rehabilitation Research (NCMRR) produced yet a third variation of the model. Here the term *pathophysiology* referred to the disease process; *impairment* to the loss of structure or function as a result of the disease; *functional limitation* to the loss or restriction of ability to perform a task in the manner or range in which it is typically performed; and *disability* to limitations or inability to perform tasks within physical or social context. Additionally, a new category, **societal limitation,** was added to address the fact that not all disablement had the individual as its origin; in fact, the ability of the individual to perform normal roles and expectations is not uncommonly a function of extrinsic societal barriers. These barriers might be physical, such as the lack of accessible buildings or transportation, or they might be social, such as societal attitudes toward individuals with disabilities.

In 2001 WHO published the new international classification system, known as ICF, introduced earlier in this chapter. The stated purposes of ICF are to (1) provide a scientific basis for understanding and studying functional states associated with health conditions; (2) establish a common language for describing functional states; (3) permit comparison of data across countries, health care disciplines, services, and time; and (4) provide systematic coding. The resultant classification system is a matrix representing the interrelationships between functioning and activity limitation. Inherent in the new classification scheme are extensive definitions as well as proposed measurement scales so that universal communication is possible. For example, under the "activities" dimension, rating scales used include the difficulty that the individual has in performing the tasks and a separate rating scale to grade the amount of assistance required to perform that task. The ICF represents the next stage in understanding the evolution of the disablement concept (World Health Organization, 2002).

Human function and disablement interact with both the individual's health condition and contextual factors like the environment. The interactions between these elements are dynamic, complex, and not always predictable. For example, the ICF describes several of these possible interactions, such as health impairment without activity limitations, activity limitations without evident impairments, and activity limitations without participation problems (2002).

Figure 1–5 illustrates the integration of the *Physical Therapy Guide to Practice* (APTA, 2001) and the *Occupational Therapy Practice Framework* (AOTA, 2002) into the models discussed previously. Discussion of specific details of these two clinical frameworks is beyond the scope of this text but should be of interest to students planning a future in rehabilitation.

Medical and Social Models of Disablement

Varieties of approaches have been proposed to understand activity limitation and disablement. The two primary views of disablement are the medical model and the social model. The **medical model** emphasizes the person, and that person's impairments, as a cause of disease, trauma, or some other health condition (World Health Organization, 2002). Within the medical model disability is a feature of the person that requires medical care provided in the form of individual treatment by professionals to "correct" the problem.

Clinicians working within the medical model will identify impairments and develop strategies to improve the individual's abilities or to help him learn to compensate for the impairments. For example, in the case of a spinal cord injury, the therapist offers activities to strengthen muscles at the same time she is training the person in new ways to complete ADL activities. Special equipment like wheelchairs and adapted vehicles are additional examples of compensations. This is the traditional approach presented in the rehabilitation literature.

The **social model** sees the society rather than the individual as the problem (World Health Organization, 2002). Within this model, "disability demands a political response, since the problem is created by an unaccommodating physical environment brought about by attitudes and other features of the social environment" (World Health Organization, 2002, p. 9). Using the spinal cord injury example again, this model would argue that the individual was disabled because he could not access local stores, public transportation, and theaters. The focus on the problem is change in social policy.

In a subtler example, the condition of attention deficit disorder has received a lot of attention in the last 15 years. This disorder has a rapidly rising incidence in the United States and Western Europe. At the same time, the incidence is relatively low in Eastern Europe, South America, and Africa. The difference in frequency of labeling this condition seems to lie in societal expectations for a child's behavior. Impulsivity, distractibility, and high activity levels are disruptive in large elementary school classrooms. Cultures that offer alternative educational and social options for children may not identify such behavior as a disability.

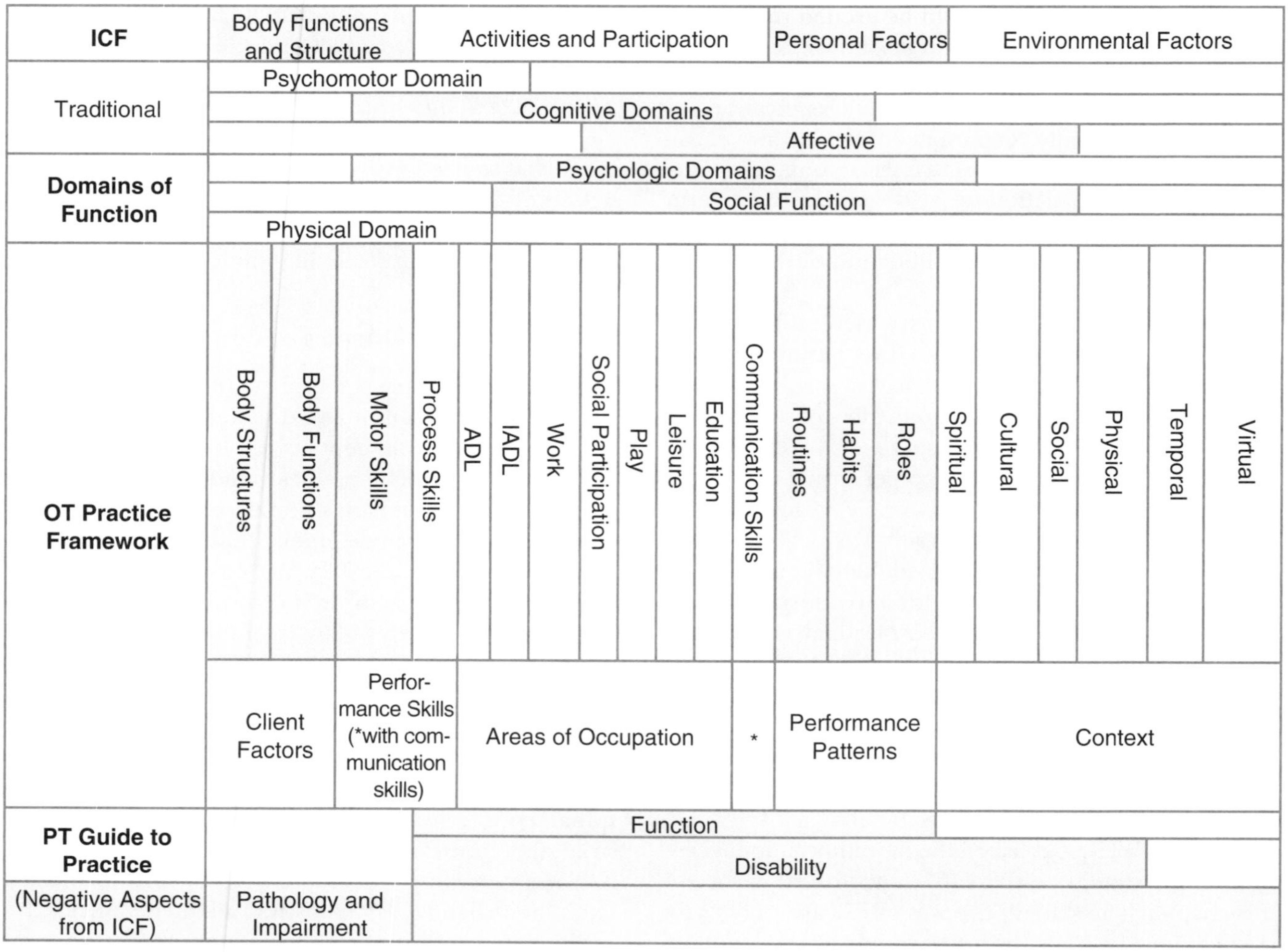

ICF	Body Functions and Structure	Activities and Participation	Personal Factors	Environmental Factors
Traditional	Psychomotor Domain			
	Cognitive Domains			
	Affective			
Domains of Function	Psychologic Domains			
	Social Function			
	Physical Domain			
OT Practice Framework	Body Structures / Body Functions / Motor Skills / Process Skills	ADL / IADL / Work / Social Participation / Play / Leisure / Education / Communication Skills	Routines / Habits / Roles	Spiritual / Cultural / Social / Physical / Temporal / Virtual
	Client Factors / Performance Skills (*with communication skills)	Areas of Occupation	* Performance Patterns	Context
PT Guide to Practice		Function		
		Disability		
(Negative Aspects from ICF)	Pathology and Impairment			

FIGURE 1–5   Relationship between Practice Frameworks and ICF Model

CLINICAL FRAMES OF REFERENCE

Rehabilitation professionals have embraced the disablement concept as a **frame of reference** for practice. A frame of reference is the theoretical perspective or viewpoint that organizes the approach to client management. The two professional groups, occupational therapy and physical therapy, have slightly different frames of reference in the management of disablement. Figure 1–5 illustrates the basic tenets of the practice frameworks for these two closely allied professional practitioners.

Occupational therapy has strong ties to both the medical and the social models of disability. In the practice guidelines for occupational therapy, a careful differentiation is made between the medical model, with its focus on the absence of disease, and the **occupational model,** with its more societal focuses on competence in performance in desired human occupations. This model views occupation as "all of the activities that occupy people's time and give meaning to their lives" (Neistadt & Crepeau, 1998, p. 5). In differing social and cultural systems, occupational therapists may reduce activity limitation through their activities at both medical and societal levels. The **Occupational Therapy Practice Framework** presented in the publication titled *Occupational Therapy Practice Framework* (AOTA, 2002) closely parallels the ICF model, especially in its unique emphasis on contextual factors.

The *Guide to Physical Therapy Practice,* published in 1997 and revised in 2001, utilizes disablement as a key concept. The disablement model referenced in the physical therapy guide is the Nagi revision as summarized by Jette (1994). It is important to relate disablement to quality of life. Jette defines *quality of life* as emotional well-being, behavioral competence, sleep and rest, energy, vitality, and general life satisfaction. Jette further posits that quality of life is impacted at the level of functional limitation and handicap (Jette, 1994).

In both professions it could be argued that clients often seek out therapists for the express purpose of improving or maintaining quality of life. Therefore, the desired therapeutic outcomes or goals should focus on functional limitations and disability rather than disease or impairments. The latter should be a focus of therapy only to the extent that pathology and impairment directly underlie the functional limitation and disability. This perspective has had major implications for rehabilitation professionals, including not only assessment and intervention, but also reimbursement factors.

SUMMARY

The study of human performance and function is vital to understanding the complex contexts within which persons seek rehabilitation or other interventions. The physical and occupational therapist must understand normal characteristics as well as identify potential person-specific concerns that may impact quality of life. This chapter has introduced the basic terminology and professional frameworks to guide the study of the human lifespan.

Speaking of

The ICF in Practice

MARYBETH MANDICH, PT, PhD
PEDIATRIC PHYSICAL THERAPIST

Many years ago, when I was a young therapist, I was working with a young man, probably 12 or 13 years old, who had spina bifida. In the fairly recent past, before I started working with him, he had given up attempts at walking. Because he was paralyzed from the waist down, he was confined to a wheelchair, and he was pretty good at getting around that way. The reason he had given up walking, it turns out, had nothing to do with energy expenditure or laziness or weight gain. The reason he had stopped walking was very simple—every time he stood up, he had a reflexive bowel movement. Now, I don't remember if this was a recently developed problem or one that he had previously, but with the onset of adolescence, he was unwilling to "pay the price" of walking.

As a brand new therapist, armed with lots of knowledge and very little wisdom, I determined that it would be an important treatment goal for this young man to regain the ability to ambulate. I had pretty good rapport with him, probably because I was so young myself, so he agreed to give it a try. Every day, he and I would leave his classroom, lock his braces up, and begin gait training. Every day, to avoid anyone else knowing his problem, I would perform the required hygiene after the inevitable bowel accident occurred. We kept this up for weeks. Eventually, however, I was forced to admit what this young man had feared—this reflexive reaction simply wasn't going to become accommodated, and, at the young man's request, we stopped the gait training.

Now, there are good reasons for encouraging walking in individuals with spinal cord injury, including congenital problems like spina bifida. Walking helps keep the bones strong. The energy used to walk helps control weight gain. Many individuals like the idea of being upright with their peers who are able-bodied.

However, I was approaching the issue with what I am now able to see in hindsight was a blatant disregard for this young man's functional abilities. I was focusing at the Body Structure and Function level, and to some extent, at the Activity level (the activity of walking). What I missed entirely was the focus on Participation. In fact, by having this young man put such an emphasis on walking, I was in fact limiting his activities and severely restricting his participation. However, in the end, it was the ability to participate with his peers that mattered most.

Continues

Speaking of Continued

What the ICF and its predecessor, the ICIDH model, have taught us is to expand our worldview in defining outcomes and setting goals for individuals with disabilities. As discussed in this chapter, it is entirely possible to have restrictions in body structure and function but not be limited in activities and participation. Conversely, it is possible to have no restriction on activity but be unable to attend a social function because of environmental or societal barriers. In order to work effectively with individuals who have disabilities, it is important to remember that activity and participation are part of normal functioning, and restoration of these abilities is part of every intervention program. This provides a mandate to the rehabilitation professional. No longer can we view our clients and patients within a single treatment area or department or gym. We have to look out to the world. We need to understand what their developmental and functional needs are in the context of their physical, social, and cultural environment. Where society puts up barriers, we need to become advocates for barrier removal.

The ICF helps us categorize and gives us a classification system to reference. But to apply the ICF correctly, we need to understand normative developmental and functional tasks across the life span. Hopefully, this text and others like it will help rehabilitation professionals learn to incorporate this frame of reference into their interventions.

REFERENCES

American Occupational Therapy Association. (2002). Occupational Therapy Practice Framework: Domain and process. *The American Journal of Occupational Therapy, 56*, 609–639.

American Physical Therapy Association. (2001). *Guide to physical therapist practice* (2nd ed.). Alexandria, VA: American Physical Therapy Association.

American Physical Therapy Association. (1997). *Guide to physical therapist practice* (1st ed.). Alexandria, VA: American Physical Therapy Association.

Bloom, B. X. (1956). Taxonomy of educational objectives: Handbook 1. *Cognitive domain.* New York: McKay.

Cech, D., & Martin, S. (1995). *Functional movement development across the lifespan.* Philadelphia: W. B. Saunders.

Jette, A. M. (1994). Physical disablement concepts for physical therapy research and practice. *Physical Therapy, 74*, 380–386.

Kamm, K., Thelen, E., & Jensen, J. (1991). A dynamical systems approach to motor development. In J. Rothstein (Ed.), *Movement science* (pp. 11–23). Alexandria, VA: American Physical Therapy Association.

Maslow, A. (1954). *Motivation and personality.* New York: Harper & Row.

McGraw, M. (1935). *Growth: A study of Johnny and Jimmy.* New York: Appleton-Century-Crofts.

McGraw, M. (1945). *Neuromuscular maturation of the human infant* (1962 reprint of 1945 edition). New York: Hafner Press, 1962.

Merriam-Webster On-line (2003). http://www.m-w.com/cgi-bin/dictionary. Chicago: Encyclopedia Britannica.

Nagi, S. (1965). Some conceptual issues in activity limitation and rehabilitation. In M. Sussman (Ed.), *Sociology and rehabilitation* (pp. 100–113). Washington, DC: American Sociological Association.

Neistadt, M., & Crepeau, E. (1998). *Willard and Spackman's occupational therapy* (9th ed.). Philadelphia: Lippincott.

Payne, V., & Isaacs, L. (1999). Introduction to motor development. In *Human motor development: A lifespan approach* (4th ed., pp. 1–25). Mountain View, CA: Mayfield.

Shumway-Cook, A., & Woollacott, M. (2001). Motor control issues and theories. In *Motor control: Theory and practical applications* (2nd ed., pp. 1–25). Baltimore: Lippincott, Williams and Wilkins.

World Health Organization. (1980). *International classification of impairments, disabilities and handicaps.* Geneva, Switzerland: World Health Organization.

World Health Organization. (2002). *ICF: International classification of functioning and disability.* Geneva, Switzerland: World Health Organization.

CHAPTER 2

Theoretical Framework for Human Performance

MaryBeth Mandich, PT, PhD
Professor and Chairperson
Division of Physical Therapy
West Virginia University
Morgantown, West Virginia

Objectives

Upon completion of this chapter, the reader should be able to

■ Define and describe the applications of theory.

■ Define and correctly apply classifications of theory.

■ Recognize and describe the contributions of key theorists according to domain of function.

■ Apply theoretical constructs to various domains of human performance.

■ Reflect on the role of theory in understanding behavior and learning.

Key Terms

accommodation	Erikson, Erik	Pavlov, Ivan
Ainsworth, Mary	formal operations	personality
assimilation	Freud, Sigmund	Piaget, Jean
Bandura, Albert	Gesell, Arnold	preoperational stage
behaviorism	Gestalt school	reinforcement
Bower, Gordon	Gibson, Eleanor	Sears, Robert
Bowlby, John	Kohlberg, Lawrence	self-actualization
Case, Robbie	Maslow, Abraham H.	sensorimotor stage
Chess, Stella	McGraw, Myrtle	Skinner, B. F.
Chomsky, Noam	modeling	temperament
classical conditioning	motor behavior	theory
concrete operations	motor development	Thomas, Alexander
developmental theory	motor learning	Vgotsky, Lev
Dewey, John	nativist school	Watson, John
empiricist school	operant conditioning	zone of proximal development

INTRODUCTION

The word **theory** has widespread usage. Most people would agree that they have a general idea of the meaning of the term. Perhaps in its broadest sense, a theory is understood to mean an explanation of a phenomenon. For example, an individual might have a theory about why a certain type of behavior occurs.

Technical definitions of the term abound. The dictionary defines a theory as "a set of propositions describing the operations and causes of natural phenomena." Thomas (2001), in the introduction to his book summarizing theories of human development, defines a theory as a proposal identifying critical variables and how these variables interact. Miller (1983) observes that a theory should meet certain criteria: It should be logically and empirically sound, meaning that it should be internally consistent as well as observationally validated. Furthermore, it should be testable, cover a broad scope of observed phenomena, and contain a manageable number of constructs and propositions.

Many of the theories that seek to explain human performance through the process of maturation are considered developmental. A **developmental theory** attempts to describe change over time (Miller, 1983). Typically, a developmental theory addresses changes that are attributed proportionately more to maturation than to environmental experience. For this reason, developmental change tends to be less sensitive than other types of change to such influences as practice, experience, and cultural variation. It is important to remember that this is in relative proportion to the influence of experience in learned behavior. The complex interplay of nature and nurture, while strongly debated in early years of developmental study, is now accepted as an assumption.

A theory is typically formed to explain a series of observations that are considered fact. However, because the theory itself is not fact, it can be disproved. Some of the theories discussed in this chapter have indeed been disproved, although they are important to know about because of their impact on the field. Others, such as that of Piaget, have been significantly altered by growth in knowledge and further study. All of the theories discussed here are under constant evaluation, with potential for rejection, revision, or strengthening.

Therapists and others who work with individuals to help them recognize their full human potential often use theory to guide their interventions. When theoretical material is organized and functionally translated into practice, it becomes a *frame of reference*. For example, one person might approach a given clinical scenario from a developmental frame of reference while another approaches the same problem from a learning frame of reference. Frame of reference describes the theoretical worldview that guides the therapeutic interaction, including both evaluation and intervention.

CLASSIFICATION OF THEORY

Theories may be classified in a number of ways. Understanding where a theory falls under a given classification paradigm helps to get a perspective of relationships among theories.

NATURE VERSUS NURTURE

As mentioned earlier, the classification of nature versus nurture reflects a historical perspective regarding the amount of influence that genetics has in determining a behavior versus the role of environmental experience. Historically, the nature-nurture argument was a focal point of developmental psychology and even philosophy. In the twenty-first century, it is accepted that behavior is inevitably a product of both nature and nurture; however, theorists continue to debate the relative contribution of each. The nature-nurture debate is also described as innate-acquired, maturation-learning, biology-culture, and nativism-empiricism debate (Miller, 1983).

QUALITATIVE VERSUS QUANTITATIVE

A *qualitative* theory says that individuals are qualitatively different at different points in the lifespan. For example, a theory that emphasizes the qualitative nature of behavior acquisition would state that behaviors at a point in time reflect maturational qualities in the individual. Until those qualities develop, the behavior cannot be represented. Qualitative theories often present behavior as developing in sequential stages. A *quantitative* theory sees development as primarily the acquisition of a number of skills; therefore, the appearance of an ability or the lack thereof is related merely to the presence or absence of a sufficient number of prerequisite exposures or skills.

STABILITY VERSUS INSTABILITY

A theory that emphasizes *stability* implies that the rules for anticipating behavior are consistent across the lifespan; hence, future behavior is predictable from current behavior. A theory that classifies behavior as *unstable* holds that different rules apply at different points in an individual's life; therefore, one must know the applicable set of rules before prediction can occur. Another classification that is sometimes used in a similar fashion is continuity versus discontinuity. *Continuity* in theory states that the same developmental laws apply across the lifespan; *discontinuity* states that there are different laws at different points in the lifespan.

REDUCTIONIST VERSUS NONREDUCTIONIST

A *reductionist* theory states that behavior is the sum of a number of smaller behavior links; a *nonreductionist* theory is one that sees behavior as a total that cannot be broken into component parts with any degree of meaning.

ORGANISMIC VERSUS MECHANISTIC

In the *organismic* model, the inherent nature of the being must be considered; that is, needs and goals and intrinsic motivations are important. Activity of the organism on the environment is a critical feature. In the *mechanistic* model, the organism is seen as "like a machine" that is acted upon by the environment. Another way to conceptualize this dichotomy is that in the organismic model the organism is active, whereas in the mechanistic model the organism is reactive (Miller, 1983; Reese & Overton, 1970).

As mentioned previously, classifying theories helps to provide some quick reference to the overall perspective taken by the theorist as well as allowing for comparison among theories. Classifications are not mutually exclusive. For example, a mechanistic theory is also likely to be reductionist, stable, and quantitative. An organismic theory is likely to be unstable, nonreductionist, and qualitative.

A final way to classify theories, which will be used here for purposes of discussion, is by the area of behavior the theory purports to address. The domains of human performance addressed in Chapter 1 are affective, cognitive, and psychomotor. These domains of performance underlie the individual's ability to function in physical, psychological, and social domains. The following theories ultimately seek to explain, describe, and predict human function in a variety of contexts by domain of performance.

AFFECTIVE DOMAIN

The affective domain includes those characteristics that underlie feeling. It includes some aspects of intelligence, which will be discussed in the cognitive domain, as well as personality and temperament. One of the most significant theorists detailing the development of personality was **Sigmund Freud.** Born in 1856 in Moravia, Freud spent most of his life in Austria, where his theory of development became the foundation of the school of psychoanalysis. Key aspects of the theory include the dynamic conflict between destructive and loving instincts. The latter came to be known as *libido.* Freud defined human mental processes according to the *id, ego,* and *superego.* The id represents the most basic instincts and drives. The ego represents intellectual activities and logical thought. The superego represents the conscience and awareness of right and wrong. Freud viewed dreams as a reflection of unconscious mental processes and used dream interpretation in psychoanalysis.

Freud saw development as qualitative and stagelike. He proposed a theory of child development based on his observations and clinical work with women suffering from hysteria. In the development of the young child, before 5 years of age, Freud identified three stages: oral, anal, and phallic. The oral stage roughly was that of infancy, concerned with feeding and oral exploration. The anal phase roughly coincided with toilet training and was concerned with gratification and the development of control. The phallic stage was the early exploration of the genitals and awareness of sexual differences. These stages were followed by a lengthy period of latency, terminating in the genital stage of adolescence and the awakening of sexuality (Puner, 1947). The resolution of these stages determines not only characteristics of sexual functioning, but also how the child relates to self and others (Miller, 1983).

Two early members of Freud's school, Alfred Adler and Carl Jung, eventually split from Freud and established their own schools of psychologic thought. Both Adler and Jung downplayed the role of sexual factors in personality. Jung's approach tended to emphasize ethics and religion, but remained true to some classic Freudian concepts such as the importance of dreams, while Adler eventually opposed most classic Freudian tenets (Puner, 1947). Adler emphasized social rather than biologic factors in explaining human motivations. He never practiced psychoanalysis, but rather employed a philosophy in which therapist and patient are on equal footing. His approach became known as *individual psychology* (Chaplin & Krawiec, 1960).

Although many of his ideas have been disproved, Freud's impact on the study of psychology was significant in several ways. Although it seems intuitive today, Freud was one of the first to realize that development was a worthwhile pursuit of study—that is, that the antecedents of adult behavior could be found in the past. Also, Freud was one of the first to devote attention to the psychology of motivation. Moreover, Freud played a role in the evolution of clinical psychology as a discipline. Prior to Freud, the role of the mental health professional such as the psychiatrist was primarily to diagnose and describe. Through psychoanalysis, Freud laid the groundwork for the notion of psychological intervention (Chaplin & Krawiec, 1960).

Among the key theorists in developmental psychology, **Erik Erikson** plays a unique role. His theory, which addresses primarily psychosocial development, was one of the few stage theories to cover the lifespan; hence, it is frequently found useful in studying human development. Like many others who had a major impact on the field of development in the twentieth century, Erikson's roots were in the Freudian tradition and, as such, are sometimes classified as "neo-Freudian." Like Freud, Erikson believed in the dynamic influences of psychological structures; however, he rejected Freud's strict biologic approach, addressing instead the sociocultural influences on development (Miller, 1983). Table 2–1

compares the basic stages described by these two important theorists.

Erikson viewed development as a series of conflicts or crises that must be resolved. These crises can be resolved in either a positive or a negative mode, which determines future function. The Erikson stages are summarized in Table 2–2.

Erikson's contributions to the field of developmental psychology were significant. As mentioned previously, the idea that developmental change occurs across the lifespan was new. Some tenets of Erikson's theory have been confirmed by research (Feldman, 1999), and his view of culture and society as important factors in shaping the individual's personality fits well with contemporary views of culture. But Erikson's theory is limited in predictive ability as well as in specific mechanisms of development (Miller, 1983; Feldman, 1999).

Freud and the neo-Freudians were essentially pursuing a psychology of motivation to answer several questions, the primary one being what drives people to act as they do. In particular, Freud's dynamic exchange among personality structures of id, ego, and superego revealed the unconscious nature of motivation. Another individual who specifically attempted to address human motivations was **Abraham H. Maslow.** Maslow's theory is organismic and is summarized by the concept of a *hierarchy of needs,* usually represented by a pyramid as shown in Figure 2–1. At the base of the pyramid are the physiologic needs, followed by safety. Then, progressing up the pyramid are love and belonging, esteem, and self-actualization. According to Maslow, a person acts according to the priority of needs at any given point in time. If a basic need, such as food, is denied, the individual will be obsessed with satisfying that need; however, as the basic needs become satisfied, the individual is free to seek the higher-level needs. Love and belonging reflect the need for intimacy and close interpersonal relationships; esteem is the need to be thought well of by self and others and relates to mastery and competence. **Self-actualization** is the need to become all that one can be (Chaplin & Krawiec, 1960). The issue of disability is an interesting one to discuss under the Maslow paradigm. According to the ICF model, there may be intrinsic and extrinsic barriers to individuals with disabilities realizing self-actualization.

Related to the study of motivation is the study of moral behavior and altruism. Psychologists wish to understand not only what developmental processes underlie the development of morality, but also what factors produce antisocial and violent behaviors. **Lawrence Kohlberg** was specifically concerned with the development of higher-level behaviors of morality and social consciousness. He identified three levels of moral thinking: preconventional, conventional, and postconventional, or autonomous (Kohlberg, 1974). In the *preconventional level,* typically represented in children aged

TABLE 2-1

Comparison of Freud's and Erikson's Theories on Dynamic Influences of Psychological Structures

Positive Outcomes of Erikson's Stages of Personality Development

1	2	3	4	5	6	7	8
Trust vs. Mistrust	*Autonomy vs. Shame/Doubt*	*Initiative vs. Guilt*	*Industry vs. Inferiority*	*Intimacy vs. Isolation*	*Identity vs. Role Confusion*	*Generativity vs. Stagnation*	*Ego Integrity vs. Despair*
The infant must form a loving, trusting relationship.	The child is motivated toward the development of functional movement.	The child is motivated by social challenges, becoming more confident.	The child is faced with peer comparisons and demands for new skills.	There is pressure to develop intimate relationships in friendships and romances.	The individual is motivated to achieve a sense of identity in adult occupational roles.	The individual is motivated toward the development of satisfaction in chosen occupational roles.	The individual is motivated to seek a sense of fulfillment and life satisfaction.

Freud's Biologic Stages

1	2	3	4	5
Oral	Anal	Phallic	Latency	Genital

Adapted from Thomas, 2001; Miller, 1983; Feldman, 1999; & Erikson, 1963.

TABLE 2–2	Summary of Erikson's Stages		

Stage	Age (approx.)	Task or Purpose	Adverse Resolution
I. Trust vs. Mistrust	Birth–1 yr	Infant learns that needs will be met; parents will return after absence; contingencies.	Fearful toward others.
II. Autonomy vs. Shame/ Doubt	1–2 yrs.	Differentiation of "self" wishes from others; learns control over basic physiologic functions and social exchange (saying NO!).	Insecurity, dependency.
III. Initiative vs. Guilt	3–5 yrs.	Begins to make or construct things in play; accepts parents as role models; "busy."	Belief that thoughts and actions are wrong, inferior, or bad.
IV. Industry vs. Inferiority	Childhood (6–12 yrs.)	Entering school; child is very proud of accomplishments.	Consistent failure may lead to a sense of inferiority.
V. Identity vs. Identity diffusion	Adolescence	Importance of peer relationships; separation from parents; tries out new roles; integration of previous resolutions.	Inability to identify roles, establish a self-identity and awareness.
VI. Intimacy vs. Isolation	Young adult	Uses identity established in previous stages; forms intimate relationships with friends, family, spouse.	Inability to form meaningful relationships; fear of commitment.
VII. Generativity vs. Stagnation	Adult	Becomes part of larger picture; wants to leave lasting mark on society through family and/or work.	Believes that life is meaningless; extreme self-absorption.
VIII. Ego Integrity vs. Despair	Older adult	Belief that life was worth living; made a lasting contribution; life is what it was—minimal regrets.	Regret for what one has done or not done.

Adapted from Miller, 1983; Feldman, 1999; & Erikson, 1963.

4 to 10, rules are obeyed primarily based on an understanding of rewards and punishment. As with all three levels, two stages are further characterized. In the first stage, rules are obeyed in order to avoid punishment, and in the second, rules are followed primarily to gain personal benefit—the concept of *pragmatic reciprocity.* In the *conventional level,* typically represented by preadolescents, rules are obeyed in order to preserve status in society as good and responsible people. In Stage 3, individuals obey rules in order to maintain the respect of others; in Stage 4 they do so in order to conform to society's rules, expressing an understanding of the importance of maintaining order in the society.

The final level is *postconventional morality.* In this level, the moral principles to which an individual subscribes are seen as transcending the dictates of a particular societal structure. In Stage 5 the individual operates on the concept of a *social contract,* an understanding of generally agreed-upon rights. In this stage,

the individual understands that personal values may dictate individual understanding of right and wrong but that there must be procedural rules founded on principles that protect all. The American Constitution reflects this stage of morality. Finally, Stage 6 consists of adherence to rules of conscience and self-chosen ethical principles (Kohlberg, 1974; Feldman, 1999).

Of course, these stages of moral thinking are inextricably linked to the development of cognitive processes that underlie these judgments, and Kohlberg states that the highest stage is unobtainable before the age of approximately 13, due to lack of development in cognitive structures. Furthermore, according to Kohlberg, not all individuals develop to the highest stage.

While some studies have findings that can be viewed as supportive of Kohlberg's theory, it has been criticized on several points. First, Kohlberg's theory is more applicable to moral judgments than to moral

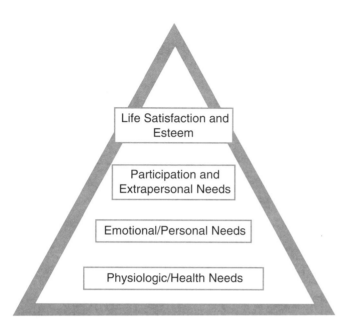

Life Satisfaction and Esteem

Participation and Extrapersonal Needs

Emotional/Personal Needs

Physiologic/Health Needs

FIGURE 2–1   Maslow's Hierarchy of Needs (adapted from Kagan, 1994, & Thomas, 2001)

behavior, meaning that individuals may make judgments reflecting the highest stage, but their judgments do not necessarily coincide with behavior. Second, Kohlberg's theory has been criticized as being descriptive only of the moral development of boys. Carol Gilligan argues that gender-related differences in child rearing relate to later differences in views of moral behavior. She believes that, for females, morality is more related to the well-being of the individual than to moral abstractions (Feldman, 1999).

Whereas **personality** represents the enduring emotional and behavioral characteristics of an individual,

temperament is conventionally used to refer to a predisposition of response (Feldman, 1999). Interest in temperament classifications resurfaced in the 1970s with the work of **Alexander Thomas** and **Stella Chess** (Kagan, 1994). In large part, dissatisfaction with the explanatory and predictive ability of either the psychoanalytic or behavioral schools led Thomas and Chess to develop a classification system for individual temperament based on nine dimensions of response: activity level, approach-withdrawal, adaptability, quality of mood or irritability, attention span and persistence, distractibility, rhythmicity, intensity of reaction, and threshold of responsiveness. The dimensions upon which analysis of temperament are based are detailed in Table 2–3. Scores on each of these dimensions may be compiled into one of three classifications of infants. These are so-called "easy" babies, "difficult" babies, and "slow-to-warm-up" babies.

Research has been done on the stability and predictive utility of these different temperament classifications (Feldman, 1999). A reason for the current significance of temperament work is based in neuropharmacology. The notion that the relative amounts of chemical neurotransmitters present in the brain in any individual at any point in time play a large role in determining an individual's pattern of behavior and response is the foundation of a great deal of research in today's laboratories. Contemporary thought regarding temperament suggests it is an ordered but changing reflection of the brain's basic chemical organization, which is both genetically and environmentally influenced (Kagan, 1994).

A discussion of the affective domain would be incomplete without some discussion of the affective elements of the human being's interactions with others in social relationships. Once again, an individual exposed early in his career to the Freudian school of thought

TABLE 2–3	Chess and Thomas's Dimensions of Temperament

- **Activity Level:** motor activity and the proportion of active and inactive periods.
- **Rhythmicity:** the predictability or unpredictability of biologic functions.
- **Approach/Withdrawal:** the individual's response to a new stimulus or a new environment.
- **Adaptability:** overall (not immediate) response to new or altered situations.
- **Sensory Threshold:** level of sensory stimulation needed to evoke a response.
- **Quality of Mood:** relative proportions of positive and negative mood behavior.
- **Intensity of Reactions:** The energy level of the person's responses.
- **Distractibility:** the degree to which outside stimuli interfere in ongoing behavior.
- **Persistence:** the continuation of an activity in the face of obstacles.
- **Attention:** the length of time an activity is pursued without interruption.

Adapted from Chess & Thomas, 1987.

developed a theory that had widespread significance. **John Bowlby** was a psychiatrist who had observed that family experience was related to emotional well-being. After World War II, Bowlby was invited to become the director of a mental health clinic. In this pursuit, he established a research division focused on the study of mother-child separation. Bowlby formulated a belief that an intimate and continuous relationship with the mother was necessary for the infant and young child to develop normal emotional attachments. He incorporated ethological work into his theory, becoming fascinated with data on imprinting and critical periods in animal development. He also presented work detailing the phenomenon of separation anxiety.

In 1950 Bowlby formed a relationship with **Mary Ainsworth** that was to further immortalize his work. Ainsworth brought her talents in methodology to the research. She worked with Bowlby in England for a while, then traveled to Uganda, where she studied the quality of mother-infant interaction. Ainsworth developed he classic *Strange Situation* experimental paradigm consisting of sequential scenarios of mother-infant play, separation, rejoining, and introduction of a stranger (Bretherton, 1994).

Ainsworth and Bowlby described three categories of attachment: secure, avoidant, and ambivalent. Infants are classified in these categories in accordance with the child's response to being reunited with the mother after separation. Securely attached children use the mother as a "home base," referencing to her when she is present. They are upset when the mother leaves and happy to see her when she returns. Avoidant children do not seek initial proximity to the mother and avoid her when she returns. Ambivalent children may have decreased exploratory behavior in the mother's presence, are distressed when she leaves, and, when she returns, alternate between a desire to be comforted and aggression toward the mother (Feldman, 1999). Ainsworth also identified the importance of the mother's sensitivity to the child's cues as one determinant of quality of attachment.

These theories of development in the affective domain have an impact on all domains of human function: physical, cognitive, and social. The domains of human function represent competence in the environment, whatever it may be. It is easy to see how that competence is related to personality, motivation and temperament, the topics addressed by these theorists.

COGNITIVE DOMAIN

The ability to function is likewise dependent on aspects of the cognitive domain—learning, language, and memory. In the ICF, these are known as specific mental functions. One of the most significant problems facing an aging population is Alzheimer's disease, which is a

dramatic deterioration of cognitive function, beginning with memory. An understanding of how cognitive functions develop, how they are impacted by the environment, and how they are sustained is important in designing learning, prevention, and remediation paradigms.

By far the best known figure in the area of cognitive development is **Jean Piaget.** Piaget's theory of cognitive development has charted the path toward understanding how human beings come to know what they know. Born in 1896 in Switzerland, he displayed an early interest in biology, publishing his first paper at the age of 10. After receiving his doctorate in 1918 at age 21 (with a thesis on mollusks), Piaget went to study at the Sorbonne in Paris, where he met Theodore Simon. Simon worked with Alfred Binet in Paris and suggested that Piaget assist in the standardization of intelligence tests by interviewing Parisian children. This experience stimulated Piaget to attempt to ascertain the nature of intelligence through meticulous empirical observation (Miller, 1983). Piaget returned to Switzerland as a director of studies at the J. J. Rousseau Institute, where he began the series of experiments that formed the basis for his theory of cognitive development.

Piaget's theory is complex and still evolving even after his death. From his background in biology, Piaget postulated two functional invariants: organization and adaptation. Organization is the tendency for integration of parts to a whole (Miller, 1983). Adaptation is a basic biologic need to permit functioning in a given environment. From adaptation, Piaget further identified the processes of **assimilation** and **accommodation,** which are integral to his theory. Assimilation is the process of changing elements of the environment so they can be incorporated into the organism's structure. The function of adaptation, illustrated in Figure 2–2, is to modify observations and experiences to fit the child's cognitive structures (Flavell, 1963). For example, when a young child labels all animals with four legs as dogs, assimilation has occurred. The child has modified the existing observation (cow, dog, horse) into the existing

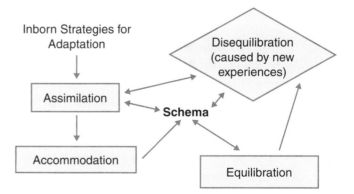

FIGURE 2–2   Adaptation and Formation of Schema as Described by Piaget (adapted from Beilin, 1994)

structure (dogs have four legs). Accommodation is changing of function in accordance with the environment (Flavell, 1963). For example, as a child learns, she might call a cow a "big dog." This shows modification of the concept of dog learned previously. In time, the child will learn to differentiate the salient features of "cow" by the process of accommodation.

The cognitive structures of Piaget's theory are known as *schema*. A schema refers to a class of similar sequences of action or mental representations that are related (Flavell, 1963; Miller, 1983). The process by which assimilation and accommodation are balanced is known as *equilibration*. Equilibration is achieved when neither assimilation nor accommodation is dominant. Conversely, *disequilibration* is when either the organism or the environment is changing and out of balance (Miller, 1983).

Piaget is a classic example of a hierarchical, or stage, theorist. He named four stages of cognitive development in which thought processes are qualitatively different from previous stages. There is some quantitative element to Piaget's theory, however, in that the number of schema and number of facts change over time (Miller, 1983). Despite the small quantitative aspect to his theory, the stages are some of the most classic elements.

The first stage is the **sensorimotor stage,** which can be divided into six substages. Although the stages are not equivalent to chronologic change, the sensorimotor stage is generally considered to run from birth to two years of age. The first substage is *reflexive,* lasting from approximately birth to one month. During this stage, the infant performs little volitional activity; most of the activity is reactive to stimuli. For example, the infant displays sucking and kicking patterns. Substage 2 is *primary circular reactions,* from approximately one to four months. Neonatal reflexes begin to be altered, so that the infant can repeat interesting actions volitionally. For example, the infant will begin to swipe or bat at objects repetitively. In the third substage, *secondary circular reactions,* the infant begins to act more upon objects, with the goal of making events that are interesting last longer. Secondary circular reactions roughly coincide with four to eight months of age. An example that is often given in this stage is picking up a rattle and shaking it. The fourth substage is *coordination of secondary circular reactions.* During this period, from approximately eight to twelve months, the infant begins to use objects instrumentally, in order to accomplish a goal. Intention is a hallmark of this stage.

Another key acquisition is first evident in Substage 4 of the sensorimotor stage: the development of the concept of *object permanence,* in which the infant knows that something continues to exist even when it is out of sight. One of the exercises infants will do to "test" this hypothesis is to drop things off the high-chair tray, visually following the object to the floor. When the parent obligingly returns the object to the tray, the infant drops it again. Through this and a number of such exercises, the infant "learns" that objects exist even when out of sight.

The second year of life is composed of two Piagetian substages, 5 and 6, lasting 12–18 and 18–24 months, respectively. In Substage 5 *tertiary circular reactions* occur, in which means and ends are combined in order to experiment with actions to determine consequences. In this stage, the child can solve problems with new means, by trial and error. A classic example would be to use a rod or stick to draw a toy that is out of reach closer. Substage 6 is *invention of new means through mental combinations.* In this stage, the child is able to mentally, without overt experimentation, devise means of manipulating the environment (Flavell, 1963; Miller, 1983; & Feldman, 1999).

The stages that follow the sensorimotor stage are **preoperational** (2–7 years), **concrete operations** (7–12 years), and **formal operations** (12 years and up). In the preoperational stage, several key aspects of cognitive development occur. The first is *symbolic function,* where the child is able to use signs and symbols to stand for something else. Piaget uses the concept of signs to refer to universally accepted signifiers that bear little or no concrete relationship to what they represent. Words are the most common signs. Symbols, on the other hand, are internal signifiers that usually have some resemblance to what they stand for. Piaget is very clear that language develops as a result of the development of symbolic function, not vice versa (Flavell, 1963).

Other characteristics of the preoperational stage include the notion of *egocentrism,* which is the inability to take another person's viewpoint. For example, when young children play hide-and-seek, they might hide in plain view, believing that because others can't be seen, others can't see them (Feldman, 1999). Another classic example of egocentrism is the Swiss mountain experiment in which toy mountain climbers are placed at various places along a mountain model. The child in this stage cannot understand how a person viewing the mountain from the other side of the table will see something different.

Still another characteristic of preoperational thought is *centration*. In centration, the child focuses on one salient aspect of a stimulus to the exclusion of others. For example, when a child looks at containers of different widths, she focuses on the width only, such that when a given amount of liquid is poured before her eyes into another container, she still does not see the volume as equal, because of an inability to decenter from focus on container width (Flavell, 1963). Children in preoperational thought cannot see the reversibility of actions. In the later preoperational stage, a transition from the more centered, rigid, and irreversible thought occurs in preparation for the transition to concrete operations.

In the period of concrete operations, the child is able to decenter, using an organized cognitive structure to organize and manipulate the environment. At this point he is capable of understanding the reversibility of actions and hence can grasp mathematical concepts of addition, subtraction, multiplication, and division. Now he grasps the concept of *identity*, that things are the same despite differences in shape or size. This permits the concept of *conservation* to evolve fully. The child in concrete operations is also able to understand relationships, such as those between distance, time, and speed (Feldman, 1999).

It is important to note that, according to Piaget, not every individual reaches the stage of formal operations. Typically, formal operations are reached when an individual has been exposed to more complexity in cognitive challenges; hence, there is some cultural bias to formal operations. Individuals who are members of a culture that places less value on math and science and greater value on agriculture may never need formal operations. The stage of formal operations is characterized by highly evolved symbolic thought and representation. Individuals who reach this stage are able to perform mental operations on abstract representations. Formal operations also permit hypothetico-deductive reasoning (Feldman, 1999).

Table 2–4 presents the basic stages described by Piaget next to those described by Erikson and Freud. This table gives some perspective on the differences between these three important theorists.

The preceding is a very brief overview of Piagetian theory, of which volumes have been written. Piaget's significance to the field of developmental psychology is enormous. It is agreed that one of his most important contributions was to make observable the study of the mind, involving cognition and learning. Previously it was believed that such topics could be approached only philosophically. Piaget's stages of cognitive development influenced educators to reevaluate their practices. His conceptualization of the child as a dynamic force in development was unique for his time, and his incorporation of both structure and function into his theory was significant.

Although Piaget's theory was rooted in biology, it incorporated the social and physical environments as key aspects of cognitive development (Beilin, 1994). In the more than half a century since his theory was first made known, it has been criticized and modified by many. One of the main criticisms of the theory was leveled at a process Piaget called *decalage* (meaning displacement), which was the idea that children do not enter a different stage of cognitive development uniformly across all dimensions. In other words, each child will show lags in some areas while moving forward in others. A developmental psychologist named **Robbie Case** has attempted to address this problem by reclassifying the stages after the sensorimotor stage and identifying substages for the latter three stages, much as Piaget did with the sensorimotor stage. Case also proposed that there is a feedback loop connecting specific contextual knowledge and general knowledge. He concluded that early cognitive function is primarily a reflection of biologic factors, but as the child ages, cultural and social influences tend to take over (Thomas, 2001).

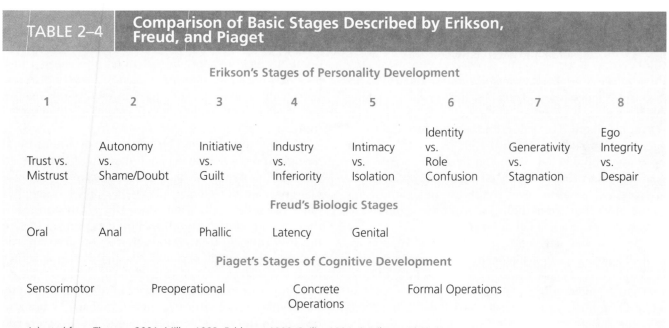

TABLE 2–4	Comparison of Basic Stages Described by Erikson, Freud, and Piaget						
			Erikson's Stages of Personality Development				
1	2	3	4	5	6	7	8
Trust vs. Mistrust	Autonomy vs. Shame/Doubt	Initiative vs. Guilt	Industry vs. Inferiority	Intimacy vs. Isolation	Identity vs. Role Confusion	Generativity vs. Stagnation	Ego Integrity vs. Despair
			Freud's Biologic Stages				
Oral	Anal	Phallic	Latency	Genital			
			Piaget's Stages of Cognitive Development				
Sensorimotor		Preoperational		Concrete Operations	Formal Operations		

Adapted from Thomas, 2001; Miller, 1983; Feldman, 1999; Beilin, 1994; & Erikson, 1963.

Another developmental theorist who studied cognitive development was the Russian **Lev Vgotsky.** Vgotsky's initial impact was not as noticeable as that of Piaget, in part because of his relatively short life (1896–1934); however, his work continues to stimulate investigation in the latter half of the twentieth century. Vgotsky differed from Piaget in his emphasis on sociocultural influences on cognitive development. This theory somewhat reflected the communist thought of the early post-revolution period, that is, the importance of communal support for the child. Vgotsky argued that in order to understand cognitive development, we need to evaluate what is significant in the cultural milieu in which the child is living. Vgotsky used the term **zone of proximal development** (ZPD) to refer to a child's being nearly prepared to comprehend a fact or perform a task such that a minimal support from others will allow her to successfully complete the task. Figure 2–3 illustrates the four stages of this process.

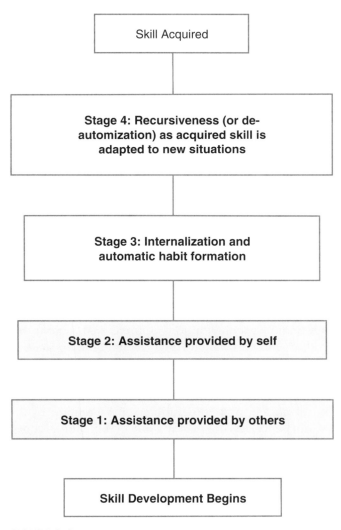

FIGURE 2–3   Vgotsky's Zone of Proximal Development (adapted from Feldman, 1999, & Thomas, 2001)

The support from others is known as *scaffolding.* Vgotsky also cited the importance to cognitive development of *private speech,* the talking to oneself that children do as they solve a puzzle, for example. He theorized that this private speech was integral to learning, but that children began to internalize this speech into mental processes by approximately nine years of age (Feldman, 1999). Psychologists have used Vgotsky's work to continue to study, among other things, the impact of culture on a child's learning and development. A psychologist named Valsiner has expanded Vgotsky's concepts, including the addition of two zones: the zone of free movement and the zone of promoted action. The *zone of free movement* refers to all the resources available to a child in an environment at a given point in time. The *zone of promoted action* refers to those actions or impulses that are promoted by the caregivers within the zone of free movement (Thomas, 2001). It is easy to see how this work is deemed invaluable in today's social and intellectual environment, which seeks to support cultural identity and diversity.

Piaget's work influenced educators in many ways, including the concepts of *active learning* and *readiness.* Vgotsky's work spawned educational innovations such as group learning and peer teaching. However, no one has had greater impact on the American educational system than **John Dewey** (1859–1952). Dewey was less of a developmental psychologist than a social psychologist and educational philosopher; however, his work had such impact on the education system that a brief overview is warranted. Like Vgotsky, Dewey believed that the cultural setting was key to understanding the human mind. Like both Piaget and Vgotsky, he believed in an empirical approach to understanding. Dewey felt that there were actually two fundamental psychologies, biologic and social, both warranting investigation. He criticized, however, the psychological laboratory as lacking relevance to the world and suggested instead that the school was the perfect "laboratory" for studying how a child learns. Dewey disagreed with Piaget on the notion that development would unfold naturally; instead, he believed that development could be directed and that education had the responsibility to shape children's intellectual development toward desired societal goals. He also disagreed with Piaget on the stage concept. Dewey believed that the school was the instrument of social progress and that the most significant outcome of education should be promotion of "growth," introducing the concept of one of education's core purposes as that of creating lifelong learners (Cahan, 1994).

The aforementioned theories had major impact on the study of cognitive development. Cognition, or mental function, is a multifaceted phenomenon, which has several related topics. Some of these include language, sensory-perceptual processing, and memory.

LANGUAGE

Piaget believed that language was a sign of underlying cognitive structure, whereas Vgotsky believed that language helped to drive and develop cognitive structures. One of the most important theorists in the study of language development is **Noam Chomsky.** Chomsky's theory of language development is classified as *nativist,* meaning that the determining mechanism for language acquisition is innate. This genetic predisposition, according to Chomsky, makes possible the learning of one or several languages that are based on universal grammar rules. The neural substrate that supports the acquisition of language was named the *language acquisition device (LAD)* (Feldman, 1999). The child's acquisition of language is viewed as a theory development, in which the child constructs the theory independent of either intelligence or experience. Chomsky argued that empirical theories of learning are inadequate to describe language acquisition, which can only be described to be an innate mental capacity tied to the universal linguistic structures (Chomsky, 1974).

Chomsky's theory is supported by several facts. First, no other organism, not even among the more highly evolved mammals such as chimps, has been successful in developing a complex language. This fact supports Chomsky's notion that the ability for language is innate and unique to humans. Second, neurobiologists have confirmed that there are areas of the human brain that are predestined to subserve the function of language. Chomsky's notion of sensitive periods, when the human is most likely to acquire language, has widespread validation.

SENSORY-PERCEPTUAL FUNCTION

The cognitive domain would not be completely discussed without giving some attention to sensory-perceptual function, which in essence is both input and product of mind. Beginning with approximately the eighteenth century, the subject of perception was addressed by such philosophers as Mill, Kant, and Hobbes, based on an interest in how people come to see the world. In the 1700s a Scottish philosopher named Thomas Reid was the first to differentiate between sensation and perception (Chaplin & Kraweic, 1960). Generally, sensation is the experience produced by stimulation of the sensory organs and is primarily a registry of information. Perception, on the other hand, uses several modes of information, including sensation, memory, and anticipation based on previous experience, to give meaning to sensory information.

The early theorists on perception were of two schools: the **nativist school** and the **empiricist school.** The nativists believed that genetic predisposition and innate abilities explained perception while the empiricists believed the formation of associations between various sensations was its origin (Chaplin & Kraweic, 1960). Helmholtz was one key theorist of the empirical camp who wrote in the mid-nineteenth century. He developed theories of hearing and color vision and believed that spatial qualities were perceived by something called *unconscious inference,* the addition to the sensory information of other information based on memory and previous experience. The association formed by all such information was what created the perception, according to Helmholtz (Chaplin & Krawiec, 1960).

Wundt was a contemporary of Helmholtz who added other analyses to the theory of perception. Also an empiricist, Wundt believed that a group of preexisting ideas and memories, which he termed an *apperceptive mass,* was applied to pure perceptions, thereby creating *apperceptions.* Thus, an apperception is an active, conscious product of mental processing, whereas the relatively simple *perception* is passive (Chaplin & Krawiec, 1960).

Titchener (1867–1927), an American pupil of Wundt's who went on to develop his theory, utilized a methodology called *introspection,* in which the psychologist analyzes self-consciousness. Titchener's theory was called a "core context" theory and had four key points. First, sensations are clustered in accordance with attention; second, the cluster of sensations is replaced by images; and third, the images provide meaning to the sensory experience. Finally, the perception, if it is common, may pass into unconsciousness and become represented in neuronal groupings (Chaplin & Krawiec, 1960).

German psychologists, including Wertheimer, Kohler, and Koffka, founded the **Gestalt school** in the late nineteenth century. The Gestalt school argued that introspection is insufficient to explain all perceptual phenomena, based on some classic experiments in which there were repetitive sensory illusions that defied the facts of the sensory experience. Gestalt psychology simply states that perception cannot be reduced to parts, but rather, the whole is greater than the sum of the parts. Figure 2–4 illustrates perceptual thinking within the Gestalt model.

Some key contributions of the Gestalt school that continue to have validity today include the notion that the individual will create a "best fit" perception in the face of inadequate or incomplete sensory data. This conclusion reflects the Gestalt belief that the perception is not a perfect or photographic representation of the world; hence, it is not merely a sum of sensations. Rather, the perception has a psychological form that represents the world but is not identical to it. The Gestalt school also pioneered the study of *figure-ground perception,* that is, the ability to pick out key points of a stimulus from the background (Chaplin & Krawiec, 1960).

Moving to a more contemporary, twentieth-century study of perception, attention must be directed to the work of **Eleanor Gibson** and her husband James. The

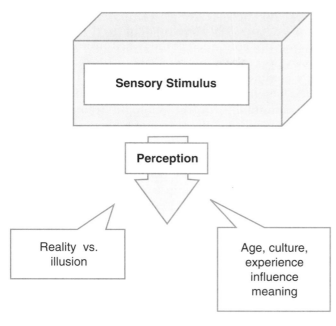

FIGURE 2–4 Principles of Gestalt Psychology (adapted from Chaplin & Krawiec, 1960)

Gibsons challenged the prior notion of associationism, saying instead that the sensory stimulation itself contained numerous meaningful elements and that perceptual learning was actually learning to pay attention or differentiate more and more information from the pattern. Eleanor Gibson did a classic visual perception experiment to support this notion. She tested seven- and nine-year-olds and adults, presenting a scribble picture of a coil, followed by other pictures, asking the subjects to identify whether they were identical to or different from the initial picture. She gave no feedback and repeated the experiment. She found the expected difference in accuracy between adults and children. However, more significantly, she found that subjects' accuracy improved over trials, indicating to her that what was occurring was that subjects expanded the salient features of the pictures over trials. For example, initially the subjects might focus on the size or shape of the coil. With repetition, all the subjects, including the children, began to take note of more features, such as direction of the coil, distance between loops, and so on.

Other features of the Gibsons' theory included the importance of information obtained through exploratory activity and the notion of *affordance,* which is the salient property of stimuli in relationship to the explorer. Gibson supported this notion of affordance in research on infant locomotor patterns. She tested two groups of infants: a group of crawlers and a group of walkers. The infants had the choice to walk over one of two surfaces— a rigid surface or a waterbed-like surface—both with the same visual pattern. The walkers consistently chose the

rigid surface, supporting the notion that for a walker, the rigidity of the surface is the salient feature.

Since the 1960s Gibson's work has focused a great deal on the development and characteristics of perception in infancy. Perhaps she is best known for her visual cliff study with Richard Walk, in which crawling infants were allowed to crawl toward their mothers on a checkered surface that had an optical drop-off. The results showed that infants of 6 to 14 months would not crawl over the visual cliff. This pioneering work of the Gibsons is anticipated to be combined with newer strategies of neurologic imaging to further our understanding of perceptual development (Pick, 1994).

MEMORY

Memory is an inherent component of cognitive function that has received greatest attention recently in the study of memory loss in aging. In the ICF framework, memory is a specific mental function. However, earlier studies focused on the development and functioning of memory from the behavioral and physiologic perspectives. Behavioral study of memory began in the nineteenth century with the experiments of a psychologist named Ebbinghaus. Ebbinghaus is perhaps best known for identifying a *retention curve* that showed the nearly immediate rapid decline in material remembered, followed by a slow deterioration. Ebbinghaus also showed that increasing the length of lists of items to be memorized increases not only the total length of time to accomplish the task, but the time per unit (Chaplin & Kraweic, 1960).

Gordon Bower, a psychologist at Stanford University, did further pioneering work in the area of memory. In particular, Bower studied the use of *mnemonics,* or memory-enhancing devices, to improve retention. Some of the mnemonic devices he has studied and documented as effective include loci, pegwords, and number-to-sound coding. The method of *loci* involves mentally putting a physical location or place to the stimulus. For example, in a shopping list, you might visualize moving through your kitchen in sequence, identifying items you need as you go. *Pegwords* means associating words, usually a list that rhymes, to numerals (1 = cat, 2 = hat). The list that is to be memorized is then tied to the pegwords in sequence. For example, if you have to get milk, you remember the cat drinks milk. Finally, *number-to-sound coding* is similar to the concept of pegwords except that letter sounds are tied to numerals. When you are given a number to remember, you simply combine the sounds into a word, even a nonsense word. Suggestions about how to remember made by Bower also include paying careful attention in registering the stimulus as the name in an introduction and also elaborating on the material mentally. For example, you might link a person's name to a rhyme or to a visual image, such as a blacksmith for Mr. Smith. Bower's work showed that the capacity to remember is much greater than the average ability to remember, and that memory skills can be taught and learned (Bower, 1974).

PSYCHOMOTOR DOMAIN

In order to discuss behaviors in the psychomotor domain, it is first necessary to establish some definitions. First, in consideration of motor function, we are looking at **motor behavior,** meaning any performance of movement that can be observed or documented (this term ignores the motor behaviors of the intrinsic muscles of the body, such as the heart, in defining motor behavior). **Motor development** is the acquisition of motor behavior that is heavily maturational in origin. Behaviors that develop tend to have a proportionally greater maturational or genetic component than learned behaviors. They also tend to have broad stability across cultures and to be less affected by environmental circumstance. **Motor learning,** on the other hand, is the acquisition of motor behavior that is more environmentally dependent. Behaviors that are learned tend to require greater environmental support, including the provision of some kind of coaching feedback. Furthermore, learned behaviors are dependent on quality and quantity of practice.

Although the categories of developed and learned behaviors are not mutually exclusive, those acquired by a developmental process, such as rolling and walking, are often called *milestones,* whereas those acquired through learning, such as jumping rope or riding a bicycle, are called *motor skills.* Measurement of acquisition time differs for the two types of behaviors. Motor development and acquisition of milestones are usually measured in months or years, whereas motor skill acquisition is measured in days or weeks.

THEORIES OF MOTOR DEVELOPMENT

In the first half of the twentieth century, significant gains were made in the theoretical underpinnings of child development. This research arose largely from a national focus, in the early part of the century, on the wars that had such an impact on the United States. The interest in child development arose around the prediction problem. When large numbers of men (and some women) entered the military, large-scale testing was carried out across a number of functions. It then became of interest to identify why individual differences in proficiency occurred and to determine if attributes could be predicted. In this climate, funding was available for large-scale studies of development, centered primarily in two places, Yale on the east coast and Berkeley on the west coast.

Arnold Gesell (1880–1961) was the director of the Yale Clinic of Child Development from 1911 to 1948, and his work continued at the Gesell Institute after his mandatory retirement from Yale in 1948. Several others, including Charles Darwin and G. E. Coghill, influenced Gesell's work. From Darwin, Gesell confirmed his commitment to the biologic framework and methodology. Coghill was an embryologist who studied the development of locomotion in salamanders, correlating the onset of motor pattern to underlying changes in neural maturation. The perspectives from Coghill's work that had a defining influence on Gesell were (1) that behavior has a characteristic pattern, (2) that the nature of that pattern reflects the underlying maturation of neural structure, and (3) that the emergence of the pattern is directly tied to the maturational process, which is genetically driven (Thelen & Adolph, 1994). Gesell's "laboratory" consisted of sophisticated cinemagraphic equipment and toys that infants and children would explore. His scientific contribution was a meticulous account of the individual child's approach to various tasks. Of course, Gesell noted individual differences in the children's performances, but he attributed these largely to innate differences.

Perhaps the most enduring contribution of Gesell's work was the publication of large-scale norms of child behavior and development. The *Gesell Schedules,* as they were called, formed the basis for numerous developmental assessments over the years. Gesell also contributed the concept of the *developmental quotient,* mirroring the intelligence quotient with a developmental age determined by a test of normative behavior in which the score was divided by the chronologic age and multiplied by 100. Because he was a pediatrician by training, in addition to being a teacher and psychologist, Gesell had a profound influence on the field of pediatrics. He was important in the establishment of the field of developmental pediatrics and in the notion that pediatricians should have some developmental training.

Gesell's theory is perhaps the most profoundly maturational of any that have been discussed here. His belief was that it was the genetically driven unfolding of the innate potential that produced acquisition of new developmental behaviors. From this belief, he formulated *laws of developmental direction.* These laws, as a group, summarized the trends of developmental milestone acquisition as follows:

1. *Development proceeds in a cephalocaudal direction.* The infant gains control progressively of the head, shoulders, down the spine, and ultimately the lower legs.
2. *Development proceeds proximal to distal.* The infant gains control of shoulder and hip before hand and foot.

3. *Development proceeds medial to lateral.* Medial to lateral development is similar to proximal to distal; for example, in the hand, development of grasp moves from ulnar (medial) to radial (lateral).

4. *Development proceeds up against gravity.* The infant progresses from completely prone to prone on elbows, then supported by hands, then supported by all four limbs, and finally standing and walking.

Other principles traced to Gesell include *functional asymmetry,* in which the infant progresses from initial asymmetry through symmetry and once again to asymmetry to develop handedness; *optimal realization,* in which the infant is able to progress despite adverse circumstances; and finally, the important principle of *reciprocal interweaving* (Thelen & Adolph, 1994), in which there is a progressive spiral reincorporation of sequential forms of behavior. Reciprocal interweaving refers to the fact that, during development, the infant will appear to show alternating dominance of antagonistic behaviors: for example, flexion-extension and approach-avoidance. However, the nondominant behavior has not disappeared but will reappear at a higher functional level (the progressive spiral). A simplistic example of this is seen in locomotor development. The infant first displays reflexive supporting and stepping responses when supported upright. These responses disappear, and the infant will enjoy a "bouncing game," withdrawing legs when placed in standing (astasia) at the age of around 5–6 months. Shortly thereafter the infant will resume standing again, but this time it is more mature in terms of postural control.

Gesell's influence on the study of child development had some unexpected negative consequences. First, his work on motor development was so persuasive in attributing development to biologic mechanisms that for several decades the processes of motor development were not considered of interest for further study (Thelen & Adolph, 1994). A second, more pervasive influence was brought about by Gesell's maturational focus. Because he believed that development was relatively unaffected by external forces, he was responsible for the "wait and see" attitude adopted by many pediatricians and child-care professionals to developmental problems. In other words, if the parent had a concern that the child hadn't yet walked, the first approach was to give the child more time, as it was believed that there was little that could be done to change the course of development. The last 20 years of study and experience have disputed these notions.

The idea of brain plasticity and the concomitant importance of early environment have driven social policy such that there is federal support for early intervention programs for infants with special needs or at risk for problems. The outcome of these programs, particularly for infants with Down syndrome, dispute Gesell's notion of the determinance of innate functions. Gesell's influence, however, was at some odds with his theoretical perspective. Gesell always recommended a nurturing and supportive environment for the infant and child, even though his perspective was that such an environment promoted unfolding of innate abilities rather than actually changing the abilities (Thelen & Adolph, 1994).

A contemporary of Gesell's who also had a lasting influence on the field of motor development was **Myrtle McGraw.** McGraw is classified as a maturationist, because, like Gesell, she was interested in correlation of change in underlying structure with change in function. However, McGraw herself was often at odds with Gesell, and the two were not collegial. McGraw differed from Gesell in that she saw the environment as having a greater influence than he did, and she believed that environment could potentially change the influences of developing structures.

McGraw was best known and probably is most cited for her famous study of two twins, Johnny and Jimmy. The purpose of the study was to determine the effect of environmental influence on motor performance. To that end, for the first 22 months of life, Johnny received a motorically enriched environmental experience, including roller-skating before one year of age. Jimmy, on the other hand, had only a minimally supportive motoric environment. The outcome of the study did not support a simplistic maturational hypothesis. For example, for some behaviors, the accelerated motor experience did not produce significant differences—as in motor milestones of sitting and walking. For motor skills such as roller-skating and riding a tricycle, differential results were obtained. Johnny learned to roller-skate very quickly, having been exposed to the skates at less than one year of age. Jimmy experienced roller-skating at 22 months of age but never became proficient; however, when skating experiences had been concluded for an interval, neither twin persisted in his skating ability.

In concluding her study, McGraw summarized key factors that affect motor development: attitude, practice, readiness, physical growth, and level of fixity (referring to how secure a skill is before practice is discontinued). She ultimately attributed the difference in motor performance between the two twins as a combination of these factors (Payne & Isaacs, 1999). Overall, the fact that there was not an immense difference in outcome between Johnny and Jimmy was seen by the scientific community as support for the biologic-maturation hypothesis, and, hence, McGraw often gets placed in that classification.

McGraw disputed a strict biologic explanation for development. She introduced the notion of *critical periods,* times when an organism is most receptive to learning a certain kind of behavior. She was explicit, however, in saying that critical periods were not exclusive, they just referred to a time when the child was most receptive and learning would be most efficient. McGraw's critical periods have been widely accepted in both education and neuroscience. One example of a contemporary application is the research table presented in Figure 2–5.

McGraw disagreed with the notion that environment had little influence on development. She believed that many of the emerging behaviors she observed had the qualities of learned components. McGraw also identified a period of disorganization and deterioration of function in times of transition to higher levels. Her theory differs from Gesell's theory of reciprocal interweaving in that Gesell never proposed an actual deterioration of function. McGraw believed such a period occurred as the underlying structures were reorganizing to support new behaviors (Bergenn, Dalton, & Lipsitt, 1994). For example, the very young infant was observed to display holding of breath and more rhythmic motions when placed in water than did the slightly older infant, who seemed to flail and struggle. McGraw viewed the seeming deterioration as a period of reorganization prior to development of true swimming behavior (McGraw, 1945). Studies of neural development and plasticity support the notion that the developing nervous system is shaping a synaptic pattern, which includes both activation and development of synapses as well as synapses becoming dormant or disappearing.

THEORIES OF MOTOR LEARNING

We have differentiated motor development from motor learning along a continuum of relative influence of the environment. Motor learning theories, therefore, constitute a very different paradigm for viewing motor behavior, with a different terminology. Motor learning will be discussed in greater detail in Chapter 3.

THEORIES OF MOTOR CONTROL

Motor control is the study of the control of posture and movement, usually emphasizing the role of the central nervous system. As with motor learning, theories of motor control may be open loop or closed loop. The typical closed-loop theory of motor control is the *reflex theory,* in which movement is elicited in response to a sensory stimulus. Consider a stretch. The resultant contraction of the muscle takes it off the stretch position, thereby eliciting a signal to stop contracting. Postural sway is a classic example of the reflex theory of motor control.

Hierarchical models of motor control had widespread acceptance from the mid- to late twentieth century, paralleling the work of Coghill, Gesell, and McGraw in describing the neural mechanisms that mediate movement. Whereas the aforementioned authors emphasized the developmental hierarchy, this model of motor control emphasized the increased role of higher centers in regulating movement as maturation

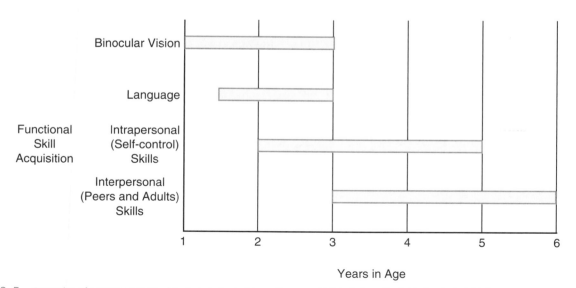

FIGURE 2–5   Examples of McGraw's Critical Periods (adapted from Bergenn, V. W., Dalton, T., & Lipsitt, L. P., 1994)
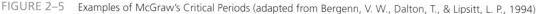

progressed. The motor patterns, primarily reflexes, that were elicited solely at the spinal level, were most primitive. As the baby matured, the mid-level of control, representing first the postural reflex patterns and then the mature postural reactions (righting, protective extension and equilibrium), developed. The behavioral manifestation of movement was believed to directly reflect the level of central nervous system (CNS) maturation. If damage to the nervous system occurred, it was believed that lower centers of control once again exerted a dominance in motor systems, and it was the task of the rehabilitation process to attempt to activate the higher levels of control.

The hierarchical model of control is no longer accepted as the definitive theory of motor control. Some reasons for its rejection include the fact that development does not perfectly reflect CNS maturation, and top-down control has been disproven. The accepted model of motor control today views a number of systems acting in parallel with elaborate multidirectional communication between neural centers. The hierarchical model of control also did not address the fact that the so-called reflexes, while dominant in the infant, are not obligatory, thereby raising the question of whether or not the reflex pattern actually exists. Finally, different responses can be elicited from the stimulation of the same neural pathways, depending on environmental context variables (Horak, 1991).

Most of today's literature emphasizes the systems theory of motor control. The dynamical systems theory, as discussed in Chapter 1, is based on a theory of physics. In systems theory, the end point, or goal, of the motor behavior is what is important. The numerous systems involved in producing movement organize themselves in such a way that the goal may be met given the constraints placed on systems by a variety of variables.

The attractiveness of the systems theory as applied to motor control is that it explains several phenomena, such as the aforementioned fact that different responses can be elicited from stimulation of the same neural pathways. In systems theory, the organization and interaction of the participating systems would change in accordance with the new environmental task constraints.

The systems theory has been challenged for terminology that is difficult to test and difficulty in operationalizing the theory (Horak, 1991). Although the systems theory is broad, other contemporary theories of motor control attempt to explain how some of the individual systems contribute to motor control. For example, in *motor program* theory, key systems guiding movements are central programs generated by CNS activity. These range from very specific neural networks called *central pattern generators,* which direct certain movement patterns, to the most sophisticated higher-level programs generated by the interaction of all CNS systems. Likewise, an ecological theory developed by James Gibson based on his perceptual work emphasizes how the active organism gears its behavior to perceptual information obtained from the environment (Shumway-Cook & Wollacott, 2001).

CONTINUOUS MULTI-DOMAIN: BEHAVIORISM

A final set of theories of performance exists that cannot be placed under a single domain. This theoretical perspective, known as **behaviorism,** covers all domains of behavior. The origins of behaviorism are in the **classical conditioning** experiments by a Russian, **Ivan Pavlov.** Pavlov documented how hungry dogs could be conditioned to salivate to the sound of a bell by pairing the sound of the bell with the presentation of meat (Feldman, 1999). Salivation was the conditioned response (CR), the sound of the bell the conditioned stimulus (CS), and the presentation of the meat the unconditioned stimulus (UCS). Pavlov's contributions to the field of psychology are founded in systematic experimentation and objective recording of results (Chaplin & Krawiec, 1960). Figure 2–6 illustrates classical conditioning. Note that the previously neutral stimulus elicits a "conditioned" response. This type of learning occurs below the level of consciousness and can be difficult to counteract.

An important feature of classical conditioning is that the subject is passive, and an outside person or event reinforces desired behavior. This has proved to be a productive model for psychological research but is less applicable in natural human environments. For therapists hoping to assist clients in positive behavior change, the strategies discussed in subsequent paragraphs utilizing an active subject are more often appropriate.

The first American to adopt the theory of behaviorism was **John Watson** (1878–1958). In 1913 Watson proposed that behavioral psychology is objective and seeks to predict and control behavior (Horowitz, 1994). Watson saw the stimulus-response relationship as the essential one between organism and environment (Chaplin & Krawiec, 1960). He is known for making the statement that if given a dozen healthy infants, by controlling the environment he could train them to become any one of a number of careers that he selected for them, including doctor, lawyer (or beggar-man and thief) (Horowitz, 1994). Watson was also known for his "Little Albert" experiment, in which he was able to condition an 11-month-old infant to be afraid of a white rat by pairing its presentation with a noxious noise. This conditioned response generalized to other stimuli, such as a rabbit, a fur coat, and a Santa mask (Miller, 1983). Watson was the extreme environmentalist; although he acknowledged some role for heredity, he saw it primarily in terms of dictating structure rather than function.

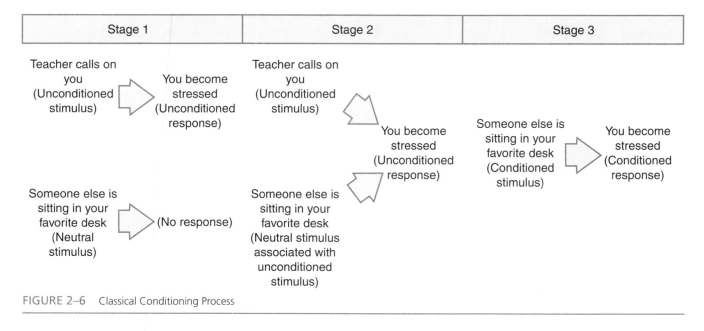

Stage 1	Stage 2	Stage 3

Teacher calls on you (Unconditioned stimulus) ➡ You become stressed (Unconditioned response)

Someone else is sitting in your favorite desk (Neutral stimulus) ➡ (No response)

Teacher calls on you (Unconditioned stimulus)

Someone else is sitting in your favorite desk (Neutral stimulus associated with unconditioned stimulus)

You become stressed (Unconditioned response)

Someone else is sitting in your favorite desk (Conditioned stimulus) ➡ You become stressed (Conditioned response)

FIGURE 2–6   Classical Conditioning Process

In the next cohort of behaviorists, Clark Hull, known for his deductive methodology, led a group at Yale. He introduced to the stimulus-response paradigm the "O" variables, which are unobservable factors. One example of such a factor is the sensory processing that occurs within the organism in response to a stimulus. Hull's learning paradigm looked something like S-O-R, in which S is the stimulus, O is the organism's processing, and R is the emitted response. Hull derived postulates describing how learning occurs. He attempted to devise precise, quantitative laws for learning (Chaplin & Krawiec, 1960). Meanwhile, at Harvard, the psychologist who came to be known as "Mr. Behaviorism" was further developing his theory. **B.F. Skinner** (1904–1990) was the most direct descendant of Watson in that he assigned the ultimate source of human behavior to the environment. Skinner's theory of **operant conditioning** relies almost entirely on the study of responses. He added to the conditioning paradigm the concept of **reinforcement,** or a stimulus produced as a result of the response, illustrated in Figure 2–7. In this model learning is conscious, and the type and rate of responses are directly related to the outcome the individual desires (earning a brownie in the example in Figure 2–7).

Skinner classified behaviors that were elicited in response to a determined stimulus, such as the food or the bell in Pavlov's experiments, as *respondents*. However, Skinner argued that the majority of behavior could not be studied from the perspective of a specific eliciting stimulus. Rather, he posited, most behaviors are emitted, meaning that specific stimuli are not identifiable. These behaviors are the *operants* (e.g., cleaning up the kitchen in Figure 2–7). Reinforcers are the result of the operant behavior. Positive reinforcers (e.g., the brownie in Figure 2–7) are desired outcomes that lead to an increase in the behavior.

Punishment is a potential consequence of a response, but Skinner describes punishment as an ineffective method of behavior control because it only temporarily eliminates the response, but not permanently. In other words, the organism learns to avoid punishment, but when the punishment is removed, the behavior is likely to recur, because the strength of the behavior, or operant, has not been affected (Chaplin & Krawiec, 1960). Skinner saw as his major scientific contribution the analysis of operant behavior, including reinforcement contingencies as related to a reinforcement schedule (Hall, 1974). Reinforcement schedules could focus on intervals (elapsed time) or ratios (number of responses required for response) and could be continuous, fixed, or variable. Using the notorious "Skinner box," which was a box with a bar that the animal pressed to receive a pellet of food, Skinner studied the effect of various reinforcement schedules on operant behavior. He also studied the contingencies under which response rate decreases as a

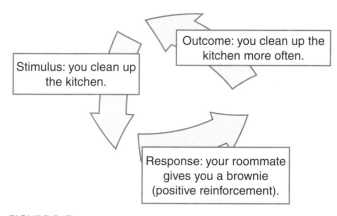

Stimulus: you clean up the kitchen.

Outcome: you clean up the kitchen more often.

Response: your roommate gives you a brownie (positive reinforcement).

FIGURE 2–7   Operant Conditioning Process (adapted from Feldman, 1999)

result of withdrawal of reinforcement. Generally, it was found that continuously reinforced behaviors were quicker to undergo extinction than those that had been variably reinforced. Extinction occurred more rapidly than forgetting, which is a time decay of the operant (Chaplin & Krawiec, 1960).

The contributions of the behaviorists, and Skinner in particular, to the study of human behavior are immense. First, they popularized the idea that empirical methods could be used to answer every question of importance in understanding human performance. Second, they had a major impact on society, especially child-rearing practices and the notion of reward and punishment. Finally, they provided scientists with a means to shape animal behavior in order to perform numerous studies on effects of manipulations on behavior.

SOCIAL LEARNING THEORY

A natural legacy of the behaviorist perspective is social learning theory, which turns its attention to how children learn the rules and behavior of social functioning. Psychologists in this field focused on three areas of socialization: aggression, dependency, and identification, which is the process of assimilating social rules regarding moral and sex-role development (Grusec, 1994). Two names inextricably linked to social learning theory are **Robert Sears** and **Albert Bandura,** who were colleagues at Stanford University, although they never collaborated on any major work. Each made significant contributions independently. The social learning theory developed by Sears had its foundation in the work of Hull; however, in the organism's functions, Sears applied the concepts of psychoanalytic theory. For example, Sears explained how the child becomes dependent on the mother. He postulated that the mother is consistently paired with the reduction of drive states, such as hunger, discomfort, and so forth, such that she ultimately becomes a reinforcer for the child. He further stated that, since the young child cannot distinguish between self and mother, the child begins to reproduce the mother's actions through imitation, which in itself becomes reinforcing (Grusec, 1994).

Eventually, social learning theorists began to decrease the emphasis on drive and look more closely at the chain of behaviors evident in a dyad or triad of interactions (Miller, 1983). This emphasis on the interaction between individuals was expanded upon later by Bandura and called *reciprocal determinism.* Sears did not view social development as occurring in stages; rather, he offered three mechanisms of explanation: learning, physical maturation, and social standards of expectation (Grusec, 1994).

Bandura's work never incorporated psychoanalytic theory; from its inception, operant principles were emphasized. However, his theory evolved over time to incorporate cognitive information processing as a key element. Bandura's legacy is perhaps most tied to the concept of **modeling,** which was how he attempted to resolve the issue of learning of novel responses. Basically, Bandura and his colleague Walters speculated that children need not be directly reinforced or punished for a behavior. Instead, a process known as *vicarious reinforcement* could occur in which the child observed the reinforcement of others' behavior and thus learned rules of reinforcement by observation. Bandura named four essential components in the process of modeling: (1) attention to the model, (2) retention of past experiences, (3) ability to reproduce the response physically, and (4) motivation to produce the response.

Bandura elaborated on the interactional dynamics of social exchange, coining the term *reciprocal determinism* for the concept that the person's actions themselves help to create or determine the environment in which social exchange occurs (Miller, 1983). Although once again maintaining its origin in the behaviorist tradition, in its final form Bandura's social learning theory is best classified as an information-processing theory, involving memory, imagery, and problem solving (Grusec, 1994).

SUMMARY

All of the theories discussed in this chapter have had a major impact on the field of psychology and the understanding of human behavior. In the preceding chapter function was divided into three categories: physical, psychological, and social. In this chapter a number of different theories have been presented regarding the nature and development of human behavior. As illustrated in Figure 2–8, theory attempts to explain human behavior, taking into account performance and contextual factors. Theory, as mentioned at the beginning of this chapter, is not fact. Therefore, theory can change, be proved or disproved. The important contribution of theory to the analysis of human function is that it leads to a set of rules that are subject to investigation. These rules also guide practice, as we've seen in the child-rearing impact of Skinner's theory and the educational impact of Vgotsky's, Piaget's, and Dewey's theories. Theories help us propose plans for interventions that will maximize human functioning; however, it is only through ongoing analysis and investigation that we will refine our ability to create interventions that optimize human potential under a number of internal and external conditions.

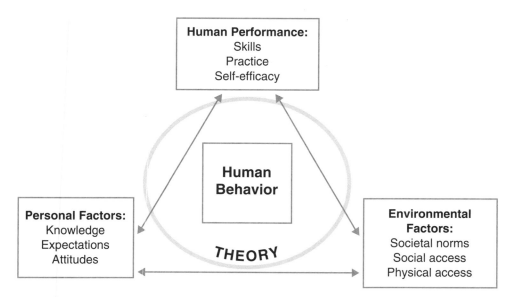

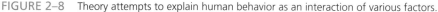

FIGURE 2–8   Theory attempts to explain human behavior as an interaction of various factors.

Speaking of

Who Really Cares About Theory?

ANNE CRONIN, PhD, OTR/L, BCP
PEDIATRIC OCCUPATIONAL THERAPIST

I like many of you, first learned about many of the theorists discussed in this chapter in my first "General Psychology" course. It was not exciting, but Pavlov and the dogs were kind of interesting. In all, it meant very little to me. Later, as a graduate student, I saw that every class seemed to have its own take on theory, and sociology theories were applied to management, and economic theories were applied to human behavior, and I plodded through them all—sometimes with interest, other times just to get through.

My first job as an occupational therapist was in an intermediate care facility for developmentally delayed adults. Part of my job was to help people transition from the institution to the community. Ricky, in his middle 30s, had been institutionalized at birth. He had severe spastic cerebral palsy, had no ability to speak, and was dependent on others in all aspects of self-care. In spite of this, Ricky was social and playful, had a wonderful sense of humor, and although untestable by traditional means, appeared to have excellent reasoning abilities. Ricky was recognized as exceptional and given special status in the institution. He had his own room and his choice of caregivers, and was allowed to share meals with the staff rather than with the other residents. Our ambitious team of young therapists and social workers worked for about two years to get Ricky equipment and build community connections. It wasn't until we started taking Ricky out to look at apartments that Ricky really understood our goal. All of us were dumbfounded as Ricky systematically "lost" the ability to use his communication device and began having bouts of aggression. We were confused and hurt by Ricky's sudden rejection of all that we had worked on.

It wasn't until I began working on my doctorate in medical sociology that the importance of theory and an understanding of Ricky came together for me. I had been keeping up with the developments in occupational therapy theory and had begun teaching occupational therapy. I was a good

Continues

Speaking of Continued

therapist, and strongly believed in the premises of my profession. Then, as I came face to face with the theories of Karl Marx, Emile Durkheim, and Karl Mannheim, I was forced to take on a societal rather than a clinical perspective. Tackling those giants in theory development, I learned how their theories had shaped beliefs and understanding, and influenced all of science for generations to come.

As I reflected on Durkheim's ideas about isolation and alienation, I understood that the challenge of a clinician is not just to collect information about people's lives and their personal expectations, but to problem-solve in a complex way that supports the individual while integrating the best your profession has to offer. I then understood that for Ricky, the institution was home. He was truly loved there and was always singled out for a lot of special attention. The community was a fearsome jungle to him. He was viewed as a freak and was avoided by others. In Ricky's view, we were replacing his home, his family, and his security with alienation and isolation. How stupid I felt. While focusing on our professional goals and values, we had lost awareness of the human being and the occupations he most valued. Ricky taught me that knowledge without perspective may result in "progress" without influencing participation in meaningful everyday contexts. Theory is a dynamic tool to help us integrate knowledge and research to address the very real human factors influencing functional performance across the lifespan.

REFERENCES

Beilin, H. (1994). Jean Piaget's enduring contribution to developmental psychology. In R. D. Parke, P. A. Ornstein, J. J. Rieser, & C. Zahn-Waxler (Eds.), *A century of developmental psychology* (pp. 257–290). Washington, DC: American Psychological Association.

Bergenn, V. W., Dalton, T., & Lipsitt, L. P. (1994). Myrtle B. McGraw: A growth scientist. In R. D. Parke, P. A. Ornstein, J. J. Rieser, & C. Zahn-Waxler (Eds.), *A century of developmental psychology* (pp. 389–423). Washington, DC: American Psychological Association.

Bretherton, I. (1994). Origins of attachment theory. In R. D. Parke, P. A. Ornstein, J. J. Rieser, & C. Zahn-Waxler (Eds.), *A century of developmental psychology* (pp. 431–471). Washington, DC: American Psychological Association.

Cahan, E. D. (1994). John Dewey and human development. In R. D. Parke, P. A. Ornstein, J. J. Rieser, & C. Zahn-Waxler (Eds.), *A century of developmental psychology* (pp. 145–167). Washington, DC: American Psychological Association.

Chaplin, J. P., & Krawiec, T. S. (Eds.) (1960). *Systems and theories of psychology.* New York: Holt, Rinehart and Winston.

Chess, S., & Thomas, A. (1987). *Know your child: An authoritative guide for today's parents.* New York: Basic Books.

Chomsky, N. (1974). Language and the mind. In *Readings in Psychology Today* (pp. 146–151). Del Mar, CA: Ziff-Davis.

Erikson, E. H. (1963). *Childhood and society.* New York: Norton.

Feldman, R. S. (Ed.) (1999). *Child development: A topical approach.* Upper Saddle River, NJ: Prentice Hall.

Grusec, J. E. (1994). Social learning theory and developmental psychology: The legacies of Robert Sears and Albert Bandura. In R. D. Parke, P. A. Ornstein, J. J. Rieser and C. Zahn-Waxler (Eds.), *A century of developmental psychology* (pp. 473–497). Washington, DC: American Psychological Association.

Hall, M. H. (1974). An interview with "Mr. Behaviorist," B. F. Skinner. In *Readings in Psychology Today* (pp. 114–119). Del Mar, CA: Ziff-Davis.

Horak, F. (1991). Assumptions underlying motor control for neurologic rehabilitation. In M. J. Lister (Ed.), *Contemporary management of motor control problems: Proceedings of the II step conference* (pp. 11–27). Alexandria, VA: Foundation for Physical Therapy.

Horowitz, F. D. (1994). John B. Watson's legacy: Learning and environment. In R. D. Parke, P. A. Ornstein, J. J. Rieser, and C. Zahn-Waxler (Eds.), *A century of developmental psychology* (pp. 233–256). Washington, DC: American Psychological Association.

Kagan, J. (1994). Yesterday's premises, tomorrow's promises. In R. D. Parke, P. A. Ornstein, J. J. Rieser, and C. Zahn-Waxler (Eds.), *A century of developmental psychology* (pp. 551–568). Washington, DC: American Psychological Association.

Kohlberg, L. (1974). The child as moral philosopher. In *Readings in Psychology Today* (pp.186–191). Del Mar, CA: Ziff-Davis.

McGraw, M. (1945). *Neuromuscular maturation of the human infant.* New York: Columbia University Press.

Miller, P. H. (Ed). (1983). *Theories of developmental psychology*. San Francisco: W. H. Freeman.

The New American Webster Handy College Dictionary (3rd ed.) (1995). New York: Penguin Books.

Payne, V. G., & Isaacs, L. D. (1999). *Human motor development: A lifespan approach*. Mountain View, CA: Mayfield.

Pick, H. L. (1994). Eleanor J. Gibson: Learning to perceive and perceiving to learn. In R. D. Parke, P. A. Ornstein, J. J. Rieser, & C. Zahn-Waxler (Eds.), *A century of developmental psychology* (pp. 527–544). Washington, DC: American Psychological Association.

Puner, H. W. (Ed.) (1947). *Freud: His life and his mind*. New York: Grosset and Dunlap.

Reese, H. S., & Overton, W. F. (1970). Models of development and theories of development. In L. R. Goulet & P. B. Baltes (Eds.), *Life-span developmental psychology*. New York: Academic Press.

Rosenblith, J. (1994). A singular career: Nancy Bayley. In R. D. Parke, P. A. Ornstein, J. J. Rieser and C. Zahn-Waxler (Eds.), *A century of developmental psychology* (pp. 499–525). Washington, DC: American Psychological Association.

Shumway-Cook, A., & Woollacott, M. (2001). *Motor control: Theory and practical applications*. Philadelphia: Lippincott, Williams and Wilkins.

Thelen, E., & Adolph, K. (1994). Arnold L. Gesell: The paradox of nature and nurture. In R. D. Parke, P. A. Ornstein, J. J. Rieser, & C. Zahn-Waxler (Eds.), *A century of developmental psychology* (pp. 357–387). Washington, DC: American Psychological Association.

Thomas, R. M. (Ed). (2001). *Recent theories of human development*. Thousand Oaks, CA: Sage.

World Health Organization. (2002). *ICF: International Classification of Functioning and Disability*. Geneva, Switzerland: World Health Organization.

Mental Functions and Learning across the Lifespan

Anne Cronin, PhD, OTR/L, BCP
Associate Professor
Division of Occupational Therapy
West Virginia University
Morgantown, West Virginia

Objectives

Upon completion of this chapter, the reader should be able to

■ Discuss ICF distinctions between specific and global cognitive functions, giving examples of each.

■ Define attention, memory functions, perceptual functions, thought functions, and executive functions.

■ Differentiate between intellectual functions and temperament.

■ Discuss the relative strengths of the psychometric approach to intelligence versus theories of multiple intelligences.

■ Differentiate between vulnerable and maintained mental abilities.

■ Discuss the goodness-of-fit model in relation to temperament and learning.

■ Define associative and nonassociative learning in the context of human development.

■ Distinguish the four types of associative learning and give developmental examples of each type.

■ Describe social learning theory in the context of human development and skills acquisition.

Key Terms

abstraction
anticipatory awareness
associative learning
attention
cognitive flexibility
comparator
consciousness
declarative learning
degrees of freedom
emergent awareness
emotional functions
executive functions
feedback
global mental functions
goodness of fit
habits
haptic awareness
immediate memory
initiation

intellectual awareness
intellectual functions
kinesthetic awareness
Knowledge of Performance (KP)
Knowledge of Results (KR)
long-term memory
memory
memory trace
mental functions
metacognition
monitoring functions
motor planning
multiple intelligences
negative reinforcement
nonassociative learning
orientation
perception
perceptual learning
perceptual trace

positive reinforcement
problem solving
procedural learning
process skills
psychomotor functions
punishment
response specifications
Schmidt, Richard
shaping
short-term memory
social learning
somatic awareness
specific mental functions
tactile perception
verbal rehearsal
vestibular perception
vulnerable abilities
visual perception
visuospatial perception

INTRODUCTION

"To achieve a meaningful and satisfying life, human beings need two primary areas of competence: the ability to form enduring interpersonal relationships and the capacity for productive activity. One classic definition of a mentally healthy person is, simply stated, one who 'has the capacity to love and to work'" (Thorne, 1999, p. 1). As you reflect on Chapter 1 of this text, in which the ICF model was compared with other formats for categorizing and defining human function, you may realize that the areas that were least clear and most difficult to define were those related to human thought. While many scientists have described aspects of mental function and cognition, the process of converting those aspects into a complex personality that is able to form stable, cooperative, and mutually supportive relationships and to make productive use of time is more difficult to describe.

The process of becoming a mentally healthy person in adult society involves both inborn potentials and the ability to learn from experience. In this discussion of learning across the lifespan, the reader will develop an appreciation of the complex interplay between sensory, motor, and social learning. Throughout the lifespan, health and temperament, developmental skills, and interpersonal aspects of the family and environment overlap and influence one another in dynamic and interactive ways (Sameroff & Fiese, 1990; Bronfenbrenner,

1986). To aid in the understanding of this process, this text will integrate constructs from many sources into the dimensions of function described in the ICF (World Health Organization, 2002).

Human learning occurs at the level of (1) the body, including innate abilities; (2) the person, including interpersonal contacts and experience; and (3) society. **Mental functions** are innate to humans and include both global functions like consciousness and specific functions like self-control. This chapter describes mental functions at the level of the body, explains how those mental functions interact at the person level, and introduces the subject of human learning strategies and aspects of learning that impact the individual's ability to function effectively in her social system.

The bodily functions that support thought and learning are described in the scientific literature in many ways. In some cases the term *cognition* is used to describe basic brain functions like the ability to attend. In other cases it is used to describe intelligence. In order to be clear in meaning, this text will use the term *mental functions* as defined in the ICF (World Health Organization, 2002). That is, mental functions are the functions of the brain and central nervous system that underlie human learning. The term includes two distinct types: global and specific. **Global mental functions** underlie the other mental activities and include consciousness, energy, and drive (World Health Organization, 2002). These functions are crucial to all human activity and are important predictive factors in rehabilitation outcomes.

Specific mental functions, such as memory, language, and calculation, are more easily quantified than the global functions and are more often a focus of intervention following brain injury. Specific mental functions include attention, memory, psychomotor control, emotional control, perception, thought, higher cognitive functions, and the mental function of sequencing complex movements (World Health Organization, 2002).

SPECIFIC MENTAL FUNCTIONS

This section focuses on the specific mental functions most commonly considered in developmental and rehabilitation settings. The ICF also lists the mental functions of language, calculation, and the experience of self and time (World Health Organization, 2002). These last specific mental functions are important to human function but are highly influenced by the context of function. The mental function of language is addressed in Chapter 5 of this text, "Lifespan Communication." The experiences of self and time are associated with cultural and social contexts and are integrated into Chapter 4, "Culture and Development."

ATTENTION

Attention has been described as " the key that opens the door to the information processing system" (Allen & Blue, 1998, p. 239). In an individual, attention is the process of detecting and orienting to important or desired environmental stimuli. It is a mental function that allows a person to focus on something while simultaneously excluding less important information (World Health Organization, 2002). The normal newborn can briefly attend to a face, a sound, or an object. This skill expands with development to include the ability to sustain a focus for the needed period of time, the ability to shift attention from one stimulus to another, and the ability to concentrate. By adolescence most people are able to divide their attention between two or more tasks and can concentrate on a single task for hours at a time. Attention is mediated by the central nervous system and is influenced by brain injury, chemical changes in the body, and emotional distress. It is necessary for learning to occur and therefore is of great importance in development and in rehabilitation (Cronin, 2001).

MEMORY FUNCTIONS

Memory functions are more complex functions than attention. In its simplest form, memory is the registering and storing of information and retrieving it as needed. Memory functions include immediate, recent, and remote memory as well as memory span (World Health Organization, 2002). This area of function also includes the skills used in recalling and learning, such as retrieval of information and remembering.

The process of memory is believed to occur in three steps. The first step, **immediate memory,** is recall of stimuli within seconds of the event (Katz, 1998). The second step, **short-term memory,** has a duration of minutes and is used to determine immediate actions or reactions (Thomas, 2001). Short-term memory may be subdivided into two *reaction tasks:* a storage task and a processing task. It appears there is little age-related decline in the storage task, which involves merely keeping the information, such as a phone number, in working memory. However, tasks that involve an interaction between processing and storage do show an age-related decline (Birren & Schaie, 2001). **Long-term memory** holds past events for indefinite periods of time.

Immediate memory, also called *sensory memory,* is the registration of information and the combining of all impinging sensations into a meaningful whole. The person who has difficulty with immediate memory does not remember spoken directions, or whether she has already added the last ingredient while cooking. Immediate memory is the ability to remember and act on information immediately preceding the present need for the information. If the event has occurred more than five minutes ago, it would be considered short-term memory (Golisz & Toglia, 2003). A person with poor recent memory forgets conversations and where they left things around the house, though they are usually able to use immediate information and act on it. Short-term memory influences the performance of many important daily tasks, since it is needed to assist in performing desired action sequences without interruption until the task is completed. This aspect of short-term memory is called *temporal sequencing* in the OT Practice Framework (AOTA, 2002).

There are also systematic classifications of memory by type. *Procedural memory* involves primarily motor skills and is less resistant to deterioration than *episodic memory.* For example, the adage that "you never forget how to ride a bicycle" applies to procedural memory. The individual does not have to search and retrieve memory of a past occurrence in order to ride a bicycle if he learned this skill at some previous time. *Episodic memory,* on the other hand, involves retrieving and acquiring information that occurred in the past, at one particular point in time. Examples of episodic memory include *prospective memory,* which means remembering to do something in the future, and *source memory,* remembering whether an event actually occurred externally or if it derived from an internal source (Birren & Schaie, 2001). Because of the aging population and the significant functional impact of diseases such as Alzheimer's, which are defined by memory loss, large amounts of research are being done on memory, and further significant gains from such research are expected.

PSYCHOMOTOR FUNCTIONS

Psychomotor functions are the mental functions of control over physical and motor skills. These control functions include the ability to originate (plan), initiate (begin) movements, monitor and adapt or adjust motions in progress, perform learned tasks automatically without conscious direction, and pace, limit, or end movement based on activity demands (World Health Organization, 2002). Psychomotor skills allow the individual to drive an automobile while listening to a conversation. All of the basic control involved in driving a car is subconscious, unless challenging road conditions occur.

The traditional differentiation of human functions presented in Chapter 1 does not identify this type of mental function. Both the ICF and the OT Practice Framework include psychomotor mental functions in the category of **process skills,** which are those skills used by the individual "in managing and modifying actions en route to the completion of daily life tasks" (Fisher & Kielhofner, 1995, p. 120). Process skills include the energy to persist, the ability to maintain an effective rate of performance, the ability to use tools and materials according to their intended purpose, and the ability to use goal-directed actions to handle tools effectively and to complete the desired task (AOTA, 2002).

Psychomotor mental functions underlie many functional limitations following brain injury or disease. Some disabilities associated with impaired psychomotor control are psychomotor retardation (very slow movement responses), agitation (excess movement without direction), posturing/catalepsy (spontaneous maintenance of postures), echopraxia/echolalia (mimicking of another's movements/speech), and stereotypy (repetitive, nondirected motor activity). These types of disorders are associated with conditions of significant mental impairment like autism and schizophrenia.

EMOTIONAL FUNCTIONS

Emotional functions include those specific mental functions related to feelings, or the affective reactions of individuals (World Health Organization, 2002). These functions include not only emotions, but the mental regulation of the appropriateness and degree of the emotion within the individual's social and environmental context. Emotions such as sadness, happiness, love, fear, anger, hate, tension, anxiety, joy, and sorrow are a part of a healthy human repertoire. The ability to appropriately assign and regulate these emotions within reasonable contexts is a mental function. Difficulty in this area includes disabilities like *lability* (poor regulation) of emotion and flattening of affect. These types of disorders are associated with human conditions like depression (mood disorders) and may be a temporary or a persistent problem.

PERCEPTUAL FUNCTIONS (special senses)

Perception is a sensation-based mental function. This is the brain's ability to recognize and interpret sensory information. Perception occurs when your sense of smell gives you information that you perceive as something burning. This complex mental function requires both attentional and memory functions to be efficient. The person must notice (attend to) the smell and remember the smell of smoke. Thus, perception is influenced by the perceiver's experience and previous knowledge (Averbuch & Katz, 1998). A new cook, for example, may be less sensitive to the smell of food about to burn than the experienced chef would be.

Perceptual functions include the mental processes of matching sensations with meaning, using the information from the individual's sensory environment. Auditory perceptions are those mental functions involved in differentiating among sounds, tones, pitches, and other acoustic stimuli (World Health Organization, 2002). Included in this is auditory discrimination, the ability to isolate an important sound in a noisy environment. Individuals with disorders in this area have difficulty making sense of auditory information. An example of this is the child who can follow written directions and sequences but is slow to understand verbal directions.

Perceptual functions provide clues to performance skills, like when to ask for information or assistance, when to initiate or terminate tasks, and the ability to look for and locate tools or other desired objects. Perception also plays a key role in being able to organize tasks and activities, to clean up after task completion, and to navigate around obstacles while performing a task. These function manifestations of perception are described as "process skills" in the OT Practice Framework (AOTA, 2002).

Visual Perception

Visual perception is the most studied type of perception. This type of mental function involves both visual identification—the matching, categorizing, and recognition of shape, size, color, and other ocular stimuli—and visual discrimination—the perception of visual details, depth, spatial relations, and directional orientation (World Health Organization, 2002). Visual perception is a key aspect of reading written language and is often the problem in dyslexia. Difficulties with visual discrimination have been important in rehabilitation fields because of the profound impact on daily function and personal safety. For example, visual discrimination allows people to determine whether the dial on the stove indicates that it is on and allows them to read a telephone number.

Olfactory Perception

Olfactory perception is the mental function involved in distinguishing differences in smells. Because of its anatomic proximity to the brain areas for stimulating alertness and emotion, it is sometimes used as a tool to help stimulate persons in a coma state. Olfactory information is processed in the midbrain rather than the cortical areas, where most other sensory information is processed. This means that olfactory perceptions can result in very strong, lasting memories that are often emotional in nature. For example, an older woman relayed to her therapist her dislike of the smell of carnations. She went on to state that there were carnations at her mother's funeral when she was five years old, and the smell of carnations always revives her grief.

Gustatory Perception

Gustatory perception is the mental function involved in distinguishing the differences in tastes, such as sweet, sour, salty, and bitter stimuli, detected by the tongue (World Health Organization, 2002). It has functional implications in aging, when diet may be compromised by changes in this perceptual function. Providing a variety of tastes to allow an enriched sensory experience is often part of the rehabilitation program for persons who have difficulty eating solid foods.

Tactile Perception

Tactile perception, the perception of touch, is an important and widely studied mental function. Tactile perception provides the individual with three main types of information: (1) **somatic awareness** information about the state of the body (touch, pressure, temperature, pain, etc.); (2) **kinesthetic awareness** about movement within the body and changes in limb position; and (3) **haptic awareness** involved in distinguishing tactual differences in texture, shape, size, and weight (World Health Organization, 2002). Tactile perception disorders can have major functional impacts on self-care and safety functions. Somatic awareness lets you know when your clothing is appropriately covering your body, kinesthetic awareness lets you know how to control your legs and trunk to sit smoothly, and haptic awareness lets you reach into your backpack for a pencil without turning your head around to look.

Visuospatial Perception

Visuospatial perception is a complex interaction of attention, visual perception, and analysis of speed and trajectory of movement. This type of perception provides information on the relative position and motion of objects in the environment (World Health Organization, 2002). Visuospatial perception interacts with tactile perception to help determine the speed of movement needed for a given activity, adjust the alignment of the body, and develop the projected action sequences needed to be skilled in sports.

Vestibular Perception

Sometimes considered a subtype of tactile perception, **vestibular perception** is the awareness of movement in terms of speed and direction. The vestibular system (also called the labyrinth system) is in the middle ear and provides information about the position and motion of the head in relation to gravity (Allison & Fuller, 2001). This system allows an individual to stand and balance without vision. Functionally, vestibular perception provides information for balance, movement, and personal protection. Thus, vestibular perception allows you to walk on uneven surfaces or down darkened stairways without relying on vision.

THOUGHT FUNCTIONS

In the ICF model, thought functions are defined as specific functions related to the presence and development of ideas (World Health Organization, 2002). In this document, thought functions emphasize the control of thought in terms of pace, content, and form. The higher-level cognitive functions described in the ICF present a construct similar to the construct called *metacognition* in the cognitive rehabilitation literature. **Metacognition** describes the use of cognitive skills and provides the basis for transfer and generalization of learned skills to daily functioning (Katz, 1998). Metacognition is the mechanism through which we plan, organize, execute, and evaluate our day-to-day activities. It has two components: monitoring functions and executive functions (Katz, 1998).

Monitoring Functions

Metacognitive **monitoring functions** include mental activities that let us think about what we are doing before, during, and after we do it (Katz, 1998). Monitoring includes intellectual awareness of personal skills, the ability to anticipate task demands or outcomes, the ability to detect errors in our work, and the ability to organize our actions to complete a desired task. Functional examples of monitoring functions are responding appropriately to environmental or perceptual cues during task performance, modifying actions or the placement of tools in response to changes in task demands or other potential problems, and adjusting the task as demands change.

Intellectual awareness is the capacity to perceive and monitor "self" in relatively "objective" terms (Golisz & Toglia, 2003). This awareness includes knowledge about the strategies we employ in our own thinking and knowledge about how our personal thoughts and feelings influence our performance and affect others. Intellectual awareness, in this context, may be considered insight into self.

Emergent and *anticipatory* awareness describe the ability to analyze and monitor a situation or task and identify what the potential strengths and weakness are likely to be (Golisz & Toglia, 2003). The game of removing one wooden block at a time from a block tower provides an example of this. The goal is to remove as many blocks as possible and still keep the tower standing. As you first slide the block, the tower wobbles. **Emergent awareness** occurs as you realize that continuing this action could topple the tower. **Anticipatory awareness** occurs when the other player covers her ears in expectation of the loud crash of blocks on the table. *Error detection,* a functional aspect of this type of monitoring function, is the individual's ability to look at his own work or the work of others, monitor the accuracy of it, and find errors (Katz, 1998). Children do this as they compare the letterforms the teacher writes to their own writing. An adult does the same thing when reviewing an invoice at work.

Organization involves monitoring something with complex features and coordinating the parts into a workable whole. This is the mental function involved in developing a method of proceeding or acting (World Health Organization, 2002). As a monitoring function, organization can be considered as task-specific—like setting out all the tools needed for a task before beginning the task, or considering what groceries need to be available to make a favorite meal. Organization can be *temporal,* as in ordering a task sequence logically from beginning to end. Organization can also be *spatial,* as in gathering and logically positioning tools and materials for a particular task.

Executive Functions

Metacognitive **executive functions** are the control, or oversight, functions of thought (Katz, 1998). These are the mental processes that organize our thoughts for action. Such thought processes are often impaired in brain injury, resulting in a person who has little self-direction. Persons with deficits in this area may think about and be able to describe all the steps in a task but not be able to start (or initiate) the task without an external prompt. Executive functions include the processes of initiating, abstraction, problem solving, cognitive flexibility, and judgment.

Initiation is the ability to start something (Katz, 1998). A person who has difficulty with initiation will know that he needs to start a task, know how to do the task, want to do the task, and still sit there without starting. If this individual is told, "Start now," he can proceed normally, until he changes activities or needs to stop and then start again. Initiation is considered an aspect of temporal organization in the OT Practice Framework (AOTA, 2002). Functionally the person should be able to self-initiate a desired task and should be able to change to a new task step without hesitation or prompting by another.

Abstraction is the mental function of considering something as a general idea, quality, or characteristic (World Health Organization, 2002). This mental function allows the individual to consider new or novel solutions to problems. Abstraction is also a creative process that allows for alternative plans of action and is therefore related to both problem solving and cognitive flexibility. These three domains—abstraction, problem solving, and cognitive flexibility—are typically considered separately but are difficult to separate in functional daily tasks, like home repair or information processing.

For example, painting a room requires coordination of many tools, space use, and sequencing, perceptual, and motor skills. At many points in this process, the painter may have to resolve unexpected and novel problems. **Problem solving,** in this context, is the ability to interpret information from the monitoring functions, like error detection, and act on that information to self-correct (Katz, 1998). This function leads to effective performance and the ability to appropriately end (or terminate) activities. This function is seen when a youngster is learning to write but finds that the paper is sliding as she moves her arm. She problem-solves by taping the paper to the table.

Cognitive flexibility is the ability to consider alternatives and change strategies or approaches to a problem (Golisz & Toglia, 2003). Cognitive flexibility allows for deviation and the consideration of alternatives in daily activities. For example, although a project's instructions state that the carpenter should use nails to hold his materials together, he may decide instead to use screws when he finds no nails in his toolbox. He has appropriately chosen another strategy to complete the task rather than discontinuing it because of a technical problem. *Judgment* is the mental function involved in making a choice when presented with options, such as is involved in making a decision or forming an opinion (Katz, 1998). Judgment requires cognitive flexibility and is used functionally in deciding how much study time is needed to pass a test, or in deciding what clothing is appropriate for the weather.

MENTAL FUNCTION OF SEQUENCING COMPLEX MOVEMENTS

Aside from specific motor control issues, there are conscious thought processes involved in the sequencing and coordinating of complex, purposeful movements. These include the idea of what the movement should do, how it should happen, and what the outcome of the movement should be. This process is **motor planning,** the ability of the brain to conceive, organize, and carry out a sequence of unfamiliar actions (Golisz & Toglia, 2003). Persons with poor motor planning have difficulty performing unlearned movements, even though they have the motor and conceptual capacity to do the new task. Motor planning involves the ability to coordinate more than one body part together to perform tasks. Experts like elite athletes and professional musicians have finely tuned motor planning that allows them to perform their expert skill seemingly without effort in a smooth and fluid manner.

MENTAL FUNCTIONS OF LANGUAGE

There are many complex thought processes associated with human communication. These will be deferred until Chapter 5, where they will be discussed in detail.

GLOBAL MENTAL FUNCTIONS

The process of everyday function is highly complex and involves the assimilation of an individual's personal resources and experience. Over the past decades researchers have made great strides in understanding human function in terms of personality, behavior, and learning. The aspects of human thought described in the ICF as *global mental functions* are those that define the individual's personality and learning style (World Health Organization, 2002). The typical infant comes into the world with the capacity for all of the mental functions identified earlier in this chapter. The global mental functions outlined in ICF are consciousness functions, orientation functions, intellectual functions, temperament and personality functions, energy and drive functions, and sleep functions (World Health Organization, 2002). This section presents a discussion of the global mental skills of intellectual functions and temperament and personality functions. While many rehabilitation specialists focus on regaining specific abilities, like the ability to walk, the individual clients' responses to their situation, their orientation, and their understanding of the therapy process will have a great impact on the efficacy of any intervention.

Consciousness is required for all other mental functions to occur. **Consciousness** is a state of awareness and alertness (World Health Organization, 2002). This mental function includes the ability to remain awake and alert. Without consciousness, the individual remains passive and dependent on others for survival. Coma is an example of a prolonged loss of consciousness.

Orientation is conscious awareness of who you are, where you are, and what time it is (Golisz & Toglia, 2003). When a person has lost consciousness for a time, return to consciousness is measured by orientation to person, place, and time. In rehabilitation, this is usually measured by a series of questions like "Where do you live? Where are you now? What year is it? Who is president? What meal did you have last?" Orientation provides the structural framework for more complex mental functions.

INTELLECTUAL FUNCTIONS

Intelligence has been studied since at least the time of Confucius, nearly 2,500 years ago (Eysenck, 1998). Generally, **intellectual functions** are those skills required for the individual to understand and constructively integrate information from all types of mental function (World Health Organization, 2002). Intellectual functions develop and change over the lifespan and are influenced by experience, environmental contexts, and learning. Many people equate intelligence with "IQ" (intelligence quotient) as derived from a standard test (Kaplan & Sadock, 1998). The scientists involved in the early efforts to measure and quantify intelligence, however, did not view intelligence as a simple or single feature. Intelligence tests were developed for the specific goal of predicting the need for special school placement for some children. Since Alfred Binet's first test was published in 1905, there has been much research and consequent improved understanding of human mental functions. Differing approaches to studying and understanding human intellectual functions have also evolved (Eysenck, 1998).

Psychometric Approaches

In the psychometric approach, intelligence is "the ability to assimilate factual knowledge; to recall either recent or remote events; to reason logically; to manipulate concepts (either numbers or words); to translate the abstract to the literal and the literal to the abstract; to analyze and synthesize forms; and to deal meaningfully and accurately with problems and priorities deemed important in a particular setting" (Kaplan & Sadock, 1998, p. 193). This approach emphasizes that there is "one general intelligence" influencing all aspects of functioning (IQ). Statistically there is very convincing evidence to support the usefulness of the IQ as a factor that correlates highly with many aspects of child and adult function (Eysenck, 1998). This approach is the most widespread and widely used in research and the scientific literature.

Psychosocial Approaches

Since the development of the first IQ tests, psychologists have disagreed about aspects of intellectual functioning (Eysenck, 1998). While the psychometric approach has greatly aided the study of human learning, proponents of the psychosocial approach argue that all aspects of human learning cannot be quantified (Sternberg, Lautrey, & Lubart, 2003). The most important of these ongoing arguments is the idea that there are many types of intelligence rather than a single intelligence factor. In developing his psychometric tools, Binet suggested that there was one predominant intelligence factor (*g*) and then several less significant special intelligences (*s*) (Eysenck, 1998). Many psychologists have since expanded on this view, proposing theories of multiple intelligences (Eysenck, 1998; Gardner, 1999; Sternberg, Lautrey, & Lubart, 2003).

Recent theorists, including Gardner (1999) and Goleman and Lama (1997), have rejected the analysis of Binet and describe **multiple intelligences** that include intelligences that cannot at present be measured psychometrically. Table 3–1 lists the seven types of intelligence described initially by Gardner as preferred learning styles. Since these multiple intelligences cannot be discretely measured, they have been challenged by scholarly research. Although challenged as a psychometric tool, the idea of multiple intelligences as a tool to enhance learning is widely accepted.

Gardner (1999) bases his definitions of types of human intelligences on qualitative observation and new technology in brain research. His theory has gained much popular attention because it appeals intuitively to those who recognize skills and abilities in people around them who perhaps did not do well in traditional schooling. Although the field of psychology hotly debates the various approaches to the identification and study of intelligence, Gardner's theory has been

TABLE 3–1	Gardner's Learning Styles Reflecting Multiple Intelligences

Linguistic Learner
- Likes to read, write, and tell stories.
- Is good at memorizing names, places, dates, and trivia.
- Learns best by saying, hearing, and seeing words.

Logical/Mathematical Learner
- Likes to figure things out, ask questions, and explore patterns and relationships.
- Is good at math, reasoning, logic, and problem solving.
- Learns best by categorizing, classifying, and working with abstract patterns/relationships.

Spatial Learner
- Likes to draw, build, design, and create things, and to play with machines.
- Is good at imaging things, sensing changes, solving mazes/puzzles, and reading maps and charts.
- Learns best by visualizing, dreaming, and working with colors/pictures.

Musical Learner
- Likes to sing, hum tunes, listen to music, play an instrument, and respond to music.
- Is good at picking up sounds, remembering melodies, noticing pitches/rhythms, and keeping time.
- Learns best by rhythm, melody, and music.

Bodily/Kinesthetic Learner
- Likes to move around, touch, and use body language.
- Is good at physical activities.
- Learns best by interacting with space and processing knowledge through bodily sensations.

Interpersonal Learner
- Likes to talk to people and join groups.
- Is good at understanding people, organizing, communicating, manipulating, and mediating conflicts.
- Learns best by sharing, comparing, relating, cooperating, and interviewing.

Intrapersonal Learner
- Likes to work alone and pursue own interests.
- Is good at understanding self, focusing inward on feelings/dreams, following instincts, pursuing interests/goals, and being original.
- Learns best by working alone, doing individualized projects, using self-paced instruction, and having own space.

embraced by many as a tool to enhance teaching and promote learning. For the student of human development, it is important to understand intelligence as a fundamental ability to perform successfully in society. The use of multiple learning styles and multidimensional teaching strategies are valuable tools in clinical practice.

Mental Functions and Abilities in Adults

In the study of adult intellectual development, the terms *vulnerable* and *maintained* abilities were coined (Sternberg, Lautrey, & Lubart, 2003). **Vulnerable abilities** are those most likely to decrease or diminish with advancing age. The most significant of the vulnerable abilities are spatial reasoning, perceptual speed, short-term memory, visual processing, and processing speed. These abilities include many process skills that assist in managing and modifying tasks in progress. The slowed performance in ADLs (activities of daily living) common to the elderly is in part due to a decline in process skills.

Maintained abilities include cultural and academic knowledge, verbal comprehension, vocabulary, number facility, and fluency of retrieval from long-term memory. Maintained abilities typically include habits. **Habits** are behaviors so ingrained in activity and context that they are performed without conscious thought. Habits "support performance in daily life and contribute to life satisfaction" (AOTA, 2002, p. 623). These abilities are typically maintained and do not diminish with age. It is for this reason that many elderly persons continue to be independent in eating and toileting following cerebral injury, whereas children with the same or lesser brain involvement are dependent in these areas. Ingrained habit patterns support previously learned behaviors in the presence of appropriate cues. Vulnerable abilities are more likely than maintained abilities to be impacted by brain injury or disease (Sternberg, Lautrey, & Lubart, 2003).

TEMPERAMENT AND PERSONALITY

Temperament is "the constitutional disposition of the individual to react in a particular way to situations" (World Health Organization, 2002, p. 42). Temperament is a collection of inborn differences among individuals that is closely associated with personality. It has been widely studied, beginning with the work of Thomas, Chess, Birch, Hertzig, and Korn (1963) in their *New York Longitudinal Study (NYLS)*. Many other researchers have added to the literature about temperament, but the characteristics of temperament described in the NYLS and shown in Table 3–2 continue to be the most widely

tested in clinical and educational settings (Carey & McDevitt, 1995).

Dimensions of temperament have been studied over time and found to be stable within individuals. This means that the temperament displayed at 5 years of age is likely to be the temperament displayed by the same individual in adulthood. Any of the nine characteristics listed in Table 3–2 that is extremely low or extremely high can be problematic for the individual. Further study of temperament has introduced the idea of "temperament risk factors." These are "any temperament characteristic predisposing a child to a poor fit (incompatible relationship) with his or her environment, to excessive interactional stress, and conflict with caretakers" (Cary & McDevitt, 1995, p. 13).

In much psychology literature temperament is associated with personality and learning style (Brandstätter & Eliasz, 2001). Learning styles, in terms of temperament and multiple intelligences, would be considered in the ICF as Personal Factors.

Goodness of Fit

An individual's temperament is not inherently good or bad. A temperament characteristic becomes negative when it is not consistent with the values and expectations of persons important to the individual. **Goodness of fit** occurs when the individual's temperament supports the demands and expectations of the environment. Poor temperamental fit is most likely to occur in childhood, because adults have a far greater degree of control over their personal environments. Some temperament characteristics are more difficult to accommodate than others (Carey & McDevitt, 1995). The elements that make particular characteristics risk factors are (1) the strength of the temperament characteristics, (2) the other characteristics of the child, and (3) the environment (Carey & McDevitt, 1995). The stronger the characteristic, the more difficult it will be to accommodate. Cultural, physical, social, personal, and temporal contexts influence whether specific characteristics contribute to activity limitations.

Stability of Temperament

Temperament is genetically driven and, as mentioned earlier, has been found to be fairly stable within an individual beyond infancy. Nevertheless, temperament is an aspect of personality and can therefore change as the individual gains experience and skills. Carey and McDevitt (1995, p. 25) state that "temperament is never fixed at any time, nor is it completely changeable in any period." Environment and learning influence how temperament is manifested.

Community and family expectations can make a difference in whether the slow-to-warm-up child, like the one in Figure 3–1, develops into a shy adult or, if

TABLE 3–2	Temperament Categories and Their Characteristics

Temperament Categories	Characteristics
Activity Level	A measure of physical motion during sleep, eating, play, dressing, bathing, and so forth.
Rhythmicity	The regularity and predictability of basic physiologic functions, such as hunger, sleep, and elimination.
Approach/Withdrawal	The nature of the individual's initial responses to new stimuli—people, situations, places, foods, toys, procedures.
Adaptability	The ease or difficulty with which reactions to stimuli can be modified. The individual's ability to accommodate the unexpected.
Intensity	The energy level of responses, regardless of quality or direction. This is how intellectually or emotionally focused the individual is; it does not relate to physical activity.
Mood	The amount of pleasant and friendly or unpleasant and unfriendly behavior in various situations. The individual's typical affect.
Persistence/Attention span	The lengths of time particular activities are pursued by the child. How long the child will work at a given task.
Distractibility	The effectiveness of extraneous environmental stimuli in interfering with ongoing behaviors.
Sensory Threshold	The amount of stimulation, such as sounds or light, necessary to evoke discernable responses in the child.

Web Questionnaires on Temperament

- An Image of Your Child: Discover Your Child's Temperament Style (infants-toddlers) (from The Preventive Ounce) at http://www.preventiveoz.org/image.html
- Guilford-Zimmerman Temperament Survey (from Pearson assessments) at http://www.pearsonassessments.com/tests/gzts.htm
- The Keirsey Temperament Sorter II (from The Keirsey Web Site) at http://www.advisorteam.com/temperament_sorter/register.asp?partid=
- Meyers-Briggs Personality Type (from Know Your Type) at http://www.knowyourtype.com/
- Personality Compass (from Personality Compass) at http://www.personalitycompass.com/

Adapted from Cary & McDevitt, 1995; Web resources.

supported in trying new situations, develops the emotional security to overcome her innate hesitation.

ENERGY AND DRIVE FUNCTIONS

Energy and Drive Functions, as described in ICF, include the physiologic and psychological mechanisms that result in the individual's energy level, motivation, appetite, craving (including craving for substances that can be abused), and impulse control (World Health Organization, 2002). Motivation is "the drive toward action" (Bonder, 1997) and believed to be a key component in successful human function. Certainly motivation is a primary predictor of a successful outcome in therapy (Ng & Tsang, 2002; Gasser-Wieland & Rice, 2002).

SLEEP FUNCTIONS

Sleep Functions are the periods of mental disengagement from one's immediate environment accompanied by characteristic physiologic changes. This disengagement is reversible; the individual can wake and regain alertness, and he can choose when to sleep or to be awake. Because of the profound impact that persistent irregularities with sleep can cause, sleep is recognized as an ADL (AOTA, 2002). Persons who cannot control sleep may have functional impairment caused by this lack of control. Narcolepsy is a condition characterized by sudden, uncontrolled bouts of sleep. These can occur without warning and make many ordinary tasks, like driving a car, life-threatening.

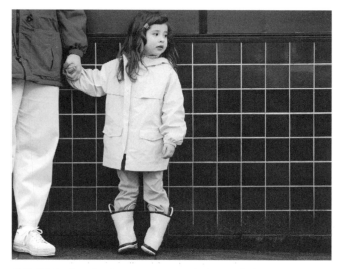

FIGURE 3–1   The slow-to-warm-up child typically has a low activity level and difficulty initiating interactions, and adapts slowly to change or unfamiliar routines. (Image courtesy of PhotoDisc®, Inc.)

OT = Therapeutic use of practice

LEARNING

Learning has been defined as "a behavioral change in a specific situation, produced by repeated experiences of the situation" (Kaplan & Sadock, 1998, p. 148). Learning has been included at the end of this chapter on mental functions because it is a composite of specific and global functions in dynamic interaction with the environment. Learning is an elemental part of mental functions, such as cognition, as well as other functions, such as motor skill performance. A primary responsibility of rehabilitation specialists is to guide learning of new and compensatory ways of functioning. Although the learning process is often considered the exclusive purview of educators, therapists must understand and facilitate it in all aspects of their work.

NONASSOCIATIVE LEARNING

In the neonate, learning is largely sensory-based and **nonassociative,** meaning it does not rely on memory or prior experiences to associate a stimulus with a sensory experience. With repeated experience of a stimulus, the individual *habituates* to it (decides that it is unimportant and no longer responds) or *sensitizes* to it (recognizes the stimulus as important and alerts to it) (Shumway-Cook & Woollacott, 2001). Nonassociative learning is important in the learning of physical and motor skills. This type of learning can result in both transient and long-term modulation at the synaptic level and is important in rehabilitation of movement disorders.

Perceptual learning is the formation of sensory memories (Shumway-Cook & Woollacott, 2001). This type of learning is a complex form of nonassociative learning. While perceptual learning does not require prior experience, it does involve memory. It is through this perceptual learning that when viewing a new skill or someone else doing a skill the individual is able to store that information for some later date when the same stimuli are present.

ASSOCIATIVE LEARNING

In **associative learning** the individual learns to predict relationships and draws on long-term memory to make associations. Several types of associative learning have been identified. These are learning based on classical conditioning and operant conditioning, as well as declarative learning and procedural learning (Kaplan & Sadock, 1998). Classical conditioning, mentioned in Chapter 2, is illustrated in Figure 3–2 but will not be reviewed here. Operant conditioning will be discussed as it relates to cognition and learning.

Operant conditioning

Operant conditioning uses a process of active trial-and-error learning. This is a learning process whereby only a "desired" response results in the subject earning a reward. Over repeated trials the subject increases the frequency of the desired behavior. The most important feature in operant conditioning is that the individual learner is active in the learning process. This active role is why operant conditioning is so useful in helping to shape and train new behavior patterns.

Positive reinforcement is a process that encompasses three features: a consequence is presented dependent on a behavior, the behavior becomes more likely to occur, and the behavior becomes more likely to occur because and only because the consequence is presented dependent on the behavior. In other words, rewarded behavior will occur more frequently.

Negative reinforcement is a process of escape, or avoidance learning. It is the reward of getting away from anything unpleasant: a hostile person, a hard job, punishment, etc. Any action by you that enables you to escape discomfort is reinforced by the relief you experience. For example, an adolescent's cleaning of her bedroom may remove parental restrictions on her social activity. Negative reinforcement removes a negative; it is not a negative consequence. In **punishment,** a negative or aversive stimulus is added. Spanking is a traditional form of punishment used to discipline children (Kaplan & Sadock, 1998). Figure 3–3 illustrates how the concepts of reinforcement and punishment are applicable to a common therapeutic situation.

Stage 1 Sight of bottle causes no response, but being fed from bottle elicits pleasurable responses such as sighs and coos

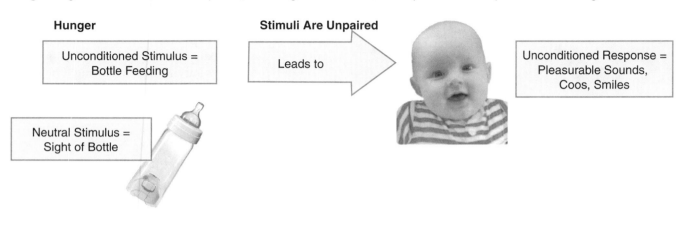

Stage 2 Sight of bottle is paired with administration of bottle

Stage 3 Now sight of bottle alone elicits pleasurable response

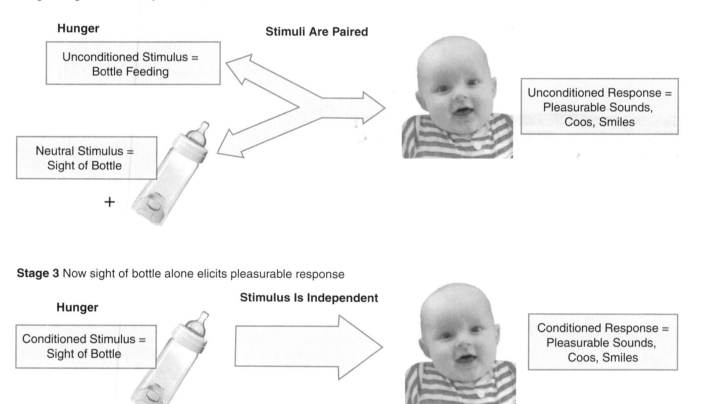

FIGURE 3–2   Example of Classical Conditioning (adapted from Kaplan & Sadock, 1998)

Shaping is a strategy used with operant conditioning that involves a deliberate and gradual plan to change behavior. This is the idea behind the popular parenting maxim, "Catch them being good." To shape behavior, the individual is reinforced for the desired behavior. For example, the first step may be to reward the child who refuses to eat vegetables for allowing a small portion of carrots to stay on his plate rather than pushing the plate or the carrots away. The next step might be for the child to take a spoonful to his mouth and smell it. Several approximations of the desired behavior will precede actually achieving the new behavior, in this case eating the carrots. Behavioral shaping has been widely adopted as a tool in both educational and medical arenas (Ceilberti et al., 1997; Arvedson, 1997; Kaplan & Sadock, 1998).

Stage 1 Child is hungry, is given milk bottle to drink, and experiences painful reflux.

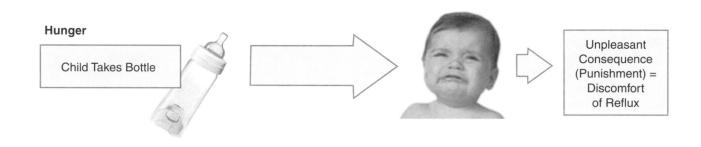

Stage 2 Child is hungry but loses interest in eating because it is unpleasant.

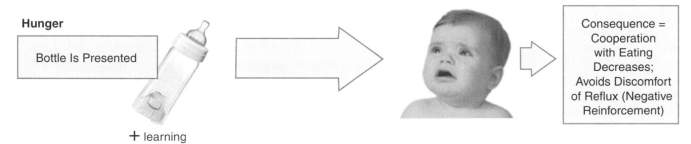

+ learning

FIGURE 3–3   This figure illustrates how the common problem of feeding avoidance is learned by infants who have reflux. To treat the avoidance behavior using operant conditioning principles, a pleasant result such as satiation or taste (positive reinforcement) needs to replace the reflux (adapted from Kaplan & Sadock, 1998).

Learning Stages

As we practice any new skill, we get faster at it, and it takes less memory and conscious effort to recall and perform. These qualitative changes are characterized by different stages in learning. Conscious effort predominates the earliest stage, **declarative learning.** The learner works out what information is relevant and what is not relevant and then breaks the task down into subtasks and individual actions.

Declarative learning is learning that the individual is conscious of and makes an effort to support. This type of learning predominates as the individual attempts a new skill at any age. Declarative learning requires both awareness of and attention to the task. The early phase of learning deals with behaviors shaped by declarative knowledge (facts and propositions). This contrasts with the later stage of **procedural learning,** with little conscious processing required. Here, thinking about what you are doing can actually be disruptive to the smooth performance of a skill learned in this stage. This phenomenon, "paralysis by analysis," is a common feature of

sport and athletic training. For instance, it is difficult to drive a car while explaining to someone else exactly what you are doing. Procedural knowledge is what we use when we have practiced until the task is automated. Here the procedures and the conditions that call for their use were learned in the declarative phase. The task no longer is inferred from declarative knowledge each time it is performed. Instead, the goal to drive the car home triggers a whole sequence of actions in an interface without having to think about each step explicitly.

MOTOR LEARNING

When an individual learns a skill, practice and active movement are obviously involved. In the course of practicing, the individual receives information about how the task is progressing. That information is **feedback,** the sensory information that is available as a result of movement (Shumway-Cook & Woollacott, 2001). Feedback that arises from the sense organs of the body is considered *intrinsic.* Feedback from the environment is *extrinsic*. Intrinsic feedback would be, for example, the "feel of the movement" or the visual result. Extrinsic feedback might come from a therapist or coach, who says something like, "You kept your head down."

Knowledge of Results (KR) is a form of extrinsic post-response feedback that tells the individual about the results of the movement with respect to the environmental goal—for example, "You walked fifteen feet today, which is five feet more than yesterday." Knowledge of results is critical to motor learning (Winstein, 1991). **Knowledge of Performance (KP)** is extrinsic feedback about the quality of movement pattern, as in the example given previously about a coach telling you that you kept your head down (Shumway-Cook & Woollacott, 2001).

Motor learning itself cannot be measured but only inferred from motor performance. There are several classic theories of motor learning. One is the *closed-loop theory*. Another way to think about closed-loop theory is feedback-dependent (hence, the stimulus-response-stimulus loop is closed). In the closed-loop theory, proposed by Jack A. Adams, sensory feedback is believed to guide the successive improvement of performance of a motor skill in the following paradigm: The individual has a **memory trace** of a movement or a movement approximation, if the movement is totally novel. When the goal is established, the person generates a **perceptual trace,** which is a working sensory motor plan based on the memory trace, modified by sensory experience or feedback. At the end of each session of practice, the new memory trace is stored. An analogy for this model is to think of word processing using a computer. You use a word processing program (the neural network) to generate a written document, which you save (the memory trace). Later, you want to edit that document, so you pull it into active memory (perceptual trace), edit it, and store it once again.

The closed-loop theory of motor learning has been criticized on two main points. First, some movements, such as throwing, occur too rapidly to be modified by feedback during the movement itself. Second, studies on animals and humans who lack input over sensory nerves have shown that capabilities to produce movement continue to exist, even though learning of new skills is severely impaired.

One of Adams's contemporaries, **Richard Schmidt,** proposed an open-loop theory of motor learning that addressed some of the limitations of closed-loop theory. In the open-loop theory, a motor response *schema* exists, consisting of a set of rules for directing movement. These rules are known as **response specifications** and as a whole, create the motor program that directs the movement through neural pathways acting on the motor neurons. During and after the movement has occurred, a number of sensory channels provide intrinsic and extrinsic feedback to the system, as described earlier. The actual sensory consequences, obtained through feedback, are compared to the expected sensory consequences, generated as part of the schema and response specifications. If an error is detected, the schema is adjusted. This theory of motor learning assigns a **comparator** with the job of comparing actual and expected sensory consequences (Shumway-Cook & Woollacott, 2001). The open-loop theory of motor learning implies that practice is best done as variable practice—that is, under a variety of conditions. Research has supported this best in young children and to a lesser extent in adults (Shumway-Cook & Woollacott, 2001).

In addition to open- and closed-loop theories of motor learning, there are theories that describe the overt aspects of motor learning in terms of characteristic stages. Fitts and Posner identified three stages of motor learning: cognitive, associative, and autonomous (Shumway-Cook & Woollacott, 2001). The cognitive stage is characterized by **verbal rehearsal,** where the individual recites, often audibly, the steps to a task. Anyone who has ever taken a dance class has participated in an example of verbal rehearsal. The early cognitive stage of learning requires that the learner initiate the movement; too much feedback or coaching in this stage can be disruptive. On the other hand, in the associative stage, feedback and coaching are very helpful in correcting and improving the motor skill. In the final, autonomous stage, the movement proceeds automatically. In fact, once a skill has been well-learned, excessive attention to the skill can result in the phenomenon known as *"paralysis from analysis,"* as discussed earlier in relation to procedural learning, where the skill worsens the more attention is paid to it. A golfer may experience this in changing a stroke, and a baseball player in the middle of a hitting slump suffers from this condition.

Another theory about stages of motor learning is based on the ongoing change in **degrees of freedom.** In motor learning, as in statistics, the term *degree of freedom* refers to the number of factors that are free to vary. In learning a task, the learner initially restricts the degrees of freedom, using a lot of co-contraction and muscle energy. As the learner acquires the skill, degrees of freedom are released, and the movement becomes more fluid and adaptable. Finally, Kim Gentile has developed a two-stage theory of motor learning. She says that in the first stage, the learner is trying to process the task demands, and in the second stage, the learner refines the movements (Shumway-Cook & Woollacott, 2001).

SOCIAL LEARNING

Social learning refers to the acquisition of behaviors within a social context. Social learning theorists like Albert Bandura, discussed in Chapter 2, posited that humans learn socially through observing others and imitating or rejecting the behavior they observe. The process of observation followed by imitation is *modeling*. Individuals are active in choosing models, and a model may present either socially positive or negative behavior (Kaplan & Sadock, 1998). For example, a mother may model food preparation for her daughter. This modeling involves the process skills of knowledge (learning use of tools and techniques), temporal organization, and organizing space and objects. In addition to the task-performance skills, parental cooking instruction also models personal and social roles and routines. As a result of such parental modeling, a common experience of new partners is the awareness that the other person does not do something "right." For example, placing clean drinking glasses upside down on the shelf is "right" because it is how the behavior of putting glasses away was first modeled.

SOCIAL ROLES

A *social role* is "the characteristic and expected social behavior of an individual" (American Heritage Dic-tionary, 2000). Roles are modeled in our environmental contexts and are subsequently ingrained in all our activities and areas of participation. Roles are especially modeled in learning environments and in apply-ing knowledge to perform learned tasks. These social roles shape communication, mobility expectations, self-care needs, domestic life, interpersonal interactions, and relationships in major life areas. It is common for occupational therapists working to help elderly men return home following a stroke to hear, "I don't need to cook; my wife will do all of that." This is an example of a deeply ingrained gender role that is functionally limiting to the older couple. The man will need constant attendance during the day, yet the spouse will be unable to resign these IADLs if her own health fails.

SUMMARY

The human system has a vast and complex mechanism for taking in stimuli from the environment and then sorting, interpreting, and storing it for future use. This chapter has introduced the names of several types of mental functions involved in the dynamic process of human development. Each of these mental functions develops and interacts throughout childhood so that by early adulthood the individual is able to make productive use of his time. The ability to be productive and the ability to form enduring relationships are considered the two most important developmental outcomes in human society. Body-level mental function components interact with the specific characteristics of each individual, resulting in distinctive personality and learning styles. These learning styles represent intrapersonal characteristics and are important to successful interpersonal functioning.

Learning continues to occur throughout life at both the conscious and the unconscious levels. It is greatly influenced by opportunity and experience in the environment, including the roles modeled and the cultural context. In adulthood, learning continues to occur, but in a more selective and specialized way. That is, learning occurs when a specific behavior is used that was observed or tried previously that results in some outcome. If the outcome is perceived as positive, the individual will use that behavior again. If the outcome is perceived as negative, the behavior is likely to be suppressed. Learning is more than the gaining of academic skills. It can be of many types, including sensory, motor, interpersonal, intrapersonal, social, and cultural.

CASE

1

Keegan

(adjusted age 10 months)

HISTORY: This child has a history of prematurity, severe gastroesophageal reflux, and bronchopul-monary dysplasia. Keegan will take a bottle only when he is sleeping. He is offered food periodically throughout the day but often refuses to eat.

CLINICAL OBSERVATION: Keegan demonstrates social and behavioral skills appropriate to his adjusted age. His mother usually feeds him as he watches a videotape. Meals take about forty-five minutes.

Continues

Keegan *Continued*

(adjusted age 10 months)

PARENT CONCERNS: Keegan is underweight and cannot be with his age group in nursery school if he doesn't eat solid foods.

PLAY OBSERVATION: Keegan demonstrated normal touch sensitivity in play. He tolerated facial touch and the oral examination well. Keegan demonstrated normal sensory skills in play and exploration. He did react to new textures in and around the mouth, indicating a sensitivity to food textures and touch. His attention skills are age-appropriate, and he follows one-step directions. Keegan is able to imitate facial expressions, gestures, and play activities.

FUNCTIONAL SKILLS: At meals Keegan has a strong, coordinated suck-swallow pattern, good lip and jaw closure, and good tongue mobility. He sits well, with good postural control, and is able to hold eating utensils. Keegan's fine and gross motor skills are normal for his adjusted age. His oral abilities appear adequate for the management of soft food. He uses some immature patterns to manage food within his mouth. These patterns reflect a lack of experience with solid food and do not suggest developmental delay.

RECOMMENDATIONS: Keegan has a learned pattern of food avoidance. The pain associated with reflux and his weak breathing have taught him that eating is unpleasant. He avoids eating and has failed to practice and develop the skills he needs to eat textured foods. He is developing well in all other areas but needs additional support in the development of self-feeding. Behavioral intervention should help Keegan accept more foods. He is beginning to finger-feed. This should be encouraged. As he gains comfort with eating, it is likely that Keegan will move directly to beginning self-feeding and will skip much of the baby food stage. This should be supported because he has the needed developmental skills for this task.

Cristina

(age 38)

HISTORY: Cristina started feeling symptoms of joint pain at age 24 but was not diagnosed with rheumatoid arthritis until she was 32 years old. Cristina is currently a 38-year-old homemaker and a college student. She is the mother of an energetic 10-year-old son and an 8-year-old daughter. She was diagnosed with rheumatoid arthritis six years ago but until her most recent flare-up was able to take care of her home and her own self-care responsibilities. After that flare-up, she told her physical and occupational therapists that her morning stiffness lasted most of the day and she was feeling "tired and miserable." She felt that she was unable to complete many of her self-care and homemaking tasks. She is having trouble finding shoes that fit, and she has a constant sense that she will fall if walking over uneven surfaces because her right ankle turns.

Continues

CASE
2

Cristina *Continued*
(age 38)

At the recommendation of her therapy team, Cristina joined a tai chi class. Studies of tai chi were associated with significant improvement in balance in all participants (Hain et al., 1999). Tai chi movement patterns are used by trained therapists as tools for both assessment and intervention. The therapist can assess misalignments that might contribute to physical limitations, and through a kinesthetic approach to learning corrected patterns can then be used in the exercise program for daily practice to help correct these problem areas. The use of mirrors, physical guidance, and a focus on the "feel" of the posture all help Cristina learn about her own body and her own movement patterns. After a 10-week tai chi class, Cristina reports not only improved balance and flexibility but decreased pain and improvement in her ability to perform daily occupations.

Speaking of

Cognitive Reserve

ANNE CRONIN, PhD, OTR/L, BCP
PEDIATRIC OCCUPATIONAL THERAPIST

Strokes (or cerebral vascular accidents) often happen to elderly family members. While the physical impairments caused by a stroke are obvious, there are commonly also impairments in cognition and learning. For most people a stroke is followed by a period of hospitalization and rehabilitation, including physical, occupational, speech, and recreational therapies. At this time the rehabilitation team works on impairments in physical function as well as impairments in participation in everyday activities. Although we always try to prepare people to return home, when the brain has been injured it is difficult to predict when and where problems with daily tasks might occur.

Some of the common issues people have after a stroke concern their short-term memory. Clients tell me things like, "I walked into the kitchen, but could not remember why I went there." Even the most "rehabilitated" report problems with doing more than one thing at a time. Although they can do many things safely and independently, when too much is going on they may have problems with tasks that are not normally hard for them. For example, one older woman who had been successfully living alone for many months was preparing a meal and at the same time trying to finish a craft project for her church bazaar. She put a potato in her microwave to cook, turned the microwave on, and then went into her sewing room to work. It wasn't until her smoke alarms went off that she realized that she had punched in 80:00 instead of 8:00 for cooking time on her microwave.

Most people have *cognitive reserve capacity* that drives many of our metacognitive functions and allows us to multitask. As people learn to overcome the problems associated with brain damage, they draw more on the remaining cognitive potential and lose their cognitive reserve.

While as therapists you will learn a great deal about common cognitive and perceptual impairments following cerebrovascular accidents, it is important to understand that cognition is a complex function. While made up of discrete abilities, mental, or cognitive, function is really an interactive whole, and impairments can be difficult to anticipate. The emphasis in therapy today is to include cognitive interventions, to work in a person's familiar environment, and to provide a "safety net" for those who have experienced brain injury and are living alone.

REFERENCES

Allen, C. K., & Blue, T. (1998). Cognitive disabilities model: How to make clinical judgments. In N. Katz (Ed.), *Cognition and occupation in rehabilitation* (pp. 225–279). Bethesda, MD: American Occupational Therapy Association.

Allison, L., & Fuller, K. (2001). Balance and vestibular disorders. In D. Umphred (Ed.) *Neurological rehabilitation* (4th ed.) (pp. 616–660). Mosby.

American Occupational Therapy Association (2002). Occupational Therapy Practice Framework: Domain and process. *American Journal of Occupational Therapy, 56,* 609–639.

Arvedson, J. (1997). Behavioral issues and implications with pediatric feeding disorders. *Seminars in Speech and Language, 18,* 51–70.

Birren, J. E., & Schaie, K. W. (2001). *Handbook of the psychology of aging.* London, England: Academic Press.

Bonder, B. (1997). Coping with psychological and emotional challenges. In C. Christiansen and C. Baum (Eds.), *Occupational Therapy: Enabling function and well-being* (pp. 313–334). Philadelphia: Slack.

Brandstätter, H., & Eliasz, A. (2001). *Persons, situations, and emotions: An ecological approach.* Oxford; New York: Oxford University Press.

Bronfenbrenner, U. (1986). Ecology of the family as a context for human development: Research perspectives. *Developmental Psychology, 22,* 723–742.

Carey, T., & McDevitt, S. (1995). *Coping with children's temperament: A guide for professionals.* New York: Basic Books.

Celiberti, D., Bobo, H., Kelly, K., Harris, S., & Handleman, J. (1997). The differential and temporal effects of antecedent exercise on the self-stimulatory behavior of a child with autism. *Research in Developmental Disabilities, 18,* 139–150.

Cronin, A. F. (2001). Traumatic brain injury in children. *American Journal of Occupational Therapy, 55,* 377–384.

Eysenck, H. (1998). *Intelligence: A new look.* New Brunswick, NJ: Transaction Publishers.

Fisher, A., & Kielhofner, G. (1995). Skill in occupational performance. In G. Kielhofner (Ed.), *A model of human occupation: Theory and Application* (2nd ed.) (pp. 113–128). Philadelphia: Lippincott Williams and Wilkins.

Gardner, H. (1999). *Intelligence reframed: Multiple intelligences for the 21st century.* New York: Basic Books.

Gasser-Wieland, T., & Rice, M. (2002) Occupational embeddedness during a reaching and placing task with survivors of cerebral vascular accident. *OTJR: Occupation, Participation, and Health, 22,* 153–160.

Goleman, D., & Lama, D. (1997). *Emotional intelligence.* New York: Bantam Books.

Golisz, K., & Toglia, J. (2003). Section II: Perception and cognition. In E. Crepeau, E. Cohn, & B. Schell (Eds.), *Willard and Spackman's Occupational Therapy* (pp. 395–416). Philadelphia: Lippincott Williams and Wilkins.

Hain, T., Fuller, L., Weil, L., & Kotsias, J. (1999). Effects of T'ai Chi on balance. *Archives of Otolaryngology Head and Neck Surgery, 125(11),* 1191.

Kaplan, H., & Sadock, B. (1998). *Synopsis of Psychiatry* (8th ed.). Baltimore: Williams and Wilkins.

Katz, N. (Ed.). (1998). *Cognition and occupation in rehabilitation: Cognitive models for intervention in occupational therapy.* Bethesda, MD: American Occupational Therapy Association.

Law, M., Missiuna, C., Pollock, N., & Stewart, D. (2001). Foundations for occupational therapy practice with children. In J. Case-Smith (Ed.), *Occupational therapy for children* (pp. 39–71). St. Louis: Mosby.

Thomas, R. M. (2001). *Recent theories of human development.* Thousand Oaks, CA: Sage Publications.

Ng, B., & Tsang, H. (2002). A program to assist people with severe mental illness in formulating realistic life goals. *Journal of Rehabilitation, 68,* 59–66.

Sameroff, A., & Fiese, B. (1990). Transactional regulation and early intervention. In S. J. Meisels and J. P. Shonkoff (Eds.), *Handbook of early childhood intervention* (pp. 119–149). New York: Cambridge University Press.

Shumway-Cook, A., & Woollacott, M. (2001). *Motor control: Theory and practical applications* (2nd ed.) Baltimore: Lippincott Williams and Wilkins.

Sternberg, R., Lautrey, J., & Lubart, T. (Eds.) (2003). *Models of intelligence: International perspectives.* Washington, DC: American Psychological Association.

Thomas, A., Chess, S., Birch, H., Hertzig, M., & Korn, S. (1963). *Behavioral individuality in early childhood.* New York: New York University Press.

Thorne, J. (1999). Factors in child development, Part I: Personal characteristics and parental behavior. In Centers for Disease Control and Prevention, *Legacy for Children #8482.* Washington, DC: U.S. Department of Health and Human Services.

Toglia, J. (2003). Section V: Cognitive-perceptual retraining and rehabilitation. In E. Crepeau, E. Cohn, & B. Schell (Eds.), *Willard and Spackman's Occupational Therapy* (pp. 607–629). Philadelphia: Lippincott Williams and Wilkins.

Winstein, C. (1991). Designing practice for motor learning: Clinical implications. In M. J. Lister (Ed.), *Contemporary management of motor control problems: Proceedings of the II step conference* (pp. 65–76). Alexandria, VA: Foundation for Physical Therapy.

World Health Organization. (2002). *ICF: International Classification of Functioning and Disability.* Geneva, Switzerland: World Health Organization.

CHAPTER 4

Culture and Development

Winifred Schultz-Krohn, PhD, OTR,
  BCP, FAOTA
Associate Professor of
  Occupational Therapy
San Jose State University
San Jose, California

Objectives

Upon completion of this chapter, the reader should be able to

- Define the terms culture, health, illness, and disease.

- Explain how understanding cultural schemas can enhance practice.

- Describe cultural differences in communication, control, and definition of self.

- Understand how developmental expectations are culturally based.

- Describe how socioeconomic factors influence development.

Key Terms

active achievement viewpoint	event schemas	person schema
authoritarianism	expressive/overt communications	poverty
collectivistic cultural group	health	race
culture	illness	restrained formal communication
cultural schemas	independent cultural group	role schemas
disease/disorder	individualistic cultural group	self schemas
egalitarianism	interdependent cultural group	
ethnicity	passive acceptance viewpoint	

INTRODUCTION

Before beginning a discussion addressing the cultural influences on development, an underlying question must be posed: Why include the topic of culture in a textbook designed to help students understand human performance across the lifespan?

Several authors have advocated the need for therapists to become culturally competent (Harris, 2000; Velde & Wittman, 2001; Wells & Black, 2000). This interest in multicultural awareness is partially generated from the recognition that the demographics of the United States are becoming increasingly diverse (Taylor, 1998; Wells & Black, 2000). But the mere fact that ethnic and cultural diversity is apparent within the United States does not justify inclusion of this topic in a textbook addressing human performance. Rather, understanding the role culture plays in a person's life offers a rationale for inclusion. One function of culture is to provide a lens to focus on significant developmental features. The identification of important developmental tasks is culturally influenced (Valsiner, 1997). One cultural group may view a baby's first steps as a significant event, whereas another cultural group places far greater emphasis on a child's ability to help with household chores or care for the family's animals (Lancy, 1996).

Development can be conceptualized as change related to the interaction of the person and the environment (Valsiner, 1989). An infant, prior to the development of object permanence, may not search for an object out of the field of vision, yet a college student may spend an extended period of time searching for her "lucky pencil" before taking a final examination. The change in interaction between the person and the environment has been viewed from a linear perspective by some researchers, particularly those who follow staged theories. This orientation toward development has been criticized as limiting the understanding of the complexity of development. Valsiner (1989) suggested that development be viewed from a "multilinear" perspective that "accounts for life experience and recognizes the possibility of multiple trajectories of development" (p. 6). This multilinear perspective provides a vantage point to examine the cultural influence on development. Development is not viewed as simply progressing along a specified trajectory but instead as the product of several interacting variables. For example, a child with sustained poor nutritional support may display decreased physical and cognitive growth.

DEFINITION OF TERMS

In the ICF, culture is a contextual factor in human function (World Health Organization, 2002). Culture is part of each individual's environmental context throughout development. The purpose of this chapter is to provide an understanding of influence of culture on human performance. As an environmental context, culture influences all areas of human activity and participation. Several terms will first be defined to aid the reader.

CULTURE

Culture is a set of "values, beliefs, attitudes, customs, language, and behaviors that are shared by a group of people and are passed down from one generation to the next" (Giger & Davidhizar, 1999, p. 3). Generally the term refers not to physical attributes possessed by an individual but rather behaviors that occur within a social context. Some authors also use this term to refer to groups of people who share common physical conditions that are linked to beliefs and values, such as being deaf and a member of the "deaf culture" (Wells & Black, 2000). The American Medical Association (1999) adds to the definition of culture by indicating that cultural experiences and knowledge are not shared with those outside the group. Culture provides group

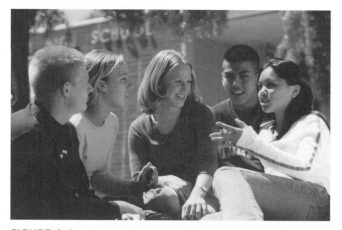

FIGURE 4–1 Colleges draw students from many cultural backgrounds and can therefore help young people understand how their cultural values differ from others. (Image courtesy of PhotoDisc®, Inc.)

members a mechanism to judge behavior, construct reality, and make decisions regarding life issues (Wells & Black, 2000). Culture also guides daily activities and tasks (McCubbin, Thompson, Thompson, McCubbin, & Kaston, 1993). These are learned behaviors that require repeated exposure to acquire. An additional characteristic of culture is its changeable nature (Downes, 1997). As individuals mature, their exposure to other cultures expands. For many college students the academic environment affords a truly multicultural experience (Figure 4–1).

RACE

Race refers to distinct biologic attributes possessed by a group of people (Giger & Davidhizar, 1999). These attributes include skin color, hair type, and bone structure (Downes, 1997). The number of racial categories varies depending on the purpose of collecting a person's racial identity. Some authors refer to three basic racial categories while others identify more categories. For example, the term *Hispanic* or *Latino* refers not to a race but to a cultural group, although it has been listed as a racial category on some reporting forms.

ETHNICITY

Ethnicity is generally used to reflect the influence of both race and culture on behavior (Downes, 1997). The ethnicity of a person may refer to shared traits, customs, language, religion, and ancestry (Canino & Spurlock, 2000; Spector, 2000). Hannah, pictured in Figure 4–2, provides an example of the confusion that surrounds race and culture. As a young African-American girl adopted by Caucasian parents, her culture is decidedly Caucasian while her race remains African American.

Blend of culture & race

DISEASE/DISORDER

Disease or **disorder** is considered a biologically based problem or condition in which a person's functional abilities have been disrupted (Downes, 1997). The World Health Organization (WHO) refers to diseases, disorders, and injuries as various health conditions and has classified these in the International Classification of Diseases, Tenth Revision (ICD-10) (WHO, 2001). Western medicine is primarily focused on the treatment of diseases instead of the effect these health conditions have on a person's ability to participate in life situations.

ILLNESS

Illness, in contrast to disease, refers to the negative changes in a person's well-being and social position within a cultural group (Downes, 1997). This term reflects Vygotsky's work that not only considers the limitations associated with a specific health condition but includes the cultural interpretation of the condition (Gindis, 1999). A young child with limited verbal skills may be diagnosed by one cultural group as language-delayed (Garcia, Mendez Perez, & Ortiz, 2000). In another cultural group, where the emphasis is on observational skills, this lack of verbal language by the child is not seen as a factor limiting social participation (Kalyanpur, 1998). From this perspective illness is not merely the presence of disease but also reflects the social and cultural interpretation of well-being.

HEALTH

Health refers to the absence of illness (Downes, 1997). The cultural understanding of well-being frames the

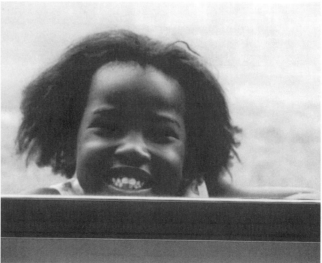

FIGURE 4–2 Hannah has an eclectic racial and cultural heritage.

concept of health. Some cultures expect an individual to engage in spiritual practice to be healthy. The behavior of spiritual practice is not universally required in the definition of health. This example is used to illustrate how the term *health* is culturally mediated, with expected behaviors to be demonstrated before an individual can claim to be healthy.

CULTURAL SCHEMAS

Schemas are ways of organizing complex information to help guide thinking (Ridley, Chih, & Olivera, 2000). **Cultural schemas** allow a therapist to systematically view the influence of culture on specific behaviors and characteristics. These schemas are divided into four areas: person, self, role, and event (Augoustinos & Walker, 1995). The areas overlap and interact with one another, as illustrated in Figure 4–3.

Person Schemas

A **person schema** refers to personal traits identified in others and predicts the social interaction between individuals based on expected behaviors (Augoustinos & Walker, 1995). This schema provides an understanding for the traits exhibited by a person. For example, the

"class clown" in a school in the United States may be seen as entertaining by classmates and as disruptive by a teacher but would not automatically be perceived as mentally ill. In another culture this behavior may be seen as severely disordered. Understanding the accepted personal schemas from a cultural group improves the interpretation of behaviors. A child who displays limited eye contact and seldom speaks to adults may not be depressed but instead be displaying respectful behavior in accordance with cultural norms (Canino & Zayas, 1997). Understanding the person schema provides the therapist with the knowledge of what personal traits are acceptable and culturally supported. These personal traits or characteristics change as the child matures. Promoting independence in self-care skills, particularly in a young child of 4 years old, may not be acceptable in all cultural groups (Zuniga, 1998). Although early independence in self-care skills may be promoted for European-American children, a Puerto Rican family may place greater emphasis on a child's social skills, particularly social behavior in public (Hanson, 1998; Canino & Zayas, 1997). Expecting a 4-year-old Puerto Rican boy to engage in dressing skills may be seen as unnecessary by his parents. These parents may be more concerned with the child's ability to properly address adults in public settings and display respect for adults.

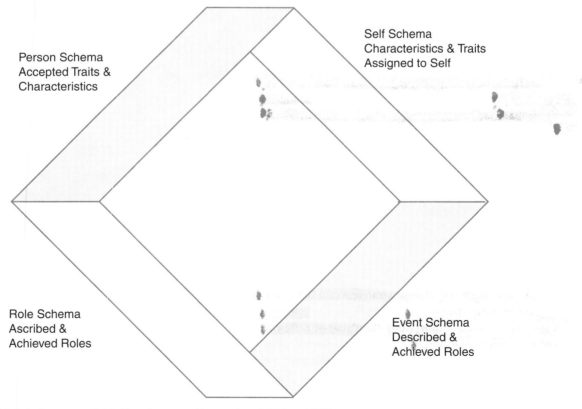

FIGURE 4–3 Cultural schemas are divided into four areas (Augoustinos & Walker, 1995).

Culturally oriented personal schemas also influence the development of language skills. In Mexican-American families, the mother is expected to know and provide for her child's needs (Garcia et al., 2000). This includes the mother's ability to read subtle nonverbal signs conveyed by the child. A diagnosis of limited expressive language skills in a 3-year-old child may be interpreted as a significant problem by a European-American clinician. Yet, in a culture that endorses the ability of a good mother to anticipate her child's needs instead of having the child ask for preferred foods or toys, this child's limited expressive language skill may not restrict participation in meaningful life events. A child who has to ask for toys and foods may actually be seen as a sign of an inattentive or inexperienced mother.

Self Schemas

The **self schema** refers to the characteristics and traits a person assigns to self (Augoustinos & Walker, 1995). These characteristics are culturally mediated and serve to define self in reflection of culturally endorsed attributes. The trait of being athletic or "good at sports" may be readily identified by boys of elementary school age as a self schema in the United States, but few, if any, of these boys would identify a characteristic of being advanced in meditation skills as an important characteristic. The presence or absence of specific skills, traits, or characteristics is culturally influenced (Sanchez, 1999). A diagnosis of mental retardation or learning disability may be seen as bringing shame on the family and can interfere with intervention plans. A therapist needs to consider that working with a teen-ager toward a goal of independent living skills may conflict with a culturally endorsed trait of interdependence on others and accepting support from the extended family members (Williams & Ispa, 1999).

Role Schemas

Role schemas refer to a person's social position within a culture and the expected behaviors of a person in that position (Ridley et al., 2000). These expectations may be based on accomplishments such as educational or athletic achievements. This type of role schema is referred to as an *achieved-status position* within a cultural group (Bonder, Martin, & Miracle, 2002). For example, a physician is expected to demonstrate certain behaviors in keeping with cultural norms. You would not expect a physician to inquire about a client's spiritual or religious practices within the United States, but health practitioners in other cultures are expected to ask about spiritual practices as part of the diagnostic process.

A role schema can also be assigned to a person according to race, gender, or age. This type of role schema is referred to as an *ascribed-status position*. In many Asian cultures, advanced age is associated with greater knowledge and wisdom, and younger people display a high level of respect and deference toward their elders. A core value of the Puerto Rican culture is respect for older people (Canino & Spurlock, 2000). This is not the dominant role schema for the elderly in the United States. Role schemas also refer to family structure and responsibilities. In some cultures an older sibling, even if only 8 or 9 years old, holds a position of authority over younger siblings and may be responsible for feeding younger siblings (Valsiner, 1997).

Event Schemas

"**Event schemas** organize sequences of well-known situations" (Ridley et al., 2000, p. 67). An example of this type of schema would be the sequence of events as a child attends the first day of elementary school (Figure 4–4). These are culturally predicted events with an order and sequence. The day may begin with dressing in new clothes reserved for the first day of school, a special breakfast, the trip to the school, locating the classroom, and meeting the teacher.

Different cultures predict different responses to events (Kalyanpur, Harry, & Skritic, 2000). This difference in expectations can lead to misinterpretations of responses during a social exchange or event. The following interaction between a therapist from a Euro-American background and a parent from a Mexican-American background illustrates this difference (Garcia et al., 2000): A meeting has been scheduled to review the results of a language evaluation on a Mexican-American child. After reviewing the test results, the therapist asks the mother if she agrees that her child has limited verbal skills. The cultural event schema for

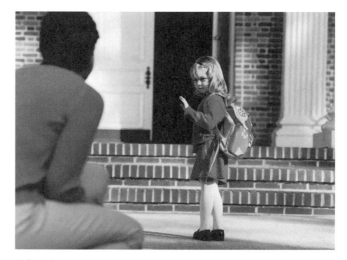

FIGURE 4–4 Culture determines the relative importance of daily events. In North America a child's first day of school often includes new clothes and special attention, signifying its importance. (Image courtesy of PhotoDisc®, Inc.)

this therapist predicts that the mother will express her own opinion regarding the child's skills even if different from the therapist's perspective. But the cultural event schema for this mother promotes social interactions that are respectful to those in authority and does not endorse open disagreement. Therefore, the mother may agree that the child has language problems, not from her actual perception of the child's limitation but in deference to the authority of the therapist.

Culturally mediated event schemas are found for social interactions such as meetings and also for many activities of daily living. Mealtime is an event that is culturally scripted and organized (Valsiner, 1997). In some African cultures, men and women do not eat together. Mealtime behavior can also serve as a framework to teach important cultural norms. Within an affluent society where food is plentiful, a child may not be expected to eat all the food offered during a specific meal. This behavior is contrasted with mealtime behavior in a country where food is scarce. A child may be scolded for not finishing his entire portion of food or may be reprimanded for not sharing what little food is available with others.

These four schemas provide a method to understand how culture can influence the construction of reality (Ridley et al., 2000). Understanding how schemas can influence development and the perception of skills is one avenue to improve cultural competence. Each schema serves as a filter to view phenomena encountered in life. Although cultural schemas are flexible and changeable, they also provide an explanatory foundation to understand people and surroundings. A therapist must consider each schema from the vantage point of the person's cultural group.

The following case is used to illustrate how schema theory can serve as a foundation in treatment. An Asian Indian family had recently immigrated to the United States. The 9-year-old daughter was riding her bicycle on the sidewalk in front of their home during the late afternoon. A drunk driver drove his car up onto the sidewalk and hit the girl, who sustained a traumatic head injury along with facial lacerations. Her parents brought her to the emergency room. She was unresponsive upon arrival and stayed comatose in the hospital for several days. A nasogastric (NG) tube was inserted for nutritional support. Approximately two weeks after the accident, she regained a minimal level of consciousness with minimal response to stimuli. During that two-week period she received occupational therapy services to address positioning, splinting needs, and sensory stimulation. Oral stimulation was also provided by the occupational therapist, but she was not given any food by mouth because of risk of aspiration.

This hospital had a policy of allowing parents to stay overnight with their children if space permitted. Parents often find this opportunity helpful as they adjust to the trauma of having a child injured or ill. In most White families, one parent, often the mother, would stay overnight for a few nights. This practice contrasts with the experience of working with families who are Asian Indian. The Asian Indian culture promotes interdependence, and often a child is cared for not only by the mother but also by several extended-family members (Ranganath & Ranganath, 1997). Consequently, in the case of this little girl, the entire family, including aunts, uncles, and grandparents, gathered in the hospital room. The event of a distressing situation required all family members to be present and support one another even if it meant sitting on the floor of a small room. Although some hospital staff initially complained of the overcrowding, all family members were allowed to stay during visiting hours. The mother and grandmother took turns sleeping in the girl's room.

The father served as the spokesperson, in keeping with the role schema for an Asian Indian family, and frequently asked questions of the occupational therapist regarding his daughter's potential for recovery. Questions regarding the use of splints while his daughter was hospitalized, the potential need for splints in the future, and when his daughter would regain full consciousness were often posed to this therapist. His manner was very quiet and controlled, in keeping with the expectations of personal conduct in the Asian Indian culture (Miller & Goodin, 1999). The family structure within the Asian Indian culture is patriarchal in nature, and deference is given to the eldest males, particularly the father. This knowledge allowed the therapist to explain information first to the father in a respectful manner and then to inform other family members. When the father was not present, the therapist would seek out the eldest male, in keeping with the cultural role expectations. Family order was maintained even in the stressful situation of having a family member who had sustained a traumatic brain injury.

As this girl regained a minimal level of consciousness, the medical team felt it was appropriate to begin oral feeds. The occupational therapist realized how important it was for the mother and grandmother to feel they had an active role in supporting the child during the rehabilitation process. Asian Indian cultural roles for a mother and grandmother include care of children, food preparation, and sacrifice for the family (Miller & Goodin, 1999). Every day these two women would return home daily to prepare substantial quantities of food and return to the hospital to feed family members and offer food to the hospital staff. Instead of using typical hospital foods of pureed potatoes or green beans to begin oral feeds, the occupational therapist consulted with the dietitian regarding a possible substitution using foods prepared by the mother and grandmother. The mother and grandmother cooked a dish of chickpeas with minimal spices and brought it to the hospital. The chickpeas could easily be pureed and the aroma was a familiar one to this little girl. Of course the mother and grandmother made an ample quantity of the chickpea dish along with several other foods. The entire family gathered in the girl's room to watch the occupational therapist give her the first few spoonfuls of food. The aroma of the food was very pleasing, and the little girl became more alert. Oral stimulation was first provided, and then the pureed chickpeas were presented for olfactory stimulation. The little girl began moving her lips. A small quantity of pureed chickpeas was offered, and the little girl was able to swallow a few small spoonfuls. Both the mother and the grandmother commented on how this girl had loved this dish and how pleased they were to be able to provide the food for her. This little girl continued to make substantial recovery in all areas and was discharged to home, eating a regular diet as well as talking and walking.

The use of cultural schemas in developing and implementing a treatment plan serves two specific purposes. First, it supports families during stressful periods and serves as a mechanism for families to adjust to change. Cultural schemas frame family roles and interaction and act as a filter to view reality. Few families have had to respond to the devastation of adjusting to a member who has sustained a traumatic brain injury. As families respond to this change, preservation of basic schemas allows the family to reorganize itself in response to the stress. Therapists can support families by recognizing the importance of a cultural foundation.

Second, the use of cultural schemas recognizes the unique strengths and abilities of the family that will be continued in the future. In the foregoing case, the cultural schemas did not promote the change in this young girl who sustained a traumatic brain injury—that was the work of the rehabilitation therapists—but the use of cultural schemas to frame intervention served as a support to the family as the members adapted to the stressor of a loved one being hospitalized. Cultural schemas are variable and flexible and yet provide a foundation to adapt to external stressors. It should be noted, however, that the described case provides an illustration of the use of schemas, not a comprehensive description of the cultural characteristics of the Asian Indian culture.

CULTURAL INFLUENCE ON DEVELOPMENT

Cultural differences must be considered when viewing the development of children (Valsiner, 1989). Culture provides a focus and a filter both to view development and to shape development. Development occurs along several continua, such as cognitive, social, adaptive, and motor (Llorens, 1969). Each of these developmental trajectories can be seen as woven together to support the infant, child, adolescent, and adult as he matures.

Differences in the development of motor skills in various countries have been attributed to cultural experiences and expectations (Hopkins & Westra, 1989, 1990; Keller, Yovsi, & Voelker, 2002; Kilbride, 1980; Super, 1976). In Kenya many parents train their infants to develop sitting and standing skills earlier than is expected by Western norms by using specific handling techniques such as holding their infants upright and stimulating the child in this position (Kilbride, 1980; Super, 1976). These accelerated gross motor skills have also been documented in Afro-Caribbean infants (Hopkins and Westra, 1989, 1990). The Afro-Caribbean mothers used specific handling techniques to foster the development of sitting and walking skills earlier than British counterparts.

Although culturally endorsed maternal practices of handling can foster motor developmental skills in infants, of equal significance is the cultural interpretation of these skills (Keller et al., 2002). German and Cameroon mothers were compared regarding their interpretation of mother-infant interaction and the infant's motor development. When watching a videotape of a Cameroon Nso mother providing motor stimulation to her 3-month-old infant, Nso women commented on the high quality of handling skills exhibited by the mother as a sign of the mother's expertise and how important it was for the mother to stimulate her infant. In comparison, German mothers made very few direct comments about the handling but instead focused on the general positive social interaction between the mother and child on the videotape. The practice of a mother providing physical handling and motor stimulation to her infant is part of the Nso culture. Competent mothers are seen as being proficient in these handling techniques. Nso infants are also expected to walk at an earlier age than German infants. In contrast, when viewing a videotape of a German mother playing with her 3-month-old infant in the supine position, many of the Nso mothers commented that the infant needed more time in the upright position and the mother did not seem to know how to stimulate the infant appropriately. German mothers, viewing the same videotape, again focused on the positive social interaction between the infant and mother instead of on the specifics of the task. The need for the mother in the videotape to physically stimulate the infant to produce motor skills was not important to these German mothers.

Children from different cultural groups have been shown to have differences in motor performance on standardized developmental instruments (Crowe, McClain, & Provost, 1999; Kerfield, Gurthrie, & Stewart, 1997). These differences have been attributed to the unique cultural expectations and the opportunity for children to engage in various activities within the cultural group. Typically developing Native Alaskan children were evaluated using the Denver Developmental Screening Test II (Kerfield et al., 1997). These children achieved many of the gross motor skills earlier than predicted by the Denver II. The authors postulated that cultural practices contributed to these differences. Native Alaskan children are provided with substantial freedom to engage in motor exploration, and older siblings are often responsible for the supervision of younger children. These older siblings exert few restrictions on motor behaviors, and this cultural practice creates the potential for Native Alaskan children to develop motor skills at an earlier age. Although some cultural practices may enhance motor development, other practices may restrict development.

Typically developing Native American 2-year-olds were evaluated using the Peabody Developmental Motor Scales (Crowe et al., 1999). Children's performance was significantly poorer on the fine motor portion of this instrument, and the authors suggested that cultural expectations again played a role in this difference. The engagement in fine motor activities, particularly for this age group, is not a cultural norm or expectation. The data collected by both Crowe et al. (1999) and Kerfield et al. (1997) highlight the need for a therapist to carefully select assessment tools to avoid cultural bias.

CONTRASTING CULTURAL CHARACTERISTICS

The way culture influences development can be conceptualized in four distinct and contrasting areas, as shown in Table 4–1 (Canino & Spurlock, 2000). These characteristics are presented as the extremes of behavioral traits, but a specific cultural group might not strongly endorse either characteristic (Coon & Kemmelmeier, 2001). A caveat is offered when discussing cultural characteristics: no example provided should be viewed as an absolute descriptor of a cultural group. There is a danger of furthering cultural stereotypes when a specific characteristic is seen as representing every person within the identified cultural group.

INTERDEPENDENCE VERSUS INDEPENDENCE

Western cultures, in particular the United States, encourage independence in children, as is demonstrated by the positive comments expressed about an attribute such as inquisitiveness (Williams & Ispa, 1999). This is an example of an **independent cultural group.** In contrast, the Hmong culture strongly endorses a sense of interdependence in children (Meyers, 1992). The characteristic of interdependence refers to the strong connections between members within a cultural group and the understanding that an individual's behavior has an impact on others. Members within such an **interdependent cultural group** rely on each other and are responsible not only for their own but for others' behavior. Thus, typical developmental assessments that expect a young child to independently explore a novel environment may be assessing skills that are perceived as detrimental to cultural norms and expectations.

Korean infants and American infants were compared regarding the amount of exploration used during play (Kim, Kim, & Rue, 1997). Although both

TABLE 4–1	Four Contrasting Cultural Characteristics	
Independent/Individualistic The individual is encouraged to pursue self-initiated interests and to be responsible for his or her own behavior. The individual's performance serves as the measure for success or failure in a task. Individual excellence is emphasized.	1	**Interdependent/Collectivistic** The group members share responsibility for behavior, and the pursuit of interests is strongly influenced by group needs. The group performance serves as the measure for success or failure. Group cohesiveness is emphasized.
Active Achievement Focus is on controlling circumstances and situations to benefit the individual.	2	**Passive Acceptance** Focus on accepting circumstances and situations as part of a natural course.
Authoritarianism Identification of a clear authority and individual freedoms are superseded by decisions made by the authority figure.	3	**Egalitarianism** Decision making is done through negotiation between members, and individual freedoms are included in the process.
Expressive/Overt Communication Public communication style openly expresses moods and feelings in addition to content.	4	**Restrained Formal Communication** Public communication style is often quiet and controlled, with limited emotional tone.

groups of infants would explore toys, "American infants used general exploration significantly more than Korean infants" (p. 190). This difference was attributed to the cultural focus of Korean mothers on interdependence instead of independence for their infants. The developmental concept of autonomy is not fully embraced in a culture that values interdependence.

The contrast in cultural orientation is also referred to as "individualistic versus collectivistic" when referring to the cultural characteristics of independence and interdependence (Brice & Campbell, 1999, p. 85). European Americans tend to be **individualistic** in their orientation and often exhibit assertive behaviors when working toward a goal (Ohbuchi, Fukushima, & Tedeschi, 1999). In contrast, Japanese are generally **collectivistic** in their orientation, avoid conflict, and are more "motivated by a concern for relationships with others" when engaged in tasks (p. 51). The pursuit of individual excellence is generally not promoted in Japan. Achieving a goal tends to be seen as the success of the group and not of the individual. This cultural orientation contrasts with that of many in the United States, where success is viewed as a personal achievement. The concept of individual rights and choice that is endorsed within a Euro-American culture contrasts with the value that many Native American cultures place on community well-being (McCubbin et al., 1993). Personal advocacy would be seen as selfish within a collectivistic cultural group. The pursuit of personal independence is not fully endorsed in collective cultures, where the development of self is defined by relationships within the family and community (Yamamoto, Silva, Ferrari, & Nukariya, 1997). The adolescent goal of independence from family must therefore be viewed from a cultural perspective and not assumed to be a universal norm (Ranganath & Ranganath, 1997). Some Asian-Indian parents expect teenagers to pursue the profession selected by their parents and agree to an arranged marriage, reflecting the interdependence within this culture. Again, these cultural characteristics are not to be automatically attributed to every person within a cultural group.

A cultural orientation toward either interdependence or independence can influence the acquisition of specific developmental skills. The task of being able to share with others has been attributed to the transition from the Piagetian preoperational to the operational stage of development, yet this skill also appears to be influenced by culture (Stewart & McBride-Chang, 2000). A comparison between Asian and Western elementary schoolchildren in regard to their willingness to share found Asian children more willing to share with peers than Western children were. Asian children were seen as influenced by a culture "where harmonious interactions are highly valued" and the needs of others are emphasized (p. 333). Although Western children and Asian children displayed similar levels of empathy toward peers, the Western children's empathy "did not translate

into a greater willingness to share with others" (p. 345). The cultural endorsement of community well-being over personal gain was seen as influential in the development of sharing skills in Asian elementary schoolchildren.

Many Chinese parents, from an interdependent cultural orientation, tend to emphasize the child's role within the community and "discourage independence and assertive behaviors under any circumstances" (Lung & Sue, 1997, p. 209). This cultural orientation results in school-aged children who may be reluctant to offer their own opinions or engage in classroom interactive discussions. As a result, a Chinese child might be inappropriately seen as withdrawn or inattentive when she is actually exhibiting appropriate culturally mediated behaviors of being respectful and quiet.

ACTIVE ACHIEVEMENT VERSUS PASSIVE ACCEPTANCE

Although "active achievement versus passive acceptance" represents a polarized view, cultures tend to endorse one of two worldviews: either that humans can change and control their destiny, or that their destiny is determined by outside forces (Downes, 1997). These contrasting viewpoints have been discussed in terms of the cultural framework used to understand the relationship between humans and nature (Bonder et al., 2002). Some cultural groups "value subjugation to nature, some value living in harmony with nature, and others value mastery over nature" (p. 35). Cultures that endorse a stance of living in harmony with nature or being subjugated to nature represent a **passive acceptance viewpoint.** This cultural orientation may view variations in body structure or function, such as mental retardation or cerebral palsy, as within the spectrum of nature and not endorse a need to change the body. In contrast to a passive acceptance perspective, a professional from a Western cultural orientation may view a young child who has a physical condition limiting participation in functional activities as in need of early intervention services to correct his health condition (Garcia et al., 2000). This **active achievement viewpoint** recommends intervention services so that the child's ability to engage in activities can be changed. Parents from a culture endorsing a passive acceptance framework may view this urgency by the professionals as confusing. Passive acceptance of the child's abilities and disabilities would negate the need for intervention services. The parents may also view the position adopted by the professionals as disrespectful toward the child by trying to change the child's behaviors and skills. Katherine Dettwyler (1994), while conducting research in West Africa, met a family who had a daughter with Down syndrome. Her conversation with this child's parents reflected their acceptance of their daughter even though the child did not speak. The parents described their daughter as happy and, like all other children, able to play and help with chores despite her limited language skills. Instead of feeling a need to change their daughter and make her speak, these parents accepted her as another member of the family.

A culture may endorse both passive acceptance and active achievement viewpoints but for different attributes (Chaing, Barrett, & Nunez, 2000). Taiwanese and American mothers of toddlers were compared regarding their beliefs about their children's behavior. All mothers were asked to report not only the frequency of various behaviors but also why they believed those behaviors occurred. American mothers attributed more of their children's positive behaviors to internal factors such as disposition and ability, while Taiwanese mothers attributed positive behaviors to external factors such as environmental support and structure. These beliefs were contrasted with beliefs about negative behaviors. Taiwanese mothers attributed negative behaviors displayed by their children—for example, hurting another child or breaking objects—to internal factors such as anger and aggressiveness. American mothers attributed these same negative behaviors displayed by their children to accidents. The results of this investigation led the authors to conclude that there is a "tendency for Americans to believe that success is a result of internal ability and failure is not one's fault" (p. 365). This cultural belief system combines active achievement and passive acceptance. American mothers reported that negative behaviors occurred as a result of external forces beyond the child's control, thus removing the responsibility from the child; yet successes were considered to be due to the child's ability. Taiwanese mothers were "more ready to blame their children and themselves for misdeeds and less willing to take credit for their positive behavior than are Americans" (p. 365). This investigation reflects the cultural norms in both societies. "Taiwanese emphasize modesty, which is in contrast to the value placed on self-confidence and high self-esteem in the American culture" (p. 365). Although active achievement is endorsed within the United States in relation to successful behaviors, there appears to be a posture of passive acceptance in regard to failure, attributing it to negative circumstances that are not the fault of the individual. Again, these examples are provided to illustrate cultural characteristics. The reader is warned not to assume that every person within a specific cultural group endorses these cultural characteristics.

AUTHORITARIANISM VERSUS EGALITARIANISM

The phrase "authoritarianism versus egalitarianism" represents a polarized stance, but some cultural groups do identify a clear authority within society while others do not. **Authoritarianism** is the preference for obedience to a clearly identified authority, with individual freedoms viewed as unimportant. A culture that endorses an authoritarian perspective often does not provide an opportunity for dissenting views or give all members equal voice in the decision-making process. Authoritarianism may also be reflected in the structure of a family in which one member makes the decisions and input from other family members is not sought out or considered. There is an additional expectation that those who are not designated as the authority figure will be submissive (Luckman, 2000). **Egalitarianism** is a preference for affirmation of the individual and allows for negotiation in authority relationships with consideration of individual differences. In an egalitarian culture, all members are included in the decision-making process. This interactional style may be mirrored in a family in which decisions require input from several members. The term *egalitarian* is also used to reflect the equal authority of members within a specific cultural group (Downes, 1997). Some cultures endorse an equalitarian view for adult family members but do not include children in the decision-making process.

In an investigation comparing parental child-rearing practices of Chinese parents in Taiwan, first-generation Chinese parents in America, and European-American parents in the United States (Jose, Huntsinger, Huntsinger, & Liaw, 2000), all parents had either preschool or kindergarten-aged children. The parents completed several questionnaires, and the families were videotaped during playtime. Both groups of Chinese parents reported exercising more control over their children and expected greater obedience when compared with European-American parents. Chinese parents also rated attributes of being calm, polite, and neat as more important than European-American parents did. Of interest was that all parents exhibited warmth and concern for the child. The authoritarian Chinese parents exhibited the same degree of warmth toward their children as the egalitarian European-American parents did.

The traditional Korean household emphasizes the authority of the father and grandfather within the family (Kim et al., 1997). This orientation has been slightly modified in the United States to include the firstborn son in a position of authority within the family. Men continue to occupy the position of authority in the family and within the community. From a perspective of the development roles, male children are often in a position of authority over female children regardless of age.

STYLES OF COMMUNICATION

Culture guides and shapes language development and communication styles (Luckman, 2000). Although there is a wide variety of communication and language styles, the two extremes of potential communication styles are presented here. On one end of the continuum is the **expressive/overt communication** style that conveys feelings, ideas, or moods in an open rather than a hidden, or controlled, manner. On the other end of the continuum is the **restrained formal communication** style that requires governing one's emotions or passions and adhering to traditional standards of correctness and without emotional content. Even the quantity of verbal interaction may be limited within this form of communication style. Several Native American groups, for example, place greater importance on a child's development of observational skills than verbal skills as a method to understand the world. This cultural emphasis has led to the misdiagnosis of language delays in bilingual Native American children by professionals trained in a Western cultural orientation (Kalyanpur, 1998).

The rate of speech and frequency of pauses during speech varies across cultural groups (Canino & Spurlock, 2000; Luckman, 2000). "Navajo children usually adopt a slow, methodical speech pattern" with frequent pauses during their statements (Canino & Spurlock, 2000, p. 13). An adult from a European-American culture may interpret this pause as completion of a statement and inappropriately move to another topic without allowing the child to finish the statement. Many Asian and Native American groups value the use of quiet vocal tone and emotional restraint when speaking, contrasted with individuals from a southern European background such as Italy. Italian verbal interaction tends to have wide fluctuations in tonal qualities, and speech is often rapid.

In Italy children are frequently engaged in lively discussions by parents, teachers, and neighbors (Schneider, Fonzi, Tomada, & Tani, 2000). Practice in verbal negotiation may assist such children in conflict resolution. An investigation compared Italian and Canadian 8- and 9-year-old children regarding their ability to resolve a potential conflict. These children were asked to share a single chocolate egg, which had an enclosed toy, with a friend. The number and variety of possible solutions were compared. The Italian children were more skilled at moving from an initial position to a final resolution of the problem than the Canadian children were. Italian children also made fewer proposals to solve the problem. The authors concluded that Italian children were more skilled at resolving a potential conflict. A culture that actively engages in verbal debate may assist the development of verbal negotiation skills.

Communication extends beyond speech to include behaviors such as eye contact, facial expressions, posture, gestures, and personal space (Giger & Davidhizar, 1999). In some Asian cultures, eye contact directed from a child to an adult is considered disrespectful (Sileo & Prater, 1998). Limited eye contact may be interpreted from another cultural perspective as a behavior associated with socioemotional problems. Facial expressions are also culturally mediated. As a symbol of respect and deference for authority, a Southeast Asian student may smile when being reprimanded by an adult. This smile indicates that the student will not harbor any anger toward the adult even when reprimanded. An adult from a European-American background might misinterpret that smile as a symbol that the student does not take the reprimand seriously and is being disrespectful. These examples serve to illustrate how cultural differences shape both the content and the style of communication.

Communication may rely heavily on the actual spoken words, as is seen in Western cultures, or may rely on a combination of nonverbal and verbal modes for communication (Downes, 1997). Korean families tend to rely less on verbal communication and more on nonverbal means (Kim et al., 1997). When British and Korean elementary school children were compared, the Korean children performed higher on tests of general intelligence and spatial skills but lower in verbal skills. The cultural emphases on verbal versus nonverbal communication may have contributed to this difference.

The degree of formality in communication style varies substantially across cultural groups (Luckman, 2000). Children in the United States may refer to adults by their first names and have casual interactions in most settings. This is contrasted with the Japanese culture, which has several levels of formality when addressing people. Children in Japan are expected to respect the status of an adult by addressing the adult in a formal manner. One arena where a degree of this formality is preserved in the United States is within the public schools. Most children are expected to refer to their teacher using a title and the teacher's last name, such as Mr. Lin or Ms. Arellano, instead of using the teacher's first name.

The socialization of mealtime conversation was investigated by comparing American and Estonian families (Tulviste, 2000). In both cultures mothers are the primary source for socialization of children. The extent and type of social interaction between mothers and teenagers revealed cultural differences. Although mothers in both countries were concerned about the social conversation skills of their teenagers during mealtime, the Estonian mothers made significantly more specific directive comments about acceptable conversational behavior. These directive comments included statements about avoiding repetitions of speech, turn-taking skills, and use of proper language. Such comments were seen as a reflection of the collectivistic cultural orientation in Estonia that endorses the responsibility of parents to control their children.

Estonian parents are responsible for socializing their teenagers in the acceptable forms of conversational patterns. These conversational behaviors are mediated by group interactions and not individual choices. In contrast, American mothers made few directive comments about speech patterns or proper language use during mealtime conversations. Conversations were focused on personal experiences and expression of feelings and moods. This difference was attributed to the individualistic nature of the American culture allowing for "freedom of choice and personal independence" (p. 553). Of interest was that teenagers from both cultures were not interested in the attempts made by their respective mothers to control their verbal behaviors or foster verbal interaction during mealtime. Teenagers from both cultures described the behavior exhibited by their mothers as intrusive and unwelcome during mealtime.

The characteristics discussed thus far are summarized in Table 4–1, which shows the different ways culture can focus a person's perspective. Although a specific cultural group may not fully adopt one characteristic over another, there is a tendency to favor one of the characteristics listed in the table over the paired characteristic. Cultural norms and characteristics can influence development in many domains of function (Valsiner, 1997). Again, one is cautioned not to assume that the examples presented are representative of every person within that cultural group. The literature cited here is not meant to foster prejudice or cultural bias but only to illustrate how the development of motor, language, and social skills can be influenced by culture.

POVERTY AND DEVELOPMENT

In addition to the influence of cultural norms and expectations on development, the level of **poverty** associated with a specific ethnic group should also be considered. Poverty is the state of not having sufficient basic resources. No culture endorses abject poverty, but poverty is present to some degree in all human societies. Members of minority social groups often have fewer material resources available and are therefore at greater risk of being poor (Spector, 2000; Wright, 2002). The effects of poverty on developmental skills have been documented (Alperstein, Rappaport, & Flanigan, 1988; Bassuk & Rosenberg, 1990; Coll, Buckner, Brooks, Weinreb, & Bassuk, 1998; Egbuonu & Starfield, 1982). Delays in motor, language, social and academic skills have been associated with the effects of poverty. Extremes in poverty, such as being homeless, have also been associated with higher levels of depression, stress, and anxiety when compared with those who

are at low-income levels but are housed (Bassuk & Rosenberg, 1990; Masten, Miliotis, Graham-Bermann, Ramirez, & Neeman, 1993).

Poverty has been described in terms of absolute and relative levels (Blackburn, 1991). *Absolute poverty* refers to severe conditions of inadequate shelter, poor nutrition, and an increased risk for delays or disability. Those who are homeless in the United States experience absolute poverty (Wright, 2002). Children who are homeless are currently the fastest growing segment of the homeless population and are more likely to have delayed development than other children (Bassuk & Rosenberg, 1990; Coll et al., 1998; Nunez & Fox, 1999). Homeless children have a much higher rate of asthma and general illness than housed children (Nunez, 2001). *Relative poverty* is a term used to describe those who can "afford some basic necessities but are unable to maintain an average standard of living" (Reviere & Hylton, 1999, p. 60). Those who experience relative poverty are also at risk for compromised health and development due to limited access to health-care services (Spector, 2000).

Children from African-American, Hispanic, and Native American households are at far greater risk to experience the effects of poverty than children in European-American households in the United States (Reviere & Hylton, 1999; Spector, 2000; Wright, 2002). There is no specific cultural trait or characteristic associated with being poor. The greatest risk factor for experiencing poverty is membership in a minority group. Members of minority groups earn less than European-Americans. Additionally, gender is related to poverty. Women, and particularly women who head families, are far more likely to experience both relative and absolute poverty (Canino & Spurlock, 2000; Reviere & Hylton, 1999). The earning power of women continues to be below that of men and, when coupled with the financial responsibility of raising children as a single parent, places families headed by women at a significant risk for experiencing poverty.

Poverty often places children in marginal environments such as overcrowded or unsafe buildings with poor nutritional support and limited access to health-care services (Canino & Spurlock, 2000). These stressors can contribute to developmental problems in several domains of function. Furthermore, the effects of poverty on development can be seen as a cyclic process (Spector, 2000). The person "lives in a situation that may create poor intellectual and physical development and poor economic production" resulting in poor earning potential for that person, thus perpetuating the experience of poverty (p. 165). In the United States poverty has been linked with an increased risk for "premature births, poor nutrition and prenatal care, and increased risk of attention deficit disorders" (Yamamoto et al., 1997, p. 45). This risk translates into children who may have difficulties meeting developmental milestones and succeeding in school.

Not all poor children display developmental delays, but their risk is greater than that for children who live in affluent households (Canino & Spurlock, 2000). The intersection of culture and economic advantages or disadvantages must be considered when addressing issues of development. The following case is presented to illustrate this concept.

Juan was a 2-year, 7-month-old boy from Puerto Rico. His family had recently moved to the Northeast from Puerto Rico for the father to pursue better employment. Juan was born with a brachial plexus injury resulting in significant loss of function in his right arm. Upon arrival in the Northeast, Juan's parents enrolled him in an early intervention program. As his occupational therapist, I was very concerned about the lack of sensation and motor control in his arm. I was also concerned about the lack of independence in self-care skills demonstrated by Juan. Although my Spanish-language skills were very limited, discussions with Juan's mother revealed that Juan did not use utensils to feed himself and he did not engage in any dressing skills. He was able to drink from a cup but preferred to use a bottle. The mother reported that Juan was healthy, and she had taken him to all his medical appointments while living in Puerto Rico, but his right arm still did not work. He had not received occupational therapy services while in Puerto Rico. Although Juan was verbal, according to his mother, and primarily spoke Spanish, he spoke only a few words during the initial evaluation session and appeared shy.

A developmental assessment revealed that Juan's fine motor skills were compromised bilaterally. He had very limited use of his right arm and hand due to decreased strength and range of motion and displayed poor dexterity on his left hand. His decreased sensory awareness of his right arm posed a potential safety risk. My initial intervention plan included play activities to stretch his right arm, along with developing basic dressing and self-feeding skills. Fine motor activities were addressed through both play and use of utensils for self-feeding. Although Juan's mother agreed to the plan, she also wanted to know how she could get his "right arm to work."

On my first home visit, Juan's parents greeted me and invited me to come into their apartment. The family lived in a small two-bedroom, one-bathroom apartment with three children, the grandmother, and both parents. The parents slept in the living room while the grandmother had one bedroom and the three children shared the other bedroom. Although Juan was the youngest child, he was also the only male child in this family. His father frequently asked if I knew how

strong Juan would become as he grew and if I could help him become stronger. Although both parents had verbally agreed that the suggested occupational therapy activities would be helpful, they reported that they did not have time to "exercise Juan's arm" even though the suggested activities were meant to be used during playtime.

My initial focus was to improve fine motor skills and motor control through the use of functional self-care tasks and play activities. The parents always agreed with my plan but then did not follow the suggested activities. During the third home visit I noticed that both the mother and the grandmother would take great pride in dressing Juan very neatly, and his older sisters would bring him toys instead of having Juan open the small toy box to get the toys himself. The cultural orientation of interdependence was revealed in many of the actions performed by this family. I began to understand that for the family to follow through with my recommendations would symbolize that the family did not provide adequate care for Juan. I was asking this family to make Juan engage in tasks that were very challenging. Although the parents agreed with my recommendations, those recommendations conflicted with the cultural stance that it would be uncaring to force Juan to use his right arm. I changed my orientation at that point. I recalled that both parents wanted Juan to be strong but did not seem concerned with Juan developing independent self-care skills. I worked with the mother and sisters to design an intervention program by which each could help Juan develop his muscles, and then explained that he should practice using his right arm to make it stronger. The practice sessions included play activities such as hammering with a toy hammer and sawing. These activities required use of both hands in activities that would be interpreted by all family members as tasks to make Juan strong.

I then progressed to activities to help make Juan's fingers strong. These activities included such tasks as pulling on his socks and shoes, but the task was now framed as an exercise to help Juan strengthen his hands. Both sisters took great delight in helping Juan become strong. The cultural orientation of providing interdependent support was used as an asset in the intervention plan. During subsequent visits Juan began to use his right hand to stabilize toys while playing and improved the dexterity of his left hand. Instead of viewing this family as noncompliant with my program, I had to reorient my program to meet the family's needs. Not all my interactions with families from different cultures have been successful, but I selected this case as an example of how recognition of cultural norms and use of those norms can be incorporated into an intervention plan to achieve a successful outcome.

SUMMARY

Understanding the unique contributions of culture on development affords a therapist greater variety and skill in developing appropriate and effective intervention plans. Culture provides both a lens and a filter to view reality. Throughout this chapter, examples have been provided to describe the interaction of cultural expectations and development. No example should be misconstrued as an absolute representation of a cultural group. Each therapist is encouraged to use the concept of cultural schemas and cultural characteristics when considering how development is viewed and the importance of various developmental stages or skills from a cultural framework. Although developing cultural competence can be seen as a lifelong pursuit, it offers an exciting and rich opportunity for therapeutic practice.

Speaking of

Culture across Borders

CRISTINA H. BOLAÑOS, PhD, OT
OCCUPATIONAL THERAPIST WORKING OUTSIDE THE UNITED STATES

I have been working as an occupational therapist in Mexico for 33 years. Although most therapists in the United States see Mexicans as a cultural group, for me Mexican culture has influenced the perception of my profession. One of the first things I learned as an occupational therapist was how the profession's status and the therapist's gender affect the kind of service you are able to provide.

When I was working as head of the Department of Occupational Therapy in a general hospital, my department was quite respected not only by the doctors but also by the therapist's coordinator, who was a physical therapist. The doctor not only referred people to me but also was actively involved in setting the therapy goals. Because I was well-educated, I was respected, but in general the women had lower status than the male doctors.

In occupational therapy school we were taught techniques that emphasized independence, function, and self-care, but we lacked insight into how the culture and the socioeconomic level could support or undermine our interventions. In our culture the family or the caregiver takes care of an ill person. Although elderly persons may be able to look after themselves, their families discourage them from maintaining their occupations. Many patients I saw who came from a high socioeconomic level were not interested at all in doing household activities. These were things that they had not done prior to their impairment, and they were not motivated to pursue them in their rehabilitation.

Later, when I moved from the physical rehabilitation area to that of pediatrics, I had more freedom and more professional respect. I was able to develop a new area of practice, working with teachers and other health professionals to facilitate the development and independence of children. In this setting I was able to develop new types of roles as consultant and researcher.

I have been involved as an educator since my early years as a clinician. My continuous challenge in this field is to help my students understand the importance of occupation competence and independence while being aware of the cultural values of our peoples and to develop an understanding that they can take care of their health through healthy occupations.

REFERENCES

American Medical Association. (1999). *Cultural competence compendium.* Chicago: American Medical Association.

Alperstein, G., Rappaport, C., & Flanigan, J.M. (1988). Health problems of homeless children in New York City. *American Journal of Public Health, 78,* 1232–1233.

Augoustinos, M., & Walker, I. (1995). *Social cognition: An integrated introduction.* Thousand Oaks, CA: Sage.

Bassuk, E., & Rosenberg, L. (1990). Psychosocial characteristics of homeless children and children with homes. *Pediatrics, 85,* 257–261.

Blackburn, C. (1991). *Poverty and health: Working with families.* Philadelphia, PA: Open University Press.

Bonder, B. R., Martin, L., & Miracle, A.W. (2002). *Culture in clinical care.* Thorofare, NJ: Slack.

Brice, A., & Campbell, L. (1999). Cross-cultural communication. In R. L. Leavitt (Ed.), *Cross-cultural rehabilitation* (pp. 83–94). London: W. B. Saunders.

Canino, I. A., & Spurlock, J. (2000). Culturally diverse children and adolescents (2nd ed.). New York: Guilford Press.

Canino, I. A., & Zayas, L. H. (1997). Puerto Rican children. In G. Johnson-Powell and J. Yamamoto (Eds.), *Transcultural child development* (pp. 61–79). New York: John Wiley and Sons.

Chiang, T., Barrett, K. C., & Nunez, N. N. (2000). Maternal attributions of Taiwanese and American toddlers' misdeeds and accomplishments. *Journal of Cross-Cultural Psychology, 31,* 349–368.

Coll, C. G., Buckner, J. C., Brooks, M. G., Weinreb, L. F., & Bassuk, E. (1998). The developmental status and adaptive behavior of homeless and low-income housed infants and toddlers. *American Journal of Public Health, 88,* 1371–1374.

Coon, H. M., & Kemmelmeier, M. (2001). Cultural orientations in the United States. *Journal of Cross-Cultural Psychology, 32,* 348–364.

Crowe, T. K., McClain, C., & Provost, B. (1999). Motor development of Native American children on the Peabody Developmental Motor Scales. *American Journal of Occupational Therapy, 53,* 514–518.

Dettwyler, K. (1994). *Dancing skeletons: Life and death in West Africa.* Prospect Heights, IL: Waveland.

Downes, N. J. (1997). *Ethnic Americans: For the health professional* (2nd ed.). Dubuque, IA: Kendall/Hunt Publishing Co.

Egbuonu, L., & Starfield, B. (1982). Child health and social status. *Pediatrics, 69,* 550–557.

Garcia, S. B., Mendez Perez, A., Ortiz, A. A. (2000). Mexican American mothers' beliefs about disabilities. *Remedial and Special Education, 21,* 90–100.

Giger, J. N., & Davidhizar, R. E. (1999). *Transcultural nursing* (3rd ed.). St. Louis: Mosby.

Gindis, B. (1999). Vygotsky's vision: Reshaping the practice of special education for the 21st century. *Remedial and Special Education, 20,* 333–340.

Hanson, M. (1998). Families with Anglo-European roots. In E. W. Lynch & M. J. Hanson (Eds.), *Developing cross-cultural competence* (2nd ed.) (pp. 93–126). Baltimore: Brookes.

Harris, C. H. (2000, March 13). Educating toward multiculturalism. *OT Practice,* 7–8.

Hopkins, B., & Westra, T. (1989). Maternal expectations of their infants' development: Some cultural differences. *Developmental Medicine and Child Neurology, 31,* 384–390.

Hopkins, B., & Westra, T. (1990). Motor development, maternal expectations, and the role of handling. *Infant Behavior and Development, 13,* 117–122.

Jose, P. E., Huntsinger, C. S., Huntsinger, P. R., & Liaw, F.

(2000). Parental values and practices relevant to young children's social development in Taiwan and the United States. *Journal of Cross-Cultural Psychology, 31,* 677–702.

Kalyanpur, M. (1998). The challenge of cultural blindness: Implications for family-focused service delivery. *Journal of Child and Family Studies, 7,* 317–332.

Kalyanpur, M., Harry, B., & Skritc, T. (2000). Equity and advocacy expectations of culturally diverse families' participation in special education. *International Journal of Disability, Development and Education, 47,* 119–136.

Keller, H., Yovsi, R. D., & Voelker, S. (2002). The role of motor stimulation in parental ethnotheories. *Journal of Cross-Cultural Psychology, 33,* 398–414.

Kerfield, C. I., Gurthrie, M. R., & Stewart, K. B. (1997). Evaluation of the Denver II as applied to Alaskan Native children. *Pediatric Physical Therapy, 9,* 23–31.

Kilbride, P. L. (1980). Sensorimotor behavior of Baganda and Samia infants: A controlled comparison. *Journal of Cross-Cultural Psychology, 11,* 131–152.

Kim, W. J., Kim, L. I., & Rue, D. S. (1997). Korean American children. In G. Johnson-Powell and J. Yamamoto (Eds.), *Transcultural child development* (pp. 183–207). New York: John Wiley and Sons.

Lancy, D. F. (1996). *Playing on the mother ground: Cultural routines for children's development.* New York: Guilford Press.

Llorens, L. (1969). Facilitating growth and development: The promise of occupational therapy. *American Journal of Occupational Therapy, 24,* 93–101.

Luckman, J. (2000). *Transcultural communication in health care.* Albany, NY: Delmar.

Lung, A. Y., & Sue, S. (1997). Chinese American children. In G. Johnson-Powell and J. Yamamoto (Eds.), *Transcultural child development* (pp. 208–236). New York: John Wiley and Sons.

Masten, A., Miliotis, D., Graham-Bermann, S., Ramirez, M., & Neeman, J. (1993). Children in homeless families: Risks to mental health and development. *Journal of Consulting and Clinical Psychology, 61,* 335–343.

McCubbin, H. I., Thompson, E. A., Thompson, A. I., McCubbin, M. A., & Kaston, A. J. (1993). Culture, ethnicity, and the family: Critical factors in childhood chronic illnesses and disabilities. *Pediatrics, 91,* 1063–1070.

Meyers, C. (1992). Hmong children and their families: Consideration of cultural influences on assessment. *American Journal of Occupational Therapy, 46,* 737–744.

Nunez, R. (2001). Family homelessness in New York City: A case study. *Political Science Quarterly, 116,* 367–380.

Nunez, R., & Fox, C. (1999). A snapshot of family homelessness across America. *Political Science Quarterly, 114,* 289–307.

Ohbuchi, K., Fukushima, O., & Tedeschi, J. T. (1999). Cultural values is conflict management. *Journal of Cross-Cultural Psychology, 30,* 51–71.

Ranganath, V. M., & Ranganath, V. K. (1997). Asian Indian children. In G. Johnson-Powell and J. Yamamoto (Eds.), *Transcultural child development* (pp. 103–125). New York: John Wiley and Sons.

Reviere, R., & Hylton, K. (1999). Poverty and health: An international overview. In R. L. Leavitt (Ed.), *Cross-cultural rehabilitation.* (pp. 59–69). London: W. B. Saunders.

Schneider, B. H., Fonzi, A., Tomada, G., & Tani, F. (2000). A cross-cultural comparison of children's behavior with their friends in situations of potential conflict. *Journal of Cross-Cultural Psychology, 31,* 259–266.

Spector, R. E. (2000). *Cultural diversity in health and illness* (5th ed.). Stamford, CT: Appleton and Lange.

Stewart, S. M., & McBride-Chang, C. (2000). Influences on children's sharing in a multicultural setting. *Journal of Cross-Cultural Psychology, 31,* 333–348.

Super, C. M. (1976). Environmental effects on motor development: A case of African infant precocity. *Developmental Medicine and Child Neurology, 18,* 561–567.

Taylor, R. (1998). Checking your cultural competence. *Nursing Management, 29(8),* 30–32.

Tulviste, T. (2000). Socialization at meals: A comparison of American and Estonian mother-adolescent interaction. *Journal of Cross-Cultural Psychology, 31,* 537–556.

Valsiner, J. (1989). *Human development and culture.* Lexington, MA: Lexington Books.

Valsiner, J. (1997). *Culture and the development of children's action* (2nd ed.). New York: John Wiley and Sons.

Velde, B. P., & Wittman, P. P. (2001) Helping occupational therapy students and faculty develop cultural competence. *Occupational Therapy in Health Care, 13,* 23–32.

Well, S. A., & Black, R. M. (2000). *Cultural competency for health professionals.* Bethesda, MD: American Occupational Therapy Association.

Williams, D., & Ispa, J. M. (1999). A comparison of the child-rearing goals of Russian and U.S. university students. *Journal of Cross-Cultural Psychology, 30,* 540–546.

World Health Organization. (2001). *International Classification of Functioning, Disability and Health.* Geneva: World Health Organization.

Wright, K. (2002). *Homeless in America.* Farmington Hills, MI: Gale Group.

Yamamoto, J., Silva, J. A., Ferrari, M., & Nukariya, K. (1997). Culture and psychopathology. In G. Johnson-Powell and J. Yamamoto (Eds.), *Transcultural child development* (pp. 34–57). New York: John Wiley and Sons.

Zuniga, M. E. (1998). Families with Latino roots. In E. W. Lynch and M. J. Hanson (Eds.). *Developing cross-cultural competence* (2nd ed.) (pp. 209–250). Baltimore: Brookes.

CHAPTER 5

Lifespan Communication

Dennis M. Ruscello, PhD
Professor of Speech Pathology and
    Audiology
Adjunct Professor of
    Otolaryngology
Department of Speech Pathology
    and Audiology
West Virginia University
Morgantown, West Virginia

Objectives

Upon completion of this chapter, the reader should be able to

◾ Describe communication, speech, and language.

◾ Summarize speech and language development.

◾ Discuss communication disorders across the lifespan.

Key Terms

augmentative/alternative
    communication (AAC)
communication
conductive hearing loss
language
language acquisition device (LAD)

language disorders
language impairment
metalinguistic awareness
morphology
phonology
pragmatics

prelinguistic period
semantics
sentence embedding
speech
speech disorders
syntax

INTRODUCTION

Communication is a broad term that encompasses the ability of humans to interact in ways that enable them to share such functions as basic needs, wants, desires, and ideas (Owens, 2001). Communication includes a broad spectrum of behaviors in several categories of the ICF. Voices and Speech Functions, a traditional domain of speech-language pathologists, is listed as a Body Function. Communication is broadly defined under Activities and Participation as "general and specific features of communicating by language, signs and symbols, including receiving and producing messages, carrying on conversations, and using communication devices and techniques" (World Health Organization, 2003, p. 12). Communication is required for functional participation and interpersonal interaction in most areas of occupation, especially education, work, and social participation.

Communication is characteristic of humans in all cultures and in all stages of development. Typically, we use language for communication purposes. That is, we express our ideas through words; however, communication can occur without some type of verbal exchange. For example, an infant may communicate needs and wants by crying. In the case of hunger, the child's caregiver reacts to the crying by providing nourishment. Other children may be delayed in the acquisition and development of communication skills and hence communicate with some type of idiosyncratic system that may include vocalizations and gestures such as pointing (Reed, 1994). Caregivers learn the meaning of such signs and attend to the wants and needs of the child.

Adults use their communication skills for a variety of functions, as we are all aware, but some incur injuries or other medical problems that adversely affect communication skills to the extent that there are limitations in their communication interactions with others (Owens, Metz, & Haas, 2000). Topics of discussion in this chapter will include the development and maintenance of communication from birth to adulthood, differences in communication, and an introduction to communication disorders that adversely affect the communication of children and adults.

COMMUNICATION

Before summarizing the development of communication, there is a need to discuss the terminology that professionals use in their discussions regarding communication and its components of speech and language. Owens (1996) has indicated that communication is a process that is part of human consciousness. As members of society, we are constantly communicating with others to share emotions, information, social interactions, and the like. Generally, we use speech and language, but, as previously mentioned, we do not have to use them for communication. Interactions such as gestures, facial expression, and overall body language may be used for communication purposes, or they may be used to supplement communication. When you see a friend, you typically provide some social greeting such as "Hi" and accompany the greeting with a smile and wave of the hand. It is obvious that communication is a very powerful tool, and competent communicators use the tool without restriction (Owens, 2001).

SPEECH

Speech is the verbal mode used for communication purposes and probably the most frequently used by the speakers of a specific language community to transmit messages. Kent (1998) indicates that speech is composed of individual sounds called *phonemes,* and these phonemes are abstractions that exist only in our minds. When we speak, we produce *allophones,* or speech sounds of the phonemes. The allophones are the actual physical realizations of the phonemes that are produced by the speaker. Phonologic rules are utilized to combine the phonemes into correct order, so that the appropriate words are produced. This discussion may sound a bit complicated, but it is not. For discussion, let's say that a speaker wants to produce the word "cat," a word composed of three phonemes. The word is generated through some mental operations that we do not totally understand in accordance with the phonologic rules of our language. The word is spoken, with the actual output that we hear being the allophones, or speech sounds of the phonemes. The consonant speech sound "k" is followed by the vowel speech sound "a" and ends with the consonant speech sound "t." A listener of the same linguistic community will recognize the sound combination as representing "cat." Our phonological knowledge allows us to generate thousands of words with different meanings.

VOICE

In addition to discussing speech in terms of phonology, or the sound system, voice production needs to be discussed, since it is an important component of speech (Owens, Metz, & Haas, 2000). A number of speech sounds are produced with voicing. This means that the vocal folds are vibrating to create a complex tone that is composed of many frequencies. Movements and positions of the lips, teeth, and tongue, together with breath support, produce various sounds. Use your hearing skills to analyze two sounds that provide a contrast between voicing and nonvoicing. If you produce the "s" sound and place your hand on your larynx (voice box), you won't feel much in the laryngeal area. Air is taken from the lungs and forced through a narrow constriction in the mouth to produce the sound. Contrast the "s" with a production of "z," because "z" is a voiced sound. You will feel vibration of the larynx as you produce the sound. Air is taken from the lungs, and through vocal fold vibration, a complex sound is produced. The larynx is an important component in the generation of speech.

Researchers such as speech-language pathologists study speech to expand the knowledge base of what is currently known. Kent (1997) indicates that speech can be studied in three different ways that include perceptual, physiologic, and acoustic study. Perceptual experiments examine the listening abilities of subjects under various conditions and listening stimuli. We use our auditory skills to receive and analyze messages that are presented by other speakers. Various measures of physiology help us to understand the actual production of allophones. Observational procedures such as X-ray are used to visualize the articulators and determine the production features of various allophones. Measurement of air pressure and airflow in the oral cavity during sound production is also employed for analysis purposes. Finally, acoustical study is utilized to quantify the parameters of sound frequency, intensity, and time.

Current technological advances allow speech researchers to analyze audio recordings of subjects and measure precisely the acoustic parameters. That is, one can quantify the physical aspects of the spoken speech signal. Collectively, these study methods have helped us add to the knowledge base, develop powerful theoretical models of speech production, and improve our assessment and treatment of persons with communicative disorders.

LANGUAGE

The American Speech-Language-Hearing Association (ASHA) Committee on Language (1983) provides a comprehensive definition of language that helps one appreciate the complexity of communication. Although it is complex, most individuals acquire language and are able to use it for communication purposes without problem. The definition of **language** is as follows: a complex and dynamic system of conventional symbols that is used in various modes for thought and communication.

Contemporary views of human language hold that (1) language evolves within specific historical, social, and cultural contexts; (2) language, as rule-governed behavior, is described by at least five parameters—phonologic, morphologic, syntactic, semantic, and pragmatic; (3) language learning and use are determined by the interaction of biologic, cognitive, psychosocial, and environmental factors; and (4) effective use of language for communication requires a broad understanding of human interaction including such associated factors as nonverbal cues, motivation, and sociocultural roles (American Speech-Language-Hearing Association, 1983, p. 44).

The definition underscores the fact that language is a multifaceted behavior that is under constant change due to a number of different factors. For example, our use of advanced technologies has resulted in the introduction of new words to our vocabularies. Concepts such as E-mail did not exist until the advent of computers, but such words have specific meanings and are part of our vocabularies. Distinct dialects have evolved, and are characteristic of certain language users among the users of a specific language (Owens, 1999). There is an idealized form of *Standard American English (SAE)*, and there are variations or dialects that are spoken by some speakers. SAE is not really a spoken standard but rather the form that is used in the publication of textbooks and heard on news broadcasts. A dialect variation such as *Appalachian English (AE)* shares most features with SAE; however, there are differences that make it distinctive. For example, a person may put things in a "poke" rather than a bag, if the person is a speaker of AE. It needs to be emphasized that dialect variations are differences and do not reflect communication impairment.

It is also important to remember that our language, like all others, is rule-governed (Kent, 1998). As a competent speaker of English, you may overlook or lack awareness of the components of language, since you learned the rules of English on an unconscious basis. Think about an aspect of language such as the rules for pluralizing different nouns. In some cases, an "s" is added to indicate plural (cat—cats), while in others there is a vowel change that signals the plural (woman—women). The point is that you learned the rules unconsciously and would typically be at a loss to list the rules for forming the plural. Contrast this with rules that you learned on a conscious basis, as in a sport. Baseball has very specific rules that players must learn in order to play the game correctly. If you do not learn the rules consciously, you have problems trying to play the game!

LANGUAGE STRUCTURE

The rules of language can be studied in relation to the five parameters: phonology, morphology, syntax, semantics, and pragmatics (Reed, 1994). Please refer to Table 5–1 for a summary of the parameters. **Phonology,** which has been discussed previously, is the rules that govern combinations of phonemes producing meaningful words. Along with morphology and syntax, phonology constitutes what is referred to as the structure of language. **Morphology** is the study of word structure, including alterations that change word meaning. There are *free morphemes,* which signal a specific meaning, and there are *bound morphemes,* which are combined with free morphemes to change meaning. For example, the word "dog" is a free morpheme that imparts a specific meaning upon a listener. If an "s" is added to the word, it becomes "dogs," and we understand that it means more than one.

TABLE 5–1	Parameters Used to Study and Quantify Language Development

Structure
  A. Phonology—sound system.
  B. Morphology—word structure.
  C. Syntax—word order.

Meaning
  A. Semantics—the meaning component of language.

Pragmatics
  A. Pragmatics—the rules and conventions for talking.

The final structural component is that of **syntax,** or the word order of our language. English speakers use word order to communicate messages with others. The sentence "I eat pizza" is a statement sentence that imparts a simple declarative message. That is, the speaker enjoys eating pizza, and the word order is very important in conveying the statement. The subject (I) is followed by a verb (eat), and the verb is followed by a direct object (pizza). In English, declarative, or statement, sentences follow a specific order in terms of the function of the different word elements. A violation of word order, such as "Eat I pizza," does not make linguistic sense to a speaker.

SEMANTIC MEANING

Semantics is the meaning parameter of language, and there are many different types of meaning that can be studied (Chafe, 1970). For purposes of this discussion, referential and relational meaning will be emphasized. *Referential meaning* is the meaning of individual words, or the word knowledge that we possess. The word "car" creates a mental image of an object that is expensive, driven by people, has doors, etc. This example illustrates that as speakers of a language we have an extensive vocabulary. Items in the vocabulary are organized and stored by the brain as a sequence of semantic features. Some researchers estimate that by completion of high school the normal adult has a vocabulary of approximately 80,000 words!

While individual words have particular referential meanings, the combination of referents in a message signals *relational meaning.* The meaning of the message is the sum total of the parts (Fillmore, 1968). If we study the utterance, "Bill hit me," as expressed by a child, we understand that the child was the recipient of some unwanted action. Each word has referential meaning, and there is the relational meaning that is coded by the combination of the words. Suffice it to say that both aspects of meaning are important to speakers as they learn and develop language.

Owens (1999) points out that other aspects of meaning are also important to the speakers of a language. For example, we also learn to use figurative language forms in place of more literal forms. When a person tells us that she is going to "throw a party," we understand that she is giving a party for a group of people. The nonliteral, or figurative, meaning is evident for a competent speaker. Similarly, metaphors and similes are semantic forms that contrast actual things with a speaker's internal representation of an image. One could say that a fast runner ran like a "scared rabbit." The semantic form conjures up the notion for a listener that the runner is very quick.

PRAGMATICS

The final element or parameter of language is that of pragmatics (Dore, 1974; Owens, 2001). Very simply stated, **pragmatics** consists of the rules for talking, or the rules governing what we say and how we say it. When we engage in a conversational interchange with another speaker, we produce utterances that are classified as speech acts. A speech act must conform to the conversational context, which is at hand. This is, an utterance or group of utterances must be appropriate for the context of the conversation. For example, "Pass me the milk" is a legitimate request to another for something. In the appropriate context, a speaker produces the utterance as a precursor to receiving the milk from another.

Prutting and Kirchner (1987) identified other aspects of pragmatic behavior to be assessed when examining conversational skills. As an example, pragmatic skills play an important role in conversation, because there is an interchange between speakers. Each contributes to the conversation and utilizes various pragmatic rules such as taking turns in the conversation, providing sufficient information, changing conversational topics, and furnishing feedback to a speaker. These are just a few illustrations of the pragmatic skills that we use as competent speakers of English. If a conversational speaker violates any of the rules, there will be a negative impact on the communication interaction. If a speaker does not take turns in a conversation, the other participant or participants cannot add relevant information and keep the conversation on track.

Language is a very complex system and there is a significant body of research that includes both qualitative and quantitative indices of language acquisition and development. A small percentage of children experience problems in the acquisition and development of the components of language. It is surprising that more children do not experience problems with the acquisition of communication skills, but communication skills develop in parallel with the other developmental domains of cognitive, psychosocial, and motor development. Moreover, researchers feel that language has a biologic basis, which makes it special to humans (Lenneberg, 1967). That is, humans are preprogrammed for language, and their interactions as developing humans facilitate the acquisition and development of language. However, in order for this wonderful process to occur, the other domains of cognitive, psychosocial, and motor development must also evolve, since they are interrelated (Owens, 2001).

CONCLUSION

Distinctions were made among communication, speech, voice, and language so that the reader would understand the perspective of professionals who carry out research in these areas and provide services to persons with communication disorders. *Communication* is a broad term that encompasses our sharing of thoughts and ideas with others. Most of the time, our communicative interactions are shared with others via language, but we can use nonverbal cues such as gesture, body posture, or facial expression exclusively or in combination with language. *Language* is a code that comprises the components of phonology, morphology, syntax, semantics, and pragmatics. The rules that govern language are learned on an unconscious basis. In summary, communication is a very powerful tool that we use introspectively and in interactions with others. A delay in the acquisition of communicative skills or a loss of skills at a later age can have serious consequences for an individual.

THEORIES OF LANGUAGE DEVELOPMENT

Before discussing language development, it is helpful to briefly summarize the major theoretical positions that have been proposed to explain the process of language development. This summary assumes a historical perspective in briefly highlighting the theories and discussing the positive aspects and limitations of each. Table 5–2 presents the different theoretical perspectives.

NORMATIVE DATA COLLECTION

Until the period of the 1950s, researchers were primarily interested in studying and classifying various aspects of language behavior. Researchers such as Templin (1957) collected normative data, and in some cases these data form the normative bases for current measures of language development. During the later years of the 1950s learning theorists considered language another behavior that was under the control of learning principles. In particular, B. F. Skinner (Skinner, 1957), whose theories are presented in Chapter 2, proposed that language acquisition was a learned behavior under operant control. It was hypothesized that the developing youngster produces various language forms, which are selectively reinforced by his caregivers. This selective shaping, the child's imitation of caregivers, and the appropriate provision of reinforcement are important variables that account for the language acquisition process (Osgood, 1963).

Critics of Skinner's theoretical proposal point out that several factors negate learning theory as a strong explanation of the language acquisition process. First, there is very little evidence in the language acquisition

TABLE 5–2	Theoretical Perspectives of Language Development Presented in Chronologic Order
1950s	1. Normative Data Collection Stage
Late 1950s–1960s	2. Operant Learning Theory
1960s	3. Psycholinguistic Theory—Structural Focus
Late 1960s–1970s	4. Psycholinguistic Theory—Semantic Focus
1980s	5. Sociolinguistic Theory—Speech Acts

literature to support the position that caregivers selectively reinforce their children. Studies of caregiver interactions do not show systematic shaping of language behaviors during the developmental period. Second, Skinner emphasizes the role of imitation in acquisition; however, imitation is not an active language acquisition strategy for many children who develop language normally.

PSYCHOLINGUISTIC THEORY— STRUCTURAL BASE

During the early 1960s psycholinguistic theory served as a model for the explanation and study of language acquisition. Rather than focusing on input and output processes that are characteristic of learning theory paradigms, researchers reasoned that language is universal among humans, and children acquiring different languages exhibit very similar acquisition strategies (Chomsky, 1959; 1965). These factors served as the foundation for suggesting a biologic basis for language acquisition. That is, humans are prewired for language. Furthermore, researchers proposed the notion that children are born with a **language acquisition device (LAD).** The LAD contains a semantic, or meaning, component and rules for constructing sentences. It is an innate mechanism that is activated through linguistic input from speakers such as the child's caregivers. Theorists were now interested in exploring the form (structure) of language, and the mental operations used to formulate spoken utterances. According to Chomsky (1957), a grammatical utterance is first a mental operation composed of a series of phrase structure rules that are created in a deep structure. At the mental operations level, phrase structure rules are thought to be universal among languages of the world. Transformational rules act to change and reorder phrase structure rules as necessary to create a surface structure, which is the spoken utterance. Transformations are specific to individual languages and operate on the universal deep structure.

The theory sounds a bit complicated, but it is really very simple. Psycholinguistic theorists are saying that

the mental operations of the mind are used in the generation of utterances. At a very basic level, all humans use the same mental operations (Deep Structure) to generate a proposed utterance. At the next stage of producing an utterance, there is another set of mental operations (Transformations), which are specific to the individual's language. The result of these operations is the spoken utterance (Surface Structure). Psycholinguistic theory helped us further understand what the child is doing or not doing during language acquisition. However, some issues cannot be explained sufficiently by the theory. For example, the language model is a syntax-based model with very little attention devoted to phonology, semantics, and pragmatics. In addition, it is difficult to explain under the theory how young children mentally process the early one- and two-word utterances that they use (Chomsky, 1968).

PSYCHOLINGUISTIC THEORY— SEMANTIC BASE

During the late 1960s psycholinguistic theorists tried to develop a more powerful model of language acquisition that emphasized the semantic, or meaning, component of a language (Fillmore, 1968). Recall that the initial psycholinguistic model included a semantic component that was part of the LAD, but the role of the semantic component was not completely developed in the original model, because it was grammar-based, not meaning-based. Bloom's research (Bloom, 1970) indicated that children produced utterances such as " Billy toy," and context information revealed different semantic relations depending on context. For example, in one context the child produced the utterance in referring to a possessive relationship of the boy's toy, while in another context the statement indicated that the boy currently had a toy. The former syntax model could not handle the same surface structure with meanings that differed depending on context. A semantic or case grammar model could handle this problem. In the examples cited, the first would be a possessive relationship (Possessor-Possessed), whereas the second would be a statement relationship (Agent-Object). In addition to the emphasis on semantic coding, researchers posited that the child's cognition is the framework for linguistic development. That is, development of the cognitive domain is an important requisite in development of the linguistic domain.

The semantic-based psycholinguistic theory advanced our knowledge base considerably (Chafe, 1970). A number of treatment approaches for children with language disorders that are currently being employed owe their development to this theory (Owens, 1999). Nevertheless, as with the other theories, there are shortcomings or flaws in the semantic-based psycholinguistic theory. The most notable is the specification of the relationship between cognitive and language development (Ginsburg & Opper, 1979). Researchers are not able to define the exact relationship between the two developmental domains. Specifically, they have not been able to establish how early cognitive concepts are translated in early linguistic utterances (McLean & Snyder-McLean, 1978).

SOCIOLINGUISTIC MODEL

The final theory to be discussed and the most recent to evolve in the 1980s is that of the sociolinguistic model of language development. The sociolinguistic premise is that the motivation or social/communicative roles of language are responsible for what we say and how we say it (Bruner, 1975). This is a much more encompassing theory than the others since it doesn't focus just on syntax or semantics, but rather on the function of the utterance in context. If a person is asked a question, she may answer "no" or provide an elaborate answer that might include several sentences of dialogue. In both cases, the function is to answer in the negative, and both ways of answering are correct, but the syntax and semantic operations differ in reaching the same goal.

Muma (1978) indicates that a speaker's goals are governed by the topic, the speaker's knowledge of the listeners, and the communicative context. Each plays an important role in coding an appropriate message. According to the theory, child-caregiver interactions are very important in language development. The child engages in early reflexive behaviors that are observed by a caregiver and acknowledged. It is through this acknowledgment that the child learns to communicate his intentions. For example, crying will result in attention from the child's caregiver and possible satisfaction of a need such as hunger. As the child develops, there is a transition from behavioral interactions to linguistic interactions, because the child realizes the power of language in influencing the behavior and actions of others.

As with the other theories, the sociolinguistic theory has its limitations in explaining language acquisition. Researchers have been unable to explain how the child learns to associate symbols with referents. That is, the child initially codes intentions through nonlinguistic means but then begins to use linguistic referents. Moreover, the theory is still evolving, and the schema for studying and classifying prelinguistic and linguistic forms are still evolving.

CONCLUSION

Theory building and empirical study of theoretical constructs are processes for either proving or disproving a particular theory. The resulting data are analyzed to determine if the data support the theory. If the data do not fit the theory, one must alter the theory, since it is not supported. Researchers have formulated a number of different theories to explain the incredible process of language acquisition. None of the theories have adequately explained the process, but each has advanced our knowledge significantly. Current thinking based on research suggests that language development has a biologic basis; however, the newborn must experiment within the environment. This social experimentation with caregivers begins at a very early age and continues as the child develops and expands language skills. As language unfolds, corresponding changes in cognitive development are also taking place, so that there is a constant interaction between the two.

PRELINGUISTIC DEVELOPMENT

Current thinking suggests that prelinguistic development forms the basis for linguistic development (Owens, 2001). The period from birth to approximately 12 months of age is the **prelinguistic period** and is characterized by the child's exploration of the environment with his caregivers. Owens (1996) points out that developmental changes in cognitive, motor, and social domains occur in parallel with prelinguistic development. When this period ends, the child begins to use words as referents, which is the hallmark of linguistic development. That is, the child produces words composed of phonemes, and the words are abstract symbols of the actual referents. For example, the sight of an approaching dog triggers the referent "doggie" from a child, thus providing evidence that the child has developed the concept of a dog and can produce a word that represents the internal concept.

FIRST THREE MONTHS

During the 1st month after birth, the human voice has a calming effect when the infant is upset. Caregivers constantly provide this stimulation, thus providing auditory and visual input to the infant. This is one of the early interactive schemes that occurs between the child and caregivers. Crying is also present and utilized by the child to signal needs such as hunger (Stark, 1986). It becomes evident to the child that crying will typically result in the satisfaction of a need; the child's caregiver provides a bottle in response to a hunger cry. The production of nonspecific vowel sounds, which are also referred to as *quasi-resonant nuclei (QRN),* are noted during times of satisfaction. The QRNs are open sounds, but they are not perceived as specific vowel sounds (Stark, Bernstein, & Demorest, 1993). Even early in infancy the child is actively engaged in interactions with caregivers.

The 2nd month of life is associated with further expansion of the infant's vocalizations. The QRN are now combined with what is perceived as back-of-the-throat sounds like "k" and "g" to produce what is known as *gooing.* Oller (1978) indicates that gooing is used during periods of satisfaction, or what we would call vocal play. The third month marks further refinement of the infant's vocalizations. The QRN are replaced by productions that appear more like the prolongations of actual vowel sounds. In times of satisfaction, the infant may produce a string such as, "Ah, ah, ah, ah," which is generally responded to by the infant's caregiver. This vocal behavior, which is known as *cooing,* is used quite frequently during this period. Other milestones during this period include turning the head toward a voice and responding vocally to the speech of caregivers (Masataka, 1995).

FOURTH THROUGH NINTH MONTHS

The 4th month is marked by additional changes in the infant's nonlinguistic productions. Consonant-vowel combinations are strung together and practiced by the infant during times of comfort and content. Babbling strings ("bah, bah, bah"), also referred to as random sound play, include sounds that are not contained in the native language (Stark, 1986). Another important landmark is the emergence of *suprasegmental features.* Suprasegmentals are features superimposed on the sound combinations produced by the infant. They give rhythm and flow to speaking (Owens, 1996). Word stress is an example of a suprasegmental feature that is used in the production of multisyllabic words. A speaker may produce a word such as "contract" with emphasis on the first syllable to mean an agreement, or produce the word with emphasis on the second syllable to indicate something that has been reduced in size.

The period from 5 to 9 months is associated with further expansion of prelinguistic behavior. The initial babbling, or repetition of similar syllable strings, is replaced by *variegated babbling,* a type of babbling that varies in terms of sound and suprasegmental pattern (Stoel-Gammon & Otomo, 1986; Stoel-Gammon, 1988).

A child may produce a string such as "Bah, bah, tah, tah, dah," with varying stress and overall inflectional patterns that are more adultlike.

Owens (2001) indicates that toward the end of this period *echolalia* emerges, a behavior that consists of the child attempting to imitate what has been said to her. Infants will often try to imitate what their caregiver says to them, and although it does approximate what was said, it is not believed that infants understand what they are imitating. The infant's processing of auditory input or comprehension is also continuing to change. For example, infants will respond to their name, and they can discriminate different emotional tones such as anger. By 6 months, infants start to recognize some words, and will "listen" when caregivers are engaged in conversation.

CONCLUSION

Changes and refinements in prelinguistic behavior continue in the time period of 10 to 12 months of age. Previous behaviors such as variegated babbling continue, but changes are also seen. One such example is the emergence of *vocables,* or protowords (Ferguson, 1978). Vocables are specific sound patterns that are specific to an infant, and they are used to represent different entities or actions. For example, a child may consistently show a toy and pair it with the production of "Eah." It is not a true word in the adult sense, but it marks a transition from vocal play and babbling to the eventual emergence of the first true words. That is, the vocable represents an actual entity in the child's mind. Toward the latter part of this period, children will be able to follow simple commands if they are paired with a visual prompt (Owens, 1996). For example, the child will wave "bye-bye" when given a motor and verbal prompt.

The first year of life is one of active exploration within the environment. Communication interactions begin immediately and are gradually refined by the child and her caregivers. When the child cries, the caregiver attends to the child by meeting some perceived need. The caregiver has assigned meaning to the act of crying, and the infant learns to respond accordingly. This constant attention and the assignment of communicative functions to actions of the child help the child in making sense of the environment. By the time infants reach 12 months of age, they can communicate with others through intentional gestures and phonologic strings of sounds that are not actual words but are the infant's representation of words. Since the sounds are used in appropriate contexts, caregivers are able to assign specific meaning to the strings of sounds. The development of communication skills in conjunction with developments in cognition primes the child for the use of the first "true" words and further expansion of the linguistic system.

LANGUAGE DEVELOPMENT

Our discussion is now shifting to the study of linguistic development in the young child. Most children acquire the basic building blocks of language within the period of 12 months to 48 months (Owens, 2001). Researchers have studied children to identify various milestones of language acquisition and have categorized the milestones in reference to stages based on chronologic age. The research paradigms have examined the components of language through the processes of comprehension and production. Recall that the components of language are phonology, morphology, syntax, semantics, and pragmatics, and the processes are understanding (comprehension) and speaking (production). Children were typically audio or video recorded while they engaged in communicative interactions with their caregivers and other children. The tapes were then transcribed and analyzed, and the linguistic behaviors studied in relation to the theory that the researcher espoused.

SINGLE-WORD UTTERANCES

Generally the first words emerge at approximately 12 months of age in most children (Hulit & Howard, 1993). This is a very important linguistic milestone, because the child is beginning to use words just as other competent speakers of the language do. The first words consist of single words used to communicate meaning relations (Schwartz & Leonard, 1984). The relations are context-based, meaning that the child talks about the here and now. The topics are those things that are perceptually available to the child. The single words are also referred to as *holophrases,* because they are thought to signal different meaning relationships.

Most of the early words consist of object names and actions. The child may be hungry and express a need for food with the action word "eat." Similarly, labels for others in the environment may be produced, such as "muhmuh" for mommie. The word shapes used by the child are simple types consisting of consonant-vowel (bye), vowel-consonant (eat), or repetitions of the simple types (muh muh). The use of holophrases is expected up to 18 months of age. Studies of comprehension or understanding indicate that the child understands more words than he actually expresses (Benedict, 1979). In addition, researchers such as Owens (2001) have suggested current thinking is that children acquire their first 50 vocabulary words as whole-word entities and are not aware of the phonology of the words. That is, children are not aware of the individual sounds that make up the phonology of words. After developing a vocabulary of 50 words, evidence suggests, children begin to crack the phonologic code and expand their vocabulary with words and word alterations that demonstrate an awareness of phonology.

TWO-WORD UTTERANCES

During the period of 18 to 24 months the child begins to produce two-word utterances. Research has shown us that the utterances at this level can best be studied in relation to the meaning that the child is trying to express (Brown, 1973). For example, the child may say "Mommy shoe," when holding one of his mother's shoes. Conversely, he may say "Mommy shoe" in the context of his mother holding a shoe. These meaning differences were first identified by Bloom (1970), and were discussed earlier in this chapter.

MORPHOLOGIC DEVELOPMENT

The next stage of development is marked by the expansion of utterance length and modulations, or changes in meaning, through the emergence of morphology (James & Kahn, 1982). Generally, the child is around 27 to 30 months of age. Children are beginning to produce phrases ("my doggie") and clauses ("my doggie eating") when communicating with others (Hulit & Howard, 1993). The appearance of phrases and clauses signals the preparation for adult sentence structure that consists of *subject-verb-object (SVO)* relationships. For example, the utterance "Billy eats pizza" is a sentence that contains a SVO relationship. Children are working toward this goal in the formation of statement sentences, and they are developing the structural knowledge to produce questions and imperative, or command type, sentences.

Various morphologic inflections also appear as children refine their knowledge of word meaning (Brown, 1973). *Inflections* are alterations to words that change meaning, and children begin to use inflectional morphemes. For example, changing a noun from singular to plural tense (hat-hats) involves the addition of an inflection and the internal semantic knowledge of pluralization. Similarly, a verb can be marked for tense by adding an inflection such as "I eat" versus "I eating." The subtle changes in words and the increases in utterance length are the products of both linguistic and cognitive growth.

One also needs to keep in mind that acquisition does not happen in a vacuum. Caregivers in the environment are constantly stimulating the child (Farrar, 1990). We know that caregivers speak to their children with less complex language, and we know that caregivers stimulate language development through various interactive techniques. Caregivers will frequently expand a child's utterances during interactions. The child may say, "drinking" while drinking, and the caregiver will follow with an expansion like "Yes, you are drinking." In other cases, the caregiver may add new information to what the child says, so that there is constant stimulation and interaction.

DEVELOPMENT OF SYNTAX

The next change in language development occurs at about 31 to 34 months of age, and encompasses additional changes in language development. Children at this level continue to add detail across the components of phonology, morphology, syntax, semantics, and pragmatics. In the previous stage, utterances could consist of either phrase or clause structure, but the majority of utterances now contain the basic structural components that include SVO relationships (Brown & Bellugi, 1964). Some of the highlights of this period are the development of questions and imperatives. Children at this stage are forming questions with the appropriate word order, such as "Can she play now?" What and where questions are also used correctly in most utterances. Imperative or command utterances like "Give me a drink" are used to request action from others.

Children can also engage in conversations, but their conversational pragmatic rules limit their conversational participation. Owens (2001) states that they can take turns in a conversation with another, but turn-taking is limited to two to three turns before topic maintenance becomes a problem. That is, the children can talk about a specific topic but not for an extended period of time. *Revision behavior,* or the ability to repair a conversation when a conversational partner is having problem with a message, is beginning to emerge, but the child's strategies are not successful (Gallagher, 1977). When engaged in a conversation, the child's caregiver might ask the child to clarify an utterance in order to repair the conversation; however, the child has not yet developed strategies such as repeating a word or the utterance, or restating the message.

SENTENCE EMBEDDING

The fifth stage in our discussion is generally observed in children between the ages of 35 and 40 months. The important linguistic feature of this period is **sentence embedding** (Miller, 1981). Embedding is a process wherein phrases and clauses are combined with other clauses to create more complex utterances. A prepositional phrase is added to an utterance, such as "Put it *under the table.*" Another example of embedding is the combining of two clauses to create an utterance that has a main clause and an independent clause. For example, the child might say "I like the boy who helped." The utterance is a complex sentence with an independent/dependent clause relationship. The independent clause is "I like the boy," and the dependent clause is "who helped." Hulit and Howard (1993) emphasize that the other components of language continue to improve, including pragmatics. Turn-taking skills improve to the level that the child can engage in a conversation and is capable of taking more than two

turns when discussing a topic. The child is learning to perceive differences in pause when conversing with a caregiver. A short pause means that an utterance is forthcoming, but an extended pause signals the cessation of an utterance.

COJOINING SENTENCES

The final stage is one of language mastery across the language components and is associated with children in the age range of 41 to 46 months (Brown, 1973). Although these children still have to refine some aspects of language, they are quite sophisticated in their production and comprehension of language. Their utterances are complete in reference to structure, and they begin to consider the perspective of the listener (Hulit & Howard, 1993). For example, a previous request for something might take the form, "Give me a pop." At this stage the child might say, "I ate my supper. Why don't you give me some pop?" Note that the child is reminding the listener that supper was finished successfully and that a reward should be forthcoming. In the previous stage, the concept of phrase and sentence embedding was discussed, and examples of such use were provided. Children continue to refine embedding, and they begin to cojoin sentences. Before this period, cojoining of items, such as "I like cookies and milk," are noted. At this stage, sentences such as "I saw the dog and I gave him a biscuit" illustrate the combining of two sentences into a single sentence. The child's preferred connector is "and," but other connecting devices such as "if" are also noted.

REFINING LANGUAGE SKILLS

It is quite obvious that children acquire the building blocks of language in a very short period of time. The process begins at birth and continues into adulthood; however, the basic foundation is formed during the preschool years. Reed (1994) notes that the school experience places the child in an environment that is rich with different experiences and interactions with others. Children continue to build their vocabulary and refine the foundation formed during the preschool years. For example, children are completing their acquisition of the sound system and expanding the domains of syntax, semantics, and pragmatics. The child's cognitive development continues to serve as a framework for speech and language. In elementary and secondary school, the child formalizes the language channels by learning to read, write, and spell. The development of literacy skills opens the child to almost limitless opportunities for learning about the world, and it also provides another medium for the expression of oneself.

METALINGUISTIC AWARENESS

Another important marker of advanced language development is the older child's development of intuitions regarding language (Paul, 2001). That is, the child can engage in introspective tasks that reflect one's knowledge of language. This ability is known as **metalinguistic awareness** and can be examined in a variety of ways. For example, one could assess phonologic awareness by asking children to identify specific sounds that are at the beginning or end of words or to generate words that rhyme with a key word. Syntactic and semantic awareness could be studied by asking the child to listen to a sentence and judge the grammaticality of the sentence.

CONCLUSION

Language development is a very complex process that is presented here in a brief and simplified manner. In a very short time children acquire a communication code that they can use with others to exchange ideas, feelings, and other communicative functions. Cognition is very important, because it furnishes the scaffolding for language development. Children develop the rules of language on an unconscious basis and gradually expand the rules. Although the major aspects of language development are completed during the preschool years, the child continues to refine the components of language into adulthood. The development of literacy is another very important milestone that represents a transition from speaking and listening to include reading, writing, and spelling. Finally, the child develops an awareness of language and can reflect on phonologic, morphologic, syntactic, semantic, and pragmatic aspects of language when necessary.

COMMUNICATION DISORDERS

Communication and language skills are integral to human function and participation in human occupations. Although complex and difficult to characterize within the ICF framework, difficulties in communication may lead to disablement as surely as do difficulties in physical or intellectual abilities (World Health Organization, 2002). Disorders in communication are the result of developmental delays or acquired problems and include individuals across the lifespan. Current estimates indicate that approximately 17 percent of the population has some type of communication disorder. About 11 percent have some type of hearing loss, and 6 percent exhibit a speech or language disorder (Castrogiovanni, 1999a; Castrogiovanni, 1999b). For purposes of discussion, communication disorders will be classified according to speech disorders and

TABLE 5–3	Classification of Communication Disorders

Speech Disorders

Speech Sound Disorders
Unknown etiology
Structural-based disorders
Sensory-based disorders
Motor speech-based disorders

Voice and Resonance Disorders
Pitch disorders
Loudness disorders
Quality disorders
Inappropriate oral-nasal coupling

Fluency Disorders

Language Impairment

Language Impairment in Children
Mental retardation/developmental disability
Autism
Hearing impairment
Specific language impairment
Neglect and abuse
Traumatic brain injury

Language Impairment in Adults
Aphasia
Fluent aphasia
Nonfluent aphasia
Traumatic brain injury
Dementia

language disorders and divided between child and adult categories when appropriate.

These divisions are traditional categorizations that permit the description of clinical subgroups. **Speech disorders** pertain to individuals with speech sound disorders (phonology), voice disorders (voice generation), and fluency disorders (stuttering), while **language disorders** refer to problems with the comprehension or production of the language components of morphology, syntax, semantics, and pragmatics. See Table 5–3 for a summary of the classification of communication disorders.

CONCLUSION

Communication disorders can be divided into speech and language disorders. Speech disorders consist of speech sound disorders, voice disorders, resonance disorders, and fluency disorders. *Speech sound disorders* occur very frequently, and in most cases the etiology of such disorders is unknown. However, there are subsets of individuals with structural or neurologic problems that are causal factors in the development and maintenance of the speech sound disorders. *Voice disorders* are classified in reference to the parameters of pitch, loudness, and quality. The causes of a voice disorder may be due to vocal abuse, a specific medical condition, or psychogenic factors. *Resonance disorders* are frequently caused by inappropriate coupling of the oral and nasal tracts. *Fluency disorders,* or stuttering, are also speech disorders, but to date, no viable cause has been established. Many children develop stuttering symptoms but outgrow the problem. Stuttering can have some very negative consequences on a person's quality of life. Research is being conducted to identify causal factors and develop a viable theory that will stand the test of empirical study.

LANGUAGE IMPAIRMENT

Language impairment is any problem in the comprehension (understanding) or production (speaking) of the language code (Reed, 1994). Recall that the code includes morphology, syntax, semantics, and pragmatics. Our discussion of language impairment will deal with children and adults separately, since the origins of their impairments differ. That is, children with language impairment experience difficulty in acquiring language, while adults have acquired the language code but lose certain language skills due to some medical condition or disease process. The difference in terms of delayed acquisition versus loss causes us to look at language impairment across the lifespan a bit differently.

A few of these disorders will be elaborated on to assist the reader in understanding the condition and the manner in which the disorder impacts function and communication.

LANGUAGE IMPAIRMENT IN CHILDREN

Paul (2001) states that most discussions of language impairment in children identify subgroups based on etiology. The different causal categories consist of mental retardation/developmental disability, autism, hearing impairment, specific language impairment, neglect and abuse, and traumatic brain injury. Accordingly, individuals from those subgroups will demonstrate language impairments that will vary as a function of the different subgroups. Keep in mind that this discussion will deal with generalities, but individual differences among children are quite evident and need to be considered (Owens, 1999). The speech-language pathologist will evaluate a child with suspected language impairment to establish a level of language function. Following assessment, a treatment program is developed to enhance existing language skills and to incorporate caregivers and significant others in a plan to improve existing language skills. Even with treatment, children with language impairment continue to have some degree of involvement across the lifespan.

Mental Retardation/Developmental Disability

Children with mental retardation/developmental disability have intelligence that is significantly below average and that manifests itself in limited functioning in areas such as communication, self-care, social skills, health and safety, and functional academics. They will exhibit language impairment of varying degrees (Paul, 2001). As children with mental retardation acquire language, they show a delay with respect to normal-aged peers. As they continue to develop, the gap between their expected language age and chronologic age increases. Expressive language is shorter in length and less complex, but all linguistic areas of structure, semantics, and pragmatics are problematic for the child with mental retardation.

Autism

Autism is a very perplexing problem that is a severe manifestation of *pervasive developmental disorder (PDD).* Autism is an impairment of social interaction, with restricted behavior and environmental interaction (Schreibman, 1988). It is generally diagnosed when the child is very young; the onset is generally before 30 months of age. Caregivers often report that the child started to develop language, but then development stopped very abruptly. A large majority of children with autism are nonspeaking, while others develop some language or exhibit echolalia. Those children who do develop some language skills frequently employ unusual or peculiar differences that reflect disparity in pragmatic language skills. Some may use echolalia, which is the immediate repetition of another speaker. In the case of autism, it is thought that the person stores and produces the utterances but does not process the utterances internally as a normal speaker would.

Hearing Impairment

As discussed under the section of speech sound disorders, hearing impairment has a significant effect on the other components of language (Reed, 1994). The severity of the language impairment will vary according to age of onset, type of loss, and degree of loss. In the case of hearing loss, the person is carefully evaluated by an audiologist to quantify the type and degree of loss. If appropriate, a hearing aid is employed to amplify speech. Note that a hearing aid will assist the person, since the aid amplifies sound; however, it does not restore a hearing loss. In the case of a severe loss, a cochlear implant is surgically placed in the cochlea, which is the end organ of hearing in the inner ear. The implant provides a means to receive speech and process it. Language impairment in an individual with a hearing impairment can be severe, with limited verbal output and poor auditory comprehension. Speakers with a hearing impairment use speech and supplement expression and comprehension of language with speech reading and manual signing.

Specific Language Impairment

The subgroup of children diagnosed as having a *specific language impairment (SLI)* do not have any cognitive, social, sensory, or motor problems that would adversely affect language acquisition. However, as Leonard (1998) points out, they show early delays in language acquisition that will continue in the event of no intervention. The lack of achievement of various linguistic milestones usually prompts caregivers to seek services when the children are young. Consequently, these children are often identified early in life and receive treatment as preschoolers, with treatment continuing into school age. Children with SLI will frequently comprehend more than they are capable of producing. They have difficulty extracting regularities from language; hence, aspects of language such as morphology are problematic. Vocabulary growth can also be a problem with these children. Finally, pragmatics, which are the rules for talking with others, are difficult for children in this subgroup to master.

Neglect and Abuse

Some children are in a family situation where there is a lack of caregiver interaction, or the children are subject to physical and/or mental abuse (Owens, Metz, & Haas, 2000). These environmental factors can have a negative impact on language acquisition. Research has established that a lack of maternal interaction has an extremely negative effect on the language development of children from homes where there is abuse or neglect (Carlson, Cicchetti, Barnett, & Braunwald, 1989). The language delays seen in this population are in all areas of language, but pragmatics is often a significant problem with these children. In particular, they have problems with conversational skills. They are not initiators in conversational interchanges, and they generally restrict their utterances when engaged in conversation with others.

Traumatic Brain Injury

The final subgroup is that of *traumatic brain injury (TBI)*, or closed head injury. These children are in the stages of language acquisition or have developed language when they incur a TBI (Blosser & DePompei, 2003). The effect on language will differ in terms of site, degree, and age of insult. In addition, cognitive deficits such as attention, memory, perception, organizational skills, and problem solving are present as the result of diffuse damage to the brain. Every year, about 1 million children and adolescents incur TBI as the result of mishaps such as car accidents. Language indicators include deficits in comprehension and difficulty with figurative language such as idioms, metaphors, and proverbs. There is concreteness to their residual comprehension of language. Another area of difficulty is that of pragmatics, particularly in the areas of conversational skills and narration. When engaged in conversation, children with TBI often go off task and lose focus. *Narratives* are verbal stories that are told to others regarding some topic and are analogous to written stories, as the speaker must introduce, maintain, and end the story. Children with TBI have problems with uniting the components of a narrative into a cohesive story because of problems with attention and focus.

AUGMENTATIVE/ALTERNATIVE COMMUNICATION

It should be noted that some children and adults with severe language impairment or those who exhibit severe motor speech disorders may never be capable of developing functional expressive speech and language skills. This problem has been an abiding issue in the profession of speech-language pathology, because many individuals have not received appropriate services. Within the past 20 years, a new assessment/treatment approach known as **augmentative/alternative communication (AAC)** has been developed. AAC is a means to provide communication in a form other than expressive speech output (Lloyd, Fuller, & Arvidson, 1997).

One common form of alternative communication is *American Sign Language (ASL)*. ASL "is a complete, complex language that employs signs made with the hands and other movements, including facial expressions and postures of the body. It is the first language of many deaf North Americans, and one of several communication options available to deaf people. ASL is said to be the fourth most commonly used language in the United States" (National Institute on Deafness and Communication Disorders, http://www.nidcd.nih.gov/health/hearing/asl.asp, accessed 8-8-03).

Its wide usage makes ASL unlike many other forms of alternative communication in that it is a true language with syntax, semantics, pragmatics, and fluency. Sign language varies by region and nationality, as does spoken language. Therefore, in addition to ASL, there is also a British Sign Language and an Australian Sign Language.

Oftentimes caregivers have the notion that the use of sign language and other forms of AAC will prevent future expressive language; however, studies indicate that using AAC increases the individual's verbal output (Owens, Metz, & Haas, 2000). Augmentative communication devices run the gamut from simple picture boards or signs to speech synthesizers via computer output. Output methods that do not require equipment, such as signing or gesturing, are classified as *unaided systems*, whereas *aided systems* use some form of either "low" or "high" technology. An example of low technology would be a communication board containing vocabulary for communication purposes.

It is one thing to design and implement an AAC system, but it is paramount that the individual and caregivers use the system just as people would engage in verbal interchanges. If pragmatic interaction skills are not taught and utilized, the AAC system will be of no communicative value to the person with the communicative disorder.

LANGUAGE IMPAIRMENT IN ADULTS

Most adults have acquired language without problem and are competent communicators with others in their language community. Language impairment in adults may be the result of a disruption of the blood supply to the brain, damage to neural tissue, or some degenerative pathological process (Owens, Metz, & Haas, 2000). Oftentimes there are other problems that co-occur with language impairment, such as sensory and/or motor deficits, memory problems, poor judgment, etc. In addition, the person may also have a coexisting motor speech disorder and possibly a swallowing disorder. It is obvious that language impairment can seriously affect a person's quality of life.

SUMMARY

This chapter was designed to furnish an overview of communication, discuss disorders that affect communication, and identify causal factors responsible for communication disorders. Communication is a fundamental human function that we use in social interactions with others. Language is that aspect of communication that enables us to share our inner thoughts and feelings, influence others, and engage in introspective talking. It has been conceptualized as comprising phonology, morphology, syntax, semantics, and pragmatics. The child acquires language through the development of cognitive-linguistic rules for pairing structure with meaning in the context of rules for communicating with others. A small number of children display developmental speech and language disorders that are of unknown origin or are related to structural or neurologic factors. Adults can also have communication disorders that are generally caused by structural or neurologic involvement. Many individuals with communication disorders have coexisting feeding disorders that require treatment. The speech-language pathologist provides services to this population; however, in many cases, appropriate management can be achieved only through different disciplines working together.

CASE
1

Jimmy

Jimmy was born approximately two months premature in a small rural hospital. The doctor who delivered Jimmy expressed concern regarding oxygen deprivation during the birth process. Despite the concerns, the youngster was placed in an incubator shortly after birth. The doctor informed the parents that Jimmy might show some developmental delays, since he was premature and there was the possibility of oxygen loss during birth. Jimmy's parents were not sure what a developmental delay was and were apprehensive about caring for the youngster.

Jimmy was discharged to his parents after a one-month stay. They noted that he seemed very irritable and was difficult to feed. He had difficulty sucking on a bottle and drooled excessively; consequently feeding required a great deal of time. When Jimmy was 6 months old, his pediatrician

Continues

CASE

1

Jimmy *Continued*

also expressed concern due to the continued presence of reflexive behaviors such as a significant tongue thrust, startle response, and overall lack of motor responding. The doctor referred the family to a hospital with a developmental evaluation center.

An interdisciplinary team consisting of a pediatrician, neurologist, physical therapist, occupational therapist, developmental specialist, speech-language pathologist, and audiologist saw the youngster. The team determined that Jimmy had mild cognitive and moderate motor delays and spastic cerebral palsy. It was recommended that the youngster be enrolled in a home-based interdisciplinary program and undergo periodic reevaluations at the center. In addition, it was recommended that the parents receive counseling to develop an understanding of Jimmy's problems and work with the home-based program personnel, so that they could also provide intervention opportunities for Jimmy.

After eighteen months of treatment by the home-based team, a reevaluation indicated that Jimmy was showing some improvements in attending behavior and body posture, was able to suck with adequate lip closure, and was taking puree-consistency foods from a spoon. His attempts at speech were not successful, so an augmentative system was developed for the youngster. An introductory picture board containing single words was developed. The words were taken from Jimmy's environment and deemed appropriate by the parents. An eye-gaze system was used, and the parents were trained to use it with Jimmy. The youngster is demonstrating progress but needs continued interdisciplinary treatment and periodic evaluations to ensure that progress is sustained.

CASE

2

Billy

Billy was 3 years old when he was seen at the University Speech and Hearing Clinic for a speech sound disorder. He was identified in a nursery school screening and recommended for a complete evaluation. His mother was interested in an evaluation, since she reported that he was "difficult" to understand. Most people don't understand Billy, including his nursery school teacher. His older brother will generally talk for him. He has no history of any developmental problems with the exception of communication. His mother had his hearing tested recently, and it was reported to be normal.

An evaluation was conducted and speech sound testing conducted. The most significant error patterns identified were those of sound omissions at the end of words and the omission of a cluster segment. For example, a word such as "bat" would be produced as "ba," and a word with a cluster like "ski" would be realized as "ki." The speech sound error pattern has a significant effect on Billy's intelligibility. An examination of the speech mechanism indicated structure and function within normal limits. Language testing indicated normal comprehension skills but a slight delay in expressive language skills. The diagnosis was a severe speech sound disorder with a mild expressive

Continues

C A S E

2   **Billy** *Continued*

language delay. The speech sound error pattern, lack of intelligibility, and mild expressive language delay indicated that treatment was necessary.

Billy was enrolled in treatment for the speech sound disorder. A minimal-pair teaching procedure was used to correct the error pattern of final-word omission. For example, word pairs like "bee-beet" were used as stimuli. Billy was first taught to discriminate among the word pairs and then taught to produce the items. He first responded to an imitation of the words and then responded to presentation of the pictures without the imitative cue. The cluster pattern was not a treatment target, because it was not developmentally appropriate. Language stimulation activities were also employed to help Billy expand his current sentence structure. His parents were taught to carry out the treatment activities at home. They were given score sheets and returned the data each week, so that the progress of the home sessions could be monitored.

After receiving two semesters of treatment at the University Speech and Hearing Clinic, Billy corrected the final-consonant-deletion error pattern. His expressive language had also improved to an age-appropriate level. His parents were instructed to continue the stimulation program, and Billy would be rechecked in six months. If cluster deletion continued, he would be enrolled for additional treatment to modify the cluster problem.

Speaking of

Assistive and Augmentative Communication (AAC) Devices

ANNE CRONIN, PhD, OTR/L, BCP
TEAM MEMBER, WEST VIRGINIA UNIVERSITY ASSISTIVE TECHNOLOGY CLINIC

Children who cannot speak are often socially isolated and frustrated. With an interdisciplinary team assessment, many of these children can use pictures or other devices and learn to communicate. Still, we find that families are often resistant to supporting the use of AAC devices. We see children in clinic who are unhappy or disruptive in school because, although they have learned to communicate nonverbally with family members, they cannot communicate with teachers and classmates. Learned helplessness can occur when the child is unable to communicate and thus has not been able to have an effect on other people. If family members are not able to interpret or respond to the child's attempts to communicate, the child may not learn that his or her actions can elicit a response. This leads to a restriction in the area of activities and participation that is far greater than the impairment might suggest.

This is a frustrating dilemma for therapists. For most children the devices really are a link to the outside world and may have little to offer families. Ironically, AAC devices require the active participation of family members—starting with assessment and continuing through the prescription, training, and day-to-day use of the device. It is often the family that is responsible for charging the battery,

Continues

Speaking of Continued

setting up the device, updating the programming, and dealing with breakdowns. There is research to indicate that in some cases AAC devices may be disruptive to family functioning, which can have an adverse effect on the individual using the device (Augmentative Communication News, 2002).

The family knows the child and the context within which the child must function. Because of this, the preferences and needs of the family should be given precedence over those of the professionals on the team. Family members are the ones who have to manage the device and who will remain responsible for the child after the current set of therapists are no longer around. Common ways that AAC devices often impact families are to (1) increase a family's time commitments and stress, (2) change family routines, and (3) alter family interaction patterns. Failure to give priority to the considerations of the family can result in the AAC system simply not being used (Angelo, Jones, & Koskoska, 1995; Hetzroni & Harris, 1996).

As clinicians, we need to support communication in all its forms and contexts. We must be sensitive to the cultural and developmental importance of communication on function and activity participation. While it is often easy to consider communication as "someone else's problem," without communication social participation is not possible. When an AAC system is recommended by the team, we must all support its use and integration into everyday activities.

REFERENCES

Angelo, D. H., Jones, S. D., & Koskoska, S. M. (1995). Family perspective on augmentative and alternative communication: Families of young children. *Augmentative and Alternative Communication, 11*, 193–201.

Augmentative Communication News. (2002). Article 3. AAC Devices: Impact on Families, accessed October 24, 2003, at http://www.augcominc.com/articles/7_6_3.html.

American Speech-Language-Hearing Association. (2002, April). *Scope of practice in speech-language pathology (2001)* (Suppl. 22). Rockville, MD: American Speech-Language-Hearing Association.

American Speech-Language-Hearing Association. (1983). Language (definition). *ASHA, 25*, 44.

Benedict, H. (1979). Early lexical development: Comprehension and production. *Journal of Child Language, 6*, 183–200.

Bloom, L. (1970). *Language development: Form and function of emerging grammars.* Cambridge, MA: MIT Press.

Blosser, J. L., & DePompei, R. (2003). *Pediatric traumatic brain injury* (2nd ed.). Clifton Park, NY: Delmar Learning.

Brown, R. (1973). *A first language: The early stages.* Cambridge, MA: Harvard University Press.

Brown, R., & Bellugi, U. (1964). Three processes in the child's acquisition of syntax. *Harvard Educational Review, 34*, 133–151.

Bruner, J. (1975). The ontogenesis of speech acts. *Journal of Child Language, 2*, 1–19.

Carlson, V., Cicchetti, D., Barnett, D., & Brauwald, K. B. (1989). The development of disorganized/disoriented attachment in maltreated infants. *Developmental Psychology, 25*, 525–531.

Castrogiovanni, A. (1999a). *Incidence and prevalence of hearing impairment in the United States: Communication facts* (1999 ed.) Rockville, MD: American Speech-Language-Hearing Association.

Castrogiovanni, A. (1999b). *Incidence and prevalence of speech, voice, and language disorders in the United States: Communication facts* (1999 ed.). Rockville, MD: American Speech-Language-Hearing Association.

Chafe, W. (1970). *Meaning and the structure of language.* Chicago: University of Chicago Press.

Chomsky, N. (1957). *Syntactic structures.* The Hague: Mouton.

Chomsky, N. (1959). A review of Skinner's *Verbal Behavior. Language, 35*, 26–58.

Chomsky, N. (1965). *Aspects of the theory of syntax.* Cambridge: MIT Press.

Chomsky, N. (1968). *Language and mind.* New York: Harcourt, Brace and World.

Dore, J. (1974). A pragmatic description of early language development. *Journal of Psycholinguistic Research, 3*, 343–350.

Farrar, M. (1990). Discourse and the acquisition of grammatical morphemes. *Journal of Child Language, 17*, 607–624.

Ferguson, C. (1978). Learning to pronounce: The earliest stages of phonological development in the child. In F. Minifie & L. Lloyd (Eds.), *Communicative and cognitive abilities—Early behavioral assessment.* Baltimore: University Park Press.

Fillmore, C. (1968). The case for case. In E. Bach & R. Harmas (Eds.), *Universals in linguistic theory.* New York: Holt, Rinehart and Winston.

Gallagher, T. (1977). Revision behaviors in the speech of normal children developing language. *Journal of Speech and Hearing Research, 20,* 303–318.

Ginsburg, H., & Opper, S. (1979). *Piaget's theory of intellectual development* (2nd ed.). Englewood Cliffs, NJ: Prentice Hall.

Hetzroni, O. E., & Harris, O. L. (1996). Cultural aspects in the development of AAC users. *Augmentative and Alternative Communication, 12,* 52–58.

Hulit, L. M., & Howard, M. R. (1993). *Born to talk: An introduction to speech and language development.* New York: Macmillan.

James, S., & Kahn, L. (1982). Grammatical morpheme acquisition: An approximately invariant order? *Journal of Psycholinguistic Research, 11,* 381–388.

Kent, R. (1998). Normal aspects of articulation. In J. E. Bernthal & N. W. Bankson (Eds.), *Articulation and phonological disorders* (4th ed.) (pp. 1–62). Boston: Allyn and Bacon.

Kent, R. (1997). *The speech sciences.* San Diego, CA: Singular Publishing.

Lenneberg, E. (1967). *Biological foundations of language.* New York: John Wiley & Sons.

Leonard, L. B. (1998). *Children with specific language impairment.* Cambridge, MA: MIT Press.

Lloyd, L. L., Fuller, D. R., & Arvidson, H. H. (1997). *Augmentative and alternative communication: A handbook of principles and practices.* Boston: Allyn and Bacon.

Masataka, N. (1995). The relation between index-finger extension and the acoustic quality of cooing in three-month-old infants. *Journal of Child Language, 22,* 247–257.

McLean, J., & Snyder-McLean, L. (1978). *A transactional approach to early language training.* Columbus, OH: Merrill.

Miller, J. (1981). *Assessing language production in children: Experimental procedures.* Baltimore: University Park Press.

Muma, J. (1978). *Language handbook.* Englewood Cliffs, NJ: Prentice Hall.

National Institute on Deafness and Communication Disorders. (2003). American Sign Language. Retrieved August 8, 2003, from http://www.nidcd.nih.gov/health/hearing/asl.asp.

Oller, D. (1978). Infant vocalization and the development of speech. *Allied Health and Behavior Sciences, 1,* 523–549.

Osgood, C. (1963). On understanding and creating sentences. *American Psychologist, 18,* 735–751.

Owens, R. (1996). *Language development: An introduction* (4th ed.). Boston: Allyn and Bacon.

Owens, R. (2001). *Language development: An introduction* (5th ed.). Boston: Allyn and Bacon.

Owens, R. (1999). *Language disorders: A functional approach to assessment and intervention.* (3rd ed.). Boston: Allyn and Bacon.

Owens, R., Metz, D. E., & Haas, A. (2000). *Introduction to communication disorders: A life span perspective.* Boston: Allyn and Bacon.

Paul, R. (2001). *Language disorders from infancy through adolescence: Assessment and intervention* (2nd ed.). St. Louis: Mosby.

Prutting, C. A., & Kirchner, D. M. (1987). A clinical appraisal of the pragmatic aspects of language. *Journal of Speech and Hearing Disorders, 52,* 105–119.

Reed, V. A. (1994). *An introduction to children with language disorders* (2nd ed.). New York: Macmillan.

Schreibman, L. (1988). *Developmental clinical psychology and psychiatry (Vol. 15).* Newbury Park, CA: Sage.

Schwartz, R., & Leonard, L. (1984). Words, objects, and actions in early lexical acquisition. *Journal of Speech and Hearing Research, 27,* 119–127.

Skinner, B. F. (1957). *Verbal behavior.* New York: Appleton-Century-Crofts.

Stark, R. (1986). Prespeech segmental feature development. In P. Fletcher & M. Garman (Eds.), *Language acquisition* (2nd ed.) (pp. 149–173). New York: Cambridge University Press.

Stark, R. E., Bernstein, L. E., & Demorest, M. E. (1993). Vocal communication in the first 18 months of life. *Journal of Speech and Hearing Research, 36,* 548–558.

Stoel-Gammon, C. (1988). Prelinguistic vocalizations of hearing-impaired and normally hearing subjects: A comparison of consonantal inventories. *Journal of Speech and Hearing Disorders, 53,* 302–315.

Stoel-Gammon, C., & Otomo, K. (1986). Babbling development of hearing-impaired and normally hearing subjects. *Journal of Speech and Hearing Disorders, 51,* 33–41.

Templin, M. (1957). *Certain language skills in children.* Minneapolis: University of Minnesota Press.

World Health Organization. (2002). *ICF: International Classification of Functioning and Disability.* Geneva, Switzerland: World Health Organization.

Lifestage Characteristics

Prenatal Development

Elsie R. Vergara, ScD, OTR, FAOTA
Occupational Therapy Program
Department of Rehabilitation
  Sciences
Sargent College, Boston University
Boston, Massachusetts

Objectives

Upon completion of this chapter, the reader should be able to

■ Identify the major contemporary issues associated with the development of the human embryo.

■ Identify the three classic periods of prenatal development—germinal (preembryonic), embryonic, and fetal—and the postconceptional ages covered within each period.

■ Describe the various classification systems used for monitoring the developmental progression of embryos and fetuses.

■ Describe the developmental changes that occur in the growing human from conception to birth across the various body systems.

■ Identify the main factors and critical, or sensitive, periods associated with atypical development, including multiple gestation, genetic alterations, congenital anomalies, and developmental disabilities.

Key Terms

behavioral states
blastocyst
cephalocaudal
chondroskeleton
ectoderm
embryo
endoderm
epiblasts
fetal viability
fetus

gestational (menstrual) age
mesenchymal cells
mesoderm
neural plate
notochord
oligohydramnios
organogenesis
ossification
pluripotent cells
polyhydramnios

postconceptional age
proximodistal
reflexes
teratogen
trimester system
trophoblast
vascularization
very-low-birthweight
  infants
zygote

INTRODUCTION

The exact moment when human life begins has been a matter of long controversy (Jones & Veeck, 2002; Richardson & Rice, 1999). Passionate ethical, moral, and religious debates over the beginning of life have been at the center of political decisions such as passage of the Human Life Bill (U.S. Senate, 1981) and the legalization of abortion. This issue has been in the forefront in the last decade as a result of the controversies surrounding genetic and stem cell research (Edwards, Gearhart, & Wallach, 2000; Jones & Veeck, 2002; Schroedel, 2000; White, 2000) and destruction or freezing of embryos conceived through in vitro fertilization (Glenister & Thornton, 2000). Although a large percentage of the U.S. population believes that life begins with conception (Pearson, 2002), others believe that life does not begin until the fertilized egg is implanted on the uterine wall or even later. Some consider the first two weeks after conception the preembryo stage, giving "special moral status" to the period beyond 14 days when the developing organism has achieved biologic individuation (Jones & Veeck, 2002). Proponents of the pro-choice movement argue that the beliefs that life begins shortly after fertilization have no scientific basis and that they are founded exclusively on religious convictions. Most pro-choice advocates believe that life does not begin until the "biological process [of fertilization] has eventuated into a human person" (Schroerlucke, 2002, p. 1). In their view this moment occurs when the fetus reaches the stage when it can live on its own without the use of life support, but there is much disagreement about the exact gestational age at which this happens. Termination of a pregnancy before the fetus is viable is therefore not considered an ethical or moral violation under the pro-choice view. In contrast, pro-life groups believe that there is convincing scientific evidence to support the notion that life begins with conception. Pro-life advocates believe that termination of a pregnancy by abortion at any point after conception is murder and should be illegal (Lipson, 1994; Willkee & Willkee, 2002). This controversy is likely to continue for years, if it is ever resolved; thus, people involved in rehabilitation services must be cognizant of the differing positions when discussing prenatal development.

The ICF classification system was not intended to be applied prenatally, but in an effort to integrate this information with the subject of rehabilitation, we will review the classification system introduced in Chapter 1. Figure 6–1 shows the areas that are specifically impacted by (or during) prenatal development. While rehabilitation therapists are not typically involved with embryos or fetuses in utero, they often work with pregnant women and with newborn infants. Moreover, rehabilitation therapists who work in neonatal intensive care units may work with infants as young as 24 or 25 weeks of gestation whose developmental patterns in many ways resemble fetuses approaching the last trimester of prenatal development. A strong knowledge base of prenatal development is crucial to understanding many of the diseases, impairments, and developmental differences in children, as well as the behavioral patterns of premature infants.

OVERVIEW

The developing human is known as an **embryo** until eight weeks following conception. Despite the lack of consensus about the beginning of human life or the ethicality of abortion or genetic research, there is considerable agreement that development of a human embryo conceived through natural means begins shortly after fertilization has occurred, within 12 to 24 hours after the

ICF	Body Functions and Structure	Activities and Participation		Environmental Factors	
(Positive Aspects from ICF)	Functional and Structural Integrity in Embryological Development	Maternal Behaviors and Environments as They Influence Embryological Development			
(Negative Aspects from ICF)	Pathology and Impairment in Embryological Development				

OT Practice Framework	Client Factors	Performance Skills (*with communication skills)	Areas of Occupation	*	Performance Patterns	Context

FIGURE 6–1   ICF Model as It Relates to Human Embryologic Development

sperm penetrates the ovum (i.e., egg cell). Fertilization, also called conception, is believed to be complete when the sperm and the ovum fuse into a single cell called the **zygote.** The exact moment when human development begins after in vitro fertilization or artificial insemination is less clear. Most people consider the moment of implantation of the fertilized ovum in the uterine wall as the beginning of human development of embryos conceived through nonnatural methods (retrieved from http://embryo.soad.umich.edu/carnStages/carnStages.html on November 23, 2002).

Emergence of the zygote marks the beginning of the first of three prenatal periods: germinal or preembryonic,[1] embryonic, and fetal. The germinal period lasts approximately two weeks from conception until the unicellular zygote has implanted in the uterus and has become an embryo, a complex multicellular organism capable of producing all of the organs and tissues of the body (called **pluripotent**). The embryonic period extends to the end of the eighth week after conception, when all of the major body structures have been formed and the embryo has developed human characteristics, at which time it can be considered a fetus. It is the period when the developing organs are most sensitive or susceptible to the effects of toxic substances or abnormal conditions (Bruer, 2001). The fetal period is the longest, extending from approximately the ninth week after conception until the moment of birth. This period involves extensive growth as well as complex structural and physiologic refinement of the tissues, organs, and systems that were formed during the embryonic period.

By the time infants are born, they will have developed all of the body structures they will ever have. Any abnormality in the structural development of an infant must have therefore occurred during the period of **organogenesis** (organ formation) in the early stages of development. Although the infant's structural development essentially ends long before she is born, much of the functional development of the structures will occur throughout the entire gestational period and even after birth. This chapter will describe the normal developmental process from conception to birth, highlighting the critical periods during which the developing infant is at greatest risk for congenital anomalies or developmental disabilities should the developmental process be interrupted or altered. A quick overview of the major developmental changes and milestones throughout the entire gestational period is found in Table 6–1.

PRENATAL CLASSIFICATION SYSTEMS

Close monitoring of an infant's prenatal development is essential to assure that the fetus is developing appropriately and to identify any deviation from typical development that may require early attention. Prenatal development is described using a variety of classification systems. Classification by menstrual, or gestational, weeks is the system most widely used by obstetricians and other clinicians to assess the maturity of an embryo or fetus and to monitor its development along the entire pregnancy. The developing infant's estimated **gestational age** is measured in weeks either from the first day of the pregnant woman's *last menstrual period (LMP)* or from the moment of conception (i.e., postconceptional age). Use of

---

[1] Some consider this stage part of the embryonic period.

TABLE 6–1	Major Developmental Changes and Milestones Throughout Gestational Period

Period After Conception	Structural and Functional Changes During Period
0 to 4–5 wks	• Fertilized egg descends from fallopian tube to uterus. • Early cell division occurs with formation of embryonic disc—zygote becomes an embryo. • Developing embryo attaches to uterine wall.
4 weeks	• Embryo divides into three layers of cells: -Ectoderm (nervous system and sense organs). -Mesoderm (circulatory, skeletal, and muscular systems). -Endoderm (digestive and some glandular systems). • Special layer of cells begin to grow into the uterine wall, where the placenta will be formed. • Special cells grow to form the amnion (water sac). • Heart tube forms; blood begins to circulate through embryonic disc tubes toward the end. • Development of neural system begins, and neural groove appears. • Intestinal tract, lungs, liver, and kidneys begin to develop. • Small buds appear on sides of body—the beginning of limbs. • By the end of this period embryo is about 4–6 mm long; head is forming; body is curled.
5 to 8–9 wks	• Bones and muscles begin to give contour to body. • Face and neck appear—human resemblance begins.
8 weeks	• Brain grows faster than rest of body; forehead becomes prominent as a result of proliferation of brain tissue. • Limb buds elongate; muscles and cartilage develop. • Sex organs begin to form. • Embryo grows to 30–50 mm in length. • Embryo becomes a fetus.
9 to 12–13 wks	• Fetal period begins. • Head continues to grow faster than rest of body.
12 weeks	• Eyelids are fused. • Sexual differentiation becomes visible. • Buds for temporary teeth emerge. • Vocal cords appear. • Digestive system begins to function; stomach and bile secretions begin. • Kidney begin to function; fetus urinates into the amniotic fluid. • Placenta passes waste products from infant to mother. • Bones and muscles continue to develop. • Spontaneous movements of arms, legs, shoulders, and fingers occur by end of the 3rd month.

Continues

TABLE 6–1	Major Developmental Changes and Milestones Throughout Gestational Period *Continued*

Period After Conception	Structural and Functional Changes During Period
13 to 16–17 wks 16 weeks 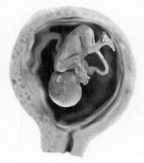	• Growth rate of lower parts of body accelerates. • Head size decreases proportionally from one-half to one-fourth body size. • Fetus is less curled. • Hands and feet are well formed, with fingernails. • Skin appears dark red (blood flows superficially) and wrinkled (lacks underlying fat). • Fingers may curl into flexion. • Reflexes become more active as nervous system maturation continues. • Strength of movement of arms and legs increases. • Fetus grows to 15 cm and weighs close to 300 g.
17 to 20–21 wks 20 weeks 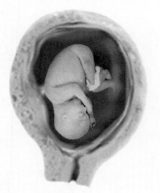	• All body structures closely resemble their final form. • Sweat glands appear and become functional. • Hair appears on scalp. • Skin continues to appear wrinkled. • Spine becomes more straight. • Spontaneous activity continues to increase. • Movements may or may not be perceived by mother. • By 21 weeks fetus measures 19 cm (about 1 ft) and weighs 460 g (approximately 1 lb).
21 to 24–25 wks 24 weeks 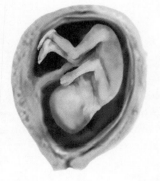	• Eyes are completely formed; eyelids open toward the end of this period. • Taste buds appear on tongue and mouth—more prominent than in the infant or adult. • Structures continue to grow; infant continues to gain weight. • By the end of this period fetus is 24 cm long and weighs over 1000 g.

Continues

TABLE 6–1	Major Developmental Changes and Milestones Throughout Gestational Period *Continued*

Period After Conception	Structural and Functional Changes During Period
25 to 28–29 wks	• Fetus is viable—may live independently, although may require temperature support.
	• Cerebral hemispheres cover almost the entire brain.
28 weeks	• Neonatal reflexes are fully developed.
	• May cry, breathe, swallow, and suck thumb.
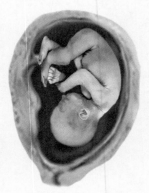	• Head hair continues to grow; body hair (lanugo) disappears.
	• By the end of this period fetus is 27.5 cm long and weighs 1500 g.
28 to 32–33 wks	• Rapid accumulation of fatty tissue occurs over the entire body.
	• Fat accumulation serves as insulation—fetus is better able to tolerate external temperature.
32 weeks	• Intrauterine crowding may decrease movement range and frequency.
	• Fetus can live independently without life support.
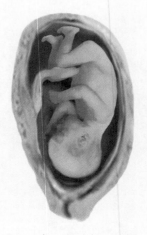	• By the end of this period fetus is 30 cm long and weighs approximately 2500 g (5 lb).
More than 32 wks	• Fetus is fully viable; grows to 36 cm and weighs over 3500 g.

the LMP, although convenient, overestimates the length of a pregnancy by about 2 weeks because it includes approximately 14 days between the first day of menstruation and ovulation, before fertilization occurs. A normal full-term pregnancy lasts approximately 40 weeks (280 days) from the LMP, or approximately 266 days (38 weeks) postconception or fertilization. Although practical and easy to calculate, estimates based on the LMP are somewhat unreliable because they depend on the woman's memory and menstrual regularity (Hadlock, 1994; Sawin & Morgan, 1996).

When fertilization has occurred in vitro or is the result of artificial insemination, gestation may be estimated based on the **postconceptional age,** not on the LMP. These two classification systems (i.e., by LMP or by postconceptional age) are used with great frequency and not always consistently; therefore, it is essential that the type of classification system used be clearly stated to avoid interpretation errors when reporting the age of a developing infant. The developmental stages presented in this chapter will be based on postconceptional age unless otherwise specified.

The most convenient classification, the **trimester system,** divides the 9 months of pregnancy into three months, counting from the date of the LMP. Many obstetricians and midwives use the trimester system because it is a simple method to monitor the pregnancy and explain to the parents the prenatal progression of their developing infant. Describing or monitoring a pregnancy by trimesters is criticized in the literature as a system that lacks precision and may be confusing (Sawing & Morgan, 1996). Arguments against the trimester system include issues such as (1) the duration of a human pregnancy (40 weeks or 280 days) is not divisible by 3, thus creating confusion regarding the time span covered within each trimester, and (2) determining the number of gestational weeks covered within a month of pregnancy is also inexact (Sawing & Morgan, 1996), Furthermore, monitoring a pregnancy by trimesters or months is somewhat artificial because it does not correspond to the embryonic or fetal milestones. Sawing and Morgan (1996) proposed a physiologically based alternate system that divides the pregnancy into four 10-week quartiles according to "natural embryonic and fetal developmental landmarks" occurring approximately every five weeks. Although somewhat more difficult to comprehend by lay people, this system has been gaining popularity since the mid-1990s.

Embryologists use a sophisticated and discrete stage system called *Carnegie stages* to classify embryos in the first nine weeks postconception, a period roughly equivalent to the first trimester (O'Rahilly & Muller, 1987). The Carnegie system describes 23 stages of maturity of an embryo based on external physical characteristics rather than the embryo's size or age (Nishimura, Tanimura, Semba, & Uwabe, 1974; O'Rahilly & Muller, 1987). A given stage number may be assigned to embryos of slightly different ages or sizes because of individual variations in growth and physical development. This maturity estimation method is highly reliable, particularly in situations where the growth of the fetus has been compromised, such as infants with intrauterine growth retardation or infants in distress. Those who wish to learn more about the Carnegie stages are referred to the University of New South Wales Web site at http://anatomy.med.unsw .edu.au/cbl/embryo/wwwhuman/Stages/CStages.htm (retrieved November 23, 2002). An outstanding presentation of pictures and videos of embryos in the Carnegie stages 13 to 23 developed by the University of Michigan is also available on-line at http://embryo. soad.umich.edu/ carnStages/carnStages.html (retrieved November 23, 2002).

FERTILIZATION

The egg cells or ova (plural of ovum) of a woman are formed prenatally during the fetal period. Ova are estimated to be the largest cells in the body (England,

1996). Primitive ova undergo their first cellular division prenatally, before the female infant is born. The daughter cells that result from the first meiotic division are called *primary oocytes.* They will be *haploid;* that is, they will have half the number of chromosomes of their parent cell. The primary oocytes that develop prenatally will remain inactive until near puberty, when a second meiotic division will occur (Moore & Persaud, 1998; Thompson. McInnes, & Willard, 1991). The second meiotic division is similar to a regular mitosis cell division, but the dividing cells will have only half the chromosomes. Before the cells divide, each chromosome will divide into two halves, or *chromatids,* thus giving rise to new cells with the same number of chromosomes as their parent cell, the primary oocyte. The new cells will be called *secondary oocytes.* The secondary oocytes will have a total of 23 chromosomes—22 chromosomes plus the sex chromosome, which will always be an X chromosome because the woman's cells do not have a Y chromosome. Those interested in reviewing a great animation of the processes of meiosis and mitosis may refer to http://biology.about.com/library/blmitosisanim.htm ?once=trueand (retrieved November 23, 2002).

As the male approaches puberty, the primitive germ cells formed prenatally that had remained dormant for years begin to multiply, grow, and divide, becoming primary spermatocytes containing the same number of chromosomes as the primitive cells. A process similar to the meiotic division of the oocytes begins, through which the number of chromosomes in the *diploid* (double chromosome) primary spermatocyte is reduced by half. This division results in the formation of two haploid secondary spermatocytes. A second meiotic division then takes place in which each of the secondary spermatocytes further divides into two *spermatids* that will eventually become mature sperm, but the number of chromosomes is not reduced during the second division. Each resulting sperm will thus have 22 chromosomes plus the sex chromosome, but, unlike the oocyte, there will be two types of sperm, one carrying the X and the other carrying the Y chromosome.

Mature sperm are believed to be the smallest cells in the human body (England, 1996). Normal sperm have an oval-shaped head, a central section, and a flexible tail. The head carries the genetic material (i.e., DNA), and the tail gives the sperm the ability to swim distances many times its size. If a sperm comes in contact with a mature oocyte and is able to penetrate it, the pronuclei of the two haploid cells will merge and the fertilized oocyte will become a unicellular diploid zygote. The type of sperm that fertilizes the ovum will determine the embryo's sex: female if the sperm carries the X chromosome and male if it carries the Y chromosome. The father's germ cell will always determine the sex of the embryo.

A woman may sometimes release two (or even more) ova within a very short period of time. If both ova are fertilized, the woman will conceive one embryo from each fertilized ovum. The product of this conception will be fraternal, or dizygotic (two-zygote), twins—or multiples in rare cases when more than one egg is fertilized. These embryos may be of the same or different sex and may look very different from each other. In the United States about two-thirds of twins are dizygotic, with the incidence of dizygotic twin pregnancies increasing with age of the mother (Moore & Persaud, 1998). The remaining one-third of the twin pregnancies result from an alteration in the division of the zygote within the first week of development. The exact mechanism by which such alterations in the division of the zygote occur is not clearly understood, but some believe that these alterations result from an incorrect encoding of the fertilized cell that signals it to become two distinct zygotes. Monozygotic twins share exactly the same genetic material because they come from the same fertilized cell. Any differences between them will be the result of environmental influences on development.

GERMINAL DEVELOPMENT: FROM ZYGOTE TO EMBRYO

The zygote is a unicellular organism that contains 46 chromosomes arranged as two pairs of 23 chromosomes—one pair coming from the mother and the other from the father. The zygote's genetic composition will be unique because it results from a combination of the genes from both parents. The cells of the zygote are believed to be pluripotent (a term introduced earlier); that is, any cell of the zygote can give rise to any cell of the embryo (Edwards et al., 2000; Polifka & Friedman, 2002). Although zygote cells are pluripotent, it is believed that by the time the zygote becomes an embryo it will bring a patterning of information that will determine which parts of the body will emerge from its different cells (Pearson, 2002). Developing cells will be constrained to become specific cells during certain periods, induced by their neighboring cells (Bruer, 2001). The possibility that removal of embryo cells for assisted reproduction or genetic testing may disrupt the development of the embryo has been argued. Most people agree that pluripotence gives the developing embryo a remarkable ability to replace cells removed or damaged during the first two weeks after conception, without any damage. If more cells are removed or damaged than what the embryo is capable of replacing, the embryo will die instead and be aborted spontaneously (Pearson, 2002; Polifka & Friedman, 2002). This is called the *all-or-none rule,* meaning that during this stage the embryo either will come out relatively unharmed or, if damage is too severe, will die. The widely accepted all-or-none rule has been recently challenged in animal studies as preimplantation exposure to **teratogens** has been associated with congenital

malformations in rodents (Polifka & Friedman, 2002). A teratogen is any agent that causes the production of physical defects in the developing embryo. Table 6–2 presents some of the known human teratogens.

First Week

Germinal development begins almost instantly after fertilization (Pearson, 2002). During the 1st week of the germinal period the unicellular zygote will become a multicellular **blastocyst.** Within the first 30 hours the zygote will undergo its first mitotic division, during which the maternal and paternal chromosomes will intermingle, and within 40 hours the zygote will already have four cells. A process of rapid cell division called *cleavage* will begin by the second day[2] through which the blastomere cells that will give rise to the embryo emerge. Cleavage will continue for 4 days after fertilization as the zygote moves downstream through the uterine tube (Graham & Morgan, 2002). Blastomere cells will become progressively smaller with each cell division. As the zygote reaches 8–9 cells, the blastomeres will begin to organize into a compact ball of undifferentiated cells called a morula. By the 4th day[3] the morula will have approximately 32 cells arranged into an inner cell mass and an outer ring, which is surrounded by a layer of cells called the *zona pellucida.* A fluid-filled cavity will begin to form in the inner cell mass, and as fluid accumulates, the inner cell mass will separate from the outer ring, forcing the inner cell mass toward one pole. This process is illustrated in Figure 6–2.

The inner cell mass, consisting of about 15 percent of the preembryo, will become the embryoblast, the cells from which the embryo and other related tissues will emerge (Pearson, 2002). The outer ring will become the **trophoblast**—the cells that will penetrate the uterine wall and give rise to the placenta and other tissues. By the 5th day the emerging structure will be called the blastocyst. When the blastocyst reaches the uterine cavity it will still be about the same size as the unicellular zygote, because its dividing cells have become half the size of their parent cell with each cell division (Moore & Persaud, 1998).

The blastocyst will begin to "hatch" as the zona pellucida disintegrates during the two days it remains floating in the uterine cavity. Once it sheds, the blastocyst will begin to grow, because it will no longer be tightly contained by the zona pellucida (England, 1996; Moore & Persaud, 1998). The "hatched" blastocyst will begin to penetrate the uterine lining at the embryonic

---

[2] There is some variability in the embryonic and fetal measurements reported in the literature. The measurements reported by Moore and Persaud (1998) are used in this chapter because of the credibility of the source.

[3] Ibid.

TABLE 6-2	Some Known Human Teratogens

Teratogens	Results
Medications	
Thalidomide	Limb reduction defects, ear anomalies
Streptomycin	Hearing loss
Tetracycline	Stained teeth, enamel hypoplasia
Valproic acid	Neural tube defects, dysmorphic facial features
Isotretinoin	Pregnancy loss, hydrocephalus, other CNS defects, small or absent thymus, microtia/anotia, conotruncal heart defects
Antithyroid drugs	Hypothyroidism, goiter
Androgens and high doses of nor-progesterones	Masculinization of external female genitalia
ACE inhibitors	Renal dysgenesis, oligohydramnios sequence, skull ossification defects
Carbamazepine	Neural tube defects
Cocaine	Pregnancy loss, placental abruption, growth retardation, microcephaly
Lithium	Ebstein anomaly
Maternal Infections	
Toxoplasmosis	Hydrocephalus, blindness, mental retardation
Varicella	Skin scarring, limb reduction defects, muscle atrophy, mental retardation
Syphilis	Abnormal teeth and bones, mental retardation
Cytomegalovirus	Growth and developmental retardation, microcephaly, hearing loss, ocular abnormalities
Herpes (primary)	Pregnancy loss, growth retardation, eye abnormalities
Herpes (active)	Vertical transmission at delivery
Chemicals	
Methylmercury	Cerebral atrophy, spasticity, mental retardation
Lead	Pregnancy loss, CNS damage
Polychlorobiphenyls (PCBs—ingested)	Low birth weight, skin discoloration
Maternal Disorders	
Insulin-dependent diabetes Mellitus	Congenital heart defects, caudal deficiency, neural tube defects, limb defects, holoprosencephaly, pregnancy loss
Hypo/hyperthyroidism	Goiter, growth and developmental retardation
Phenylketonuria	Pregnancy loss, microcephaly, mental retardation, facial dysmorphism, congenital heart defects
Hypertension	Intrauterine growth retardation
Autoimmune disorders	Congenital heart block, pregnancy loss
Reproductive Toxins	
Cigarette smoking	Pregnancy loss, low birth weight
Hyperthermia	Neural tube defects
Chronic alcoholism	Growth and developmental retardation, microcephaly, craniofacial dysmorphism
Therapeutic radiation	Growth and developmental retardation, microcephaly

Adapted from Genetic Drift (1995); Teratogen Update, 12: Fall, accessed October 28, 2003, at http://www.mostgene.org/gd/gdvol12h.htm.

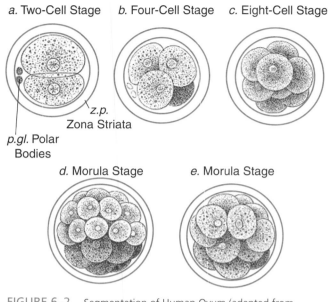

a. Two-Cell Stage   b. Four-Cell Stage   c. Eight-Cell Stage

z.p.
Zona Striata

p.gl. Polar
Bodies

d. Morula Stage   e. Morula Stage

FIGURE 6–2   Segmentation of Human Ovum (adapted from Bartleby, 2003, *Fertilization of the human ovum,* accessed October 28, 2003, http://www.bartleby.com/107/5.html)

pole of the inner cell mass around the 6th day after fertilization. The trophoblast will grow and separate into an inner layer and an outer mass as it becomes attached. The outer mass of the trophoblast will form tentacle-like projections that penetrate the intrauterine wall and extend toward the point of attachment of the embryonic pole. The inner layer will form the placental structures. Toward the end of the 1st week after fertilization, the outer mass will start producing enzymes that disintegrate the tissues around the implantation site, enabling the blastocyst to implant deeper into the uterine wall (Moore & Persaud, 1998). Pregnancy formally begins with the completion of implantation (Graham & Morgan, 2002).

Atypical implantation of the blastocyst may occur during the 1st week. The most common abnormality is implantation of the blastocyst in the inferior portion of the uterus, a condition called *placenta previa.* Premature separation of the placenta accompanied by severe bleeding often occurs when the embryo has implanted low in the uterus. Another, more serious implantation abnormality is *ectopic implantation.* In this case the blastocyst becomes implanted outside the uterus, usually in the intrauterine tubes. Tubal rupture and other serious complications from ectopic pregnancies are common and will cause severe bleeding, placing the mother's life at high risk. Other implantation abnormalities are rare (Moore & Persaud, 1998).

Second Week

The beginning of the 2nd week is characterized by rapid division and differentiation of the trophoblast, accompanied by quickly progressing implantation of

the blastocyst. This process requires adequate hormonal support and the release of protein-dissolving trophoblast enzymes, which erode the tissues around the implantation site, enabling deeper penetration of the blastocyst into the uterine wall.

As implantation continues, during the first part of the 2nd week the inner cell mass of the blastocyst will begin to form a new cavity that will be lined with a layer of cells called *amnioblasts.* Amnioblasts will form the amniotic tissues. The lining layer becomes the amnion and the cavity the amniotic cavity. The inner cell mass of the preembryo will reorganize into a flat, bilaminar structure of somewhat differentiated cells called the *embryonic disc.* The layer of the disc that is farthest from the amniotic cavity will form the primary yolk sac. Yolk sac cells will form a layer of connective tissue called the *extraembryonic mesoderm* that will encircle the amnion and the yolk sac. Simultaneously, many small cavities will begin to appear in the trophoblast near the embryonic pole. These cavities will begin to accumulate maternal blood, marking the beginning of what will later become the utero-placental circulation system. By the 10th to the 12th day a rudimentary network of arteries and veins will have formed, initiating a primitive blood circulation process that will nurture the embryonic disc.

By the 12th day the blastocyst will have penetrated fully into the uterine wall. The trophoblast around the embryonic pole that will later become the placenta will begin to look like a sponge. Toward the end of the 2nd week the primary chorionic villi of the placenta and a membrane called the *chorionic sac* will begin to be formed from the trophoblast. The chorionic sac will eventually enclose the embryo, the amniotic sac, and the yolk sac.

Completion of implantation by the end of the 2nd week marks the end of the germinal period and the beginning of the embryonic period. By this time, the embryo will have a flattened appearance with thickening of a small area of the embryonic disc. This thickened area will become the *prechordal plate*—the area from which the mouth and some head structures will emerge. Identification of abnormalities in the developing embryo, particularly chromosomal alterations, is becoming more available; however, the risk and reliability of some of these procedures remain questionable. Preimplantation diagnosis is a preferred alternative to prenatal (fetal) diagnosis for couples at risk for transmitting a genetic disorder (Kanavakis & Traeger-Sinodinos, 2002).

EMBRYONIC DEVELOPMENT

The embryonic period begins with the 3rd week postconception and continues throughout the 8th week. It is a period of active cell proliferation, migration, and differentiation. It is the period when all of the tissues and organs of the body will be formed, and when exposure to teratogens will be most devastating to the developing embryo (Moore & Persaud, 1998; Sawin & Morgan, 1996). Teratogens may alter many processes during this period including cell migration, programmed cell death, gene expression, and tissue formation. The type of anomaly that may occur from teratogen exposure is determined by gestational timing of exposure, dose, duration, and nature of the teratogen (Graham & Morgan, 2002; Polifka & Friedman, 2002). Development will progress from the cephalic to the caudal ends of the embryo, with head and upper trunk structures forming and becoming functional several days before lower trunk and leg structures. By the end of the 8th week the embryo will have a human resemblance. It will have rudimentary eyes and eyebrows, ears, arm buds with hands, fingers, leg buds with feet, and toes. The embryo's head will be proportionately much larger than the rest of the body. From this point on, the developing organism will be called a **fetus.**

Third Week

A key feature of the third week is the organization of the embryonic disc into three layers: endoderm, mesoderm, and ectoderm. The **endoderm** is the germ layer from which the digestive system, many glands, and parts of the respiratory system are formed. The **mesoderm** is the germ layer that forms many muscles, the circulatory and excretory systems, and the dermis, skeleton, and other supportive and connective tissues. The **ectoderm** is the primary embryonic cell layer from which the skin, the nervous system, and other structures will evolve. All of the organs and tissues of the developing infant will emerge from these three layers of cells. By the end of the third week the embryo will have the rudiments of important body structures that have emerged from one or more of these layers.

Differentiation of the embryonic disk into the three layers begins when cells from the layer that forms the floor of the amniotic cavity proliferate and migrate to form a line in the center of the embryonic disc called the *primitive streak.* As cells accumulate, the primitive streak will elongate, move inward (infold), and form three distinctive areas: the primitive groove (an indentation along the primitive streak), the primitive node (a raised area at the cephalic end), and the primitive pit (an indentation in the primitive node) (Moore & Persaud, 1998). The embryo takes an elongated shape as these three structures are formed, allowing identification of cephalic (head), caudal (tail), dorsal (posterior), and ventral (anterior), and right and left surfaces. Cells will continue to multiply rapidly and migrate in all directions, generally from the center of the embryo toward the periphery.

A group of cells called **mesenchymal cells** will migrate away from the primitive streak to form connective tissue around the primitive groove. At the same time other cells called **epiblasts** will migrate toward the roof of the yolk sac to form the endoderm, one of the germinal layers. The epiblast cells remaining after the mesenchymal cell migration will form the ectoderm, another germinal layer. The third germinal layer, called the *intraembryonic mesoderm,* will be formed between the endoderm and the ectoderm layers, also from mesenchymal cells. Intraembryonic mesoderm cells will subsequently migrate toward the periphery of the embryonic disc to merge with the extraembryonic mesoderm, which had emerged during the previous week around the embryo, the amniotic sac, and the yolk sac. The mesoderm will become a widespread layer of cells that will give rise to blood cells, blood and lymphatic vessels, muscles, bones, and other tissues. The primitive streak will disappear around the beginning of the 4th week after it stops producing mesoderm cells. Although each of the germinal layers will give rise predominantly to specific organs and systems, cells from the different layers will many times be involved in the formation of the various organs.

Mesodermal Structures

The mesoderm is the middle layer of the embryonic disc. It will give rise to muscle, bone, cartilage, and connective tissues, as well as the cardiovascular, reproductive, and other internal organs. Mesenchymal cells first migrate upward between the ectodermal and endodermal layers to form a hollow chord at the embryo's midline that will soon evolve into the **notochord,** a rodlike structure around which the vertebral column will form. The notochord gives rudimentary stability to the embryo, and it is also believed to serve as "the primary inductor" of early embryonic development (Moore & Persaud, 1998).

A portion of mesenchymal cells will migrate along the notochordal process to merge at the cephalic end near the prechordal plate. These cells will become the cardiogenic mesoderm from which the heart and other vascular tissues will originate. The embryonic blood vessels and the endocardial heart tubes appear first, but by the end of the week the tubes will have fused into a hollow bulge that will begin to function as a rudimentary heart. This hollow bulge will connect with the emerging embryonic blood vessels and will begin to beat and pump blood by the end of the week, thus becoming the first functional system in the embryo. The chorionic villi and other structures that will constitute the placental circulatory system will also begin to emerge from the mesoderm, and by the end of the week the embryo will have primary stem villi connected to a rudimentary placental structure (Sawin & Morgan, 1996).

Toward the end of the week the intraembryonic mesoderm on each side of the notochord will begin to form pairs of bead-shaped buds called *somites*. The somites will emerge in a **cephalocaudal** direction (relating to a head-to-tail direction along the long axis of the body) and will differentiate into two types, each giving rise to different types of structures: dermomyotome (skin and muscles) and sclerotome (bones). Somites will remain conspicuous through the 5th week. The number of somites present is often used to estimate the embryo's gestational age during this period.

Two other structures will also emerge from the mesoderm during the 3rd week: the *intraembryonic coelom,* which will form the embryo's internal cavities, and a small area at the most caudal end called the *cloacal membrane,* which will later give rise to part of the intestines and the anus.

Ectodermal Structures

The ectoderm is the outermost layer of the embryonic disc that gives rise to the nervous system, skin, teeth, various glands, and other related tissues. Ectodermal cells adjacent to the notochord will begin to organize into a thickened elongated area that will become the **neural plate,** the structure from which the central nervous tissue will originate. As the neural plate broadens and extends rapidly along the notochord, it will begin to form an indentation along its longitudinal axis called the *neural groove.* The lips of the neural groove will become the neural folds. As seen in Figure 6–3, as the neural plate continues to fold in, the neural folds will merge at the midline to form the *neural tube.* As cell proliferation continues, the neural tube will begin to separate from the superficial layer of the ectoderm. As it separates, a group of ectodermal cells will begin to migrate between the neural tube and the superficial ectoderm to form the *neural crest.*

The neural crest soon separates into two areas of cells, one on each side of the embryo's midline, that will form the peripheral and autonomic nervous systems. As the neural plate continues its rapid expansion, the embryo will gradually lose its flattened shape, adopting the curled, or flexed, posture it will maintain until birth. This process begins during the 3rd week and continues through the 4th week. It is called the *cephalocaudal folding of the embryo.* The outermost cells of the ectoderm will begin to differentiate into epidermal cells while nervous system development continues.

Endodermal Structures

The endoderm will give rise to most of the digestive, urinary, and respiratory structures (Graham & Morgan, 2002). As cephalocaudal folding progresses, two pockets will appear in the endoderm, one at the cephalic end and one at the caudal end. These pockets represent the areas where the foregut and the hindgut will develop. Toward the end of the 3rd week and the beginning of the 4th week the primordial gut tube will be formed from the portion of the yolk sac that remains inside the embryo, as the endoderm and the endoderm-lined yolk sac folds in. By around day 19 or 20 the embryo will also begin to fold lengthwise. This process is called *lateral folding of the embryo.* Lateral folding is the result of expansion of the paraxial mesoderm and the emerging somites.

By the end of the 3rd week the embryo will have a distinguishable human resemblance. Although it will still be mostly flat, it is beginning to curl. It will have clearly identifiable cephalic, caudal, dorsal, and ventral surfaces. Several structures will be evident, including the bulge of the developing heart and inner organs; the oropharyngeal membrane at the cephalic end; the neural plate extending along the dorsal region; the somites at the mid-dorsal section; and the cloacal membrane and plate at the caudal end. The embryo will have four to twelve somites by the end of this period. It will remain connected to the yolk sac through the yolk stalk (Moore & Persaud, 1998).

Fourth Week

The first part of the 4th week marks the beginning of the organogenesis phase, during which all of the embryo's organs and the internal cavities will be formed. The embryo will become strongly curved by the end of the 4th week as a result of its cephalocaudal folding; the cephalic fold will be deeper than the caudal fold as a result of the cephalic-to-caudal developmental progression. The embryo's ventral surface will close during the 4th week from the combination of lateral and cephalocaudal folding. As the embryo continues to fold ventrally, the space between the embryo and the yolk sac will decrease, and the connection between the intraembryonic and extraembryonic coeloms will be reduced to a small duct. The stalk that connects the intraembryonic and extraembryonic structures will give rise to the umbilical cord.

Brain tissue will grow and begin to differentiate rapidly during the 4th week, as the upper two-thirds of the neural tube wall enlarges. By the middle of the week the brain will consist of three vesicles: forebrain, midbrain, and hindbrain. The forebrain will be the most prominent vesicle at this stage. The forebrain is the most anterior of the three primary regions of the embryonic brain, from which the cerebral hemispheres will arise. The cerebral hemispheres are the two halves of the brain cerebrum. These hemispheres make up the largest part of the brain. The middle of the three primary divisions of the brain is the midbrain of the embryo. The most posterior of the three primary divisions of the embryo's brain is the hindbrain. The spinal cord will begin to form as the walls of the neural tube become thicker and begin to close as a result of the merging of the lateral folds along the dorsal midline.

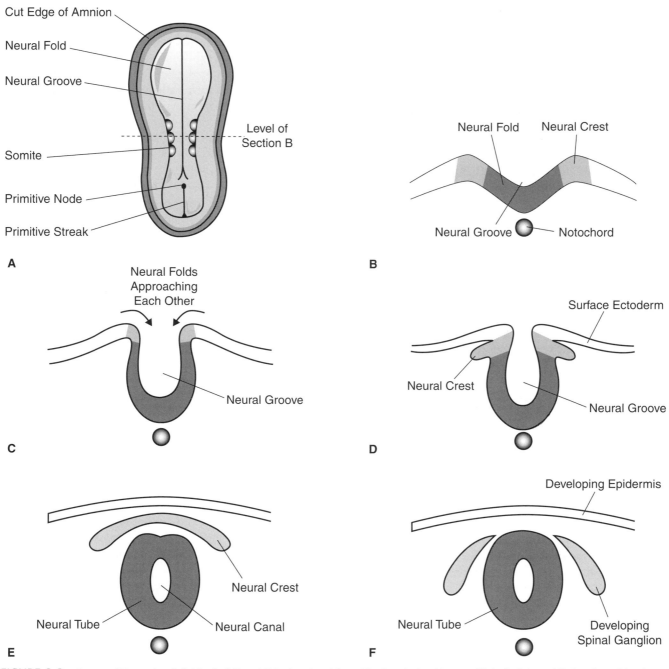

Cut Edge of Amnion

Neural Fold

Neural Groove

Somite

Primitive Node

Primitive Streak

Level of Section B

A

Neural Fold   Neural Crest

Neural Groove   Notochord

B

Neural Folds Approaching Each Other

Neural Groove

C

Surface Ectoderm

Neural Crest

Neural Groove

D

Neural Crest

Neural Tube   Neural Canal

E

Developing Epidermis

Neural Tube   Developing Spinal Ganglion

F

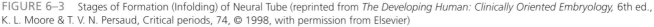

FIGURE 6–3   Stages of Formation (Infolding) of Neural Tube (reprinted from *The Developing Human: Clinically Oriented Embryology,* 6th ed., K. L. Moore & T. V. N. Persaud, Critical periods, 74, © 1998, with permission from Elsevier)

This is an extremely critical stage, where developmental alterations may cause neural tube defects such as spina bifida or anencephaly (absence of brain).[4] When it begins to form, the developing spinal cord occupies the entire length of the emerging spine, but by the time the infant is born it will end at the level of the upper lumbar vertebras, because the spine will have grown longer than the spinal cord. Peripheral nerves, consisting of motor and sensory neurons, will begin to grow rapidly toward the end of the 4th week from the ventrolateral sides of the developing spinal cord and from occipital neural crest cells. The ventral motor neurons will appear first. These are the neurons that activate muscle cells. Motor neuron development is followed by the appearance of dorsal sensory neurons. Dorsal sensory neurons are nerve cells that conduct impulses from a sense organ to the central nervous system. The axons of the motor fibers will grow fast, seeking out and

---

[4] The incidence of *neural tube defects (NTD)* has decreased significantly since preconceptional and periconceptional folic acid supplementation has been in use. Conversely, exposure to folic acid antagonists increases the NTD risk (Hernandez-Diaz, Werler, Walker, & Mitchell, 2001).

migrating toward specific muscles. Sensory fibers will grow more slowly. The emerging nerves will migrate toward and into the limbs as the limbs are developing. It is believed that chemical markers at the target organ attract and direct nerve axons to establish correct connections (Sperry, 1963, as cited in Bruer, 2001). Axons that connect with the incorrect structure will not become functional and will eventually degenerate.

The cephalic end of the embryo will begin to resemble a human head as the forebrain grows and the oropharyngeal membranes and heart tube migrate ventrally. At this stage three pharyngeal arches will emerge from the oropharyngeal membrane on the ventral surface of the embryo immediately below the forebrain. These arches will give rise to the maxilla, mandible, pharynx, larynx, face, mouth, tongue, and other orofacial structures. The thyroid, the first gland to emerge, will also begin to develop around this time from the pharyngeal arches. The otic pits (primitive internal ears) and a thickened area where the eyes and retinas will emerge will appear around the 26th day. The ventral opening at the cephalic end of the neural tube will close by the 25th or 26th day, whereas the caudal opening of the neural tube will close approximately two days later, around the 28th day. Limbs will also begin to appear around the 4th week. Limb development will progress in cephalocaudal and **proximodistal** directions. Arm buds will appear around day 26, but leg buds will not appear until approximately the 28th day; proximal segments will emerge before distal segments.

The 4th week is also an important developmental period for cardiorespiratory structures. The heart tube will elongate and curve into an "S." The cardiovascular system will continue to branch out into the developing organs and the lymphatic system begins to emerge. Several respiratory structures—larynx, trachea, bronchii, and lung buds—will begin to differentiate as the laryngotracheal groove emerges at the ventral aspect of the developing pharynx. Initially the laryngotracheal tube will have a direct connection with the pharynx.

At this stage, most of the gut hangs from the posterior wall of the emerging peritoneal cavity. The first sign of the formation of the gastrointestinal system is the emergence of liver buds at the caudal end of the foregut. The liver will grow rapidly over the following days to occupy a large area of the ventral bulge. The stomach will begin to form shortly after as a small dilatation at the lower end of the foregut.

By the end of the 4th week the embryo will be somewhat cylindrical and about 4 mm long, will have well-defined body cavities and a tail at its caudal end, and will have approximately 26 to 28 pairs of somites (Moore & Persaud, 1998). Other cells will continue to differentiate into the various organ systems, but the cardiovascular system is the only system that will be considerably functional by the end of the 4th week.

The most common congenital anomalies associated with this developmental period are epigastric hernias (abdominal organs growing into the amniotic cavity, outside the abdominal wall) and spina bifida (defect in the center of the spinal column). Epigastric hernias will result from failure of the ventral fusion of the lateral folds, whereas spina bifida is caused by failure of the dorsal fusion of the neuropores and lateral folds. Tracheo-esophageal fistulas may also occur if the trachea and the pharynx fail to separate adequately (Moore & Persaud, 1998).

Fifth and Sixth Weeks

These two weeks are characterized by major differentiation and growth of many organs and structures. By the 5th week the placental circulation system will be functional, carrying oxygen and nutrients from the mother to the fetus through the umbilical cord (Graham & Morgan, 2002). The head will experience the greatest growth during this period because of the cephalocaudal progression of development. By the 5th week the brain will have divided into five vesicles; the cerebral hemispheres will form from the most cephalic vesicle of the forebrain and will gradually cover other brain structures. Brain waves can be recorded as early as the beginning of the 6th week (Hamlin, 1964). Cranial nerves will also begin to emerge between the 5th and the 6th weeks. The cranial nerves are composed of twelve pairs of nerves that emerge from brain tissue.

Primitive eyes covered by eyelids will appear between the 5th and the 6th weeks, as well as auricular hillocks and primitive external ear canals (Moore & Persaud, 1998). The mouth area will also be clearly identifiable by the 5th week. An enlarged area of the frontonasal processes of the pharyngeal arches will become the nasal placodes from which the nose will later emerge. By the 6th week the nasal placodes from each side will merge at the midline, creating the primordial lower lip. The palate will also begin to form between the internal surfaces of the developing maxilla as the nasal prominences merge, but its development will not be complete until the 12th week. The nasal pits will deepen to form the nasal sac and nostrils.

During the 5th week the upper limbs will look like paddles, with digital rays appearing distally on the hand plates. By the end of the 6th week the upper limbs will have a complete cartilaginous skeleton and rudimentary elbow joints. Footplates will begin to emerge by the 6th week, but will become more prominent by the 7th week.

Critical developmental changes in most of the body organs and systems will occur during the fifth and the sixth weeks. Emergence of the heart septum—a membranous structure between the two heart atria or between the two heart ventricles—initiates the division of the heart into atrial and ventricular chambers. All four chambers of the heart will be formed by the 7th week. Development of the respiratory system will include branching of the lung buds into two bronchial buds, as well as appearance of a rudimentary pleural cavity and a primordial diaphragm. The developing lungs and heart will descend into the thorax region by the end of the 6th week. The cardiovascular system will be functioning fairly well by this stage, but the respiratory system will not become functional until much later, because most of its development will occur toward the end of the fetal period.

The developing stomach bulge will expand during the 5th and 6th weeks and rotate clockwise until it assumes its mature position around the 8th week. During the 6th week the intestines are elongating much faster than the abdominal cavity is enlarging, forcing a loop of the intestines to herniate into the umbilical cord. The intestines remain herniated until the 10th week, when they spontaneously begin to rotate into the abdominal cavity when space becomes available.

The most common congenital anomalies likely to occur around the 5th and 6th weeks include cleft lip and cleft palate. Lip and palate defects occur when the placodes and related structures fail to fuse at midline. Cleft palate defects may also occur at later stages, because the palate continues developing into the 12th week. Other abnormalities in the development of the pharyngeal arches include "U"-shaped cleft palate, retrognathia (retracted jaw), micrognathia (small jaw), and nasal airway abnormalities. Disturbed neural crest development may result in esophageal atresias as well as abnormalities of the heart and the great vessels (Otten et al., 2000). Other common developmental anomalies that may occur during this period include cardiac septal defects, limb anomalies, and abnormalities associated with persistent herniation or malrotation of the intestines.

Seventh and Eighth Weeks

One of the most important developments toward the end of the 7th week is the formation of cartilage and the beginning of **ossification** in the developing upper body. Ossification is the formation of bone or the conversion of fibrous tissue or of cartilage into bone. Craniofacial bones will emerge from neural crest cells that had migrated earlier into the pharyngeal arches. The vertebras and ribs will emerge from sclerotome somites. Most flat and long bones will emerge from mesenchymal cells that had organized earlier into sheaths of connective tissue or into cartilage formations.

Ossification begins with mesenchymal cells differentiating into osteoblasts (bone-forming cells) and osteoid tissue. Bones will primarily form from calcium phosphate accumulating in the osteoid tissue between the osteoblasts or, in the case of the long bones, in primary ossification centers of the cartilage formations. The clavicles and upper limbs will calcify first. Ossification of the vertebras and the lower limbs will occur later, during and after the 8th week. The trunk and limbs will elongate as their pre-bone structures calcify. The embryo will adopt a less curved appearance as bones begin to form around the spine. Bones will continue to ossify throughout the entire fetal period as well as postnatally.

Wrist joints will appear around the 7th week as limb development continues to progress proximo-distally. Notches will form between the digital rays of the hand plates, initiating the development of the fingers. By the end of the 7th week the embryo will have hands with wrists and webbed fingers as well as fan-shaped feet with emerging toes. The webs between the fingers and the toes will have disappeared within a week. At that point, all joints of the body will resemble the adult form and the limbs, including hands and feet, will have their adult appearance.

By the 7th week the embryo's heart will have primitive aorta, carotid, subclavian, and pulmonary arteries. The primordial pharynx will have elongated and established connections with the mouth and the esophagus. The cloaca will separate into two tubes: urogenital (giving rise to urogenital structures) and anorectal (giving rise to the rectum and anal canal). A layer of cloacal membrane ectoderm at the end of the developing anal canal will perforate to form the anal opening. Nonfunctional kidneys will have moved to their permanent location by the 8th week.

By the end of the embryonic period, the embryo will be approximately 5 cm long and will have a well-defined large head (approximately one-half the embryo's crown-to-rump length) and a smooth neck. Facial characteristics present will include low-set ears with distinguishable auricula, widely separated eyes, eyelid folds above and below the eye, forward-facing nostrils, and a complete upper lip. The embryo will have all of its rudimentary organs, well-formed limbs, and arteries, veins, nerves, cartilage, and muscles growing into the various body parts and systems, providing nutrition and functional support to the emerging structures. It will have three circulatory systems: umbilical or placental, embryonic, and vitelline. The umbilical or placental system will disappear at birth; the vitelline system will become part of the portal (liver) system; the embryonic system will mature into the infant's cardiovascular system. Each circulatory system will have its own network of arteries and veins.

The 5th through the 8th week is also the most sensitive period in the development of the limbs. Exposure to teratogens during this period will affect the limbs or part of the limbs that will be developing at the time of exposure. Upper limbs and proximal segments of the limbs will be affected earlier, whereas lower limbs and distal segments will be affected during the 7th and 8th weeks. Intermediate segments of a limb may be affected less frequently, resulting in absence or reduction of one or more bones.

FETAL DEVELOPMENT

The end of the 8th week and the beginning of the 9th week signal one of the most important milestones in prenatal development. It is that particular moment when the developing embryo begins to look clearly human and is considered a fetus. It is the point beyond which arguments about the beginning of human life decrease (Richardson & Rice, 1999). It is also the moment beyond which exposure to teratogens will not necessarily cause widespread or lethal damage, because all of the organs and body systems have already been formed. Short-duration exposure to teratogens may cause placental functional deficits and fetal growth restriction more than birth defects (Graham & Morgan, 2002). Any birth defect caused by mild to moderately harmful teratogens after this period will likely be localized to a specific part of the body; large or prolonged exposure or highly harmful teratogens may cause fetal death. The differential impact of teratogens at different times, in accordance with critical periods of maturation of various systems, is summarized in Figure 6–4.

The fetal period is one of rapid fetal and placental growth as cell proliferation and hypertrophy or hyperplasia continue (England, 1996; Moore & Persaud, 1998). Between 9 weeks postconception and term age the fetus will grow from about 5 cm to 36 cm (crown-to-rump length) and will increase in weight from about 8 g to 3400–3600 g (Moore & Persaud, 1998).[5] From the 10th through the 20th week the fetus will grow primarily in length, but after the 20th week weight gain will predominate, whereas the rate of length growth will begin to decline. Organ and tissue differentiation will continue, particularly during the first four to eight weeks of the fetal period. Bones will continue to ossify and remodel throughout the entire fetal period (The Human Embryology Website, www.met.uc.edu/embryology). The rate of growth of the head will decrease as the rate of growth of the extremities increases, beginning to give the fetus a more proportional appearance.

Although fetal development is most often obstetrically monitored by trimesters counting from the last menstrual period, the developmental milestones that occur during this period are best described in blocks of 4 to 5 weeks, counting from the moment of conception (Sawin & Morgan, 1996). The following sections highlight the most important developmental changes in the fetus from the 9th week through term age.

Ninth through Twelfth Week

During the period of the 9th through the 12th week, the fetus will continue to grow, body parts will become more detailed, and various body processes and systems will become functional. Crown-to-rump length will double between the 8th and the 12th weeks. After the 9th or 10th week fetal growth and development may be monitored using ultrasound imaging, making it possible to identify a number of structural and functional anomalies in the fetus or the placenta. A well-formed cartilaginous skeleton (**chondroskeleton**) may be identified at the lowest portion of the skull, the spine, ribcage, scapulas, and extremities by the 10th to 11th weeks (Jirasek, 2001). Cartilaginous ribs may be visible under the skin. Ribs will grow first toward the ventral midline, fusing with the costal cartilages toward the end of this period. By the 12th week the primary ossification centers will have appeared in the skull and all long bones. The head will continue to grow somewhat faster than the rest of the body, therefore remaining disproportionately large by the 12th week. The upper limbs will approximate their proportional full-term length in relation to the rest of the body, but the lower limbs will remain proportionately shorter by the end of the 12th week.

By the 9th week the hands and feet will be well developed. Between the 9th and the 12th weeks fingernails will begin to form (toenails will emerge later). The eyelid folds will fuse and will remain fused until the end the 24th week. The ability to swallow will emerge, enabling the fetus to ingest amniotic fluid for nourishment and lung development. The kidneys will develop lobes and connecting tubules and begin to function. Fetuses will begin to produce urine around the 9th week; by the 12th week they will be urinating into the abdominal fluid. External genital organs, particularly the penis, will be well defined by the 12th week, thus making it possible to distinguish the sex of the fetus through ultrasound.

During this time, there is continued vascularization. **Vascularization** is the growth of blood vessels into a tissue or organ with the result that the oxygen and nutrient supply is improved. Fetal-placental circulation will improve because of the continued development of vascularization. The placenta will also begin to remove waste products urinated by the fetus into the amniotic fluid.

---

[5] There is some variability in the embryonic and fetal measurements reported in the literature. The measurements reported by Moore and Persaud (1998) are used in this chapter because of the credibility of the source.

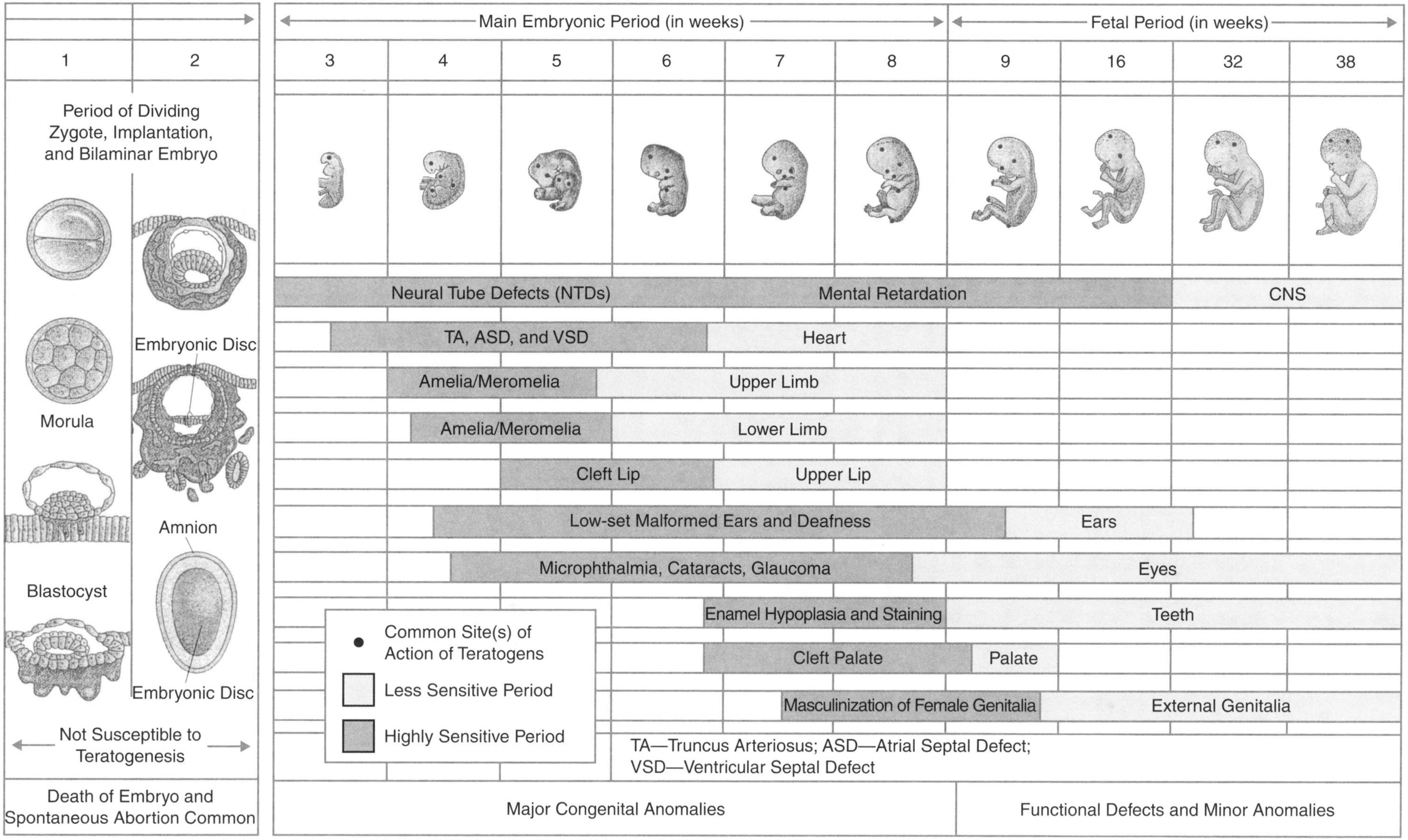

FIGURE 6-4 Summary of Critical Periods in Prenatal Development (reprinted from *The Developing Human: Clinically Oriented Embryology*, 6th ed., K. L. Moore & T. V. N. Persaud, Critical periods, 548, © 1998, with permission from Elsevier)

Blue denotes highly sensitive periods when major birth defects may be produced.

Thirteenth through Sixteenth Week

Fetal growth will be very active during the period of the 13th through the 16th week. The rate of growth of the head will have slowed down considerably in relation to the caudal structures and lower limbs. By the 16th week the entire body will be more proportional, and the legs will approximate their full-term proportional length. Enhanced coordination as a result of neuromuscular system refinement enables the fetus to reach a number of important motor milestones throughout this period, including moving the eyes slowly, bringing a hand to the mouth, and, less commonly, sucking the thumb (England, 1996). **Reflexes,** particularly withdrawal, will strengthen as the nervous system matures. Although the fetus is much more active, the mother may still not be able to perceive the fetal movements (Binnholz, 1981). Improvements in the sensory component of the nervous system will enable the fetus to hear and feel discomfort.

Blood vessels will be superficial and clearly visible under the thin skin (England, 1998). By the 13th week, blood will begin to reach the lung epithelium as a result of ongoing capillary proliferation (Sawin & Morgan, 1996). Ossification will also be very active during this period, enabling the identification of many bones through ultrasound by the 16th week (Sawin & Morgan, 1996).

Seventeenth through Twentieth Week

Fetal changes occurring during the period of the 17th through the 20th week are not as remarkable as those of previous stages. One of the highlights toward the end of this period is the mother's ability to perceive the more robust movements or her fetus. The rate of growth of the fetus will have decreased markedly. By the end of the 20th week all body structures will have approximated or reached their final position and size proportions and will resemble their full-term appearance. The skin of the fetus will be covered with fine hair called *lanugo,* and a layer of a greasy paste called *vernix caseosa.* The vernix caseosa will protect the fetus from injury to the skin (Moore & Persaud, 1998). Another important development during this period is the emergence of adipose tissue and heat-producing brown fat (Moore & Persaud, 1998). Brown-fat accumulation will enable the fetus to maintain body heat toward the end of the fetal period (England, 1996). Accelerated lung maturation is still another important development of this period, preparing the fetus for survival. By the end of the 17th week, all elements of the lungs will be present, although nonfunctional.

Fetuses suspected of or at high risk for having congenital heart disease may be diagnosed as early as 18–20 weeks postconception, when the heart is no bigger than a thumbnail, with a specialized diagnostic procedure called *fetal echocardiography* (Schonberg & Tift, 2002). Infants with congenital heart disease often have other congenital or genetic anomalies or malformations (Schonberg & Tift, 2002). These infants often undergo chromosomal and high-resolution ultrasound diagnostic studies in utero to identify other potential anomalies and to establish an early intervention plan to address the presenting conditions. *Magnetic resonance imaging (MRI)* may be used after the 20th week to diagnose fetal anomalies with greater precision when diagnosis through ultrasound is uncertain (Schonberg & Tift, 2002). Examples of conditions that may be diagnosed with MRI include a variety of brain abnormalities and amount of lung tissue present in fetuses whose lung development is compromised, such as those with diaphragmatic hernias (Schonberg & Tift, 2002).

Another diagnostic procedure that can be effectively used to identify abnormalities in the developing embryo as early as 7 weeks postconception is *transabdominal embryofetoscopy.* Although this type of study increases the risk of spontaneous abortion, the use of thin-gauge needles has decreased this risk considerably (Quintero, Abuhamad, Hobbins, & Mahoney, 1993). Furthermore, the benefits of early diagnosis often offset the slightly higher miscarriage risk the procedure may carry.

Twenty-first through Twenty-fifth Week

Several key milestones occur during the period of the 21st through the 25th week, the most important one being the enhanced probability of survival for infants born prematurely after the 23rd week who are provided with intensive life support. Survival before 21 weeks postconception and of infants weighing less than 500 g is rare. One of the factors improving survival after 22 weeks is the accelerated weight gain, during which the fetuses nearly double their weight. Enhanced lung development and the beginning of the production of *surfactant* (a substance that promotes alveolar functioning) around the 22nd week will further enhance the fetus's chances of survival (Sawin & Morgan, 1996); however, infants will continue to have a high mortality rate by the 26th week because of respiratory and central nervous system immaturity. Moreover, many infants who survive premature birth at such early ages will develop secondary disabilities.

By the 21st week the eyes will be completely developed and primitive rapid eye movements may be observed. By the end of the 25th week the fetus will have eyebrows and open eyelids with eyelashes. Taste buds will have emerged on the tongue and mouth. The skin will continue to appear thin, wrinkled, and reddish. The volume of amniotic fluid will increase as the kidneys develop and the fetus' ability to urinate into the amniotic cavity improves. Decreased production of urine by obstruction of the urinary tract or other factors will diminish the amount of amniotic fluid that accumulates, resulting in a condition called **oligohydramnios** (Graham & Morgan, 2002). Oligohydramnios occurs most frequently during the third trimester and may have other causes, such as placental insufficiency (Moore & Persaud, 1998). Oligohydramnios may cause a number of fetal abnormalities, the main ones being pulmonary hypoplasia (underdevelopment) and compression of the umbilical cord, which may cause serious damage to the fetus, including death (Moore & Persaud, 1998). The fetus's ability to swallow amniotic fluid will also be improving during this time. Any problem that interferes with the fetus's ability to swallow will cause a condition called **polyhydramnios,** manifested by excessive accumulation of amniotic fluid. Both of these conditions will affect the fetus's development toward the end of the pregnancy.

Twenty-sixth through Twenty-ninth Week

The period of the 26th through the 29th week is characterized by increased weight gain, fat accumulation, and accelerated maturation of the respiratory and central nervous systems. The fetus will gain about 700 g (roughly 1½ lb) of weight and by the end of the 29th week will weigh approximately 1700 g (over 3½ lb). Infants born before the 28th week will probably weigh under 1500 g and therefore will be classified as **very-low-birthweight infants.** These infants have a higher risk of neonatal complications (Sawin & Morgan, 1996).

Pulmonary maturity will accelerate by the 28th to the 29th week. Neural regulation of respiration will be well established, and the lungs will be sufficiently developed to breathe air, should the infant be born prematurely. A fetus is considered viable when it is sufficiently developed to live outside of the uterus. **Fetal viability** at this stage will be much improved, and risk for disability will be lower, but the prematurely born infant will still require temperature support because of limited subcutaneous fat and immature *thermal regulation.* Thermal regulation refers to the fetus's ability to maintain body temperature outside the womb environment. Because this is a transitional phase for the respiratory system, respiratory problems associated with minor delays in maturation in infants born prematurely around this period are not uncommon. The risk for other neonatal complications, particularly serious ones, will be low after the 28th week. As illustrated in Figure 6–5, the external support for immature body systems in the premature infant is provided in a specialized medical environment that is very different from the uterus.

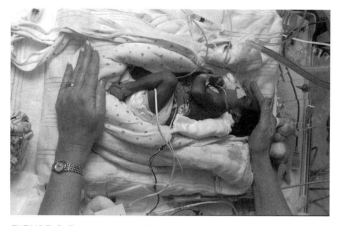

FIGURE 6–5   Premature Infant Care

By the 29th week the fetus will have all of the external characteristics of full-term infants, including full-term body proportions, open eyes, a head full of hair, fingernails and toenails, and less wrinkled skin because of increased subcutaneous fat. The fetus will still be covered with lanugo and a thick coat of vernix caseosa, but the skin will appear thicker and less reddish than during the previous period. All of the neonatal reflexes will be present, although not fully developed. The fetus will be able to cry audibly.

Thirtieth through Thirty-fourth Week

Weight gain will continue at an accelerated pace, and by the 34th week the fetus will have reached another important weight-related milestone: that is, the 2500 g (5½ lb) mark, when an early-born fetus will no longer be considered premature by weight. Infants born between the 30th and the 32nd weeks will likely require transitional temperature support because thermal regulation may not be completely developed, but the probability of surviving without problems will be high. Thermal regulation will be better established by the end of the 32nd week of gestation; thus, most infants born after this point will need only minimal transitional temperature support, if any, and will survive without complications. In contrast, 50–65 percent of infants born before 34 weeks postconception or weighing under 1800 g will have respiratory difficulties and frequent respiratory pauses called *apneic episodes* (Gomella, 1999). If prolonged or very frequent, such apneic episodes may compromise the infant's well-being. The incidence of apnea, however, has declined since the 1990s with the introduction of preventive neonatal therapies such as caffeine and surfactant administration. Infants who have difficulty coming out of an apneic episode may require stimulation (e.g., tactile, auditory, vestibular). Periodic breathing is another common respiratory pattern of premature infants born before 34 weeks of gestation. Periodic breathing usually causes no problems unless pauses are frequent and prolonged. The maturity of the fetus at 34 weeks is comparable to that of the full-term neonate. The fetus will look like a smaller full-term infant, with a head full of hair, pinkish and smooth skin, and a plumpish appearance resulting from increased subcutaneous fat accumulation toward the end of the period.

Thirty-fifth through Thirty-eighth Week (Full-Term)

The fetus will gain approximately 900 g (approximately 2 lb) during the period of the 35th through the 38th week. Fat will accumulate at a rate of 14 g per day in the final weeks of the pregnancy (Moore & Persaud, 1996), providing the infant with much improved insulation and less need of temperature support. Chemical thermoregulation will be improved. Intrauterine fetal body movements will decrease considerably as the fetus approaches term age. The incidence and duration of movement bursts will remain stable, but they will be more spaced apart (Ten Hof et al., 2002). Although the decrease in body movements has been traditionally attributed to intrauterine crowding or greater quiescence, recent evidence suggests that motor activity decreases because of developmental maturation (i.e., greater stability and motor control), rather than either increase in quiet states or space restriction (Ten Hof et al., 2002). A similar decrease in motor activity is observed in infants born prematurely as they approach term age. Reflex development will continue to evolve until approximately the 35th week, but by the 36th to the 37th week the infant should display all neonatal reflexes.

Within a few seconds after birth, infants must begin to breathe on their own and must shift from fetal circulation to adult circulation. Crying immediately after birth facilitates lung expansion and the beginning of respiration. The shift from fetal to adult circulation will require closure of the ductus arteriosus and the foramen ovale, two openings that enabled circulating blood to bypass the lungs in utero. The *ductus arteriosus* is the passageway that exists between the pulmonary trunk and the aorta that normally closes within the first few hours after birth. Most infants born after the 35th week will have no difficulty transitioning to adult circulation, but in some cases the ductus arteriosus will remain open for one or more days. In most instances it will close spontaneously, but in some cases a simple surgical procedure to ligate the ductus will be necessary.

Once adult circulation is established, most infants will demonstrate physiologic stability comparable to the full-term infant's, including thermoregulatory and cardiorespiratory responses. After 36 weeks of gestation, respiratory difficulties are rare. Respiration rates become more regular and slower as the fetus approaches term age, but infants born with very low birth weights will usually have higher respiration rates when they reach term age than will the full-term newborn. Heart rate of prematurely born infants also tends to be higher at term age than for the full-term newborn.

Infants born beyond 35 weeks will respond in similar ways to the full-term newborn in most respects. **Behavioral states** will be well-defined, with clearly identifiable sleep and wake states ranging from deep sleep to crying, and smooth transitions between states. Behavioral states are among the most important aspects of behavior in the newborn infant and may be defined as the infants' level of arousal mediating the responsivity to environmental inputs.

Infants born after 34 weeks will be able to escalate to a full cry when upset, but healthy infants born before states have been established will tend to cry less frequently and less intensely when they reach term age than the healthy full-term newborns will. Although full-term infants will be able to cry when hungry or in discomfort, infants born prematurely may need close monitoring because they may have difficulty demanding care or expressing their needs through crying or fussing. Quiet alertness will be much improved as the infant approaches term age. By 36 weeks, most newborn infants will be able to sustain attention for a sufficiently prolonged period to engage in social interaction with a caregiver or to focus on a nonhuman stimulus for brief periods. The ability to socially interact will make the full-term infant an active participant in family and society life.

SUMMARY

Prenatal development is a very complex process. This chapter merely summarizes the most relevant aspects of prenatal development for the rehabilitation therapist. Emphasis is given to critical periods in development during which alterations in development could result in conditions that interfere with development. Behavioral differences of infants born prematurely are described because of their importance to therapists in neonatal and early intervention practice.

CASE

1

Jeanine

MARYBETH MANDICH, PT, PhD
PEDIATRIC OCCUPATIONAL THERAPIST

Jeanine is a 36-year-old woman who is pregnant for the third time—this time with twins. She didn't start trying to get pregnant until she was 34 years old, and she has had two miscarriages since then. She is thrilled that she is past the 20-week point in this pregnancy. Overall, she has felt fairly good—hardly any morning sickness, although in the first trimester, she was a little tired. She did everything she could do to protect this pregnancy: ate well, didn't smoke or drink, and got plenty of rest. At her 22-week doctor visit, the doctor said she had oligohydramnios evident on ultrasound. The fetuses were showing signs of distress in ultrasound heart rate monitoring. Jeanine was sent home with a form to monitor fetal movement and told to call her doctor to check in. However, before she could do that, she started to have labor contractions. She came to the hospital, and they bought some time in stopping the contractions with medication; however, about 10 days later, Jeanine delivered 24-week gestation twins: Robbie and Rachel.

The twins were in critical condition for the first few weeks as their lungs were so underdeveloped. They were given artificial surfactant. The twins' size was appropriate for gestational age, which the doctors said was a good sign. When Jeanine first saw her babies, two days after they were born, she cried. They didn't look real to her. They were so small they could fit in the palm of her husband's hand. While they were on the ventilator, they looked very floppy and sick. The nurses attempted to keep them in a flexed position through use of blanket rolls. They couldn't cry because of the ventilator, but they did have spontaneous movements and facial grimaces.

As the weeks progressed, Robbie and Rachel seemed to have a will to live. However, they continued to face struggles. Because of the long time on the ventilator, they both developed bronchopulmonary dysplasia. Like most premature infants, each had a patent ductus arteriosus and a heart murmur, which the cardiologist monitored. They were not very physically attractive babies because they lacked body fat, and their heads were molded somewhat and elongated in the anterior-posterior direction (flattened). Everyone noticed how Robbie liked to be swaddled. It decreased his fussiness and improved his respiratory status. However, no matter what the nursery staff did, Rachel seemed irritable. One day, after the babies were off the ventilators, the nursery staff decided to lay them in the same isolette for a trial. Rachel scooted close to Robbie, who placed his body in contact with hers. Rachel had improved physiologic status due to diminished stress. It was as if the babies were used to being in contact in utero, and when they could reestablish that familiarity from the womb, it made them much calmer.

This case study illustrates what happens when a fetus becomes a baby too soon, when all the body systems are still at a fetal level of maturation, but the environment is very intense and includes everything from gravity to lights and stimulation. For infants as young as Robbie and Rachel, nurseries often implement a minimal-stimulation protocol to minimize the time the babies are touched or handled. Likewise, where possible, attempts are made to avoid extremely bright lights and loud sounds. Every attempt is made to position the babies in flexion, as they would be in utero but are too weak to assume at birth. The long-term effects of such extreme prematurity are constantly studied, and the fact that these babies are kept alive at all is a miracle. Most babies born prematurely do surprisingly well by school age, depending, of course, on how early and how little they were initially. Therapists work to provide an environment that minimizes the trauma to these infants, who by all rights should still be in utero.

Speaking of

Genetics and Biology

ANNE CRONIN, PhD, OTR/L, BCP
PEDIATRIC OCCUPATIONAL THERAPIST

As aspiring therapists and health care providers, you may wonder why you need to learn the biology of what goes on before the person is born, and certainly before the person is your patient. One reason why a basic understanding of prenatal development is needed for contemporary practice is that the rapid improvement in medical technology allows infants to survive at increasingly early times in their gestation, and these children born too soon need therapy support. Another compelling reason is that such knowledge is a tool for understanding and organizing the exponential increases in understanding of human genetics. In clinical settings you will meet both children and adults who have been labeled as having a "genetic disorder" that is rare, newly identified, and/or has no clinical documentation of its functional impact. For example, birth defects common to the early weeks of gestation, during the formative period for the neural tube, are anencephaly, cepholocele, and the chiari malformations associated with hydrocephalus. These are profound disorders with a pervasive influence on functional performance.

Additionally, disorders may be specific to an embryologic cell layer, and this is valuable knowledge for the therapist to have. Cystic fibrosis is a genetic disorder of the endoderm germ layer. Although cystic fibrosis is primarily perceived as a respiratory disorder, the endoderm is actually the cell layer from which the digestive system, many glands, and parts of the respiratory system are formed. Reflecting this, children with the disease typically have digestive as well as respiratory problems. Artthrogryposis multiplex congenital is a disorder of mesodermal development that results in insufficient and atypical development of the muscles, skin, skeleton, and connective tissues.

While it may be difficult for a clinician to know and remember all of the possible genetic conditions and their functional manifestations, an understanding of prenatal development provides an invaluable tool for clinical reasoning as you address the needs of your clients.

REFERENCES

Birnholz, J. C. (1981). The development of human fetal eye movement patterns. *Science, 213,* 679–681.

Bruer, J. T. (2001). A critical and sensitive period primer. In D. B. Bailey, J. T. Bruer, F. J. Symons, & J. W. Lichtman (Eds.), *Critical thinking about critical periods* (pp. 3–26). Baltimore: Brookes.

England, M. A. (Ed.) (1996). *Life before birth* (2nd ed.). London: Mosby-Wolfe.

Glenister, P. H., & Thornton, C. E. (2000). Cryopreservation— Archiving for the future. *Mammalian Genome, 11,* 565–571.

Graham, E. M., & Morgan, M. A. (2002). Growth before birth. In M. Batshaw (Ed.), *Children with disabilities* (pp. 53–70). Baltimore: Brookes.

Hadlock, F. P. (1994). Fetal growth. In M. R. Harrison, M. S. Golbus, & R. A. Filly (Eds.), *Ultrasonography in obstetrics and gynecology* (3rd ed.). Philadelphia: W. B. Saunders.

Hamlin, H. (1964). Life or death by EEG. *Journal of the American Medical Association* (October 12, 1964), 190: 112–114.

Hernandez-Diaz, S., Werler, M. M., Walker, A. M., & Mitchell, A. A. (2001). Neural tube defects in relation to use of folic acid antagonists during pregnancy. *American Journal of Epidemiology, 153,* 961–968.

Jirasek, J. E. (2001). *An atlas of the human embryo and fetus—A photographic review of human prenatal development.* New York: Parthenon Publishing Group.

Jones, H. W., & Veeck, L. (2002). What is an embryo? *Fertility and Sterility, 77,* 658–659.

Kanavakis, E., & Traeger-Synodinos, J. (2002). Preimplantation genetic diagnosis in clinical practice. *Journal of Medical Genetics, 39,* 6–11.

Lipson, T. (1994) *From conception to birth: Our most important journey.* Newtown, Australia: Millennium Books.

Moore, K. L., & Persaud, T. V. N. (1998). *The developing human: Clinically oriented embryology* (6th ed.). Philadelphia: W. B. Saunders.

Nishimura, H., Tanimura, T., Semba, R., & Uwabe, C. (1974). Normal development of early human embryos:

Observations of 90 specimens at Carnegie Stages 7 to 13. *Teratology, 10,* 1–5.

O'Rahilly, R, & Muller, F. (Eds.) (1987). *Developmental stages in human embryos.* Washington, DC: Carnegie Institution of Washington, Publication 637.

Otten, C., Migliazza, L., Xia, H., Rodriguez, J. I., Diez-Pardo, J. A., & Tovar, J. A. (2000). Neural crest–derived defects in experimental esophageal atresia. *Pediatric Research, 47,* 178.

Pearson, H. (2002). Developmental biology: Your destiny from day one. *Nature, 418,* 14–15.

Polifka, J. E., & Friedman, J. M. (2002). Medical genetics: 1. Clinical teratology in the age of genomics. *CMAJ-JAMC, 167,* 265–273.

Quintero, R. A., Abuhamad, A., Hobbins, J. C., & Mahoney, M. J. (1993). Transabdominal thin-gauge embryofetoscopy: A technique for early prenatal diagnosis and its use in the diagnosis of a case of Meckel-Gruber syndrome. *American Journal of Obstetrics and Gynecology, 168,* 1552–1557.

Richardson, M. K., & Reiss, M. J. (1999). What does the human embryo look like, and does it matter? *The Lancet, 354,* 246–248.

Sawin, S. W., & Morgan, M. A. (1996). Dating of pregnancy by trimesters: A review and reappraisal. *Obstetrical and gynecological survey, 51,* 261–264.

Schonberg, R. L., & Tifft, C. J. (2002). Birth defects, prenatal diagnosis, and fetal therapy. In M. Batshaw (Ed.), *Children with disabilities* (pp. 35–52). Baltimore: Brookes.

Schroedel, J. R. (Ed.) (2000). Is the fetus a person? A comparison of policies across the fifty states. Ithaca, NY: Cornell University Press.

Schroerlucke, G. How one clergyperson arrives at a pro-choice view on abortions. An essay written by Rev. Gilbert Schroerlucke, retired United Methodist Clergy. Retrieved November 23, 2002, from http://members.iglou.com/gils/oneclerg.htm.

Ten Hof, J., Nijhuis, I. J. M., Mulder, E. J. H., Nijhuis, J. G., Narayan, H., Taylor, D. J., Westers, P., & Visser, G. H. A. (2002). Longitudinal study of fetal body movements: nomograms, intrafetal consistency, and relationship with episodes of heart rate patterns A and B. *Pediatric Research, 52,* 568–575.

Thompson, M. W., McInnes, R. R., & Willard, H. F. (Eds.) (1991). *Thompson and Thompson genetics in medicine* (5th ed.). Philadelphia: W. B. Saunders.

White, G. B. (2000). What we may expect from ethics and the law. *American Journal of Nursing, 100,* 114–117.

Willkee, D, & Willkee, J. C. (Eds.). Why can't we love them both? Chapter 11—The human embryo. Online books. Retrieved November 23, 2002, from http://www.abortionfacts.com.

CHAPTER 7

The Newborn

MaryBeth Mandich, PT, PhD
Professor and Chairperson
Division of Physical Therapy
West Virginia University
Morgantown, West Virginia

Objectives

Upon completion of this chapter, the reader should be able to

▪ Describe the developmental tasks of the neonate, including physiologic and behavioral dimensions.

▪ Discuss the impact of the birth of a baby on the family.

▪ Describe the characteristics of premature at-risk newborns and contrast these with those of the term neonate.

▪ Describe the challenges the birth of a premature newborn places on the family.

Key Terms

anencephaly
anticipatory grief
attractor well
asymmetrical tonic neck reflex (ATNR)
biologic risk
bronchopulmonary dysplasia (BPD)
cerebral palsy
cocaine-exposed infants
cognitive competencies
conceptional age
cultural practices
ductus arteriosus
efficacy
engrossment
entrainment
environmental risk
fetal alcohol syndrome (FAS)
foramen ovale
gag reflex
gastroesophageal reflux
gender issues
HIV-exposed

hypoxic ischemic encephalopathy (HIE)
interactive behaviors
iIntegration
interuterine growth retardation
intraventricular hemorrhage (IVH)
jaundice
kangaroo care
kernicterus
labyrinthine righting reactions
meconium
minimal-stimulation protocols
Moro reflex
myelination
Neonatal Intensive Care Unit (NICU)
neonatal neck-righting reaction
neonatal period
neonate
neurogenesis
neuromotor behavior
oral motor reflexes
palmar grasp reflex
patent ductus arteriosus (PDA)

persistent fetal circulation
periventricular leukomalacia (PVL)
phasic bite reflex
physiologic immaturity
placing reactions
plantar grasp reflex
positive support reaction
postconceptional age
postural control reflexes
preterm infant
primitive stepping
protective factors
pulmonary hypertension
reflex
respiratory distress syndrome (RDS)
retinopathy of prematurity
rooting reflex
small for gestational age (SGA)
societal-level risk factors
suck-swallow reflex
suckling
synaptogenesis
tonic labyrinthine reflex

INTRODUCTION:

The birth of an infant is an irrevocable and life-altering event. Based on increasing knowledge of the competencies and behaviors of the human fetus, we know that birth represents not the beginning of human behaviors but rather a continuation of behaviors already emerging in utero. However, the challenge for the newborn is adaptation to an immensely altered environment. This challenge to adaptation is significant for the term newborn. The baby must take over the functions of respiration and nutrition previously supplied by the placenta. The baby must begin to function in an environment characterized by gravity and a wide variety of stimuli. Many body functions and some aspects of body structures, as outlined in the ICF framework, are developing in the newborn infant.

Furthermore, the baby is now capable of participating in social exchange with parents and others. For the family as well, the birth of an infant is an enormous adaptive challenge. The ICF model addresses functions of the individual, but also makes links to the influence of attitudes, supports, and relationships in the environment. Environmental issues are very dynamic during the newborn period. Although many parents approach childbirth with the professed belief that nothing will change after the baby is born, this attitude rarely persists beyond the first few days of parenthood.

These developmental life tasks are challenging in the normative term birth experience. However, because of the medical ability to save infants who are increasingly younger and sicker, more infants are facing the challenges of prematurity and at-risk birth. Since the early 1970s, the impact of preterm, at-risk birth on infants and their families has been extensively studied. A large number of professionals are involved in supporting these infants and their families in making transitions as easily as possible. It is important for professionals to understand, therefore, both the challenges facing the term and at-risk newborn.

THE TERM INFANT

The term infant in the space of an instant must take a first breath and begin to adapt to an environment that is extremely different from the aquatic environment of the womb, in which gravity is eliminated, physiologic support is largely provided, and all sorts of environmental stimuli are filtered through the amniotic fluid. For the most part, term infants make this transition quite effectively over the first few hours and days of life. The first four weeks after birth are known as the **neonatal period,** and the baby is commonly referred to as a **neonate.** The transitions of the neonatal period encompass all domains of function.

BODY FUNCTIONS

A number of physiologic systems must respond to the demands of birth. Perhaps most notable is the cardiopulmonary system. In utero the lungs are not necessary to provide oxygen to the fetus, since the majority of oxygenation occurs through the placental circulation. Therefore, the fetal circulatory system bypasses the lungs for the most part (see Figure 7–1). This bypass is called the *right-to-left shunting of blood,* meaning that the blood passes from the right side of the heart directly to the left without passing into the pulmonary circulation. This right-to-left shunting of blood occurs through two major valves. The first, the **foramen ovale,** is an opening between the two atrial chambers of the heart. The second, the **ductus arteriosus,** is the passageway that exists between the pulmonary trunk and the aorta (Lindsay, 1996).

Normally, the ductus arteriosus closes within the first few hours after birth and the foramen ovale within the first two weeks. Occasionally, these pathways do not close off normally, resulting in a persistent postnatal shunting of blood and an associated failure of the pulmonary vascular beds to open and permit sufficient perfusion of the lungs. This condition is known as **persistent fetal circulation** and the associated condition of **pulmonary hypertension.** Persistent fetal circulation is most commonly seen in the slightly **preterm infant,** 34–38 weeks old. It is a medical emergency and must be treated aggressively for the infant to survive. Failure of the ductus arteriosus to close is known as **patent ductus arteriosus (PDA)** and is a condition often seen in premature infants. In most cases the ductus closes with maturation (Shepherd, Hanshaw, & Lane, 1999)

Another system that experiences dramatic change postpartum is the liver and its hemopoetic activity. Because of this change, most newborns experience an increase in bilirubin levels in the blood at 24 to 72 hours after birth. This increase in bilirubin causes the infant's skin to have a yellowish cast, known as **jaundice.** Normally, the bilirubin level increase is benign and never approaches levels that would cross the blood-brain barrier. However, bilirubin levels are routinely monitored postpartum, and if the levels increase to a certain point, intervention is warranted.

The most conservative interventions involve placing the infant in direct sunlight. Occasionally breastfeeding is temporarily suspended, since if there is a maternal infant blood type incompatibility, this can contribute to the jaundice. The more aggressive intervention involves placing the infant under phototherapy lights in the blue spectrum or on phototherapy crib pads. The phototherapy light helps metabolize the bilirubin. Excessive bilirubin levels lead to a condition called **kernicterus.** When the bilirubin levels reach the point where the blood-brain barrier is crossed, certain parts of the brain are particularly susceptible. In particular, the basal ganglia, buried deep in the cerebral hemisphere, are susceptible in kernicterus, and before the current era of management, damage to this area resulted in children who had a type of cerebral palsy known as *choreoathetoid* (Long & Toscano, 2002). **Cerebral palsy** is the most common congenital (present from birth) disorder of childhood. It affects muscle tone and coordinated movement, and can result in problems with eating, bladder and bowel control, breathing, and learning. Although the choreoathetoid type of cerebral palsy has become rare in the western world, it is still occasionally seen, particularly as a sequelae of extreme prematurity.

Of course, the issue of nourishment is another challenge for the neonate. Within the first few hours of life, the infant normally takes its first feeding. Even immediately postpartum, the infant will often, if laid upon its mother's chest, attach to the breast and begin to suck. The mother produces a nutritive substance called *colostrum* for the first 48–72 hours after birth. This substance is viscous, clear, and full of antibodies that are passed from mother to infant. Normally, if the mother is breastfeeding, her milk comes in after the first few days. Much has been written about the value of breast-feeding.

The process of elimination, or voiding, also undergoes change in the first few days postnatally. Initially the infant voids a thick, tarry substance known as **meconium.** This substance is normally voided in utero as well but is absorbed in the amniotic fluid. Meconium staining of the amniotic fluid is one sign of fetal distress, and it is possible for infants to swallow the meconium during labor and birth. This is called *meconium aspiration,* and it is a condition that can result in asphyxia and brain damage if not recognized and treated (Shepherd, Hanshaw, & Long, 1999).

DEVELOPMENT OF BODY STRUCTURES

The area of **neuromotor behavior** is probably the most prescriptive of the neonatal characteristics. The relative immaturity of the neonate's central nervous system is a function of the fact that while neurogenesis has largely been completed by the fifth gestational month, the

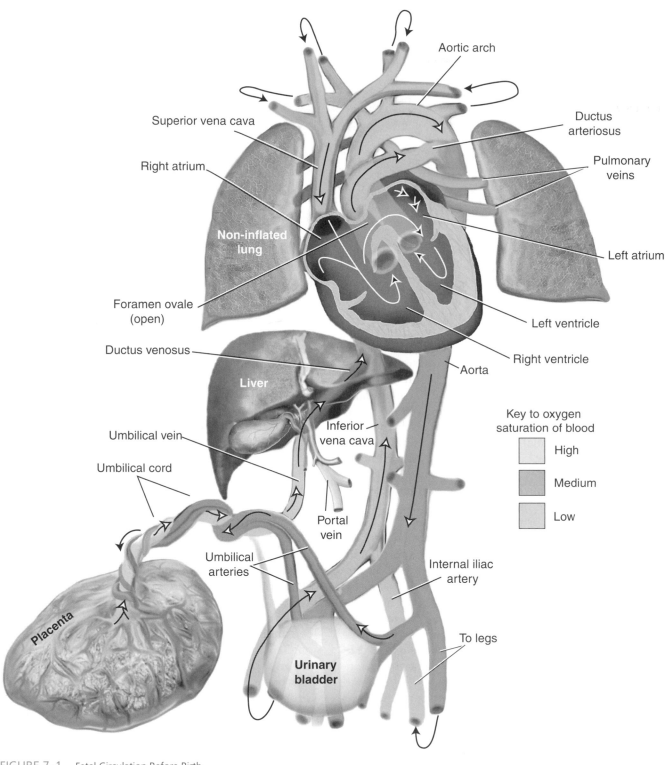

Aortic arch

Superior vena cava

Right atrium

Non-inflated lung

Foramen ovale (open)

Ductus venosus

Liver

Umbilical vein

Umbilical cord

Umbilical arteries

Placenta

Ductus arteriosus

Pulmonary veins

Left atrium

Left ventricle

Right ventricle

Aorta

Inferior vena cava

Portal vein

Internal iliac artery

Urinary bladder

To legs

Key to oxygen saturation of blood

High

Medium

Low

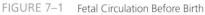

FIGURE 7–1   Fetal Circulation Before Birth

establishment of the complex structure of the CNS is beginning. **Neurogenesis** is the process by which new nerve cells are generated. *Myelin* is the fatty substance that covers and protects nerves. **Myelination** is the developmental process of building a myelin sheath on the nerves to insulate the fibers and ensure that messages sent by nerve fibers are not lost en route. A related process, **synaptogenesis,** is the building of specialized junctions at which a nerve cell communicates with a target cell. Myelination and synaptogenesis are only in relatively early stages at birth (Eliot, 1999). Because of this immaturity, the newborn infant has a fairly limited and stereotypic repertoire of motor behavior.

Work done on **anencephalic** infants (infants born without a cerebral cortex) in the early part of the twentieth century showed that these infants displayed much of the same motor behavior as term neonates. For this reason, a large number of developmental studies reflected the maturationist view of neonatal behavior. This view, espoused by such renowned names in the field of infant study as Myrtle McGraw and Arnold Gesell, states that the behavior of the newborn is a direct reflection of the parts of the central nervous system (CNS) that are functionally capable of directing this behavior (Goldfield & Wolff, 2000). Because many of the motor behaviors seen in the neonate are processed at the spinal cord and brainstem levels, it was thought that the normal newborn was largely a subcortical creature. It was not until the neurobehavioral studies of the latter part of the twentieth century revealed the immense variability and function of the neonate's behavioral repertoire that the view of the neonate as functioning at subcortical levels was rejected.

Likewise, for motor behavior, the maturationist view held that motor behavior developed hierarchically in conjunction with the progressive maturation of the higher brain centers. Over the past two decades the traditional reflexive, hierarchical frame of reference has been challenged by the premise that neonatal motor behavior is best explained by a systems theory of motor control (Horak, 1991; Thelen & Spencer, 1998; Goldfield & Wolff, 2002). In systems theory, behavior at any given point in time is emergent and depends on the interaction of a number of systems, both intrinsic and extrinsic to the organism. In the case of the neonate, systems theory challenges a large number of assumptions about motor behavior (Goldfield & Wolff, 2002). Work by Thelen and Heriza suggests that the manner in which neonatal motor behavior has traditionally been studied and characterized is valid only for the environmental constraints in which the behavior occurs. For example, the neonate is clearly capable of kicking when supine and performing a stepping pattern when supported in an upright position. Thelen and Fisher found that the only difference in these patterns is the posture in which they are produced (Thelen & Fisher, 1982; Heriza, 1991).

NEONATAL REFLEXES

The neonatal reflex was traditionally considered the building block of neonatal motor behavior (Goldfield & Wolff, 2002). A **reflex** is defined as a stereotypic obligatory response to a given stimulus. Newer theorists challenge the concept of reflexes, stating that very few normal behaviors actually meet the strict definition of reflex. A conceptual descriptor of motor behavior in the neonate that reflects the contemporary notion of systems is the term **attractor well.** An attractor well is a preferred pattern of movement. A very deep attractor well is reflected by a motor pattern that is highly predictable in being elicited in response to a given stimulus. Many neonatal motor behaviors would fall under this classification.

As the infant matures and motor behavior repertoire expands, the infant experiments with a number of motor strategies to accomplish functional movement. The motor behavioral repertoire becomes less predictable and more variable. Eventually, through processes of maturation and learning, the baby will develop preferred strategies to accomplish functional tasks. The preferred strategies are attractor wells that are not as deep as those of early life, where little variability in strategy is possible.

An analogy for this is to consider a marble on a flat surface. When the surface is tilted, the marble moves in any direction in response to the tilt. If the surface is topographically changed to have peaks and valleys (wells), the marble will move toward the well, but in different circumstances, it can vary its path. However, if the attractor well is very deep, the marble will nearly always find that well, irrespective of the stimuli around it (Shumway-Cook & Woollacott, 2001). These very deep attractor wells typify the motor behavior of the newborn. However, the old terminology of *reflexes* is commonly used in the literature and in the clinical environment. Therefore, the so-called *neonatal reflexes* are described separately as follows in the ensuing discussion. Keep in mind that current research is challenging the stereotypic and obligatory nature of the normal patterns of movement, going so far as to say that these aforementioned characteristics are signs of abnormality. Rather, these patterns previously thought of as reflexes are highly preferred strategies that are not obligatory in that they can be altered under various circumstances, such as internal and external environmental characteristics (Goldfield & Wolff, 2002).

One final concept is extremely important in understanding the role of these neuromotor patterns that have traditionally been called reflexes. That is, many of the patterns seen in the term newborn must be **integrated** to permit more complex and mature neuromotor patterns to develop. Integration means that the reflexive pattern is no longer a highly predictable or preferred pattern. Maturation of the nervous system in combination with environmental experience and practice promotes the development of more variable patterns of neuromotor behavior that underlie functional accomplishments (Eliot, 1999). It is very important to understand, though, that while integration means the reflex is no longer a dominant feature of infant behavior that is easily visible, the pattern itself has not been erased from memory. In fact, the pattern of the neonatal reflexes can be brought out in stressful situations as well as when the nervous system sustains damage. The reemergence of these patterns following neurologic damage such as stroke or head injury presents a challenge to therapists in positioning and handling clients. Therefore, it is important to learn the typical stimulus-response characteristics of these patterns, not only to understand normal infant development but also to understand how to intervene in a therapeutic situation.

Oral Motor Reflexes

Among the earliest reflex behaviors observed are the reflexes associated with eating and swallowing. **Oral motor reflexes** are those reflexes specific to the muscle actions of the mouth and oral area. Several oral motor reflexes are present in the healthy newborn. See Table 7–1 for a summary of reflex activity in the neonate.

Suck-Swallow Reflex.

Of all the neonatal motor behaviors, the most basic is the one associated with the intake of nourishment, or the **suck-swallow reflex.** First appearing around the 28th week of gestation, this pattern is well established by birth. The stimulus to elicit this pattern is downward pressure on the tongue and the response is a rhythmical sucking movement. The early oral motor behavior of the neonate is differentiated from the more mature patterns developed by the end of the first postnatal trimester. The neonate tends to respond with a total forward and down movement of lips, tongue, and jaw followed by a backward and upward retraction. Thus, the neonate is actually pressing the nipple or teat to the hard palate and using a process of positive pressure, or expression, to obtain milk. The amount of negative pressure or suction that the neonate can generate is limited because of weakness of the lip, tongue, and cheek musculature. This neonatal pattern of movement is called **suckling.** Over the first few months of life, the infant begins to develop the ability to disassociate lip, tongue, and jaw movement and create negative pressure, or suction, in the intra-oral cavity. When this occurs, the pattern more resembles a mature pattern and is known as *sucking.* The normal suckling pattern of the neonate is highly rhythmical and is characterized by a burst of several sucks followed by a pause. The rhythmicity of this pattern is important, and dysfunction in developing this pattern is often a problem for premature infants in making the transition to oral feeding. Typically, the suck-swallow pattern is linked, with a burst of sucks followed by a swallow (Goldfield & Wolff, 2002).

Phasic Bite Reflex.

The neonate has a **phasic bite reflex.** This reflex is elicited by pressure on the gums, with a normative response being an up-and-down motion of the jaw that often accompanies the feeding behavior. A sustained bite in response to touch in or near the mouth, which the infant is unable to release, is a *tonic bite reflex,* and is never normal. This type of abnormal pattern may be indicative of CNS damage, as in perinatal asphyxia (Kedesky & Budd, 1998).

Gag Reflex.

The **gag reflex** develops later in utero than the primary feeding reflexes, not making its appearance until the 34th week of gestation. The gag reflex is elicited by touch of the posterior half to third of the tongue or the soft palate/uvula region. The normal response is a gagging pattern. The gag reflex plays an important role in feeding development in preterm infants. Because of its relatively late appearance, it is one factor associated with the standard caregiving practice of avoiding oral feeding in preterm infants until they have reached approximately the 34th gestational week (Kedesky & Budd, 1998).

Rooting Reflex.

Another neonatal behavior associated with feeding is the familiar **rooting reflex** (see Figure 7–2). The rooting reflex is elicited by perioral touch. The stimulus is to stroke on either side of the infant's cheek. A normal response is to turn toward the stimulus. If the upper lip is stroked, the infant extends the head. If the lower lip is stroked, mouth opening occurs. This reflex is the vestige of early patterns allowing newborns of other species born with their eyes closed to seek out the maternal teat (Kedesky & Budd, 1998; Hepper, 2002).

Tonic Labyrinthine Reflex.

Tonic postural reflexes are activated by head and neck movements and influence the distribution of muscle tone throughout the body. The **tonic labyrinthine reflex** plays a role in mediating the strong early patterns of flexion seen in the newborn (see Figures 7–3 and 7–4). The sensory trigger for this reflex is head position. When the infant is prone, systemic flexion is facilitated; and when the infant is supine, systemic extension is facilitated. Thus, the effect of the tonic labyrinthine reflexes is to pull the infant into gravity (Hepper, 2002).

Labyrinthine Righting Reactions.

From the moment the infant enters a gravity environment, the tonic labyrinthine reflexes are in competition with the development of antigravity behaviors, mediated by the

TABLE 7–1	Summary of Reflex Activity in Neonate

I. The primitive gravity-dependent influences of the tonic labyrinthine reflexes compete with the very early development of the labyrinthine righting reaction.

(TLR) Tonic Labyrinthine Reflex (Prone, Supine)

Onset	Prenatal
Integration	6 months
Position	1. Prone 2. Supine
Procedure	Observe the child's tone and posture in prone and supine positions. Child in prone, lift head; evaluate presence of flexor tone. Child in supine, pull to sit, noting presence of extensor tone.
Response	Prone, flexor tone dominates; child will not lift head.
	Supine, extensor tone dominates; child will not flex in pull to sit.
Significance	Persistence will preclude ability to roll and to develop anti-gravity behaviors.

Labyrinthine Righting Reaction

Onset	Birth to 2 months
Integration	Persists through life
Position	Hold child vertically under the arms, tilting child in space.
Procedure	Tilt child's body in all directions.
Response	Head orients to vertical position and is steady, maintained in proper orientation to environment.
Significance	Persistence will prohibit antigravity behaviors; this is the starting point for the Landau reflex.

II. The hands are predominantly flexed; grasping (finger and toe flexion) is dominant.

Palmar Grasp Reflex

Onset	Birth to 2 month
Integration	4–11 months
Position	Place child supine with head in midline and hands free.
Procedure	Place index finger into the infant's hands with pressure over the metacarpal heads.
Response	Fingers will flex around the examiner's.
Significance	Cannot utilize volitional reach and grasp until integrated.

Plantar Grasp Reflex

Onset	Prenatal
Integration	9 months
Position	Place child supine with head in midline and legs relaxed.
Procedure	Place firm pressure against volar aspect of foot, directly below toes.
Response	Plantar flexion of toes occurs.
Significance	Indicates an immature attempt to maintain stability; should disappear in standing, coinciding with mature postural equilibrium.

III. The newborn is born with certain reflexes ensuring survival.

Rooting Reaction

Onset	Prenatal
Integration	3 months
Position	Place child supine with head in midline.
Procedure	Using your finger, stroke the perioral skin at the corner of the mouth, moving laterally toward the cheek, upper lip and lower lip.
Response	Infant turns head toward stimulus; if to lower lip, mouth tends to open.
Significance	Is rarely absent when infant is not satiated; absence may indicate CNS depression.

Continues

TABLE 7–1	Summary of Reflex Activity in Neonate *Continued*

Suck-Swallow Reflex

Onset	Prenatal
Integration	2–5 months
Position	Place child supine with head in midline.
Procedure	Place finger or nipple into the infant's mouth.
Response	Rhythmic suckling movements occur; lips, tongue, and jaw move synchronously, first down and forward, then up and back.
Significance	Rarely suppressed in a nonsatiated infant; absence may indicate CNS depression.

IV. The infant's motor abilities in postural control and mobility are composed of some of the following additional characteristic patterns.

Traction Response

Onset	Prenatal
Integration	2–5 months
Position	Place child supine with head in midline.
Procedure	Grasp child's wrists and pull toward sitting position.
Response	Flexion of shoulders, elbows, wrist, and fingers occurs.
Significance	Persistence will inhibit voluntary use of arms.

Moro Reflex

Onset	Prenatal
Integration	5–6 months
Position	Place child supine with head in midline.
Procedure	Support infant's head and shoulders with hands and allow head to drop back 20–30 degrees with respect to trunk, stretching neck muscles.
Response	Abduction of the upper extremities with extension of the elbows, wrists, and fingers occurs, followed by subsequent adduction of the arms at the shoulders and flexion at the elbows.
Significance	Is part of any standard neurologic assessment of the newborn; although frequently the adduction component is variable, total absence of this reflex is usually indicative of neurologic abnormality.

Galant's Response (Incurvation of the Trunk)

Onset	Prenatal
Integration	By end of first trimester
Position	Place infant prone (in horizontal suspension) over your hand.
Procedure	Stroke with pressure along a paravertebral line.
Response	Trunk curves with shortening on the stimulated side.
Significance	May be useful in early evaluation of children with spina bifida to determine where trunk muscles are innervated.

Neonatal Neck Righting

Onset	Prenatal
Integration	Second trimester as mature neck righting develops
Position	Place child supine with head in midline.
Procedure	Lift and turn child's head to side.
Response	Child's body follows "like a log," i.e., nonsegmentally.
Significance	Often persists in the presence of spasticity; will prohibit normal de-rotative rolling.

Continues

TABLE 7–1 **Summary of Reflex Activity in Neonate** *Continued*

Asymmetric Tonic Neck Reflex (ATNR)

Onset	Birth to 2 months
Integration	4–6 months
Position	Place child supine.
Procedure	Have child turn head to one side.
Response	Extension of the arm and leg to which the face is turned occurs, along with flexion of the opposite limbs, producing an apparent "en guarde" fencing posture.
Significance	In normal development, probably is responsible for early linkages between eyes and hands. Is not uncommonly apparent in the motor behavior of adults and children with CNS damage; when present and obligatory, prevents symmetrical behaviors, hand to mouth, and may contribute to the development of scoliosis.

Placing Reactions (Arms and Legs)

Onset	Arms = birth; legs = prenatal
Integration	First trimester
Position	Hold child upright, in vertical suspension.
Procedure	Brush the dorsum of child's hand or foot against tabletop.
Response	The limb lifts in flexion, then is followed by extension as if to place it on the table.
Significance	Seen in CNS damage.

V. Movement patterns of the lower extremities are strongly reciprocal and reflect the spinal cord organization of the agonist/antagonist relationships between flexors and extensors. Central pattern generators (clusters of neurons which fire in alternate sequence) may be involved.

Flexor Withdrawal

Onset	Prenatal
Integration	First trimester
Position	Place child supine with head in midline and legs relaxed.
Procedure	Apply noxious stimulus, such as pinprick, to sole of foot.
Response	Stimulated leg reacts with flexion at hip, knee, and ankle, withdrawing the extremity.
Significance	A withdrawal to a painful stimulus persists throughout life; however, it becomes localized to just a jerk of the ankle; the reflex is correctly named for the total withdrawal of the limb and is integrated in early life.

Crossed Extension

Onset	Prenatal
Integration	First trimester
Position	Place child supine with head in midline.
Procedure	Hold one leg straight; apply firm pressure or noxious stimulus to sole of foot.
Response	Flexion, adduction, and then extension of the *opposite* leg.
Significance	Represents spinal cord neural networks that will lay the foundation for reciprocal pattern of locomotion.

Neonatal Positive Supporting

Onset	Prenatal
Integration	First trimester
Position	Support infant in vertical suspension with your hands under arms and around trunk.
Procedure	Allow feet to make contact with support surface.
Response	Co-contraction of lower extremity muscles occurs, with limb support of minimal body weight.
Significance	Indicates normal muscle tone; if persists, may be associated with high muscle tone, as in spastic diplegia.

Spontaneous Stepping

Onset	Near birth
Integration	First trimester
Position	Support child as in vertical suspension as described above, but lean infant's body weight forward.
Procedure	Hold infant upright in vertical suspension, touching feet to support surface. Lean infant slightly forward to elicit stepping.
Response	Alternating stepping movements occur.
Significance	May persist, as in spastic diplegia.

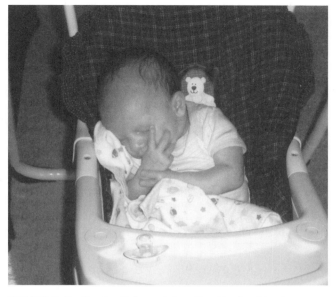

FIGURE 7–2   Rooting Reflex as Infant Gets Hand to Mouth

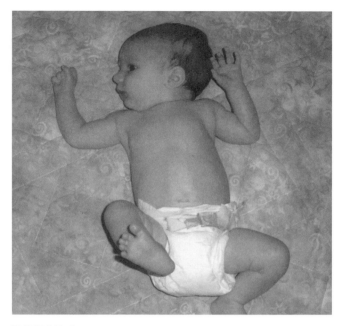

FIGURE 7–4   Resting Posture in Supine—Still Flexed but More Inclination toward Extension

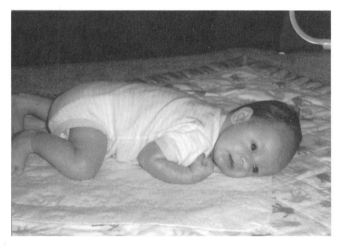

FIGURE 7–3   Resting Posture in Prone—Position Dominated by Flexion

labyrinthine righting reactions. The righting reactions as a group are a number of upper brainstem–mediated responses that either align the body with respect to gravity and/or the support surface or rotate the body parts into alignment with each other, thereby permitting the individual to change positions, as in rolling. The labyrinthine righting reaction is the first to appear. The stimulus for this reflex, as in the tonic labyrinthine reflex, is position of the head or body in space. However, in this case, the response is an antigravity response, allowing the infant to lift up into extension when prone or lift into flexion from the supine position. At birth, the labyrinthine righting reactions are barely evident but can be seen when the infant is held in prone suspension and can lift its head into alignment with the body. Alternatively, parents see evidence of

labyrinthine righting when they lay their newborn facedown and the baby slightly lifts and turns his or her head to the side. Often, the amount of head righting evident is variable in accordance with the arousal level of the infant. Infants who are agitated or crying may lift their head up farther. Another test of early labyrinthine righting is to pull the newborn to a sitting position (Swaiman & Ashwal, 1999). Normally the head lags back into extension for most of the pull to sit; however, as the infant approaches the supported sitting position, there are brief attempts to bob the head erect (see Figure 7–5).

Over the first six months of life, the labyrinthine righting reaction totally subsumes the tonic labyrinthine reactions such that by six months, the infant can fully extend in prone and will lift the head to help in the pull-to-sit maneuver.

Neonatal Neck Righting.   The first of the rotary righting reactions to develop is the **neonatal neck righting reaction,** which is also present at birth. This is an immature example of the rotary righting reactions. The task accomplished by rotary righting reactions is to allow the infant to transfer from one postural set to another (i.e., prone to supine). The neonatal neck righting reaction is immature in that when the infant's head is turned passively, the body follows "like a log," rotating in a nonsegmental fashion. Because of the lack of antigravity control at birth, combined with immature rotary righting reactions, the neonatal neck righting is not sufficient to complete a roll from supine to prone position. Rather, it will allow the infant to roll from back to

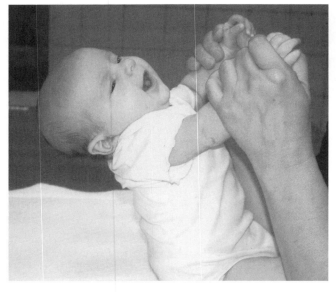

FIGURE 7–5   Head Lag in Pull-to-Sit

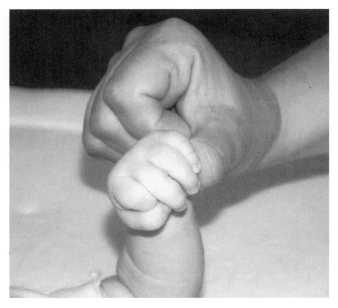

FIGURE 7–6   Palmar Grasp

side and vice versa. The truly mature rolling pattern is not seen until approximately 4 months of age.

Grasp Reflexes.   The grasp reflexes are highly predictable in the newborn. Most obvious is the **palmar grasp reflex** (see Figure 7–6). This pattern occurs in response to pressure in the palm, usually by the examiner placing a finger in the infant's palm. The response is that the infant's fingers curl around the examiner's finger, appearing to grasp. The **plantar grasp reflex** is similar, but the stimulus is a pressure across the metatarsal heads just under the toes (see Figure 7–7). The response is grasping of the toes (Hepper, 2002). This pattern is seen later as the infant tries to stand. The plantar grasp reflex represents a very primitive attempt at balance.

Placing Reactions.   The **placing reactions** are also present in both hands and feet. The stimulus to these reactions is to stroke the back of the hand or top of the foot as against a tabletop. The infant will lift the limb in flexion, then extend the limb as if to place it on the table.

Standing Reactions.   Two key patterns are seen in standing. One is the **postural support reaction.** When the infant is held in vertical suspension and the feet are placed on the surface, the positive support reaction mediates extension through the lower limbs. If the infant is subsequently tipped slightly forward, she will spontaneously and reciprocally flex one leg and extend the other in alternating patterns. This is called **primitive stepping** (see Figure 7–8). Both of these patterns occur without true weight bearing and must be integrated to permit true weight bearing and walking to occur (Hepper, 2002).

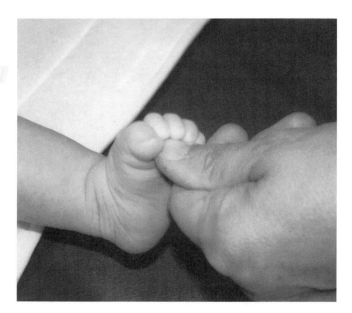

FIGURE 7–7   Plantar Grasp

Moro Reflex.   A key pattern used in all neonatal assessment to determine neurologic integrity is the **Moro reflex** (see Figure 7–9). In the Moro reflex, the infant's head is dropped backward, stimulating the vestibular system of the inner ear. The response to the stimulus is abduction of the arms, followed by adduction of the arms across the chest (Hepper, 2002). The Moro is also a very predictable aspect of normal newborn behavior. Total absence of this reflex is a sign of neurologic problems. Asymmetry of the Moro may indicate a problem such as a brachial plexus palsy or stroke.

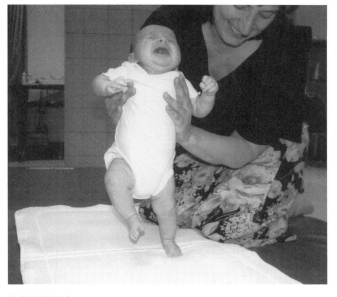

FIGURE 7–8   Primitive Stepping Pattern

Asymmetrical Tonic Neck Reflex.   The normal term newborn rests asymmetrically. That means the head is turned to one side or the other, virtually never remaining in the midline. Beginning at birth and peaking over the first 2 months of life, a typical postural set is mediated by the **asymmetrical tonic neck reflex (ATNR)** (see Figure 7–10). The stimulus for the ATNR is turning the head to one side. The response is very typical. The upper and lower limbs on the side toward which the infant is looking (i.e., the face side) extend. The upper and lower limbs facing the back of the head (the skull side), flex. This creates a postural set symbolic of the en guarde position in fencing, so the pattern is

sometimes referred to as the *fencing position* (Hepper, 2002). The ATNR is believed to play a role in establishing linkages between the dominant hand and the eyes, since it tends to be stronger to the right in most infants. An obligatory ATNR or persistence of the ATNR beyond 4–5 months of age is an unfavorable neurologic sign. The ATNR must be integrated to permit more mature behaviors, such as hands to midline and hands to mouth to emerge.

NEONATAL MOTOR BEHAVIOR

The reflexive patterns of behavior just described dominate the newborn's motor behavior. Functionally, at birth the newborn's motor behavior is fairly limited and gravity-dependent. It may be summarized as follows. In prone position, the newborn is able to lift the head and turn it from side to side. Flexion is noted in upper and lower limbs. In supine, the head is typically turned to the side. Reciprocal kicking is noted. The infant will direct hand to mouth with varying degrees of success. In pull-to-sit, there is total head lag, but when the infant is held supported in sitting, the head will bob erect into a neutral position. In supported standing, there is some acceptance of weight, but the standing pattern is immature and the weight is largely supported.

It is easy to see that if neuromotor behavior alone is considered, it could be assumed that the infant's nervous system is extremely immature. It used to be thought that the higher cortical centers were not active in the newborn infant, since many of the reflexive patterns as described previously are present in anencephalic infants. However, studies of other aspects of newborn infant behavior do not support that assumption.

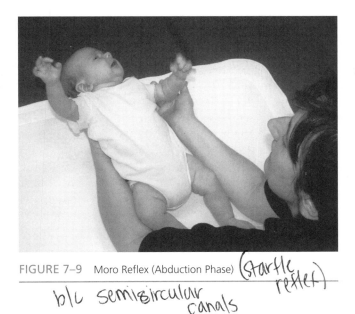

FIGURE 7–9   Moro Reflex (Abduction Phase) (startle reflex)

b/c semicircular canals

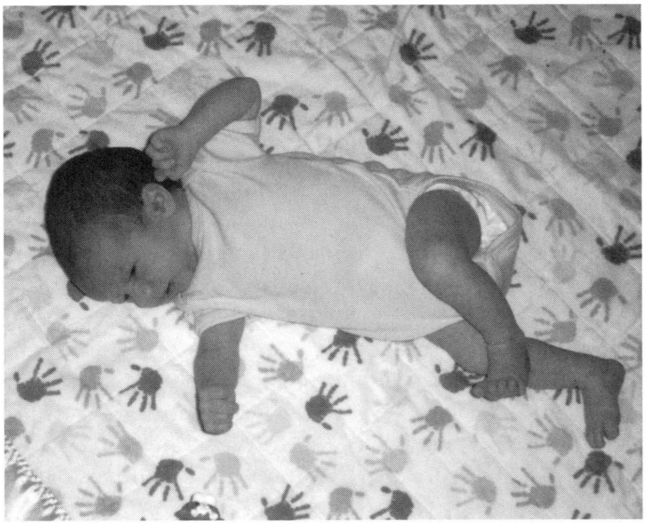

FIGURE 7–10   ATNR Pattern in Supine Position

BEHAVIORAL STATE AND SENSORY FUNCTION

One of the most important aspects of behavior in the newborn infant is the concept of behavioral state. *Behavioral state* may be defined as the infant's level of arousal mediating the responsivity to environmental inputs. The notion of behavioral state can be studied at two levels. The first level is physiologic and includes such data as analyzing the brain activity of the infant. The second is behavioral, analyzing the infant's behavioral response to stimulation (Wilhelm, 1993).

Physiologic studies of infant behavioral state utilize data such as the study of brain wave activity through electroencephalograms (EEGs). Basically, there is an attempt to identify clusters of brain activity that are differentiated from other clusters and that correlate with level of arousal. From these studies, it has been found that the first signs of behavioral state organization are not seen until the infant reaches 32 weeks gestational age. Between 32 weeks and term, there is increasing organization of characteristic cycles such that by term, three identifiable states are seen. These loosely correspond to wakefulness, rapid eye movement (REM) sleep, and non–rapid eye movement (NREM) sleep (Freudigman & Thoman, 1994). Other states are termed transitional.

Behavioral state as measured from the infant's behaviors such as responsivity to stimuli has become the benchmark for all assessment of term infant behavior. First classified for evaluative purposes by the neurologist Prechtl in 1974, six behavioral states have been identified. The concept of behavioral state was further defined and incorporated into the Neonatal Behavior Assessment Scale (BNBAS) (Brazelton & Nugent, 1995). Since the widespread incorporation of behavioral state into that assessment, common definitions for the behavioral states are as follows, always indicated by the Roman numerals preceding them.

Behavioral State I is deep sleep, corresponding to NREM sleep. There is no eye movement, there are no spontaneous startles, and the infant is difficult to rouse. *Behavioral State II* is active, or REM, sleep. In this state, startles are elicited. The infant may make spontaneous movements but will settle down quickly. In *Behavioral State III* the infant is in transition from sleep to wakefulness. One eye may be open, or both eyes may partially open. The infant appears to rouse but then seems drawn back into sleep. *Behavioral State IV* is extremely significant because of its importance in establishing social relationships and early learning. This state is called *quiet alert* and is the optimum behavioral state for evaluation (see Figure 7–11). In this state the infant does not have a great deal of extraneous body movement. He is visually attentive and will fixate on a stimulus. *Behavioral State V* is active alert. The infant maintains

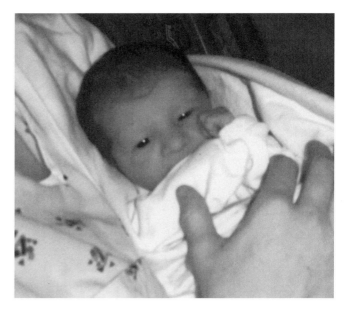

FIGURE 7–11   Newborn in Behavior State IV

eyes open, but extraneous body movements interfere with sustained attention. *Behavioral State VI* is crying. The infant is aroused but is crying and therefore does not engage in interaction.

An infant's behavioral state determines her responsiveness to different stimuli; therefore, it is extremely important that assessments be done as close to Behavioral State IV as possible. An infant may appear abnormally unresponsive during an exam if the entire exam is carried out in nonoptimal behavior states (Brazelton & Nugent, 1995).

As the preceding discussion implies, the behavioral assessment of state is largely dependent on the infant's response to sensory stimulation. The term newborn has all senses functioning, although some are relied upon more than others. The sense of smell is highly developed in the term newborn. Studies have shown that as early as the first week of life, the infant can distinguish breast milk from her mother soaked on a breast pad from that of other women (Schaal et al., 1980). Likewise, the sense of taste appears to develop fairly early. Studies have shown that infants display preferences for different tastes. In a study by Mendella and Beauchamp (1996), when vanilla was added to either breast milk or formula, infants sucked longer and consumed more milk. These authors concluded their study by suggesting that one additional benefit of breastfeeding was that infants are exposed to a rich experience of foods that may help familiarize the infant with dietary habits of a given culture.

The sense of touch is very well developed in newborn infants. The somatosensory cortex, which processes touch information, is the most mature of the sensory cortical areas at birth (Lundy-Ekman, 1998). Klaus et al. (1970) described the immediate postpartum behavior of infant-mother dyads. They reported that mothers typically initiated a period of massage of their newborns, beginning on the extremities and ending with palmar contact on the trunk. The importance of touch to the mother-infant relationship was first proposed in the classic Harlow study, which showed that infant monkeys would prefer a cloth-covered surrogate to a wire-covered surrogate that dispensed food (Harlow, 1958). The prominent infancy researcher Tiffany Field has studied the effects of massage on premature infants and found that massage can enhance weight gain and improve sociobehavioral responses. Massage has also been shown to positively affect the performance of neonates on habituation items of the Brazelton Neonatal Behavioral Assessment Scales (NBAS) (Scafidi, Field, & Schanberg, 1993). There are, in all likelihood, tangible hormonal responses to tactile stimulation. Mooncy et al. (1997) reported that when preterm infants were allowed to rest naked on their mother's breasts, beta-endorphin levels dropped significantly from a control condition. This seems to indicate that physiologic indices of stress may be impacted by tactile stimulation. In summary, the tactile system is fairly well functioning in the term newborn at birth, and provision of sensory input over that system appears to enhance the well-being of sick or distressed infants.

Related to the sense of touch is the vestibuloproprioceptive sensory modality. This modality mediates the responsivity to position and movement. Of all sensory experiences, perhaps none is as practiced at birth as this, for the infant has been moving in an aquatic environment for some months. Once exposed to the extrauterine environment of gravity, the infant's motor responses are primarily the source of inferences about the functioning of this system. For example, the Moro and labyrinthine reactions occur in response to vestibular inputs. The classic work of Korner and Thoman (1970) showed that the infant's level of arousal was affected by positioning, with the upright position promoting a more alert state. Rocking, which has long been a way to quiet a fretful infant, is also a vestibular mediated sensory experience.

The two sensory systems that have received the most attention in infant research are those of vision and hearing. With respect to vision, prior to the mid-twentieth century it was believed that for all intents and purposes, the newborn infant was blind, because of the inability to form meaningful perceptions (Lamb & Campos, 1982). Fantz reported breakthrough studies on visual perception in infants in the 1960s. These classic studies showed that newborn infants had clear visual preferences. For example, infants preferred black-and-white patterned stimuli to gray and a facial stimulus to a neutral stimulus (Fantz, 1961; Fantz, 1963). Subsequently, it was suggested that it was the high contrast inherent in the face pattern, not the face itself, that was appealing to newborns (Lamb & Campos, 1982). However, more recent work continues to contribute to the premise that there is something about the human face that has intrinsic appeal to the newborn. Walton, Bower, & Bower (1992) reported that by 1–2 days of age infants seem to recognize images of their mother's face as compared with the face of a stranger by changes in the infant's sucking response. These same authors have reported that infants seem to be able to discriminate the mother's face and recognize it through a variety of rotations and transformations (Walton, Armstrong, & Bower, 1997). Slater et al. (1998) have reported that early in the 1st week of life, infants seem to look longer at faces judged to be attractive by adults.

It is also pertinent to understand some of the limits of an infant's vision. For example, it is known that visual acuity at birth is not the same as that of a normal adult, i.e., 20/20. Because of difficulties in accurately determining visual acuity in newborns, there is a range of estimated acuity somewhere between 20/300 to 20/800 (Cohen, DeLoache, & Strauss, 1979). Another way to view the research on visual acuity in newborns is that they see best objects that are about 8 to 12 inches from their face, about the distance of the mother's face when cradling the infant in a traditional *en face* feeding position.

Another area of research on infant vision that has received recent attention is the ability of the infant to perceive color. For some period of time, studies on color preference were confounded by brightness, a problem that was resolved in more recent studies which control for the brightness variable (Cohen, DeLoache, & Strauss, 1979). It is fairly well established, however, that infants react to colors as early as 4 months of age. This research, like the studies on visual acuity, is difficult to determine definitively in the newborn. One general summary statement about newborn color preference can be made. It is clear that, in combination with the previous findings about infants preferring stimuli of high contrast, the traditional pastel colors of the newborn nursery have little appeal to newborns. Adams et al. (1994) studied newborns and reported that they could clearly discriminate the red color only from a nonchromatic patch of consistent luminescence. As a result of this consensus, a number of toys for infants made up of black, white, and red have been marketed.

A summary of neonatal visual abilities is as follows. First, the neonate clearly has the ability to see, process, and react to visual stimuli, although this ability is not fully mature at birth. Neonates prefer high contrast in visual stimuli and seem to prefer the human face. They are able to discriminate the maternal face within the 1st week of life. In order to optimally stimulate the infant, the object should be held relatively close (8–12 inches) from the infant's face. Finally, neonatal color vision is very limited. It seems to first be evident in the red portion of the spectrum.

In addition to vision, the hearing capabilities of the newborn infant have been studied extensively. Unlike vision, the auditory system has been extensively stimulated in utero, with the most common sounds being those of the mother's heartbeat and the swish of blood flow through the placenta. However, as reported earlier, the fetus clearly responds to auditory stimuli in the external environment, including the mother's voice. Studies have shown that newborns can distinguish between their mother's and a stranger's voice (DeCasper & Fifer, 1980; Spence & Freeman, 1996). Furthermore, the ability to distinguish voices occurred even when the mother's voice was filtered, taking out the high-frequency sounds that assist in the detection of meaningful speech (Spence & Freeman, 1996). Newborns can detect a whispered voice as well but are unable to distinguish between voices when they are whispered. Newborns did not appear to be able to distinguish or prefer the father's voice (DeCasper & Prescott, 1984), a finding that was interpreted to support the idea that learning of the maternal voice occurs in utero. It has also been reported that newborn infants can discriminate pitch (Nazzi, Floccia, & Bertocini, 1998). Sounds can also be soothing to newborns. Five-day-old infants were subjected to one of three conditions: white noise, heartbeat sounds, or silence during a heel-stick procedure. It was found that infants in both of the stimulus conditions (white noise and heartbeat) showed less reactive response to the invasive procedure (Kawakami et al., 1996).

Integration across several senses also appears to occur in the newborn. Meltzoff and Borton (1979) demonstrated that infants who experienced tactile exploration of a certain shape of pacifier displayed a visual preference for that pacifier later. There is also evidence that the newborn can imitate behaviors that are already within his behavioral repertoire. In the classic work on neonatal imitation done by Meltzoff and Moore (1977), infants were shown to imitate common movements such as tongue thrusting and mouth opening. Infants have also been shown to imitate facial expressions in a study by Kaitz et al. (1988). Morrongiello et al. (1998) have shown that infants as young as 2 days could seemingly learn audiovisual pairings and reacted when the expected pairings did not occur.

As evidenced by the preceding studies, the normal newborn actually shows a quite sophisticated behavioral repertoire in terms of responding to various aspects of the environment. From the time of birth the human newborn is processing and reacting to information from the environment.

INTERACTIVE BEHAVIORS

Not only is the term newborn responsive to stimuli in the environment, she is able to engage in social interactions with animate stimuli. All active behaviors that are directed at gaining the attention of others are called **interactive behaviors.** Abilities such as the imitation of behaviors are part of such interactions. The newborn's interactive abilities also play a key role in the development of social attachments, as to the parents. Immediately postpartum, the mother and infant undergo characteristic behaviors that seem to have the rhythmicity associated with all social interactions. For example, when two adults are speaking to one another, the speaker will not only verbalize but also make facial gestures and body movements. The listener will not speak but shows engagement in the exchange through various body movements and facial gestures. When the speaker is finished, the person who listened will typically engage in a verbal response, and the roles of the interaction are reversed. At birth, a rudimentary variation of this social exchange appears to be present (see Figure 7–12). This linked behavioral exchange has been called **entrainment.**

The famous developmental psychologist John Bowlby proposed in the 1950s that the infant has innate social capabilities (Karen, 1994). Condon and Sander (1974) described the entrainment of the infant's movements with the mother's voice with infants only a few hours old. In their classic study, these authors observed films of infants during the presentation of taped speech. They found that there was a relationship between distinct limb movements and speech.

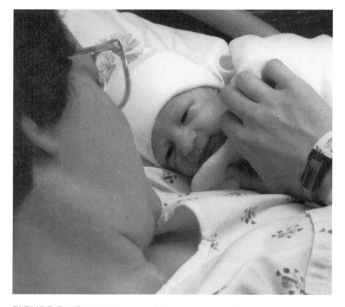

FIGURE 7–12   Newborn and Postpartum Mother in Entrainment

Klaus and Kennell suggest (1982) that the responses or signals put forth by the infant during entrainment are important elements in the formation of attachment. Brazelton (1963) says that these early communications with the infant help the parents begin to see their newborn as an individual and to adjust their own behaviors to the infant's signals. This premise of the importance of early social interaction with the neonate is challenged by the often necessary separations that occur during a preterm or at-risk birth, which will be discussed later.

COGNITIVE AND LANGUAGE DEVELOPMENT

The traditional areas of developmental accomplishment, cognition and language, are, for obvious reasons, difficult to definitively characterize in the neonate. We have discussed in Chapter 3 some of the **cognitive competencies** of the newborn, including the abilities of discrimination and recognition. Newborns have also been shown to respond to both classical and operant conditioning. Some studies have suggested that newborns can remember stories that they heard read aloud prenatally (DeCasper & Fifer, 1980). As discussed in Chapter 5, it is important to make a distinction between speech and language. *Language* is typically defined as a representation of cognitive structure. *Speech,* on the other hand, is only one mode of expression of language, using the vocal and oral mechanism. It is obvious that speech is mostly absent in the newborn, whose vocalization repertoire consists primarily of crying and sounds made during suckling. The extent of understanding the language of the newborn is more complicated and related to cognition. It appears that newborns are able to perform some of the functions of receptive language. However, expressive functions remain limited and are primarily of the nonverbal form of exchange.

ENVIRONMENTAL AND FAMILY ISSUES

The birth of a child is a significant life event. Svejda et al. (1982) suggests that one of the tasks of the first 4 weeks of life is the establishment of *biorhythmicity.* Anyone who has brought a newborn home from the hospital knows how completely the normal rhythms of life are disrupted for the first weeks. This, in combination with the normal hormonal fluctuations of the postpartum mother, usually creates some element of stress. In fact, the birth of a child has sometimes been referred to as a "life crisis." Subsequently, authors have used less dramatic labels for the so-called transition to home, but there is no one who would suggest that there is not

some element of stress in the situation. Rarely are the parents getting enough sleep, as the aforementioned biorhythms are in the process of being established. The postpartum mother is experiencing tremendous swings in hormones, which usually allow her to function through the transition but in some cases may result in more severe disturbances, such as *postpartum depression.* Fathers, on the other hand, are adjusting as well. They may feel the additional financial burdens of the new baby. A heightened sense of family responsibility may be felt. In addition, first-time fathers worry about factors such as the well-being of their wife and the new baby, how well they will make the transition to fatherhood, and how their relationship with their wife will change over time (McNall, 1976).

Cowan et al. (1978) suggested that irrespective of parental philosophy about gender roles, more traditional roles tend to emerge in the early postpartum weeks, with mothers spending more time with their infants in caregiving. However, Parke and Lamb both pioneered research on fathers and reported that fathers are capable of establishing attachments to their infants at around the same time as the mothers (Lamb et al., 1982). Furthermore, studies by Parke (1979) have shown that fathers are capable of responding to their infant's cues, interpreting infant signals, and feeding their infants effectively (see Figure 7–13). The term **engrossment** has been used to describe the sense of absorption, preoccupation, and interest that fathers have in their newborn (Greenberg & Morris, 1974).

In families where there are other children at home (i.e., the mother is multiparous), the postpartum adjustment of necessity must include the siblings (see

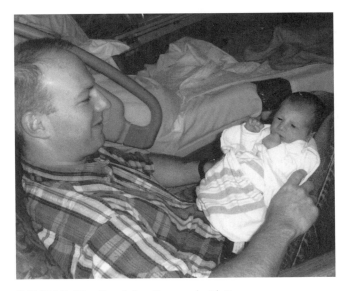

FIGURE 7–13   New Father Engrossed with Son

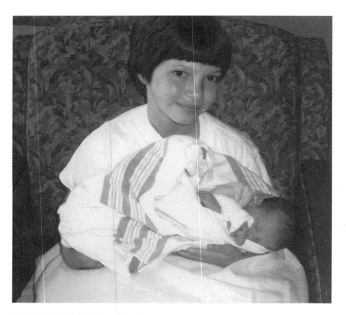

FIGURE 7–14   New Big Sister

Figure 7–14). Trause and Irvin (1982) summarize the research on sibling adjustment. For the most part, becoming a sibling is seen to be traumatic. A study by Legg, Sherick, & Wadland (1974) reported that most of the new siblings reported feeling negative emotions such as jealousy. There appears to be an age effect in that the younger the child, the more significant the problems.

Trause et al. (1981, 1977) were responsible for the early documentation of the return of dependence behaviors in new siblings under the age of 3. Despite this often challenging transition, in by far the majority of cases the family adaptation to the newborn occurs successfully, and the infant is integrated into the rhythms of family life.

GENDER AND CULTURAL ISSUES

Culture and gender issues are difficult to isolate specifically to the neonatal period. Most studies examine more than the neonatal period. With respect to gender, the preceding discussion identified some of the effects of parental gender on typical patterns of interaction with the newborn. What about the gender of the infant? **Gender issues** illustrate cultural practices. In some cultures the birth of a male infant is much more highly prized than the birth of a female infant. In Western cultures, traditional parents (defined as the father as the primary breadwinner and the mother as primary caregiver) tend to interact more with sons than with daughters. However, in one interesting study,

Lamb et al. (1982) reported that in nontraditional Swedish families, parents tended to interact more with daughters. The authors speculated that parents in nontraditional families possibly overcompensated for their perception that girls were traditionally given less attention than boys.

Cultural practices affect not only the birth process but the immediate postpartum period as well. The infant is shown to respond preferentially when the mother has ingested culturally typical food. This may be a way of acclimating the infant to normative food preferences for a given culture. There are also cultural differences in caregiving of the neonate. In some cultures, leaving the infant to cry for longer periods of time is valued to develop independence. In other cultures, such as American, infants are quickly picked up and soothed, rocked, and subjected to calming voices in speech and song. Japanese infants are said to have a more quiet temperament. Finally, contact with the parents is very different between cultures. In some cultures the infant is almost never physically separated from the mother, being carried on cradleboards and pouches. In Eastern cultures it is not uncommon for the infant to sleep with the parents, not only immediately after birth but for some time thereafter.

THE AT-RISK INFANT

Processes of neonatal development and the transition to extrauterine life are complicated in the normal circumstances surrounding birth. However, a number of infants fall into the category of "at-risk," which even further complicates this early period. Risk is traditionally thought of as arising from either biologic or environmental factors. **Biologic risk** is related to factors in the infant or the mother that are known to have potentially adverse consequences for the infant (Shonkoff & Phillips, 2000). Such risk factors include genetic problems, disease or disability in the mother or infant, maternal age, maternal smoking or drug use in pregnancy, **intrauterine growth retardation (IUGR),** and prematurity. IUGR describes infants who are born with low birth weight (less than 2500 grams) and are also **small for gestational age (SGA).** The SGA infant is an infant born at less than the 10th percentile for weight based on gestational age (Shepherd, Hanshaw, & Lane, 1999). **Environmental risk** is related to factors in the infant's environment that may have a potentially adverse effect on the infant, such as low socioeconomic status (SES), inadequate parental caregiving, neglect or abuse, poor nutrition, etc. (Shonkoff & Phillips, 2000).

Unfortunately for the infant, biologic and environmental risk factors often correlate. For example, there are definite biologic risks for the infant of a teenage mother who smokes during the pregnancy; however, environmental risks such as poor nutrition, low SES, and inadequate parental caregiving are not uncommonly associated with this scenario. Thus, biologic and environmental risk factors often combine and escalate the effects of each other to the detriment of the infant. **Protective factors** are those factors that help to ameliorate the risks. They may be either environmental (family support) or consitutional (physical attractiveness) (Shonkoff & Phillips, 2000).

Prematurity and associated sequelae will be dealt with at length in subsequent paragraphs. A brief review of some of the other risk factors is as follows. Obviously, **societal-level risk factors** such as teenage pregnancy and maternal drug and alcohol abuse are often discussed. The risk factor in a teenage pregnancy is first and foremost biologic. The immature physical development of the mother may affect the pregnancy, resulting in an infant that is born too small or too early. Likewise, the teen mother may not have adequate nutrition, both before and during the pregnancy. Few teenagers are conscious of eating a healthy diet, not only for them, but to sustain another life. Once the infant is born to a teenage mother, the baby is frequently brought home to the maternal home. Grandparents are often extended caregivers in the family system. The father may not be part of the family. If the father does try to assume a paternal role, he is frequently struggling to support the family financially. For teenage parents, who have their own developmental tasks to conquer, mastery of the superimposed task of parenting is often difficult to impossible.

SUBSTANCE ABUSE

By far the majority of research on risk has been done on the issue of substance abuse by the mother during pregnancy. The two general categories of substance abuse are alcohol and drugs. The effects of prenatal exposure to alcohol are well known and may be classified by effect. The first, and most serious, is *fetal alcohol syndrome (FAS)*. This syndrome is associated with characteristic physical features, microcephaly (small head), and often mental retardation. The second is called *fetal alcohol effects syndrome (FAES)*. In this case, the alcohol abuse by the mother was not as severe in either amount or duration as in the preceding case. Nevertheless, the infants may have softer neurologic signs, such as learning and attention problems or lowered IQ (Pierog, Chadavasu, & Wexler, 1977). The amount of alcohol required to produce these syndromes is surprisingly small, as little as 2 to 3 ounces per day (Moore, 2003).

Prenatal drug use has also been shown to affect the developing fetus, as manifested in the behavior of the newborn. The drug receiving the most emphasis in recent study is cocaine. Studies have clearly demonstrated short-term effects of maternal use of cocaine. **Cocaine-exposed infants** often show behavioral irritability, difficulty in quieting, and poor feeding (Phillips et al., 1996). Whether or not there are long-term effects on the infant of maternal cocaine abuse are less clear, but the preponderance of evidence suggests that most effects are in the neonatal period and that long-term effects, if any, are subtle. Furthermore, long-term effects of maternal cocaine abuse are difficult to separate from other socioeconomic variables.

Other drugs that have been studied include street drugs such as heroin. Infants born to mothers who are heroin addicts typically must go through drug withdrawal and display associated symptoms such as rapid breathing and irritability (Householder et al., 1982).

SMALL FOR GESTATIONAL AGE

The term *small for gestational age (SGA)* is used to describe infants born at less than the 10th percentile for weight. When infants are born low birth weight (less than 2500 g), and are also SGA, the term *intrauterine growth retardation (IUGR)* is used to describe the outcome. The consequences of IUGR have primarily been shown to relate to attentional and activity disorders; however, the outcome appears to interact with the support in the postnatal environment. In other words, environmental risk appears to bring out the tendencies for attentional disorders in infants who are IUGR, but a supportive environment may help minimize the consequences (Robson & Cline, 1998). IUGR reflects poor fetal nutrition during pregnancy. One common cause of IUGR is maternal smoking, which deprives the fetus of oxygenation.

HIV-EXPOSED

Over the past two decades the incidence of infants infected with HIV has increased dramatically, creating an international health crisis, particularly in some parts of the world, such as sub-Saharan Africa. The mechanism of transmission of the disease is believed to be from mother to infant through the placental circulation. Alternatively, fetal contact with the mother's blood and body fluids through vaginal delivery is another means of transmission. Infants who contract the HIV virus from the mother are considered HIV-exposed and have a high probability of developing full-blown pediatric AIDS in the first two years of life; however, identification in the neonatal period is not common because the presence of maternal antibodies may block identification (Rainville, 1999). If the virus is identified in the mother during pregnancy, it has been shown that drug therapy can decrease the likelihood of fetal infection (Grose, 1996).

THE PRETERM INFANT

The definition of term infant and preterm infant is a direct estimate of the duration of the pregnancy, dated from the mother's last menstrual period. This is called *gestational age*. Gestational age, or **postconceptional age,** is the common terminology associated with dating the age of the preterm infant. An infant is defined as preterm if born before the 37th week of gestation. A term pregnancy is considered 38–42 weeks gestation. The week discrepancy (37–38 weeks) is attributed to various classification systems. Prematurity must be considered in conjunction with birthweight. A birthweight less than 2500 g is considered *low birthweight (LBW)*. Therefore, many premature infants are also low birthweight. Infants weighing less than 1500 g at birth are considered to be *very low birthweight (VLBW),* and infants weighing less than 1000 g are considered to be *extremely low birthweight (ELBW)* (Shepherd, Hanshas, & Lane, 1999).

CHARACTERISTICS OF PRETERM INFANT

The preterm infant differs from the term infant in many important ways. First, there is the obvious **physiologic immaturity.** The most important body system in considering physiologic immaturity is the lungs. The development of the lungs in the last postnatal trimester in utero is in large part what enables the successful transition to extrauterine life at term birth. Conversely, when the infant is born too soon, the immaturity in the lungs creates a condition known as **respiratory distress syndrome (RDS).** Nearly all preterm infants have this condition, which is attributable to a lack of surfactant. A major improvement in care of preterm infants in the 1990s was the development and routine administration of an artificial surfactant, which helps to promote maturation of the lungs. Still, one of the more common adverse outcomes of prematurity is the development of a chronic lung condition known as **bronchopulmonary dysplasia (BPD).** BPD is a progressive scarring of the lungs creating a emphysematous-like function. The etiology of BPD is multifactorial, but probably related to prolonged ventilation of immature lungs; therefore, infants who do not wean well from the ventilator are considered to be at risk for this condition (Long & Toscano, 2002).

Other aspects of physiologic immaturity include the cardiac system. As stated earlier, the circulatory system in utero is one that involved a right-to-left shunt of blood, bypassing the lungs, which are not needed in the fetus since it receives all oxygenation through the placenta. Patent ductus arteriosus (a prolonged opening of the ductus) is not uncommon. This condition usually resolves itself with maturation but occasionally requires surgical intervention. Another condition exists when the shunting of the blood persists beyond the perinatal period. This is known as **persistent fetal circulation** (discussed earlier in this chapter), and is treated by aggressive oxygenation through special ventilators or through extracorporeal membrane oxygenation (ECMO). Because persistent fetal circulation is associated with diminished blood flow through the lungs, the vascular resistance in the lung capillary beds stays extremely high, creating a condition known as **pulmonary hypertension.**

The gastric system is also immature in the preterm infant. In particular, the sphincter that holds food in the stomach is often underdeveloped and weak. Thus, after the infant finishes feeding, the stomach contents can reflux into the esophagus, creating a heartburn-like condition known as **gastroesophageal reflux (GER)** (Long & Toscano, 2002). This condition is extremely common in premature infants and can produce behaviors such as incoordination in swallowing, feeding aversion, and arching. Since therapists often work with feeding problems in the nursery, these behaviors are important to identify. Treatment for GER ranges from very modest interventions to very aggressive. Typically, the first intervention attempted when GER is suspected is thickening of the feeds. Also, keeping the infant in a semi-upright position, by elevating the bed or placing the infant in a sling on a reflux board, is helpful. Antacid medications are also routinely prescribed. Finally, there is a surgery called a *Nissen procedure* that can be done to tighten the sphincter.

The musculoskeletal system of the preterm infant is noticeably different from that of the term infant, as can be seen by just walking into a room where infants are lying in their isolettes. The preterm infant is predominantly hypotonic prior to approximately 34 weeks gestational age. The development of muscle tone progresses from lower extremities to upper, in a caudal-cephalic direction. Claudine Amiel-Tison characterized the development of the preterm infant across three dimensions: passive tone, active tone, and reflex tone. Passive tone primarily defined the resting postures and resistance to passive movement of preterm infants. *Active tone* described normal righting reactions in horizontal and vertical suspension, and *reflex tone* described the postnatal evolvement of reflexes (Amiel-Tison, 1968). The tests of passive muscle tone are still in common use today and reflect the development of muscle tone. The skeletal system of the preterm infant is very malleable. This is especially important because if careful positioning is not done, the preterm can develop an elongated skull in the sagittal plane. This condition is sometimes referred to as *craniofacial molding.* Likewise, tightness in the shoulder girdle and external rotation of the hip can persist for some time after hospital discharge.

The nervous system of the preterm infant is also immature and can be susceptible to insult. One type of insult that is not uncommon results from a lack of oxygen due to asphyxia and is known as **hypoxic ischemic encephalopathy (HIE).** Fragile blood vessels near the ventricles of the brain can rupture, causing **intraventricular hemorrhage (IVH).** Another adverse outcome for the vulnerable nervous system is **periventricular leukomalacia (PVL),** characterized by necrosis and cavitation of the white matter of the brain. PVL may develop following a vascular insult such as IVH or in isolation, presumably due to some insult to the neural tissue (Long & Toscano, 2002).

The neurologic immaturity of the normal preterm infant can manifest itself in several ways. The preterm infant is more tremulous than the term infant, and *clonus,* a reflex that is a rhythmic alternation of muscular contraction and relaxation in response to quick stretch, is commonly seen. Specifically, behavioral states as a reflection of neurologic maturity are different in preterm versus term infants. Researchers have known for some time that sleep-state development in the preterm infant does not approach that of the term infant until after 32 weeks gestation, as recorded by EEG. In fact, active sleep patterns do not emerge until approximately 35 weeks gestational age and quiet sleep patterns until 37 weeks (Dreyfus & Brisac, 1970). Developmentalists such as Als have built upon the work of T. Berry Brazelton, expanding the concepts of the Brazelton assessment to attempt to describe the interactive maturity of the premature infant. Als described five developmental subsystems that are undergoing maturation through the synergy of a number of differing external and internal factors. These subsystems are autonomic (physiologic functioning), motor, state organization, attention or interaction, and regulatory. Als went on to describe the behaviors of the infant that signal engagement or disengagement across the various subsystems (Als, 1986). Early in the care of the preterm infant, the term *infant stimulation* was routinely used to describe environmental interventions aimed at promoting neural maturation as evidenced by maturing behavioral response. With greater understanding of the physiologic demands on the immature infant, the concept of infant stimulation has been largely abandoned in favor of the concept of *developmental care.* Developmental care is intervention that has the dual purpose of reducing aversive stimulation and promoting optimal behaviors through provision of opportunities for engagement with the environment (Young, 1996).

Finally, the visual system of the preterm infant is fragile and susceptible to compromise. One common problem associated with prematurity is **retinopathy of prematurity (ROP),** caused by ischemia, or lack of blood flow to the eyes. It can result in visual impairment and blindness (Mechoulam & Pierce, 2003). ROP is related to excessive oxygen levels that can lead to abnormal patterns of retinal vascularization and destruction of vascular endothelial cells (Claxton & Fruttiger, 2003). Currently, common treatments for ROP include laser surgery to remove the abnormal vascularization and promote normal vascular growth.

CHARACTERISTICS OF PRETERM INFANT ENVIRONMENT

Preterm infants are cared for in a very special environment known as the **neonatal intensive care unit (NICU).** NICUs are typically considered Level III nurseries, meaning that they have the ability to resuscitate infants. The intensive care in an NICU really refers to intensive nursing care. The nurse-to-infant ratio in a typical NICU is very low. Typically, after the infant "graduates" from intensive care, he moves on to a step-down unit (NSDU, or Neonatal Step-Down Unit), where the nurse-to-infant ratio is higher.

The necessities of medical caregiving in these nurseries create a very abnormal environment for the preterm infant, who normatively should be in a totally flexed position in a dark, aquatic environment. This environment provides multisensory stimulation. The lighting in an NICU is high, and in many cases there is no diurnal cycling of the lights as would occur in a normal environment. The high light has been suggested to affect the developing retina (Glass, 1990). In addition, studies have shown that infants react physiologically to the lighting in the environment. Gordon-Shogan and Schumann (1993) found, in a study using infants as their own controls, that rapid increases in lighting were associated with decrease in oxygen saturation. Many investigators have reported that when light-dark cycles are implemented, preterm infants tend to improve in physiologic and behavioral parameters (Young, 1996).

Noise is also an issue in the NICU. The noise in the nursery is largely caused by medical equipment. The isolette does not protect the infant from these noise levels, which have been likened to that of light traffic or machinery; however, noise levels in the nursery can peak at levels consistent with a busy airport. As in the case with light, the noise levels in the nursery have been shown to adversely affect both behavioral and physiologic parameters (Young, 1996).

Finally, patterns of caregiving involving somatosensory stimulation are unique in the NICU. Not surprisingly, the preterm infant is more likely to be touched for medical procedures (such as drawing blood, adjusting lines and leads) or physiologic caregiving (diaper change, positioning, turning) than in a social context (rocking, rubbing, skin-to-skin contact). Like other forms of stimulation, the typical handling of these infants can produce physiologic distress, including oxygen desaturation, apnea, decreased heart rate (bradycardia), and increased respiratory rate.

Minimal-Stimulation Protocols

The compilation of evidence of infant distress from handling has resulted in the common application of **minimal-stimulation protocols.** In these protocols, caregivers attempt to cluster caregiving procedures such that the infants have the ability to settle into quiet behavioral states and rest between disturbances (Young, 1996). Some studies have shown that by careful handling of preterm infants, including attention to positional support and infant behavioral cues, the amount of time in fretful behavioral states, with its associated physiologic costs, is reduced (Becker, Brazy, & Grunwalk, 1997). Another popular area of research, as mentioned earlier, is the effect of providing supplemental tactile stimulation such as massage on the preterm infant (Scafidi, et al., 1993; Field, Scafidi, & Schanberg, 1987). Another form of intervention in the NICU designed to promote more normative patterns of sensory and social stimulation is the concept of **kangaroo care,** where the infant is laid inside the parent's clothes in skin-to-skin contact. This procedure, conceptualized in Sweden, has been suggested to promote a thermal homeostasis for the infant without having to introduce abnormal stimulation through machines. Other advantages of kangaroo care are the skin contact and the social bonding with the parents (Bosque, 1995).

SOCIAL EFFECTS OF PRETERM BIRTH

In the 1970s, due to the work of a number of researchers, including Klaus and Kennell, the importance of parental contact with the infant in the immediate postnatal period was conclusively demonstrated (Klaus & Kennell, 1982). These studies have significantly changed labor and delivery room practices as well as hospital care by promoting the need of the infant and parents to have time together in the immediate postpartum period. However, these findings beg the question of the situation that is typical in preterm birth. In the preterm birth, the infant is typically resuscitated if necessary, shown to the mother, and whisked away to the NICU. The NICU is frequently in a different hospital, and the infant is transported by ambulance or helicopter, leaving the postpartum woman behind. Even in the relatively optimal situation where the NICU is in the delivery hospital, the medical needs of the infant result in maternal-infant separation almost immediately.

Parent-neonate separation is a prevalent problem associated with preterm birth. The short-term consequences of this separation are well documented. Parents of preterm infants report a wide range of psychological responses. One of these typical responses, **anticipatory grief,** occurs when parents are afraid that the infant will not survive, so engage consciously or subconsciously in protective behaviors. Examples of such behaviors might be choosing not to take advantage of visiting with their baby, delaying the naming of the infant, and not wanting to talk about the baby (Sweeney & Swanson, 2002).

Another response that is widely reported is a sense of lack of efficacy. **Efficacy** is the personal sense that you are competent and effective in your life roles. The mother of the preterm infant is seeking to reinforce her efficacy as a caregiver. Efficacy is reinforced when she is able to take care of her infant, including feeding, as well as to calm her infant when crying. Infants with irregular biorhythms or difficult temperaments, or who are poor feeders, do not promote these feelings of efficacy in their mothers, and this can lead to additional stress. Because these infants have so many medical needs that are attended to by professionals, the parents may feel detached and that they cannot take care of their baby. They report feeling as if the baby belongs to someone else. The separation that the parent of the preterm experiences is physical, as well as geographical. By physical separation, we mean that the medical caregiving equipment prevents the parent from holding, touching, and talking to the baby as would otherwise be done. Despite these short-term consequences, many parents of preterm infants do ultimately attach to their infant and place the NICU experience in perspective.

Professionals working with families in this vulnerable situation can help minimize the stress on the infants and families. Nurseries that provide a welcoming atmosphere to families, allowing them to stay at their infant's bedside, promote attachment. Professionals should be careful to instruct the parents in how to care for their infants and support parents in their early attempts at caregiving. It was shown by Culp, Culp, and Harman (1989) that parents who observed their preterm infant's performance on developmental assessment showed less anxiety and improved confidence in their ability to deal with their infant's cues. It has been shown that coping behaviors of parents of preterm infants can be enhanced by providing them with information and emotional support (Cusson and Lee, 1994). There are many ways that professionals interacting with preterm babies and their parents can promote positive interactions. These include helping parents to recognize their infant's cues, helping them with support groups after discharge, and teaching parents about play and caregiving strategies (Holloway, 1997).

SUMMARY

Much of the focus on the newborn centers on the maturation of body structures and body functions. The ability to participate as a family member emerges as the infant develops control over his physiologic functions. The life tasks associated with the neonatal period for both the newborn and the family are quite dramatic and cross all domains of behavior. It is remarkable that in most cases the challenges of birth and the neonatal period are successfully met with relatively little difficulty. There are, however, situations of both biologic and environmental risk that can negatively affect this life transition. Professionals working with neonates to promote positive outcomes for all concerned often focus on individuals in the infant's environment to foster the development of healthy and supportive relationships.

CASE 1

Elise

Elise is a 36-year-old woman. She waited to get pregnant and then sustained two miscarriages before having a baby, Joshua, who was born at 26 weeks gestation. The time in the neonatal intensive care unit was very difficult. Elise stayed away from her husband in the Ronald McDonald House of the teaching hospital where Joshua was born. That caused some family stress because her husband, John, wanted to be there and got frustrated at Elise's "hormonal" and emotional reports. Joshua had respiratory distress syndrome, and bronchopulmonary dysplasia developed. He was put on medicine for reflux. He had a small intraventricular hemorrhage (Grade II) on the right.

Elise was very frustrated by the fact that she couldn't hold Joshua. When she was finally allowed to try to feed him by mouth, two months after he was born, he displayed arching and fussy behavior, and she felt as if she couldn't take care of her own baby.

Eventually, Joshua's problems resolved, and he was discharged from the nursery, but he had to receive oxygen and be on a breathing monitor. The first few weeks at home, Joshua seemed to have no development of rhythmic patterns of sleeping and waking. He cried a good bit, and his voice sounded pathetic and raspy. When Joshua went back for his clinic visit 2 weeks after discharge, he hadn't gained any weight.

Joshua was discharged when he was approximately 40 weeks gestational age, but by that time he was chronologically 3½ months old. Elise wondered if Joshua was delayed because he didn't do anything that a 3-month-old baby would do. The pediatrician suggested a referral to an early intervention program to give Elise some support.

The therapist associated with early intervention did a developmental assessment when Josh was adjusted-age 1 month and found that his behavior was approximately that of a newborn. He seemed tired and listless and had a very significant head lag. The therapist suggested some positioning strategies and showed Elise how to swaddle Joshua. Some sensory techniques were attempted to try to calm him. The therapist showed Elise how attentive Joshua was to her face and voice when he was in a quiet behavioral state.

Over the next 6 months, Joshua was weaned off oxygen. He began to display the motor behaviors of his adjusted age. The therapist continued to come to the home and give suggestions about activities to do with Josh. Overall, however, John, Elise, and Josh are now doing much better and enjoying each other very much.

Speaking of

Practice in the NICU

MARYBETH MANDICH, PT, PhD
PEDIATRIC PHYSICAL THERAPIST

My first experience working with these special babies came when I was in graduate school. I walked into the Neonatal Intensive Care Unit (NICU) and was totally overwhelmed. The first baby I saw was large by today's standards—probably around 2000 g. But the baby looked so small to me! I remember picking up the baby to test head control and all the alarms went off. I nearly dropped the baby, and I thought I had done something really terrible.

Since that time, I have had a fascination with the world of these tiny babies born too soon. They should be in a flexed position, in a dark, aqueous environment, listening to their mother's heartbeat and muted voice. Instead, these babies are placed in the intensive care environment of lights, sounds, pinpricks, and monitors. I have always wondered what the world seems like to them and, also, what effects it has on them both immediately and long-term. It seems incomprehensible to me that this aberrant environment could not have some sort of impact on the baby.

One of the studies we did a few years ago really emphasized what I mean. As a therapist, I am interested in making life better for these infants, helping them to function in the environment. We did a study of infant swaddling and found that, as a result of something as simple as swaddling, the babies had a more positive behavior state for a greater proportion of the time. Likewise, it reduced their incidence of apnea and bradycardia. Something so simple, which caregivers have done for infants the world over, actually appears to have medical benefit. I listened to Dr. Kennell many years ago (of the Klaus and Kennell theory of maternal-infant bonding). He was discussing the positive effects on labor and delivery of having a woman, called a *duenna,* there to support the mother. The effects were remarkable. He later commented that if these effects had been a drug, everyone would want to know where to get it. But because it was a human intervention, people were hesitant to believe the results.

I think the same applies to the NICU. The simplest intervention can make life better for these babies. For that reason, I can't stop searching for those tiny things that we can do to help these precious little ones.

REFERENCES

Adams, R. J., Courage, M. L., & Mercer, M. E. (1994). Systematic measurement of human neonatal color vision. *Vision Research, 34,* 1691–1701.

Als, H. (1986). A synactive model of neonatal behavioral organization: Framework for the assessment of neurobehavioral development in the premature infant and for support of infants and parents in the neonatal intensive care environment. In J. K. Sweeney (Ed.), *The high-risk neonate: Developmental therapy perspectives* (pp. 3–53). New York: Haworth Press.

Amiel-Tison, C. (1968). Neurological evaluation of the maturity of newborn infants. *Archives of Disease in Childhood, 43,* 89–93.

Becker, P. T., Brazy, J. E., & Grunwalk, P. C. (1997). Behavioral state organization of very low birthweight infants: Effects of developmental handling during caregiving. *Infant Behavior & Development, 20,* 503–514.

Bosque, E. M. (1995). Physiologic measures of kangaroo versus incubator care in a tertiary-level nursery. *Journal of Obstetrical, Gynecological and Neonatal Nursing, 24,* 219–226.

Brazelton, T. B. (1963). The early mother-infant adjustment. *Pediatrics, 32,* 931–938.

Brazelton, T., & Nugent, J. K. (1995). Neonatal Behavioral Assessment Scale. *Clinics in Developmental Medicine (No. 137)* (3rd ed.). Philadelphia: J. B. Lippincott.

Claxton, S., & Fruttiger, M. (2003). Role of arteris in oxygen induced vaso-obliteration. *Experimental Eye Research, 77(3),* 305–311.

Cohen, L. B., DeLoache, J. S., & Strauss, M. S. (1979). Infant visual perception. In J. Osofsky (Ed.), *Handbook of infant development* (pp. 393–438). New York: John Wiley & Sons.

Condon, W. S., & Sander, L. (1974). Neonate movement is synchronized with adult speech: Interactional participation and language acquisition. *Science, 183,* 99–101.

Cowan, C., Cowan, P., Coie, C., & Coie, J. D. (1978). Becoming a family: The impact of a first child's birth on the couple's relationship. In W. Miller & L. Newman (Eds.), *The first child and family formation.* Chapel Hill: University of North Carolina Press.

Culp, R., Culp, A. M., & Harmon, R. J. (1989). A tool for educating parents about their premature infants. *Birth, 16,* 23–26.

Cusson, R. M., & Lee, A. L. (1994). Parental interventions and the development of the preterm infant. *Journal of Obstetric Gynecologic & Neonatal Nursing, 23,* 60–68.

DeCasper, A. J., & Fifer, W. P. (1980). Of human bonding: Newborns prefer their mothers' voices. *Science, 208,* 1174–1176.

DeCasper, A. J., & Prescott, P. (1984). Human newborns' perception of male voices: Preference, discrimination and reinforcing value. *Developmental Psychology, 17,* 481–491.

Eliot, L. (1999). *What's going on in there? How the brain and mind develop in the first five years of life.* New York: Bantam Books.

Fantz, R. L. (1961). The origins of form perception. *Scientific American, 204,* 66–72.

Fantz, R. L. (1963). Pattern vision in newborn infants. *Science, 140,* 296–297.

Field, T. M., Scafidi, F., & Schanberg, S. (1987). Massage of pre-term newborns to improve growth and development. *Pediatric Nursing, 13,* 385–387.

Freudigman, K., & Thoman E. (1994). Ultradian and diurnal cyclicity in the sleep states of newborn infants during the first two postnatal days. *Early Human Development, 38(2),* 67–80.

Glass, P. (1990). Light and the developing retina. *Documenta opthalmologica, 74,* 195–203.

Goldfield, E. F., & Wolff, P. H. (2002). Motor development in infancy. In A. Slater & M. Lewis (Eds.), *Introduction to infant development* (pp.61–82). Oxford, England: Oxford University Press.

Gordon-Shogan, M., & Schumann, L. L. (1993). The effect of environmental lighting on the oxygen saturation of pre-term infants in the NICU. *Neonatal Network, 12,* 7–13.

Greenberg, M., & Morris, D. (1974). Engrossment. The newborn's impact upon the father. *American Journal of Orthopsychiatry, 44,* 520–531.

Grose, C. (1996). Viral infections of the fetus and newborn. In W. E. Nelson, R. E. Behrman, R. M. Kleigman, & A. M. Arvin (Eds.), *Nelson's textbook of pediatrics* (pp. 523–527). Philadelphia: W. B. Saunders.

Harlow, H. F. (1958). The nature of love. *American Psychologist, 13,* 673–685.

Hepper, P. G. (2002). Prenatal development. In A. Slater & M. Lewis (Eds.), *Introduction to infant development* (pp. 39–60). Oxford, England: Oxford University Press.

Heriza, C. (1991). Motor development: Traditional and contemporary theories. In *Contemporary management of motor control problems* (pp. 99–126). Alexandria, VA: American Physical Therapy Association.

Holloway, E. (1997). Parent and occupational therapist collaboration in the neonatal intensive care unit. *American Journal of Occupational Therapy, 48,* 535–538.

Horak, F. B. (1991). Assumptions underlying motor control for neurologic rehabilitation. In *Contemporary management of motor control problems* (pp. 11–27). Alexandria, VA: American Physical Therapy Association.

Householder, J., Hatcher, R., Burns, W., & Chasnoff, I. (1982). Infants born to narcotic-addicted mothers. *Psychological Bulletin, 92,* 453–468.

Kaitz, M., Meschulach-Sarfaty, O., & Auerbach, J. (1988). A re-examination of newborns' ability to imitate facial expressions. *Developmental Psychology, 24,* 3–7.

Karen, R. (1994). Astonishing attunements: The unseen emotional life of babies. In *Becoming attached: Unfolding the mystery of the infant-mother bond and its impact on later life* (pp. 347–359). New York: Time-Warner Books.

Kawakami, K, Kurihara, H., Shimizu, Y., & Yanaihara, T. (1996). The effects of sounds on newborn infants under stress. *Infant Behavior and Development, 19,* 375–379.

Kedesky, J. H., & Budd, K. S. (1998). Assessment of environmental factors in feeding. In *Childhood feeding disorders* (pp. 79–114). Baltimore: Brookes.

Klaus, M. H., & Kennell, J. H. (1982). *Parent-infant bonding.* St. Louis: C.V. Mosby.

Klaus, M. H., Kennell, J. H., Plumb, N., & Zuehlke, S. (1970). Human maternal behavior at first contact with her young. *Pediatrics, 46,* 187–192.

Korner, A., & Thoman, E. (1970). Visual alertness in neonates as evoked by maternal care. *Journal of Experimental Child Psychology, 10,* 67–78.

Lamb, M. E., & Campos, J. J. (1982). Sensory and perceptual development. In *Development in infancy: An Introduction* (pp. 57–91). New York: Random House.

Lamb, M. E., Frodi, A. M., Hwang, C. P., Frodi, M., & Steinberg, J. (1982). Effect of gender and caretaking role on parent-infant interaction. In R. Emde & R. Harmon (Eds.), *The Development of attachment and affiliative systems* (pp. 109–118). New York: Plenum Press.

Legg, C., Sherick, I., & Wadland, W. (1974). Reaction of preschool children to the birth of a sibling. *Child Psychology & Human Development, 5,* 3–39.

Lindsay, D. (1996). *Functional human anatomy* (p. 447). St. Louis: Mosby.

Long, T., & Toscano, T. (2002). *Handbook of pediatric physical therapy* (2nd ed.). Philadelphia: Lippincott Williams & Wilkins.

Lundy-Ekman, L. (1998). *Neuroscience: Fundamentals for rehabilitation.* Philadelphia: W. B. Saunders.

McNall, L. K. (1976). Concerns of expectant fathers. In L. K. McNall & J. T. Galeender (Eds.), *Current practice in obstetrics and gynecology.* St. Louis: C.V. Mosby.

Mechoulam, H., & Pierce, E. A. (2003). Retinopathy of prematurity: Molecular pathology and therapeutic strategies. *American Journal of Pharmacogenomics, 3(4),* 261–277.

Meltzoff, A. N., & Borton, R. W. (1979). Intermodal matching by human neonates. *Nature, 282,* 403–404.

Meltzoff, A. N., & Moore, M. K. (1977). Imitation of facial and manual gestures by human neonates. *Science, 198,* 75–78.

Mendella, J., & Beauchamp, G. K. (1996). The human infant's response to vanilla flavors in mother's milk and formula. *Infant Behavior & Development, 19,* 13–19.

Moore, K. (2003). Human birth defects. In K. Moore, T. Persaud, & W. Schmitt (Eds.), *The developing human* (7th ed.) (pp. 167–201). Philadelphia: W. B. Saunders.

Morrongiello, B., Fenwick, K., & Chance, G. (1998). Crossmodal learning in newborn infants: Inferences about properties of audiovisual events. *Infant Behavior & Development, 21,* 543–554.

Nazzi, T., Floccia, C., & Bertocini, J. (1998). Discrimination of pitch contours by neonates, *Infant Behavior & Development, 21,* 779–784.

Parke, R. M. (1979). Perspectives on father-infant interaction. In J. Osofsky (Ed.), *Handbook of infant development* (pp. 549–590). New York: John Wiley & Sons.

Phillips, R. B., Sharma, R., Premachandra, B. P., Vaughn, A., & Reyes-Lee, M. (1996). Intrauterine exposure to cocaine: Effect on neurobehavior of neonates. *Infant Behavior & Development, 19,* 71–81.

Pierog, S., Chandavasu, O., & Wexter, I. (1977). Withdrawal symptoms in infants with fetal alcohol syndrome. *Journal of Pediatrics, 90,* 630–633.

Rainville, E. B. (1999). Prenatal and perinatal risk factors. In S. M. Porr & E. B. Rainville (Eds.), *Pediatric therapy: A systems approach* (pp. 22–60). Philadelphia: F. A. Davis.

Robson, A., & Cline, B. (1998). Developmental consequences of intrauterine growth retardation. *Infant Behavior & Development, 21,* 3331–3344.

Scafidi, F. A., Field, T. M., & Schanberg, S. M. (1993). Factors that predict which pre-term infants benefit most from massage therapy. *Developmental & Behavioral Pediatrics, 14,* 176–180.

Schaal, B., Montaganer, H., Hertling, E., Bolzoni, D., Moyse, A., & Quichon, R. (1980). *Les stimulations oflactives dans les relations entre l'enfant et la mere. Reproduction, Nutrition, Development, 20,* 843–858.

Shepherd, J. T., Hanshaw, J. K., & Lane, S. J. (1999). Working in the neonatal intensive care unit. In S. M. Porr & E. B. Rainville (Eds), *Pediatric therapy: a systems approach* (pp. 313–378). Philadelphia: F. A. Davis.

Shonkoff, J. P., & Phillips, D. P. (2000). *From neurons to neighborhoods: The science of early childhood development.* Washington, DC: National Academy Press.

Shumway-Cook, A., & Woollacott, M. (2001). *Motor control: Theory and practical applications* (2nd ed.). Philadelphia: Lippincott, Williams & Wilkins.

Slater, A., VonderSchulenburg, C., Brown, E., Badinock, M., Butterworth, G., Parsons, S., & Samuels, C. (1998). Newborn infants prefer attractive faces. *Infant Behavior & Development, 21,* 345–354.

Spence, M., & Freeman, M. (1996). Newborn infants prefer the maternal low-pass filtered voice, but not the maternal whispered voice. *Infant Behavior & Development, 19,* 199–212.

Svejda, M. J., Pannabecker, B. J., & Emde, R. N. (1982). Parent-to-infant attachment: A critique of the early "bonding" model. In R. Emde & R. Harmon (Eds.), *The development of attachment and affiliative systems* (pp. 88–93). New York: Plenum Press.

Swaiman, K. F., & Ashwal, S. (1999). *Pediatric neurology: Principles and practice* (3rd ed.). St. Louis: Mosby.

Sweeney, J. K., & Swanson, M. W. (2001). Low birth weight infants: Neonatal care and follow-up. In D. Umphred (Ed.), *Neurological rehabilitation* (4th ed.) (pp. 203–258). St. Louis: Mosby.

Thelen, E., & Fisher, D. M. (1982). Newborn stepping: An explanation for a "disappearing" reflex. *Developmental Psychology, 18,* 760–775.

Thelen, E., & Spencer, J. P. (1998). Postural control during reaching in young infants: A dynamic systems approach. *Neuroscience and Biobehavioral Reviews, 22* (4), 507–514.

Trause, M. A., & Irvin, N. A. (1982). Care of the sibling. In M. Klaus & J. Kennell (Eds), *Parent-infant bonding* (pp. 110–130). St. Louis: C. V. Mosby.

Trause, M. A., Boslett, M., Voos, D., Rudd, C., Kennell, J. H., & Klaus, M. H. (1977). A birth in the hospital: The effect on the sibling. Abstract #70 in *Pediatric Research, 11,* 383.

Trause, M. A., Voos, D., Rudd, C., Klaus, M., Kennell, J., & Boslett, M. (1981). Separation for childbirth, The effect on the sibling. *Child Psychology & Human Development, 12,* 32–39.

Walton, G. E., Armstrong, E. K., & Bower, T. G. R. (1997). Faces as forms in the world of the newborn. *Infant Behavior & Development, 21,* 537–543.

Walton, G. E., Bower, M. J., & Bower, T. G. (1992). Recognition of familiar faces by newborns. *Infant Behavior & Development, 15,* 265–269.

Wilhelm, I. (1993). Neurobehavioral assessment of the high-risk neonate. In I. Wilhelm (Ed.), *Physical therapy assessment in early infancy* (pp. 35–70). New York: Churchill Livingstone.

Young, J. (1996). *Developmental care of the premature baby.* London: Bailliere Tindall.

CHAPTER 8

Infancy

MaryBeth Mandich, PT, PhD
Professor and Chairperson
Division of Physical Therapy
West Virginia University
Morgantown, West Virginia

Objectives

Upon completion of this chapter, the reader should be able to

- Describe the developmental tasks of the infant across all domains of performance.

- Name the major behavioral milestones of each period of infancy.

- Describe the characteristic reflexes and reactions associated with each period of infancy and discuss how these relate to motor behavior.

- Discuss the interaction between domains of performance, such as the relationship between object permanence and stranger anxiety.

- Identify why a thorough knowledge of developmental sequence is important for therapists.

- Identify and discuss the social roles of the infant, including a thorough definition and discussion of the concept of attachment and its implications.

- Define developmental delay and discuss its significance.

Key Terms

abnormal development	lateral pincer grasp	raking
astasia	locomotor pattern	righting
balance	mature rotary neck righting	stereotypy
body-on-body righting	myelin	stranger anxiety
body-on-head righting reaction	optical righting reaction	superior pincer grasp
cruising	plasticity	symmetrical tonic neck reflex
developmental delay	posture	(STNR)
equilibrium	postural control	synapse
equilibrium reactions	postural set	toddling
hypotonia	prehension	transfer pattern
inferior pincer grasp	protective reactions	

INTRODUCTION

The term *infancy* is used here to describe the period of life from birth through 12 months of age. It is a time of rapid physical growth as well as rapid developmental maturation. The newborn is largely dependent, although able to exert more control over the environment than once was thought. However, by the end of infancy, the child shows significant environmental mastery across multiple domains of behavior. The near total gravity-dependency and limited mobility of the newborn are replaced at 1 year by an ability to move from place to place and manipulate objects in the environment. The limited communication skills of the newborn are replaced at 1 year of age by the purposeful use of language as a communication skill. Finally, by 1 year of age, the infant has adopted a clear social role, with characteristic temperament and a style of interaction with both family and others.

The processes that underlie this change in the 1st year of life are both intrinsic and extrinsic. The normally developing infant will experience maturation and growth in all body systems. However, it is the incredibly rapid maturation of the *central nervous system (CNS)* that is especially important in the first year of life. This CNS maturation supports much behavioral change over the 1st year (Eliot, 1999). Despite the important role played by innate functions, the effect of the environment is not to be underestimated (Scarr, 1992). The role of environment in infancy is evident in many ways. First, cross-cultural study of different caregiving practices demonstrates their impact on infant development (deVries, 1999; Shonkoff & Phillips, 2000). Second, studies of infants who have had negative environmental experiences through deprivation, abuse, or overstimulation confirm the fact that such experiences negatively

impact developmental acquisition of behavior (Hakimi-Manesh, Mojdehi, & Tashakkori, 1984; Chang & Merzenich, 2003; Teicher et al., 2003). Finally, many studies, both animal and human, confirm the interaction effect of environmental experiences and neural maturation (Eliot, 1999; Johnston et al., 2001).

The 1st year of life is a remarkable and fascinating time in the human lifespan. Professionals working with children who are developing normally or who have special needs derive great satisfaction from the opportunity to have an impact on the human potential represented by the infancy period.

PHYSIOLOGIC CHANGE AND GROWTH OVER THE 1ST YEAR

In the 1st year of life, growth continues at a very rapid rate. The average male infant grows 6.75 inches (17.2 cm), and the average female grows 3.25 inches (7.1 cm). These measurements represent an increase in length of approximately 50 percent (Payne & Isaacs, 1999). The average male infant weighs 7.5 lbs (3.27 kg), while the average female infant weighs 7 lbs (3.23 kg) (Payne & Isaacs, 1999). Infants tend to lose some of their birthweight in the first postnatal days and return to birthweight by the end of the second week. By 5–6 months birthweight has doubled, indicating a rate of growth of approximately 1 ounce per day. In the second half of infancy, weight gain slows down to about ½ ounce per day. By the end of the first year, typically, birthweight has tripled (Payne & Isaacs, 1999). The newborn's head is a greater proportion of the body than at 1 year.

The newborn's heart rate ranges from 120 to 140 beats per minute but slows over the 1st year to approximately 80 to 100 beats per minute. Blood pressure in the infant is also lower than in the adult. Normative blood pressure at birth is around 80/55, and the systolic pressure increases gradually so that at 1 year normal blood pressure is approximately 95–100/55 (Choukair, 2000).

THE 1ST YEAR OF LIFE: AN OVERVIEW

The 1st year of life is commonly subdivided into periods of 2 to 3 months. These periods are defined by characteristic accomplishments. In this text, development during the first 12 months is organized into four

time frames, each consisting of 3 months. These periods of 3 months are defined as early infancy (birth–3 months), middle infancy (4–6 months), late infancy (7–9 months), and infancy transition (10–12 months). Within each period, accomplishments are categorized and discussed according to domains typically associated with development. These domains are gross motor, fine motor/adaptive behavior, person-social behavior, and cognitive-language. A summary of development over the 1st year across these periods may be found in Table 8–1 (Long & Toscano, 2002; Infant Development, retrieved on March 28, 2004 from http://www .envisagedesign.com/ohbaby/develop.html).

TABLE 8–1	Summary of Development During 1st Year of Life

EARLY INFANCY: Birth through 3 Months

Gross Motor	Fine Motor	Oral-Motor	Cognitive-Language	Personal-Social
Present: ATNR; tonic labyrinthine; labyrinthine righting Behavior: • Lifts head in prone (NB) • Lifts head 45 degrees (1–2 mo.) • Lifts head 90 degrees (2–3 mo.) • Increasing extension at rest • Predominantly asymmetrical (NB) • Total head lag in pull-to-sit (NB), which decreases (1–3)	Present: ATNR; palmar grasp reflex; upper extremity traction Behavior: • Hands closed most of the time with spontaneous opening (NB) • Hands swipe at mouth (NB) • Inserts hand in mouth and sucks (1) • Hands open (1–3) • Grasps object placed in palm briefly	Present: Suck-swallow reflex; phasic bite reflex; rooting Behavior: • Suckling pattern • Bottle/breast-fed • Vigorous suck • Coordinates suck, swallow, and respiration	Behavior: • Cries • Coos • Vocalizes when not crying • Chuckles	Behavior: • Cries to communicate • Calms to human face and voice • Visual tracking Not across midline (NB) Across midline 180 degrees (3 mo.) • First smile (2–3 mo.)

MIDDLE INFANCY: 4–6 Months

Gross Motor	Fine Motor	Oral-Motor	Cognitive-Language	Personal-Social
Integrated: All primitive reflexes ATNR, TLR, palmar grasp, stepping, supporting Appears: Body-on-body righting Rotary neck righting Protective extension down and forward Prone equilibrium	Integrated: Palmar grasp Behavior: • Hands are closed at rest less of the time • Hands to midline in play (4) • Grasps object placed in palm (4)	Integrated: Rooting reaction Phasic bite reflex Behavior: • First spoon feeding: Upper lip not active (4) • Disassociation of lips, tongue, jaw begins with true sucking (4)	Behavior: • Secondary circular reactions—infant acts on environment to prolong interesting experiences • Disyllabic utterances • Increase in sounds produced	Behavior: • Early play • Infant shows delight • Laughs and chuckles

Continues

TABLE 8–1	Summary of Development During 1st Year of Life *Continued*

MIDDLE INFANCY: 4–6 Months   *Continued*

Gross Motor	Fine Motor	Oral-Motor	Cognitive-Language
STNR Behavior: • Rolls prone to supine, supine to prone (4–6) • Full prone extension (6) • Lifts head and helps in pull-to-sit (5) • Midline behavior: hands and feet to mouth • Sits propped (5–6) • Supported standing with weight bearing	• Predominantly ulnar palmar grasp (5–6) • Reaches (5–6) • Rakes (5–6)	• Voluntary suck: increased negative pressure in oral cavity (4) • Upper lip activates in removing food from spoon	• Babbling begins (5–6)

LATE INFANCY: 7–9 Months

Gross Motor	Fine Motor	Oral-Motor	Cognitive-Language	Personal-Social
Integrated: STNR Appears: Protective extension; side (7–8); backwards (9–10); sitting equilibrium (7–8) Behavior: • Sits erect independently (7–8) • Commando crawls (7–8) • Assumes sitting (8–9) • Pushes to hands and knees (8–9) • Rocks in hands and knees (8–9) • Quadruped may begin (9)	Behavior: • Radial palmar grasp (7) • Lateral pincer grasp (8–9) • Voluntary release	Behavior: • Eats well from spoon (7) • Early solids, uses munching pattern (7–9)	Behavior: • Babbles clear vowel-consonant sounds • Secondary circular reactions (4–8) change to coordination of secondary reactions (8–9) • Aware of ability to manipulate environment • Object permanence develops	Behavior: • Shows anger and fear • Will protest if caregiver leaves • Demonstrates early signs of caregiver attachment • Becomes an "emotional being"

TRANSITIONAL INFANCY: 10–12 Months

Gross Motor	Fine Motor	Oral-Motor	Cognitive-Language	Personal-Social
Appears: Equilibrium quadruped (9–10); Standing (11–12)	Behavior: • Inferior pincer grasp (10–11) • Pincer pad-to-pad grasp (11–12)	Behavior: • Eats solids with tongue lateralization	Behavior: • First true word (11–12) • Babbles more sounds	Behavior: • Shows an attachment style • Stranger anxiety

Continues

TABLE 8–1	Summary of Development During 1st Year of Life *Continued*

TRANSITIONAL INFANCY: 10–12 Months *Continued*

Gross Motor	Fine Motor	Oral-Motor	Cognitive-Language
Behavior: • Assumes and maintains quadruped (10) • Creeps on hands and knees (10–11) • Pulls to stand (10–11) • Cruises at furniture (10–11) • Walks with two hands held, then one hand held • Walks independently	• Superior pincer tip-to-tip grasp (12)	• Appearance of diagonal and rotary jaw movement	• Object permanence more secure • More sophisticated means-end relationships

EARLY INFANCY: BIRTH TO 3 MONTHS—AN OVERVIEW

The first 3 months of life are a transition period for the infant (and the family). The changes that occur over the first 3 months are cumulative but not dramatic. The infant is laying the groundwork for the remarkable achievements of the ensuing months. In motor development, there is increasing postural extension and increasing ability in antigravity control, especially of the head and arms. The arms develop and begin to explore space. Early communication progresses from crying to gurgling and cooing. The infant gets to know Mom and Dad and begins to clearly express preferences. The infant's cognitive development is mostly manifested through attention, visual fixation and following, and habituation to familiar stimuli.

GROSS MOTOR DEVELOPMENT

As previously discussed, the newborn's movements are heavily influenced by the deep *attractor wells* of behavior otherwise known as *reflexes*. Antigravity behavior in prone is limited at birth to lifting and turning the head from side to side (Figure 8–1A). Over these first months, this ability improves significantly, so that by 4 months of age, the head can be lifted up to 90 degrees, and the infant is able to look around. Concurrent with this improved head control in prone, the infant's arms begin to prop, so that by 4 months, her elbows are

tucked under her body, and she lifts up on elbows to look around (Figure 8–1B). These abilities coincide with the diminishing influence of the tonic labyrinthine pattern in prone and the increasing labyrinthine righting abilities.

In supine, the newborn is once again gravity-dependent. Grasping his forearms and pulling him to a sitting position while assessing the righting of his head usually tests the amount of antigravity control he has from the supine position. At birth, in the pull-to-sit, there is nearly complete head lag (Figure 8–2), but by 4 months of age the infant shows minimal head lag.

Once the newborn is sitting, her head will fall forward on her chest, but brief periods of righting are seen; however, by the end of early infancy, sitting with head stable and upright is seen (Figure 8–3A).

In the upright position, when the baby is held in vertical suspension, righting against gravity likewise develops over the first 3 months of life. At birth, the influence of the supporting reaction produces a successive extension of the lower limbs without true weight-bearing support. The newborn when held in supported standing also displays a rhythmic alternating stepping movement (Figure 8–4). These stepping patterns are similar in kinematic characteristics to the patterns of supine kicking, and it has been proposed that early kicking and stepping are similar patterns differing only in postural set in which they occur (Thelen & Fisher, 1982). Using Thelen's terminology, patterns such as kicking/stepping have been referred to as stereotypies. A **stereotypy** is an intrinsic nonpurposeful movement

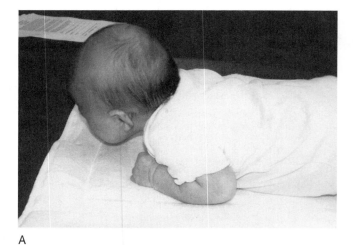

A

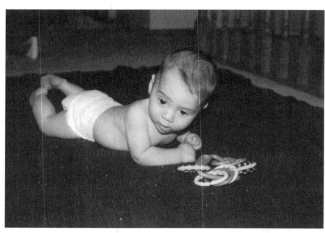

B

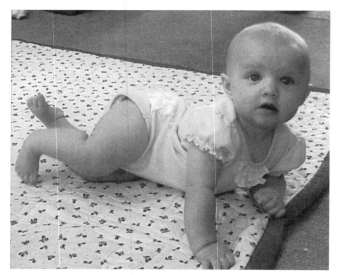

C

FIGURE 8–1   Maturation of Prone Behavior: A, 1–2 Months; B, 3–4 Months; C, 4–5 Months

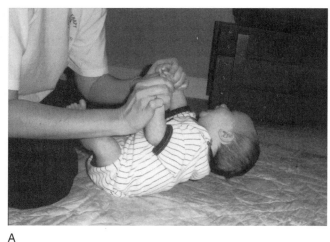

A

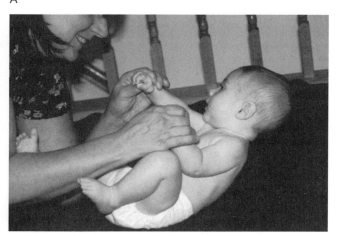

B

FIGURE 8–2   Decrease in Head Lag in Pull-to-Sit: A, Newborn; B, 5 Months

pattern that repeats itself. It appears to be intrinsic and therefore does not depend on sensory feedback to be elicited (Payne & Isaacs, 1999).

FINE MOTOR DEVELOPMENT

The development of hand function ultimately serves the function of **prehension.** Prehension is the use of the hands for grasping, holding, and manipulation of objects. In order to accomplish a prehensile task, several components are necessary. These include the ability to approach the object in space, known as *reach;* the ability to position and close the hand around the object, known as *grasp;* the ability to move the object while it is held, known as *manipulation;* and the ability to release the object when desired (Duff, 1995). These different components of fine motor control mature variably over the first year, with grasp being one of the earliest functions, beginning as a reflex and progressing to increasing volition. At birth the hands are predominantly

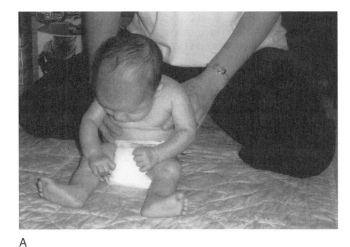

A

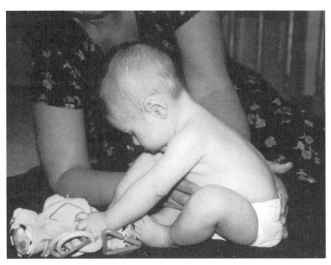

B

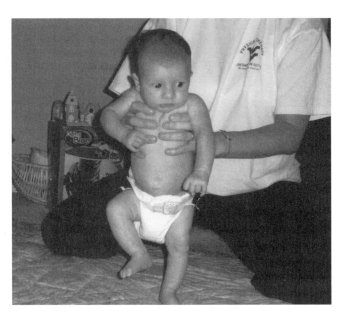

FIGURE 8–4   Reflexive Stepping Behavior in Newborn

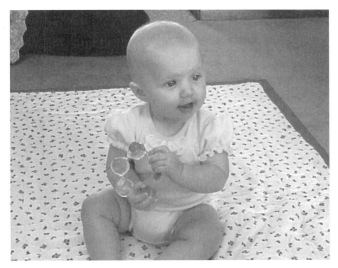

C

FIGURE 8–3   Maturation of Sitting Behavior: A, Newborn (Supported); B, Increasing Extension at 4–5 Months; C, Sits Erect at 6–8 Months

fisted, but the pattern is never obligatory in the normal case. The infant's hands will open spontaneously. In addition, the infant will swipe at the mouth, sometimes inserting the entire fist in the oral cavity. Typically, it takes a few months for the infant to truly engage in thumb-sucking behavior, although occasionally this is seen perinatally. Throughout the first 3 months, he increasingly keeps his hands open, so that by 4 months of age, his hands are open most of the time.

In the newborn, grasp is reflexive and nonfunctional. The newborn's fingers will close around an object when pressure is applied across the metatarsal heads, but there is no volitional release and hence the object cannot be held for any purposeful use. This grasp reflex is shown in Figure 8–5. It gradually diminishes over the first few postnatal months.

Likewise, at birth there is no purposeful reaching pattern, although there is believed to be a kind of reaching called *visually triggered reaching*. This means that early in life the infant is able to see a target and will attempt to approach the target with her arms (Shumway-Cook & Woollacott, 2001). The newborn has semidirected swipes, usually at the mouth, as described previously. By 3 months of age, she has more directed swipes, batting at objects placed above the head in preparation for true reach; however, the hands are largely open as the arm is extended, making grabbing of the object impossible. Thelen describes these waving motions of the arms as an example of a stereotypy involving upper extremities (Payne & Isaacs, 1999). Near the end of early infancy, the infant begins to be able to sustain grasp on an object placed in the hand.

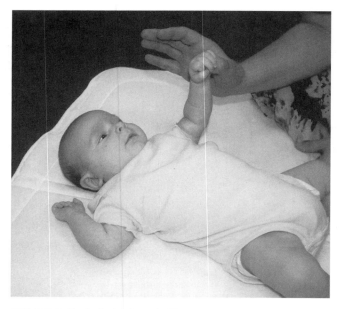

FIGURE 8–5   Reflexive Grasp in Newborn

ORAL-MOTOR DEVELOPMENT

The neonate demonstrates the suckling pattern, as described in Chapter 7. The suckling pattern exemplifies the developmental principle of general-to-specific in that there is little disassociation of lips, tongue, and jaw in this pattern. Likewise, the neonate shows the reflexive behaviors described previously of phasic bite, suck-swallow, and gag. Most infants are bottle- or breast-fed through the first months. Even if cereal is introduced in this period for medical reasons or reasons of convenience, it is often mixed with the formula in the bottle. The young infant is not an efficient spoon-feeder. The major occurrence in oral-motor behavior between birth and 3 months is the increasing volitional aspects of the suck-swallow pattern. There is better lip closure, and the infant will demonstrate mouth opening and anticipatory behaviors as the bottle approaches his mouth (Koontz-Lowman & Lane, 1999). Concurrent with these changes, there is an increase in negative pressure in the oral cavity, which is the beginning of the transition to a mature suck pattern.

COGNITIVE AND LANGUAGE DEVELOPMENT

The production of sound is related to oral-motor development in that the muscle control developed early in feeding also underlies the production and differentiation of sounds. At birth the infant's primary means of communication is the cry. During crying, the mouth is open and the tongue is observed to shape and cup, much as it does in feeding. With increasing control of lips, tongue, and jaw through the first few months, the infant begins to vocalize. The earliest vocalization, occurring around 1–2 months of age, are cooing and gurgling sounds usually used to indicate pleasure during feeding. By the end of the early infancy period the infant is typically using open-mouth, monosyllabic utterances (Long & Toscano, 2002).

Cognitive development in the 1st year of life is difficult to assess and is largely judged indirectly through observation of behaviors. From a Piagetian perspective, the first 3 months of life comprise the reflexive stage and primary circular reactions. In the *reflexive* stage of the first month, infants respond to the world based on prewired responses to stimulation, as in the sucking reflex when an object is placed in the mouth. However, as the infant enters the stage of *primary circular reactions,* the hallmark of repeating interesting actions occurs. This may start very simply, as the infant might begin to repeat actions such as sucking or looking at hands in order to maintain an interesting phenomenon.

Historically, it was initially thought that infants had very little cognitive capability—in fact, the tradition was to view the infant as functioning at a subcortical level of the nervous system, primarily due to observation and interpretation of motor behavior. However, research done beginning in the mid-twentieth century has changed this view significantly. During the fetal period, between 100 and 200 billion nerve cells or neurons are formed (Feldman, 1999). The first 2 years of life are critical for brain development. During that period the nerve cells establish elaborate connections with each other, called synapses. A **synapse** is the junction across which a nerve impulse passes from an axon terminal to a neuron, muscle cell, or gland cell. The pattern of synapse formation is related to environmental experience in both human and animal studies (Eliot, 1999). The first 2 postnatal years are thought of as a time of synaptic sculpturing, with the formation of new synapses being only one important component. Another important component is the dormancy or disappearance of other synapses and neurons, according to their pattern of use. Therefore, provision of a nurturing and supportive environment for infants is extremely important in determining their ability to maximize their innate potential.

In addition to the formation and disappearance of synapses, the nervous system also changes in another significant way in early life. The processes of nerve cells are encased in a fatty, or lipid-based, substance known as **myelin.** Myelin helps speed nerve conduction, and the first 2 years of life are the time when most of the myelin develops. In addition to adequate environmental stimulation, adequate nutrition is also especially important in the first 2 years of life, since an inadequate diet can disrupt the formation of myelin, thereby negatively influencing neural and behavioral development (Eliot, 1999).

In light of new knowledge about the nervous system, as well as newer, more sophisticated studies of infant development using experimental paradigms such as habituation and physiologic monitoring, much more information is available about what the infant "knows." In early infancy, visual acuity and visual tracking improve. By 4 months of age, the infant is able to visually track across midline consistently. He continues to prefer patterns with high contrast, such as black and white, but by the end of the period, there is indication that he can make distinctions between lights of different wavelength and begin to perceive color in groupings similar to those of adults (Teller & Bornstein, 1987). Using a checkerboard with various numbers of squares, a number of researchers have demonstrated that infants prefer patterns of increasing complexity with increasing age (McCluskey, 1981). In general, it is also thought that over the first few months, the infant begins to respond less with a defensive reaction to a novel stimulus—such as a light, unexpected touch—and more with an approach, or orienting, response (Resiman, 1987).

PERSONAL-SOCIAL DEVELOPMENT

At birth the newborn will show emotions, especially distress due to physical discomfort. Over the first 3 months, she will begin to show increasing periods of positive affect, including turning toward a pleasurable stimulus (Sroufe, 1996). By the end of the period, she is clearly showing social pleasure by smiling. Infants are able to differentiate between their mother and a stranger within the first weeks of life (Masi & Scott, 1983). Infants in the first few months are capable of imitating activities that are already in their behavioral repertoire, such as opening of the mouth or sticking out the tongue.

Temperament and interaction style are relatively stable aspects of infant behavior. Infants have been classified as *externalizers,* who have a great deal of facial expression and low physiologic reactivity, and *internalizers,* who have a relatively flat affect but are highly physiologically reactive (Field, 1990). Chess & Thomas have developed a classification of three main temperament types: easy, difficult, and slow-to-warm-up. An *easy* baby shows curiosity in novel situations, high rhythmicity in behaviors such as sleeping and eating, and moderate emotional intensity. In contrast, a *difficult* baby will have moods that are more negative and be less adaptable in general. A *slow-to-warm-up* baby shows less activity and is relatively calm; however, this baby would approach a novel situation with withdrawal and shows more negative affect than the easy baby (Feldman, 1999). The sensitivity and reactivity to people and events in the environment that constitute temperament here been

shown to be relatively stable over time and hence are probably heavily attributable to innate processes (Field, 1990).

MIDDLE INFANCY: 4–6 MONTHS— AN OVERVIEW

The period of 4–6 months of age is one of major change in motor behavior. In gross motor behavior, the infant learns to master antigravity control in both prone and supine. The first independent sitting occurs, as does the first transfer of postural set from prone to supine and supine to prone. The infant develops functional use of the hands, and is able to reach and grasp an object with a characteristic palmar grasp. Near the end of the period, the infant may be beginning to transfer objects from hand to hand. In language, a greater variety of sounds is produced, including disyllabic utterances. The infant begins babbling during this period. Cognitive development is seen in activity on the environment, especially activity designed to prolong interesting phenomena. These are the secondary circular reactions. By 6 months, the infant is developing object permanence. In personal-social development, he expresses joy and delight and engages in early play activities, such as peek-a-boo (Table 8–1).

GROSS MOTOR DEVELOPMENT

In the middle infancy period there is a significant change in gross motor ability, both in terms of posture and in terms of mobility. Because motor behavior rapidly grows more sophisticated, it is worthwhile to discuss some terminology that will be helpful in describing further motor development. Motor behavior is generally the result of muscle contraction. Exclusive of smooth and cardiac muscle, which will not be discussed here, motor behavior usually produces two functional consequences: holding or moving. **Posture** is the alignment of the body at any given point in time, including both biomechanical and neuromotor elements. **Postural control** is the ability to maintain the body in a position by keeping the center of gravity over the base of support or returning it over the base of support following displacement, for the dual purposes of orientation and stability (Payne & Isaacs, 1999; Shumway-Cook & Woollacott, 2001). There are two classifications of postural control—static and dynamic. *Static postural control* is the ability to sustain or hold a quiet position, whereas *dynamic postural control* is the ability to maintain alignment of body parts during movement.

Balance is another word for postural stability, which is when the body is maintained in equilibrium at rest (static equilibrium) or during movement (dynamic equilibrium) (Shumway-Cook & Woollacott, 2001). **Postural set** is the alignment of body parts at any given point in time. The process of bringing the body parts into alignment is known as **righting** (Van Sant, 1995). The process of reestablishing the center of mass over the base of support once displaced is known as **equilibrium.**

Postural patterns control the alignment of the center of mass over the base of support and the relative alignment of body parts. Mobility patterns perform one of two functions. The first type of mobility pattern is a **transfer pattern.** A transfer pattern permits the person to transfer or translate from one postural set to another, as in going from lying down to sitting up or from prone to supine. A **locomotor pattern** moves, or translates, the entire body through space, as in crawling or walking. At birth the infant's motor repertoire is very limited. Postural control is reflected only in very brief periods of righting the head in the postural sets of prone and sitting. Also, at birth there are no mobility patterns of either the transfer or locomotor types. The infant is very dependent on the caregiver for these functions. We have seen how over the first 3 months of life, the infant's postural control develops in various postural sets so that by the beginning of the 4th month, he is able to prop up in prone on elbows, lifting the head and maintaining control. In supported sitting, he is able to maintain the head in a stable position, and in pull-to-sit, his head no longer lags. There is increasing symmetry in the supine posture as well. By the beginning of the 4th month, he can bring hands to midline and keep the head in midline to explore them. However, through the end of this period, he is still dependent in transfer and locomotor patterns.

In the 4th through the 6th month, the infant makes dramatic gains in motor ability across all the dimensions described. In this period, all the early dominant patterns of posture and movement, characterized by deep attractor wells, such as the tonic labyrinthine, asymmetrical tonic neck, grasp, stepping, and grasp reflexes, have been integrated. As this occurs with maturation of neuromotor and musculoskeletal systems, more functional motor behavior is permitted. Some characteristic patterns develop that underlie these new abilities, many of which appear at 4–6 months of age.

A series of righting reactions mediated by the CNS appear fully in the period of 4–6 months. The purpose of these righting reactions as a group is first of all to orient the head (and body) in space and the body parts with respect to each other and, second, to rotate the body parts into alignment with each other. The first, labyrinthine righting, has been defined as movement of the head into alignment with gravity in response to position in space, as detected by the vestibular system of the inner ear. Labyrinthine righting appears at birth in the limited abilities of the infant in antigravity

control, but it is fully mature by the 6th month. A related reaction, **optical righting,** serves the orientation function of postural control, by positioning the head in response to the visual environment. The **body-on-head righting reaction** rotates the head into alignment with the body or the surface on which the body is lying. These righting reactions all serve a postural function, whereas the other two righting reactions are known as *rotary righting reactions,* which serve a mobility function. The early neonatal neck righting reaction is replaced by **mature rotary neck righting** in this period. The stimulus for rotary neck righting is rotation of the head and neck, in which the body de-rotates back into alignment. **Body-on-body righting** is similar, but in this case a rotary stimulus is applied along the long axis of a limb segment, and the body de-rotates into alignment. Figure 8–6 illustrates body-on-body righting as rotation among body parts.

As a group, these righting reactions are present in the period of 4–6 months and reflect changes in neural maturation. Traditional thinking was that the emergence of these reactions was a determinant factor in the coincident emergence of postural control. However, contemporary thought in the systems model identifies changes in the neuromuscular response patterns as only one of several reasons for changes in behavior underlying milestone acquisition. Other factors to be considered include changes in the musculoskeletal system, maturation of sensory systems, and development of organizational strategies to process sensory input and development of internal representations to map these inputs. There is sound preliminary evidence that the emergence of milestones as traditionally reported is related to the postural set assumed in testing—in other words, that postural set interacts with the motor skill, and that when infants are

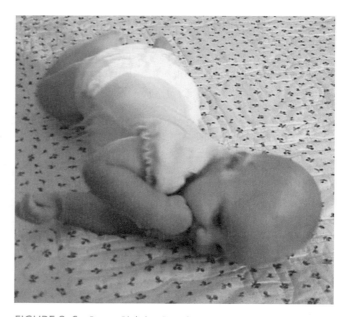

FIGURE 8–6   Rotary Righting Reactions

put in different postural sets, the skill that may be observed is different. Simply put, an infant may be able to demonstrate reaching easier in supported sitting than in supine. Furthermore, there is evidence that some of the postural reactions can respond to training (Shumway-Cook & Woollacott, 2001). Taking all current information into account, it appears that the development of the postural reactions, such as righting, plays a role in the acquisition of motor milestones; however, the role represents just one component of a complex system and is not as determinant as was once believed.

There are two other sets of postural reactions that contribute to balance. The first are the **protective reactions.** Protective reactions are also known as *parachute reactions,* indicating that these reactions provide a safety response for the child. The stimulus that elicits these reactions is consistent—a displacement of center of mass such that the body cannot recenter over the base of support. In this case the arms come out in extension to catch or protect the proximal body parts. The parachute reactions develop in a prescribed sequence, the first one being in response to downward displacement at approximately 5 months of age, followed by the anterior protective extension response at about 6 months of age (Shumway-Cook & Woollacott, 2001; VanSant, 1995)

The final set of postural reactions, which serve the function of balance, are the **equilibrium reactions.** These reactions, unlike the protective reactions, come into play in an attempt to reestablish the center of mass over the base of support in displacement. They have a very characteristic appearance. When a person's center of mass is displaced, the trunk responds by curving sideways against the direction of the displacement. Meanwhile, the limbs on the side that the displacement occurs are increasing their tone for weight bearing. The opposite arm and leg abduct. These equilibrium reactions also develop sequentially, with the prone reaction the first to appear at approximately 5–6 months of age (Shumway-Cook & Woollacott, 2001).

In terms of motor behavior, then, the infant's behavior is no longer dominated by primitive patterns with deep attractor wells. The righting reactions have all developed, as well as protective extension forward and down and the earliest equilibrium reaction. One observable change is increasing antigravity postural control. From 4 months, when the infant is able to prop on elbows, the infant begins to lift up even higher in prone, propping on hands by 4–5 months of age (Figure 8–1C). By 6 months of age, when held in horizontal (prone) suspension, the infant performs total antigravity extension, traveling through the hips. This pattern is known as the *Landau reaction* (Figure 8–7), which is at least in part a combination of the postural righting reactions (Shumway-Cook & Woollacott, 2001). This mastery of total antigravity control is

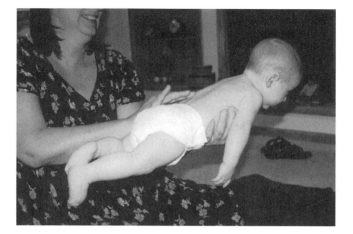
FIGURE 8–7 Landau Reaction at Approximately 5–6 Months

considered critical in some therapies, and is also known as the *pivot prone pattern* or *prone extension pattern.*

The infant's antigravity control in supine also changes dramatically from 4 to 6 months. By 4 months, the infant can keep the head in midline and engage hands, but by 5 months or so, she can also bring feet to midline and will often play with hands and feet to mouth (Figure 8–8).

This ability reflects increasing antigravity or flexor postural control in supine. Likewise, when the infant is pulled to sitting beginning at about 5 months, he actually anticipates that movement and lifts his head in an attempt to help (Figure 8–2B). Antigravity control also manifests itself in sitting. The infant's spine, initially rounded in supported sitting during early infancy, now begins to show extension. At 4 months, the extension of neck and cervical spine is evident, but by 6 months, the extensor posture has traveled into the thoracic and lumbar spines, showing the normal lordotic curves in the cervical and lumbar spine (Figure 8–3B). The first independent sitting typically occurs around 5 months of age. This sitting uses the arms for support, with the infant's legs positioned Indian style. One final "reflex" of postural tone appears in this period. This is the

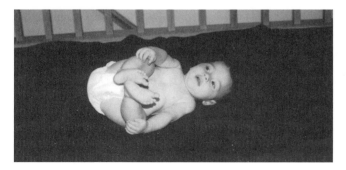
FIGURE 8–8 Hands-to-Feet Behavior at 4–5 Months

symmetrical tonic neck reflex (STNR). Like its ATNR counterpart, the stimulus for the STNR is position of the head as detected by joint receptors in the neck. However, in this case, the head is flexed or extended. The response is for the arms to follow the postural attitude of the head and the legs to do the opposite. For example, when the neck is flexed, the arms flex and the legs extend. When the neck is extended, the arms extend and the legs flex. As shown in Figure 8–9, it is easy to see how the posture of the latter position relates to the earliest independent sitting (head extended, arms extended, legs flexed).

In standing, the infant performs an interesting transition during 4 to 6 months. Recall that the earliest standing is heavily reflexive, with the infant requiring a great deal of extrinsic support and bearing little true body weight. In the transition to upright control and true weight bearing, the infant early in this period displays **astasia,** which means "without stance." In this pattern the infant draws up legs and feet when attempts are made to place her in supported standing (VanSant, 1995). Parents will often interpret this pattern as the infant wishing to play a "jumping" game. During middle infancy, astasia disappears, and there is true weight bearing with an increasingly erect stance (VanSant, 1995).

With respect to mobility patterns of transfer, the infant in middle infancy develops the first ability to change from one postural set to another with rolling. Rolling occurs in prone when the infant, who has been experimenting increasingly with postural control in prone on elbows by shifting weight, actually shifts weight enough to accomplish a complete transition,

combined with the increasing rotation of body segments.

Traditional milestones for American infants give the first roll as occurring from prone to supine at 4–5 months and subsequently supine to prone at 5–6 months (Figure 8–10). Cultural practice may influence this sequence, however, as American babies are now spending more time in supine due to the "Back to Sleep" public health initiative. This initiative was aimed at reducing the incidence of *sudden infant death syndrome (SIDS),* because major epidemiologic studies show that countries where people have always placed infants in supine to sleep have a lower incidence of SIDS than do countries where infants are placed prone.

Davis et al. reported on a prospective study of 351 infants who slept in either prone or supine positions. This study found that earlier attainment of motor milestones was associated with prone sleeping, including rolling prone to supine, sitting propped, creeping, crawling, and pulling-to-stand. However, there was no significant difference according to sleep position in the age of walking (Davis, Moon, Sachs, & Ottolini, 1998).

In summary, it seems that there is a variability in attainment of early postural and mobility milestones that is affected by sleep position, but that this age of attainment does not adversely affect developmental outcome. In any case, by 6 months of age, the infant is rolling freely from prone to supine and back. Locomotor patterns that move the body through space have yet to develop; however, a precursor pattern often appears during this period. This pattern is a prone or abdominal pivot in which the infant raises up on hands,

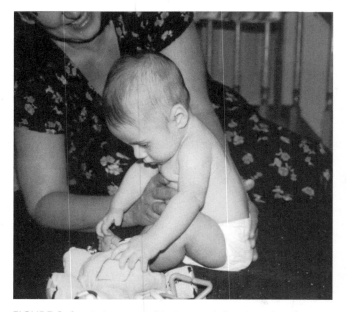

FIGURE 8–9 Sitting Propped in Symmetrical Tonic Neck Reflex Position

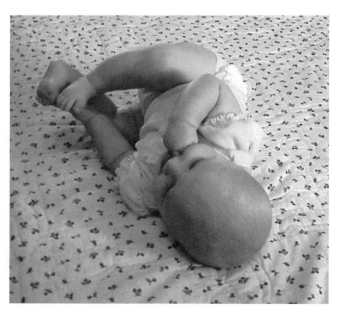

FIGURE 8–10 Rolling

and turns in a circle, bending the arms and legs on one side of the body.

FINE MOTOR DEVELOPMENT

There is also remarkable change in the function of the arms and hands in the second period of middle infancy. At 4 months the infant begins to display a greater variety of hand movement patterns. He is able to grasp and hold on to objects placed in the hand. At 5 months, he can grasp a one-inch cube with a *primitive squeeze grasp,* using all the fingers without active use of the thumb. In this primitive squeeze grasp, the wrist is usually flexed, which occurs because the hand is often extended beyond the object, which is approached laterally, with all fingers closing around the object to the palm (Shumway-Cook & Woollacott, 2001). By 6 months, the infant is grasping with a similar palmar grasp, but with wrist neutral. Typically these early grasp patterns are oriented primarily to the ulnar side of the hand. In addition, sometime around 5–6 months the infant begins to show the pattern of **raking,** in which a small object such as cereal or a raisin is approached with open hands and fingers, which cover the object like a rake, then attempt to sweep the object into the palm by closure of fingers. By the end of the period, some investigators indicate that infants can perform a primitive transfer of a cube from one hand to another. This is an early indicator of release, because one hand can release the object as the other grasps it (Duff, 1995). By 6 months, the infant is usually able to hold the bottle with both hands as well.

Reaching also becomes much more functional at this time, with the appearance of visually guided reaching. Whereas *visually triggered reaching* is important in the initiation of reach by prospectively seeing an object and initiating reaching, *visually guided reaching* is feedback-dependent. Visually guided reaching requires the coordination of proprioceptive information from the hands with the visual inputs (Figure 8–11). Visually guided reaching develops in the second period, concurrent with improved postural and upper extremity control (Shumway-Cook & Woollacott, 2001). This means that by 6 months of age, the infant is able to reach and obtain an object such as a cube that is offered.

ORAL-MOTOR DEVELOPMENT

The oral-motor pattern used for sucking from the bottle is changing in middle infancy. Because lips, tongue, and jaw no longer move as a complete unit, or are disassociated, the jaw is able to stabilize for the nipple, with the lips forming a tight seal. This generates increased negative pressure in the oral cavity, and the pattern becomes true sucking as opposed to the suckling pattern of early

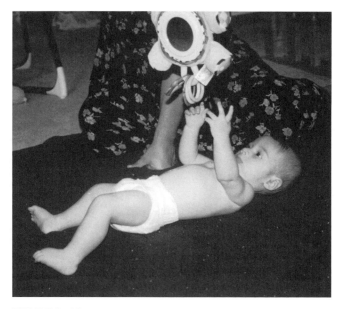

FIGURE 8–11   Reaching (for Toy)

life, which depends largely on positive pressure or expression. Likewise, the sucking pattern comes under voluntary control around 4 months of age.

It is around 4 months that the first spoon-feeding is offered, usually infant cereal. The infant approaches the first spoon-feeding with an immature repertoire of movement, stroking the tongue forward and back out of the mouth in an attempt to manage the bolus of food. The upper lip is initially not active in scraping the food off the spoon; rather, the caregiver usually scrapes the spoon off the upper gums to remove the bolus. Using this rather inefficient pattern, a great deal of the food is often lost onto the chin. By the end of this period, 6 months of age, the upper lip becomes active to sweep food off the spoon, and spoon-feeding becomes more efficient. By this time the infant's diet includes stage-one baby foods, which are of consistently pureed texture. The infant will also demonstrate food preferences at this time.

The first teeth often appear at around 6 months (Kedesdy & Budd, 1998). In part depending on this acquisition, solid food may be offered to the infant. If this is done, the infant is able to bring the food to mouth and perform an early munching pattern, using an up-and-down jaw motion. Likewise, it is highly variable whether the infant has been presented a cup this young, but if the infant has, an attempt to suckle liquid from the cup with ensuing liquid loss is usually the result.

COGNITIVE/LANGUAGE DEVELOPMENT

The sounds that are emitted in this period of middle infancy have a much greater variety and typically begin to be bisyllabic rather than monosyllabic babbling.

Initially infants babble the sounds heard in all languages, but they begin to refine their babbling to the speech sound of their own language by 6–7 months. Sound becomes a form of secondary circular reaction, which is the Piagetian period encompassing 4–6 months. In secondary circular reactions the infant volitionally repeats activities that produce interesting results. Unlike primary circular reactions, which are primarily focused on the infant, secondary circular reactions are focused largely on the environment, as the infant learns that things can be controlled. For example, during this stage, infants begin to notice that the sounds they make influence what happens in the environment; therefore, they repeat interesting sounds (Feldman, 1999). Infants also engage in outright laughter during social exchanges.

The cognitive acquisitions of the 4–6 month infant also include repetitive actions on objects in the environment. The infant may squeeze, pat, or shake an object in order to produce interesting sounds. Near 6 months the infant begins to experiment with the object permanence concept. *Object permanence* is the realization that objects continue to exist once they are outside the direct visual field. By 6 months the infant is able to obtain a partially hidden object and may begin to experiment with object permanence by purposefully dropping something and watching to see what happens.

PERSONAL-SOCIAL DEVELOPMENT

In the 4–6 month period, the infant, as already stated, will express delight, laughter, and joy during social exchange (Figure 8–12). There is early play across affective, vocal, and motor dimensions (Sroufe, 1996). The reciprocal exchange in interactions, which was rudimentary in the early months, is now fully developed. It is during this period that games like patty-cake and

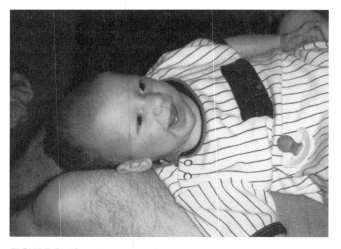

FIGURE 8–12 Infant Is Social Participant and Expresses Pleasure

peek-a-boo usually begin. Although the infant's role is mostly of delighted observer at this early stage, these are important aspects of early play. In addition, in this period infants show a clear preference for parents or caregivers, although when the caregiver leaves, the infant is easily distracted and consoled (Lamb & Campos, 1982).

LATE INFANCY: 7–9 MONTHS: AN OVERVIEW

In late infancy the infant is able to manipulate objects with hands while in a stable sitting position. She also develops the first mobility pattern, allowing translation from place to place. Grasp becomes refined enough to pick up small objects, and she is able to hold two objects at once, as well as transferring objects from hand to hand. The infant displays clear babbling sounds, typically including "Mama" or "Dada," or both, but the sounds are not yet discretely applied to the appropriate person. The infant can begin to use tools to manipulate, and object permanence is a key cognitive construct that is developing in this period. Concomitant with the development of object permanence, the infant begins to show increasing distress when the caregiver leaves or when a stranger appears. The infant is now an emotional being.

GROSS MOTOR DEVELOPMENT

The period of late infancy is one in which the infant makes great strides in transfer and locomotor ability, establishing security in postural sets that are progressively up against gravity. At the beginning of this period the infant is able to perform the abdominal-pivot locomotor pattern but is not able to crawl from one place to another. Around 7 months of age, he develops the ability to crawl with belly on the floor. This belly-down type of locomotion is known as *belly crawling* or *commando crawling* (named after the type of locomotor pattern used by soldiers). This is the first true locomotor pattern.

In terms of postural set, the infant at the beginning of this period was already sitting, but arms were used as props or supports. Around 7–8 months of age, she develops the ability to sit upright without using hands for support (Figure 8–3C). This subsequently allows the hands to be free for manipulation when sitting. The development of sitting erect coincides with the appearance of the sideways protective reactions, and the sitting equilibrium reactions develop shortly thereafter. The infant will be able to sit erect for a while before posterior protective extension reactions develop, usually around the 9th month (Figure 8–13).

As evident in Figure 8–14, the maturation of sitting balance allows the infant to lean forward and return to

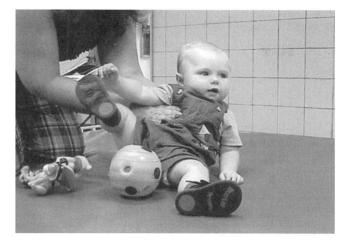

FIGURE 8–13   Protective Extension Side/Back

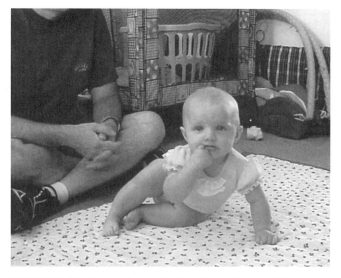

FIGURE 8–15   Rotary Pattern Used to Get to Sitting Position

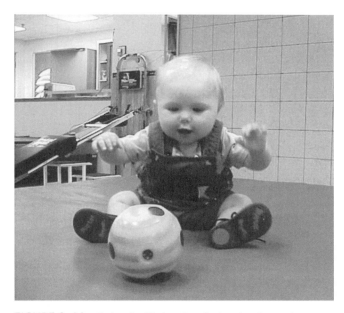

FIGURE 8–14   Sitting Equilibrium Permits Leaning Forward

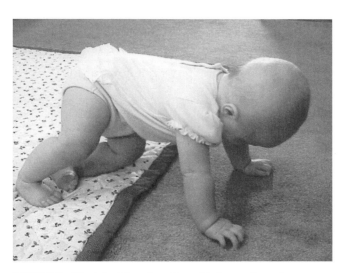

FIGURE 8–16   Infant Experimenting with Assumption of All-Fours Position

upright without balance loss. Note also that he is able to sit erect before he is able to assume the sitting position.

The transfer from lying to sitting positions usually occurs around the 8th month, and is heavily rotary in nature (Figure 8–15). The infant's limited abdominal muscle strength, in addition to body shape, precludes symmetric sit-up patterns at this early age.

In prone, while the early locomotor pattern of crawling is being perfected, the infant is also progressively pushing up against gravity. She pushes up on hands and attempts to flex the hips and knees under the body. Initially, this is a crude attempt, and she often falls forward onto her arms; however, gradually she is able to coordinate the demands of the quadruped position (Figure 8–16). These demands include a stable

horizontal trunk with flexion at hips, knees, and shoulders, but extension of elbows and wrists. Often, as the infant seeks stability in the all-fours, or quadruped, position, it will appear as if he is rocking forward and backward (Figure 8–17). This quadruped rocking is practice of graded eccentric and concentric closed kinetic chain muscle activity, which is representative of the sort of activity demanded of the lower limb for gait. The ability to perform a locomotor pattern in quadruped develops usually around 9–10 months.

The terminology that is associated with these early locomotor patterns is unfortunate. To the lay public, the quadruped locomotor pattern is often referred to as crawling; however, developmentalists use the term *creeping* to describe the all-fours pattern, and *crawling* is reserved for the earlier belly-down pattern (Payne &

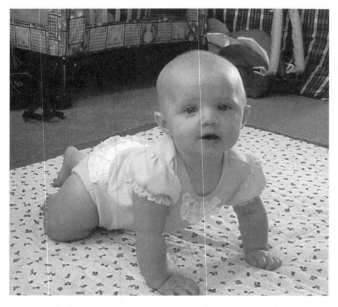

FIGURE 8–17   Infant Who Has Mastered All-Fours Position

Isaacs, 1999). A simple convention for individuals working with children to use is simply to describe the pattern more fully, as in "belly-down crawling" and "all-fours creeping" to avoid confusion.

FINE MOTOR DEVELOPMENT

The fine motor development of late infancy is especially significant with respect to prehensile function of the hands. It is during this period that two important phenomena occur: one is disassociation of thumb and fingers, with increasing activity of the thumb, and the second is a progressive movement radially of grasp functions. Around 7 months of age the infant's palmar grasp begins to move radially, with the force of the grasp occurring more on the radial than the ulnar side of the hand. By about 8 months the infant is able to refine the raking pattern of the 6-month-old and can grasp a small object such as a raisin with the pad of the thumb to the side of the index finger. This may be thought of as a **lateral pincer grasp.** This use of the thumb in opposition provides humans with the myriad sophisticated hand activities that are characteristic. It has been said that 40 to 70 percent of normal hand function is provided by the opposition of the thumb (Duff, 1995).

Another key element of hand function in this period is release. Voluntary release occurs in the 7–9 month period, and the infant will begin to enjoy games that involve placing objects in containers and then dumping them out to start the game over again (Duff, 1995). The disassociation of the fingers allows the infant to isolate the index finger, and during this period

she will poke at a small object of interest (Koontz-Lowman & Lane, 1999). This isolation of the index finger is also used for pointing, which can serve as a form of communication. The combined effect of these developments in fine motor function is the ability to play and manipulate toys (Figure 8–18).

ORAL-MOTOR DEVELOPMENT

In the period of late infancy, solid foods are introduced. The infant is quite effective in eating from a spoon, and the upper lip is active. The activity of the upper lip in general produces a stronger seal on the bottle. Overall, there is increasing disassociation and control of lips, tongue, and jaw. The infant mouths almost every object that is presented, in part in an effort to decrease discomfort associated with teething. Cup drinking is still inefficient, although there is less liquid loss. As mentioned previously, the first solid food is presented in this period. The infant can hold the soft cracker or teething biscuit and bring it to his mouth, holding his jaw closed over the soft solid until a piece is bitten off. Chewing is nonrotary, and jaw movement is an up-and-down movement known as *munching*. This munching pattern is in part a reflection of the fact that the tongue is not yet actively lateralizing, or moving food from side to side in the mouth. If food is placed in the mouth laterally, however, the infant is able to lateralize the tongue, and some rotary-diagonal jaw movement appears (Koontz-Lowman & Lane, 1999).

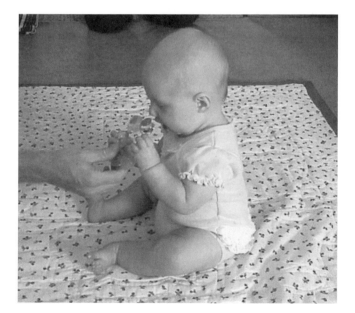

FIGURE 8–18   Proximal Gross Motor and Advancing Fine Motor Control Allow Playing with Toys

COGNITIVE-LANGUAGE DEVELOPMENT

In late infancy language development has progressed to clear babbling of the sounds of the spoken language. In English, "Ma-ma" or "Da-da," or both, are usually heard, although often not yet applied specifically as names of the parents. As mentioned earlier, the first sounds represent primary circular reactions, in which the infant will repeat an interesting sound just to hear it again. Babbling in part represents secondary circular reactions. The infant continues to experiment with interesting sounds, and begins to use the sounds to control the environment. This raises an interesting question regarding language development. It takes nearly 1 year for the first true word to be uttered. What takes the infant so long to attain this milestone? There are two potential sources of complexity in language development that impact the length of time it takes to acquire words. The first is the *phonology,* or the complexity of the sound production. It has been estimated that more than 70 muscles and eight to ten body parts must be directed under neural control to utter a one-syllable word (Acredolo, Goodwyn, Horobin, & Emmons, 1999). The second source of complexity is the *cognitive structure development* that underlies the purposeful use of patterns of sound as language. During this time, the infant passes from secondary circular reactions into a coordination of secondary schema.

This phase of coordination of secondary circular reactions is marked by several key factors. Beginning at about 8 months, with the onset of this stage, the infant begins purposeful manipulation. As part of this stage, the infant will push one toy out of the way to reach another toy that is lying underneath it (Feldman, 1999). Object permanence begins to develop in earnest in this period. For example, the infant will search for a toy that is hidden while he is watching. The development of object permanence also has large implications for personal-social milestones, including demonstration of negative affect around strangers. These two major changes—searching for hidden objects and becoming upset around strangers—represent a large behavioral shift that indicates an increasing ability on the part of the infant to coordinate present and past events using memory processes (Sameroff & Cavanagh, 1979).

The 7–9-month-old infant also is developing in sensory-perceptual areas. For example, in the classic "visual cliff" experiment, infants were allowed to crawl over a plexiglass surface with a checkered pattern underneath. At some point, the pattern drops away from the surface, giving the illusion of the "cliff." Infants as young as 6–7 months would not crawl over the cliff (Gibson & Walk, 1960). Further studies have shown that the development of depth perception is related to the cortical developments that support binocular vision (Eliot, 1999).

PERSONAL-SOCIAL DEVELOPMENT

The concept of object permanence is a major cognitive foundation for the development of attachment and for reactivity to strangers, which begins in this period of late infancy. Before this time, the infant demonstrates an "out of sight, out of mind" worldview with respect to parents or other caregivers leaving. This worldview begins to change at about 7 months of age, and infants begin to protest the departure of specific people, especially parents. At this time they are initially unwilling to be consoled by substitutes, a behavior that has been called *separation protest* (Lamb & Campos, 1982).

Another factor that influences personal-social development in late infancy is the increasing mobility of the infant. Before 7 months, the infant would be unable to attempt to sustain contact by any means other than crying. However, in this period, she has some form of prone locomotion, so it is possible to try to follow the parent or caregiver upon leaving. This behavior of trying to maintain or prolong contact with the caregiver will emerge fully in the next phase.

During this period, the infant will become more fully engaged as a social being. He will interact with other infants by attempting to touch them and by increasing vocalizations. He will also purposefully initiate interactions with the caregiver, explore the caregiver by touching his or her face, and attempt to manipulate interactions (Sroufe, 1996).

By 9 months, the infant is an "emotional being" (Sroufe, 1979). This term reflects the fact that the infant now has become sensitive to the meaning of events. The infant from 7 to 9 months will begin to demonstrate the emotion of anger. For example, anger may be expressed when an expected consequence does not occur. Fear, as mentioned previously, also begins to appear in this period, particularly when a stranger is introduced. The fact that the infant shows distress to specific stimuli, will use affect as a motivation, and will seek help for maintaining an interesting game or experience all support the idea of this major developmental milestone of becoming an emotional being occurring in this phase.

INFANCY TRANSITION: 10–12 MONTHS—AN OVERVIEW

At the beginning of the transition period from the 10th to the 12th month, proficiency in quadruped mobility is developing. By the end of this period, at 12 months, the infant typically takes the first steps. It will take some time before gait and postural mechanisms mature to adult-like patterns. Grasp is secure, and the infant can pick up even the smallest object. She is independent with finger-feeding and drinks from a cup. The first word is also said sometime in this period. She also displays clear maternal or caregiver attachment behaviors at this time, and stranger anxiety is a typical phenomenon.

GROSS MOTOR DEVELOPMENT

The infancy transition period represents the culmination of an extremely rapid progression of gross motor milestone acquisition. At the beginning of infancy transition, the infant has successfully pushed into the all-fours, or quadruped, position and rocks. As he gains stability in this position, the ability to sustain quadruped emerges, followed shortly by the locomotor pattern of hands-and-knees creeping. Not all children progress through this period. One study reported that 82 percent of normal infants used creeping on all fours as their pre-walking locomotor pattern. Other patterns identified included *shuffling* in a sitting position, rolling, and belly-crawling. About 7 percent of infants did not demonstrate any pattern before they initiated walking.

Some of the infants who did not use the all-fours locomotor pattern showed a transient hypotonia, especially those in the belly-crawling, sitting, and shuffling classifications. **Hypotonia** is a condition of diminished state of muscle tension and diminished resistance of muscles to passive stretching. These hypotonic infants walked later than the infants who performed quadruped creeping or who skipped the phase entirely (Robson, 1984).

From these and similar data, it may be concluded that it is not necessary to pass through the quadruped creeping phase in order to develop standing and walking. However, failure to do so, especially if using the alternative patterns, may be associated with delayed onset of walking. Furthermore, some children who have impaired motor control may show a preference to avoid the quadruped creeping pattern; despite that fact, the pattern has elements that might prove to be of therapeutic benefit. For example, children who would benefit from this pattern in particular are children with Down syndrome, who need to develop the rotary movement and graded control, and children with hemiplegia, who need to develop bilateral weight bearing.

Shortly after the child begins to creep, she will get to a piece of furniture and initiate a pull-to-stand. She should ideally pass through the half-kneel position in order to reach standing. Infants will often explore this ability to pull-to-stand when waking up in the middle of the night. As shown in Figure 8–19, they will pull up at crib or playpen rails.

Interestingly, the infant will be able to pull-to-stand before being able to lower and will often cry the first few times this occurs. It will not take infants long to figure out how to get down, but until they do, parents may

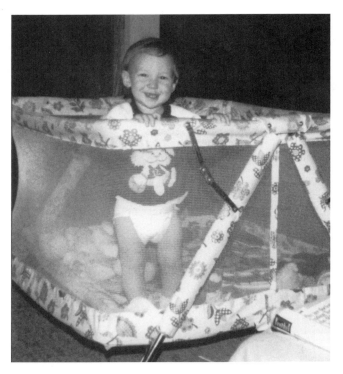

FIGURE 8–19   Infant Demonstrating Result of Pull-to-Stand and Readiness to Cruise

be distressed to find that the infant who was formerly sleeping through the night now awakes and pulls-to-stand, crying for the parent to come to the rescue once successfully standing.

After pulling-to-stand, the infant will typically move sideways around furniture. This pattern is called cruising. **Cruising** is a locomotor pattern that uses an abduction, lateral shift mobility pattern with extrinsic postural support. Gradually, the infant typically begins to free one hand from the support surface and moves between pieces of furniture, such as coffee table and couch. Meanwhile, parents are typically "walking" with infants by this time, holding first two hands and then one hand to provide support. The 10–12-month-old will be demonstrating true weight bearing through the legs but does not yet have the postural control for independent gait.

Sometime around the 1st birthday, the infant takes the first independent steps. Bipedal gait is the definitive locomotor pattern for humans. The early infant gait does not have the smoothly coordinated, effortless appearance of mature gait. In fact, early gait is so distinctive that it even has a unique name applied, **toddling,** and these early walkers are called by the associated name, *toddlers.* Several features characterize toddling, or immature gait. The upper extremities are held up and out from the body in abduction. There are several reasons given for this pattern of the arms. It has been suggested that this is a "readiness" pattern, to catch the infant should he fall. It has also been suggested that this pattern represents the effort to maintain an upright trunk in extension when postural control is still immature. The lower trunk is in extension, with lumbar lordosis. Associated with this lordosis is protuberance of the infant's belly. This pattern is associated with the relatively inactive abdominal musculature at the end of the first year. The lower limbs are abducted in a wide base of support. This increased base of support is a common compensation for immature balance reactions (Figure 8–20).

As the infant takes early steps, the cadence is often rapid, because there is inadequate control for sustained unilateral stance. Hence, the appearance is almost as if the infant is falling from one leg and catching with the other (Figure 8–21). It will take approximately another 2 years of practice before the infant's postural and mobility patterns in gait resemble those of the adult (Sutherland et al., 1980).

Normal adults have a series of so-called strategies they use to sustain postural control. These include an *ankle strategy,* in which the ankle musculature contracts in response to a backward or forward displacement. This strategy helps move the center of mass over the base of support and comprises the typical postural sway seen in quiet stance. The ankle strategy is used when the displacement is small and the standing support surface is firm. A second strategy is the *hip strategy,* which is used when the standing support surface is soft or is smaller than the base of support provided by the feet.

The hip strategy is also used in larger or faster displacements. The *stepping strategy* allows the person to step and reestablish the base of support. This is used when the disturbances are large, so that the base of support cannot be recovered. These three strategies are an example of *muscle synergies,* defined as the functional coupling of groups of muscles that operate together as a unit (Shumway-Cook & Woollacott, 2001).

It has been found that after 3–6 months of walking experience, toddlers demonstrate the hip strategy; however, the amount of abdominal muscle activation in this strategy is less than that of the adult until 7–10 years of age (Woollacott et al., 1998). Likewise, it has been found that it takes 1–3 months of walking experience before the toddler is able to successfully use a stepping strategy for balance recovery (Roncesvalles et al., 2000).

FINE MOTOR DEVELOPMENT

The increasing opposition of the thumb and the movement of grasp distally to the fingertips characterize the infancy transition period. Beginning at about 10 months, the infant can further oppose the thumb so that it approximates the volar surface of the index finger. This is known as an **inferior pincer grasp.** Control moves through the phase distally, first to the pad of the index finger. The pad-to-pad opposition of thumb and index finger is considered a pincer grasp. The most discrete and controlled grasp is between the tip of the

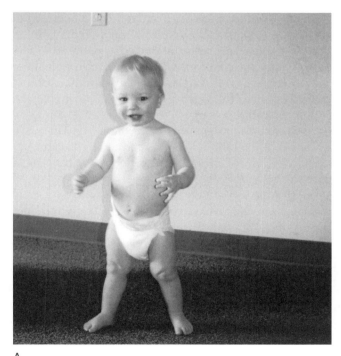

A

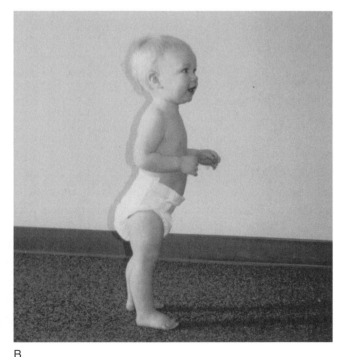

B

FIGURE 8–20   Front and Side Views of Typical Infant Standing Posture at 1 Year

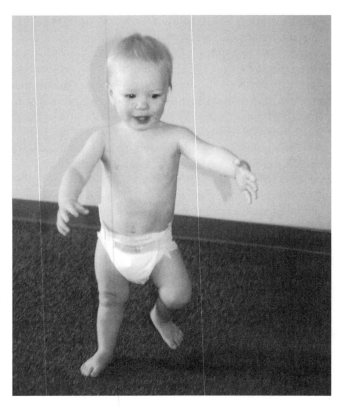

FIGURE 8–21 Walking at 1 Year

thumb and the tip of the index finger, such as one might use a needle in sewing. This **superior pincer grasp** appears around 1 year of age (Duff, 1995).

With increasing manipulatory ability supported by developments in other domains, including cognitive, the infant begins to demonstrate adaptive skills. *Adaptive skills* may be considered those skills that permit the infant to perform self-care. Usually by 1 year of age, the infant begins to take off clothing, often starting with socks. He will hold out arms to assist with dressing.

ORAL-MOTOR DEVELOPMENT

Infants from 10 to 12 months develop proficiency with solid foods, feeding themselves with fingers. The chewing pattern is more mature, with a mix of up-down and rotary/diagonal components. The infant at this time is able to drink independently from a "sippy" cup. Although the infant at 12 months is quite proficient with removing food from the spoon or fork, parents are still often hesitant to allow her to try to self-feed using utensils. In the case of the spoon, the infant still cannot efficiently scoop the food onto the spoon and, if presented a spoon already filled, will pronate and wave it around just as often as getting it to the mouth. In the case of the fork, it is easier for the infant to get the food on the fork by spearing it; however, most parents are concerned that

infants will jab themselves with the tines. Often, however, the infant in this period will begin to show a desire for independence with some of these activities.

COGNITIVE-LANGUAGE DEVELOPMENT

It is in this transition period that the first word usually emerges. Typically, by 12 months, the infant specifically applies "Mama" and "Dada" to the appropriate people and may have one or more additional words. Often, these early words are names for pets, siblings, or other family members. This phase encompasses the cognitive phase of coordination of secondary circular reactions begun in the previous phase. The infant's ability to manipulate using tools continues to be refined. He will spend long periods playing games such as putting blocks in a plastic milk bottle and dumping them out. Object permanence continues to become more secure. The infant routinely searches for hidden objects; however, he can still be fooled. For example, if someone hides a toy under one cup with him watching but subsequently moves the object, he often continues to focus on finding the object in the first hiding place (Feldman, 1999).

PERSONAL-SOCIAL DEVELOPMENT

In this transition phase, attachment behaviors are clearly developed. The child's emotional, cognitive, and physical maturity enable her to use the mother as a "secure base" from which to explore the world (Sroufe, 1996). The child at 10–12 months will fall into one of the three classifications of attachment behavior: securely attached, avoidant, or insecurely attached. The *securely attached infant* will seek to maintain proximity with the caregiver (in this case, let's say it is the mother) and will react with negative emotion when she leaves. When the mother returns, the infant will go immediately to her. When the mother is present, the infant will leave her to explore the room, referencing back to her visually or approaching her at intervals, as if to make sure she is still there.

Avoidant infants do not seek proximity to the mother, and when she returns, they tend to ignore her. Ambivalent infants will seek contact with the mother and become distressed when she leaves, but when she returns, these infants may display anger at her and resist comforting.

A recently added category of attachment is *disorganized-disoriented.* In this category, the infants will show inconsistent behavior that is often self-contradictory. These infants may be the least securely attached (Feldman, 1999).

It is also in this stage that infants will show true **stranger anxiety,** which has been developing over the past several months. This is differentiated from the *stranger protest* in that stranger anxiety has an anticipatory quality to it. The infant may react negatively to strangers, as in a clinic room, before the stranger has actually approached the infant and while the parent is still present.

IMPORTANCE OF DEVELOPMENTAL SEQUENCE

This chapter has presented an overview of the sequence of acquisition of key behaviors in the 1st year of life. There are several key points to remember. First, the exact time of milestone acquisition is highly variable and less important than the sequence itself. In the case of motor development, although the sequence is predictable and appears to have a large innate component, it is not unaffected by environmental experience. Relatively small changes in cultural and care-giving practices can produce small variations in timing and sequence of milestone acquisition, such as the United States initiative of the "Back to Sleep" program, as described previously (Davis, Moon, Sachs, & Ottolini, 1998).

Cross-cultural studies of development have also shown that caregiving practices can affect the pattern of development (Cintas, 1988); however, in most cases, the ultimate outcome of walking around 1 year of life is unchanged. Motor development may be thought of as relatively "privileged," meaning that a wide range of caregiving practice can be tolerated without a negative effect on the developmental outcome (Eliot, 1999). This is an important factor in cases where infants may have to be casted or have other kinds of constraints for a few weeks or months in the first year. Otherwise, normal children should not demonstrate significant delays as a result of this intervention. These observations do not imply, however, that motor development cannot be adversely affected. In studies of infants who were raised in extremely deprived environments, such as orphanages in third world countries, motor development may be seriously affected. The reason for the problems of these infants may be multifactorial, and include nutrition.

A number of studies have shown that the quality of the attachment developed in the 1st year of life relates to types of relationships the infant forms later in life (Feldman, 1999). Securely attached infants are believed to have learned how to regulate emotional arousal and how to depend on others for assistance when needed (Sroufe, 1996). Across all domains of development, the importance of a supportive and nurturing environment in the first year of life to future functioning cannot be overstated.

Traditionally, individuals who want to assess the performance of infants in the 1st year of life use the developmental sequence of milestone acquisition. The infant's capabilities are compared against the norms, and an assessment is made of whether or not his performance falls in the range of normal variability. Failure to fall within the normative range of milestone acquisition is labeled as **developmental delay.** Developmental delay is less a diagnosis than a descriptor. In other words, developmental delay says only that the child is slow in acquiring milestones; it does not imply a specific etiology of delay. For example, developmental delay may be due to a known condition such as Down syndrome, or it may be identified in a former premature infant with risk factors but no known specific cause for delay.

Developmental delay may be global or focal. In the former case, delays in all areas of development are noted, as in the case of the child with Down syndrome. Conversely, the delay may be restricted to only some areas, such as motor or language development. The determination of the areas of deficit helps in determining etiology. Thus, if the infant's delay is restricted to language, it would be imperative to determine if the child has a hearing impairment. If the delay seems to be most significant in the motor areas, a problem such as cerebral palsy may be the reason. Cerebral palsy, by definition, is not a diagnosis. Rather, it is a description of clinical sequelae resulting from a defect of lesion of the brain in early life that are manifest in primarily neuromotor systems with secondary impact on musculoskeletal and other systems (Wilson-Howie, 1999).

Developmental delay may be distinguished from **abnormal development.** Developmental delay is primarily a quantitative concept—i.e., it refers to how many of the normative milestones an infant has acquired—whereas abnormal development refers less to the quantitative than the qualitative aspects of development. For example, an infant who had a mild stroke might be at the slow end of normal ranges in timing of milestone acquisition, but the qualitative aspects of movement make the parents worry that something is wrong. An infant with a diagnosis of mental or psychiatric impairment might show an abnormal quality of attachment behavior.

Of course, abnormal development and developmental delay often coexist, as in the case of the infant with cerebral palsy. These infants will show stereotypic patterns of posture and movement that look abnormal, and they are bound by these patterns so that acquisition of milestones does not occur on time. It is also important to remember that not all developmental conditions can be diagnosed immediately in infancy. For example, a child with cerebral palsy may acquire early milestones within the normative range but fall off later in the 1st year.

Finally, there is a transient developmental delay. In this case the infant fails to acquire early milestones but catches up later in the 1st year. Transient delay is often seen in infants who had a difficult perinatal course, and it seems that the brain as well as other body systems take some time to recover. Transient delay is not equivalent to the observation that premature infants tend to develop according to their gestational rather than chronologic age. Therefore, when assessing the developmental milestones of the premature infant, the convention is to adjust the infant's age for prematurity. Subtracting the number of weeks the infant was premature from the infant's chronologic age obtains the adjusted age. Thus, an infant who was born 8 months ago is that chronologic age. However, suppose that infant was a 28-week-gestation premature infant. Since a term pregnancy is dated at 40 weeks, that infant is 12 weeks, or 3 months premature. Therefore, the adjusted age and associated normative milestones would be at the 5-month level. Adjustment for prematurity is traditionally done in developmental assessment until the infant has reached 2 years of age.

These examples demonstrate the importance of therapists and other professionals working with infants to know the normative patterns and sequences of development in the 1st year. The developing brain is highly plastic, due to the rapid synaptogenesis and the extensive myelination that occurs in the first 2 years of life. **Plasticity** is a term used for the brain's ability to make structural and functional changes in response to the environment. The current standard of intervention is based on the fact that the earlier a problem is identified, the greater the likelihood that intervention will have a positive effect, because of maximizing the neural resources available to the child due to plasticity. There is a large and ever growing literature regarding animals and humans that shows the importance of early environment and experience to the synaptic sculpturing of the developing brain (Eliot, 1999).

SUMMARY

The first year of life rivals only the fetal period in its rapidity of developmental change, and from the aspect of behavior, it is the most dynamic period of change across the human lifespan. In gross motor development, the infant progresses from being relatively dependent on external support for something as simple as head control to being able to walk independently. In fine motor development, she progresses from a nonfunctional reflexive grasp to being able to pick up the smallest of objects. In oral motor development, the 1st year marks progress from a total diet of liquid taken by bottle or breast to a slightly modified mature diet, including drinking liquids from a cup and finger-feeding diced solids. Communication and language skills progress in the 1st year from being limited to nature and extent of crying to one or more single words, including identification of parents by name. Finally, in personal-social development, as the infant becomes a toddler, he has typically developed attachment to one or several primary caregivers and is an active participant in social relationships. To watch an infant progress from the relatively dependent newborn to the curious, active toddler who exerts mastery over a wide array of skills is truly one of life's most exciting opportunities for professionals, parents, and families.

CASE

1

Meghan and Amy

Sheila and Terri are good friends, and they each had a baby within 6 weeks of each other. They were very excited to be pregnant together and were sure that their babies would grow up to be "best friends." They both had baby girls. However, Sheila's baby, Meghan, who was born first, was a model baby from the start. Meghan was sleeping through the night by the time she was 2 months old. By 4 months, she was rolling over and beginning to sit up. By 6 months, she was sitting well, and shortly after that, she started to turn into a semi–hand-and-knees position. By 8 months of age, she was creeping on hands and knees, and by 10 months of age she was walking. Meghan had a vocabulary of four words at 1 year and was a very social child.

On the other hand, Terri's little girl, Amy, was a very difficult child. She was irregular in all her patterns and clearly had a difficult temperament. For the first 2 months, Amy cried nearly all night

Continues

CASE

1

Meghan and Amy *Continued*

long, and Terri and her husband were up trying to quiet her until the early hours of the morning, not getting very much sleep themselves. Amy hated to be on her stomach, and the only position where she was semi-happy was in her infant swing, where she spent a lot of time those first months. At 6 months of age, Amy was rolling from her back to her stomach, but not stomach to back. She was barely sitting propped. By 8 months of age, Amy would sit and play with toys briefly, but nothing interested her for long. Amy did not start pulling-to-stand until she was close to 1 year of age. She was saying only "Ma-ma" and "Da-da" at 1 year of age.

Sheila and Terri and their spouses were having dinner one night. After they got home, Terri's husband commented that he was worried because Amy seemed "slow." He wondered why Amy wasn't walking yet. Terri burst into tears and said she felt like she was a failure as a mother.

This case study illustrates the individual variability in infants. Meghan, who was an infant with an easy temperament, was developing at an accelerated rate. Amy, on the other hand, had a difficult temperament and was a more demanding child. She was less open to new experiences and more demanding of caregiver attention. But both children were developing normally. It would be important to make sure that Terri and her husband could appreciate Amy's uniqueness and recognize that Meghan's relative acceleration will make very little difference over time.

CASE

2

Manuel

Julie and Tim have been unable to have children. They are very excited when they find out they have been approved to adopt a child from an orphanage in a South American country. They gather their resources and fly to pick up their new son, Manuel. There is no medical history available. Manuel is about 10 months old when they adopt him.

They bring Manuel back to the United States. He is a very quiet baby. He lies quietly and rarely cries. Manuel is barely sitting forward propped. He has a head lag in pull-to-sit. Manuel refuses to eat anything, taking only the bottle. He occasionally makes babbling sounds, but he has very little affect. He does not get upset, no matter who is holding him. Manuel will reach and grasp toys but drops them after a brief period of exploration.

Julie and Tim are very worried. Although they already love little Manuel, they were assured that the baby they were adopting was "normal" and did not have any kind of neurologic problem. The pediatrician has an MRI done, and there is no brain damage. Julie and Tim ask about a referral to early intervention. When the early-intervention team visit Julie and Tim, they conclude that there are definite delays; however, without knowing Manuel's medical history (whether he was term or preterm), it is difficult to determine the severity of the delays. The early-intervention team encourage Julie and Tim to provide a rich, supportive environment for Manuel. They explain brain plasticity and suggest that there is a good chance that Manuel will respond to their activity suggestions.

By 18 months of age, Manuel seems like a different child. He is clearly attached to Julie and Tim and has four to six words. He is walking well and eating solids. Although they continue to work especially on Manuel's language development, they are thrilled with their little boy and feel they have seen first-hand the effect of environment on development.

Speaking of

The Parent-Infant Bond

SUSAN LYNCH, MD
NEONATOLOGIST, DIRECTOR OF WEST VIRGINIA UNIVERSITY NEONATAL FOLLOW-UP CLINIC

As a pediatric resident, you tend to view your work in terms of illness and acute care. Your concerns are focused around how to identify and treat sickness in children. You learn how to recognize an ear infection, and how to select the correct antibiotic to treat that infection. Neonatologists like myself complete a fellowship in which we are faced with the responsibility of learning a huge body of science and the sometimes overwhelming task of incorporating this knowledge into day-to-day care of premature and sick infants. Again, the focus is on sickness. You learn to make acute, even emergent decisions. You put an immense effort into becoming the best you can be at taking care of babies—once again, however, focusing primarily on the well baby–sick baby continuum.

As years go by and I develop more perspective, I realize that as daunting and as rewarding as taking care of sick infants is, the real meaning of what I do is reflected in families. Every year, I never cease to be amazed by the strength of the parental bond, the ability of mothers and fathers to selflessly love and care for their infants. I believe these abilities sometimes surprise even parents themselves.

Often, after particularly poignant interactions with parents, I find myself quietly reflecting on this attribute. For example, it is not uncommon for me to see a mother, sitting at the bedside of her critically ill infant day after day, laying her head down and sleeping on the corner of the bed to get some rest. Recently, I had to deliver some bad news to a father about his infant's condition, and he responded by saying, "We were told that we could never have children due to my wife's illness. Our son is a gift from God and we know he would not take away such a gift. We know he will be okay."

You can read about and study attachment and bonding. But until you have experiences such as those I have described, you can't begin to appreciate the power of that relationship between parent and infant. Each family, unique in its beliefs and traditions, welcomes the infant and nurtures the infant, thereby creating a new relationship or bond. The strength of that bond in terms of love and dedication never ceases to amaze and inspire me.

REFERENCES

Acredolo, L. P., Goodwyn, S. W., Horobin, K. D., & Emmons, Y. D. (1999). The signs and sounds of early language development. In L. Balter & C. Tamis-LeMonda (Eds.), *Child psychology: A handbook of contemporary issues* (pp. 116–139). Philadelphia: Psychology Press.

Chang, E. F. & Merzenich, M. M. (2003). Environmental noise retards auditory cortical development. *Science, 300(5618)*, 498–502.

Choukair, M. (2000). Blood chemistry/body fluids. In G. K. Siebert & R. Iannone (Eds.), *Harriet Lane handbook* (pp. 119–180). St. Louis: Mosby.

Cintas, H. M. (1988). Cross-cultural variation in infant motor development. *Physical & Occupational Therapy in Pediatrics, 8*, 1–20.

DeVries, M. W. (1999). Babies, brains and culture: Optimizing neurodevelopment on the savanna. *Acta Paediatrica Supplement, 88(429)*, 43–48.

Duff, S. V. (1995). Prehension. In D. Cech & T. Martin (Eds.), *Functional movement across the lifespan* (pp. 313–353). Philadelphia: W. B. Saunders.

Elbert, T., Pantev, C., Weinbruch, C., Rockstroh, B., & Taub, E. (1995). Increased cortical representation of the fingers of the left hand in string players. *Science, 270*, 305–307.

Eliot, L. (1999). *What's going on in there? How the brain and mind develop in the first five years of life.* New York: Bantam Books.

Feldman, R. S. (Ed). (1999). *Child development: A topical approach.* Upper Saddle River, NJ: Prentice Hall.

Field, T. (1990). *Infancy.* Cambridge, MA: Harvard University Press.

Hakimi-Manesh, Y., Mojdehi, H., Tashakkori, A. (1984). Short communication: Effects of environmental enrichment of the mental and psychomotor development of orphanage children. *Journal of Child Psychology and Psychiatry and Allied Disciplines, 25(4),* 643–650.

Infant Development. (2003). Accessed October 9, 2003, from http://www.envisagedesign.com/ohbaby/develop.html.

Johnston, M. V., Nishimura, A., Harum, K., Pekar, J., & Blue, M. E. (2001). Sculpting the developing brain. *Advances in Pediatrics, 48,* 1–38.

Kedesky, J. H., & Budd, K. S. (1998). Assessment of environmental factors in feeding. In *Childhood feeding disorders* (pp. 79–114). Baltimore: Brooks.

Koontz-Lowman, D., & Lane, S. J. (1999). Children with feeding and nutritional problems. In S. Porr & E. B. Rainville (Eds.), *Pediatric therapy: A systems approach* (pp. 379–423). Philadelphia: F. A. Davis.

Lamb, M. E., & Campos, J. J. (1982). *Development in infancy.* New York: Mosby.

Long, T., & Toscano, T. (2002). *Handbook of pediatric physical therapy* (2nd ed.). Philadelphia: Lippincott, Williams & Wilkins.

Masi, W. S., & Scott, K. G. (1983). Preterm and full-term infants' visual responses to mothers' and strangers' faces. In T. Field and A. Sostek (Eds.), *Infants born at risk: Physiological, perceptual and cognitive processes* (pp. 173–179). New York: Grune & Stratton.

McCluskey, K. A. (1981). The infant as organizer: Future directions in perceptual development. In K. Bloom (Ed.), *Prospective issues in infancy research* (pp. 119–136). Hilldale, NJ: Lawrence Erlbaum Associates.

Payne, V. G., & Isaacs, L. D. (1999). *Human motor development: A lifespan approach.* MountainView, CA: Mayfield.

Resiman, J. E. (1987). Touch, motion and proprioception. In P. Salapatek and L. Cohen (Eds.), *Handbook of infant perception: From sensation to perception* (Vol. I) (pp. 265–303). Orlando, FL: Academic Press.

Robson, P. (1984). Prewalking locomotor movements and their use in predicting standing and walking. *Child Care, Health and Development, 10,* 317–330.

Roncevalles, M. N. C., Wollacott, M. H., & Jensen, J. L. (2000). The development of compensatory stepping skills in children. *Journal of Motor Behavior, 32,* 110–111.

Scarr, S. (1992). Developmental theories for the 1990s: Development and individual differences. *Child Development, 63(1),* 1–19.

Shonkoff, J. P., & Phillips, D. P. (2000). *From neurons to neighborhoods: The science of early childhood development.* Washington, DC: National Academy Press.

Sameroff, A. J., & Cavanagh, P. J. (1979). Learning in infancy: A developmental perspective. In J. Osofsky (Ed.), *Handbook of infant development* (pp. 344–392). New York: John Wiley & Sons.

Shumway-Cook, A., & Woollacott, M. (2001). *Motor control: Theory and practical applications* (2nd ed.). Philadelphia: Lippincott, Williams & Wilkins.

Sroufe, L. A. (1996). *Emotional development: The organization of emotional life in the early years.* New York: Cambridge University Press.

Sutherland, D. H., Olshen, R., Cooper, L., & Woo, S. (1980). The development of mature gait. *Journal of Bone & Joint Surgery, 62A,* 336–353.

Teicher, M. H., Andersen, S. L., Polcari, A., Anderson, C. M., Navalta, C. P., & Kim, D. M. (2003). The neurobiological consequences of early stress and childhood maltreatment. *Neuroscience and Biobehavioral Reviews, 27(1–2),* 33–44.

Teller, D., & Bornstein, M. (1987). Infant color vision and color perception. In P. Salapatek & L. Cohen (Eds.), *Handbook of infant perception: From sensation to perception* (Vol. I) (pp. 185–236). Orlando, FL: Academic Press.

Thelen, E., & Fisher, D. M. (1982). Newborn stepping: An explanation for a "disappearing reflex." *Developmental Psychology, 18,* 760–785.

VanSant, A. (1995). Development of posture. In D. Cech & T. Martin (Eds.), *Functional movement development across the lifespan* (pp.275–294). Philadelphia: W. B. Saunders.

Wilson-Howie, J. M. (1999). Cerebral palsy. In S. Campbell (Ed.), *Decision making in pediatric neurologic physical therapy* (pp. 23–83). New York: Churchill Livingstone.

Woollacott, M., Burtner, P., Jensen, J., Jasiewics, J., et al. (1998). Development of postural responses during standing in healthy children and in children with spastic diplegia. *Neuroscience and Biobehavioral Reviews, 22,* 583–589.

Family and Disability Issues through Infancy

Dianne Koontz-Lowman, EdD, OTR
Assistant Professor
Department of Occupational Therapy
Virginia Commonwealth University
Richmond, Virginia

Objectives

Upon completion of this chapter, the reader should be able to

- Describe the basic premises and the components of family systems theory.

- Discuss the impact of disability on the family system.

- State the stages of the development of attachment in infancy.

- List Greenspan's stages of emotional development.

- Discuss the functional aspects of the caregiving relationship for both the infant and the caregiver.

- List the characteristics of successful caregiver-child interactions.

- Explain to caregivers why it is important to closely observe and respond to their infants' cues.

- List the possible impacts of having a sibling with a disability.

- Describe how risk factors might impact families.

- Identify potential protective factors and resources available to assist families at risk.

Key Terms

attachment

bonding

boundaries

caregiver-child interactions

cohesion

coping styles

family-centered intervention

family functions

family life cycle theory

family structure

family subsystems

family systems theory

ideological style

risk factors

sibling subsystem

transitions

INTRODUCTION

Children are born into families. Their first relationships, their first group, and their first experience with the world are with and through their families. The ICF considers a *contextual factor* in human function, influencing and potentially either supporting or impeding function (World Health Organization, 2002). Children grow and develop in the context of their family (McGoldrick, Heiman & Carter, 1993). Children referred for therapy services come to the evaluation with this family. Professionals working with families of children with disabilities have come to realize that the child's development cannot be separated from the context provided by the family. Through families, children learn about themselves, their world, their values and standards, and relationships. In addition, the family represents the most long-lasting relationships children have throughout childhood (Humphry & Case-Smith, 2001). Any intervention with the child ultimately impacts the family (Winton & Winton, 2000).

Over the past century professionals have considered parents in the following ways: as the source of the child's disability, as organization members, as recipients of professionals' decisions, as teachers, and as members of advocacy organizations. In their current role, families are viewed as educational decision makers and collaborators (Turnbull & Turnbull, 1997). Professionals have come to realize the importance of collaborating with all family members, not just the child's parents, to plan for and develop successful intervention programs. Family members are critical members of the planning team, functioning as equal partners with therapists, administrators, and teachers. The challenge for therapists is to collaborate with the team in designing an intervention plan that builds on the family's strengths and addresses the family's needs (Mattingly & Lawlor, 2003).

Family-centered intervention can be described by the general principles shown in Table 9–1. Some components of family-centered intervention include the following: (1) families are mandated members on state-level advisory boards that make decisions about the provision of early intervention services; (2) the family's concerns, priorities, and resources drive the development of the individualized intervention plan; and (3) families play an important role in the assessment and evaluation of their child (Winton & Winton, 2000). For these reasons it is critical that therapists understand families. This chapter will provide an overview of family systems, including an introduction to how the birth of a child with disabilities might influence the family systems.

Consider the following vignette: As a new therapist working with families of young children with disabilities, you are aware of the need to ask the caregiver what goals are important to her. You hold an initial evaluation meeting with Margarita Sanchez, a young mother whose third child was just recently diagnosed with cerebral palsy. Mrs. Sanchez lives in a small apartment with her husband, his mother, and three children, ages 6 years, 5 years, and 11 months. After a successful meeting, you set up a therapy schedule where the mother will bring the 11-month-old to your clinic every Wednesday at 3:00 P.M. Mrs. Sanchez does not come to the next therapy session.

FAMILY SYSTEMS

As a social system, the family is a group of individuals with interrelated occupations. Each member of this interrelated group has his or her own needs that may or may not be congruent with the needs of the other members, or with the family as a whole. **Family systems theory,** originated by Murray Bowen, recognizes that a family is greater than the sum of its parts (Kaplan & Sadock, 1998). In family systems theory, drawn from the general systems model introduced in Chapter 1, individual actions and beliefs impact on every member of the family. For example, an individual's idea about what constitutes "good" parenting, like being highly restrictive about contact with persons outside the cultural group, will impact the child's sense of identity and comfort in social situations.

TABLE 9–1	Principles of Family-Centered Intervention

The following guiding principles are based on the belief that family-centered intervention seeks to build and promote the strengths and competencies present in all families:

- The family is the constant in the child's life while the service systems and personnel within those systems fluctuate.
- Young children are uniquely dependent on their families for survival and nurturance.
- Each family has its own structure, roles, values, beliefs, and coping styles.
- Intervention systems and strategies must honor the racial, ethnic, cultural, and socioeconomic diversity of families.
- Families must be able to choose the level and nature of intervention involvement in their lives.
- Professionals must reexamine their traditional roles and practices and develop new practices in response to family needs when necessary.
- Family/professional collaboration that promotes mutual respect and partnerships is the key to family-centered intervention.

Adapted from McGongiel, M. J., Kaugman, R. K., & Johnson, B. H., 1991.

As outlined in Table 9–2, a basic premise of family systems theory is that the individual members are so interrelated that any experience or problem affecting one member will affect all members of the family (Humphry & Case-Smith, 2001; Turnbull & Turnbull, 1997).

Viewing the child and family as part of a system has given therapists a new perspective on working with families. This systems perspective clarifies some issues and highlights the complexity of working with families of children with disabilities. For example, as seen in the vignette at the beginning of this chapter, therapists have been puzzled by why parents, typically the mother, often do not comply with the treatment plan. The systems perspective encourages the therapist to look at all the factors that might have influenced the mother's actions, including having to meet the older two children as they arrive home from school at 3:00 (Beckman, 1996). The following discussion of family systems will involve an understanding of the components of family systems (family structure, functions, interactions, and life cycle) highlighted in Table 9–3 (Peeks, 1997; Turnbull & Turnbull, 1997).

FAMILY STRUCTURE, OR WHO IS IN THE FAMILY?

The family defines who is a member of their family and the role of each family member. **Family structure** refers to the variety of characteristics that make the family unique, such as membership characteristics, cultural style, and ideological style (Seligman & Darling, 1997). These structural characteristics influence interactions and communications among family members (Lynch & Morley, 1995). An important reason for understanding family structure is to determine who is the head of the household (Humphry & Case-Smith, 2001). Family systems have

rules, spoken or unspoken, that define who has the authority in different situations. A spoken rule might be, "No one eats until after the blessing." An unspoken rule might be that no decisions are made until the father is consulted (Winton & Winton, 2000). In the opening vignette the intervention schedule might not have been approved by the decision maker of the family (in this case, perhaps the father or the paternal grandmother).

Membership Characteristics

Membership characteristics are variables such as, but not limited to, the number of children, the number and marital status of the parents, the relationship to extended family members, and the presence of live-in family members unrelated by blood or marriage (Turnbull & Turnbull, 1997). The structure of the family may shape their response to a child with disabilities. Larger families may be less stressed or have more resources available to them. Having other children may remind the parents that their child with disabilities is more like his brothers and sisters than different. Similarly, if two parents are participating in care, more supports and resources are available to deal with the stressors of raising a child with disabilities (Turnbull & Turnbull, 1997). Grandparents (Figure 9–1) can be a strong source of support by providing respite and/or financial assistance (Case-Smith, 1998).

Families today are more diverse, both structurally and culturally, than at any time in our nation's history. Single parents, adoptive or foster parents, grandparents, or same-sex partners, as well as married couples today may head families. Parents may postpone having children until their forties. Teen pregnancy is also common in some subcultures (Darling & Baxter, 1996). Given the pressures of raising a child alone, some single parents have limited resources, time, or energy to

TABLE 9–2	Basic Premises of a Family Systems Model

1. The family defines who is in their family.
2. A family is a group of individuals with interrelated occupations; changes in one family member's occupational performance potentially impacts all members. Simply stated, what affects one member of the system affects the whole system.
3. A family system must be understood as a whole, and it is more than the sum of the abilities of each member.
4. Families are made up of subsystems that are defined with their own patterns of interactions.
5. Like all systems, families have "rules" that define order and hierarchy, or who has power and authority. These rules may be spoken or unspoken.
6. The family's ideological style is based on family beliefs, values, and coping behaviors.

Adapted from Humphry & Case-Smith, 2001; Peeks, 1997; Turnbull & Turnbull, 1997; Winton & Winton, 2000.

TABLE 9–3	Key Components of a Family Systems Model

Family Structure
Who Is in the Family?

Mother and father
Blended family
Single parent
Extended family members
Multigenerational family
Foster family

Family Interactions
Who Talks to Whom?

Subsystems
Marital
Parental
Siblings
Cohesion
Adaptability

Family Functions
Why Do We Have Families?

Economic
Health function
Socialization function
Educational function
Affection function
Recreational function

Family Life Cycle
How Do Families Change Over Time?

Developmental stages
Couple
First child
Young children
Elementary school age
Adolescents
Children as adults
Transitions

Adapted from Turnbull & Turnbull, 1997.

devote to being involved in intervention. However, other single parents or teen mothers have a wide circle of extended family members for support (Case-Smith, 1998; Turnbull & Turnbull, 1997).

Ideological Style

Ideological style refers to the family's beliefs, values, and coping behaviors (Seligman & Darling, 1997). As discussed in Chapter 4, different racial, ethnic, and religious groups have different values, norms, and beliefs regarding child rearing, the roles of fathers and mothers within families, discipline, the importance of development of the child's independence, and other issues. Understanding the family's beliefs about disabilities (e.g., punishment, injustice, genetics, God's will, fate) and what and who can influence the future (e.g., control is within family, control is in the hands of others, or the future is uncontrollable) is critical to understanding the family. These beliefs are contextual factors

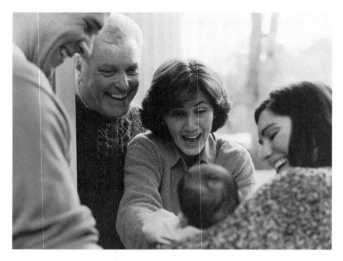

FIGURE 9–1 Grandparents are an important part of many family systems. (Image courtesy of PhotoDisc®, Inc.)

that impact the family members and their reactions to intervention from professionals outside the family system (Barnell & Day, 1996; Lynch & Morley, 1995).

Coping styles are the way families "contend with difficulties and act to overcome them" (*American Heritage*, 2000). Coping styles can be both internal and external. Internal strategies include *passive appraisal* (problem will resolve itself over time) and *reframing* (making adjustments to live with the problem). External strategies include social support, spiritual support, and professional support (Seligman & Darling, 1997; Turnbull & Turnbull, 1997). Considering the available resources, demands of the disability, and the family's coping style, the team can determine resources needed to enhance the family's ability to adapt.

FAMILY FUNCTIONS, OR WHY DO WE HAVE FAMILIES?

Why do groups of individuals come together to form a family? Families exist to meet the individual and collective needs of each member. The tasks that families perform to meet these needs are called **family functions.** Some categories of family functions include affection, self-esteem, socialization, economics, daily care, health care, recreation, and educational/vocational issues (Turnbull & Turnbull, 1997). Basic functions of families include dealing with economic issues and daily-care needs of the members, such as housing, food, and safety. The family is the first place a child experiences affection that bonds the family together. As will be discussed later in this chapter, the development of attachment between a caregiver and a child is critical to development. From a family systems perspective, attachment between and among family members is a priority

function. Cultural influences may dictate how families develop emotional commitments and display affection. No matter how displayed, this attachment among family members helps the members figure out who they are and their worth (Humphry & Case-Smith, 2001; Turnbull & Turnbull, 1997).

Family Time Use, Routines and Habits

How do families with limited time and energy select priorities among competing functions? As discussed in Chapter 2, Maslow described a *hierarchy of needs*. If a family is struggling to meet physiologic or safety needs, there is less energy available to meet needs related to esteem and self-actualization. Consider the following vignette written by a parent of a child with significant disabilities:

> I remember the day when the occupational therapist at Jody's school called with some suggestions from a visiting nurse. Jody has a seizure problem, which is controlled with . . . drug can cause the gums to grow over the teeth . . . the nurse . . . recommended, innocently enough, that the children's teeth be brushed four times a day, for five minutes, with an electric toothbrush. . . . Although I tried to sound reasonable on the phone, this new demand appalled me. I rehearsed angry, self-justifying speeches in my head. Jody, I thought, is blind, has cerebral palsy, and is retarded. We do his physical therapy daily and work with him on sounds and communication. We feed him each meal on our laps, bottle him, change him, bathe him, dry him, put him in a body cast to sleep, launder his bed linens daily, and go through a variety of routines, designed to minimize his miseries and enhance his joys and his development. (All this in addition to trying to care for and enjoy our other young children and making time for each other and other careers.) Now you tell me that I should spend fifteen minutes every day on something that Jody will hate, an activity that will not help him to walk or even defecate . . . Well, it's too much. Where is that fifteen minutes going to come from? What am I supposed to give up? Taking the kids to the park? Reading a bedtime story to my eldest? Washing the breakfast dishes? Sorting the laundry? . . . Because there is not time in my life that hasn't been spoken for, and for every fifteen-minute activity that is added, one has to be taken away (Featherstone, 1980, pp. 77–78).

Recreation and leisure time are important for individuals and for families. Shared recreation forms the basis for many family traditions. As was the case in the foregoing vignette, professionals sometimes emphasize educational/therapeutic activities more than recreation activities, and parents are asked to do more at home than the family system can handle. Parents need to know that doing something fun with their children is just as important as doing something educational. Therapists can assist by scheduling therapy and educational programs to help families engage in recreational activities (Humphry & Case-Smith, 2001; Seligman & Darling, 1997). There will be more discussion on the topic of family time use, routines, and habits in later chapters.

FAMILY INTERACTIONS, OR WHO TALKS TO WHOM?

A number of interdependent members make up a family. In order to understand and work effectively with the family, the therapist must understand the relationships and interactions between the members. As shown in Table 9–3, important components of these family interactions are the concepts of subsystems, boundaries, cohesion, and adaptability.

Family Subsystems

While it is true that the family system must be understood as a whole and is more than the sum of the members, there are interacting component parts, or subsystems, within the family. Major **family subsystems** might include

- Marital subsystem: marital partner interactions
- Parental system: parent and child interactions
- Sibling subsystem: child and child interactions
- Extrafamilial subsystem: interactions with extended family, friends, professionals, etc.

The makeup of subsystems is determined by the structural characteristics of the family and by the current life cycle stage. Considering the subsystems can be helpful when planning intervention. For example, if there is a sibling subsystem of teenager brother and preschooler with disabilities, it would be important to include the older brother in planning. However, any potential strategies need to be considered within the context of all subsystems so that intervention with one subsystem does not negatively impact another. Talking to all members of the family is critical (Humphry & Case-Smith, 2001; Seligman & Darling, 1997).

Cohesion

Whereas subsystems within a family describe who will interact, **cohesion** refers to how family members interact. In family systems theory, **boundaries** are lines of demarcation between individuals who are inside or outside a subsystem. Boundaries may be open or closed, referring to the interaction with people outside the

subsystem (Turnbull & Turnbull, 1997). Family cohesion refers to the emotional bonding within members of the subsystem; cohesion ranges from highly enmeshed on one end of the continuum to highly disengaged on the other end of the continuum. Balanced families have an equilibrium between enmeshment and disengagement; the boundaries between subsystems are clearly defined, and family members feel both a close bonding and a sense of autonomy. Highly enmeshed families have weak boundaries and can be overinvolved. Overprotective families may have difficulty letting go of a child with a disability. On the other hand, disengaged families have rigid subsystem boundaries characterized by underinvolvement. In a disengaged family, a member (such as the father or grandparents) may withdraw from interactions (Seligman & Darling, 1997). For a professional interacting with the family, it is important to view cohesion within a cultural framework and to provide or refer the family to services appropriate for the family.

Adaptability

Family adaptability refers to the family's ability to plan and work together when change and stress occur. On opposite ends of the adaptability continuum, families who are rigid do not easily change, whereas families who are chaotic appear to be inconsistent. Families who are rigid have a high degree of control and structure, with interactions governed by specific rules. The power hierarchy and roles are clearly delineated. For example, if the mother is the primary caregiver for the children and a disability adds more demands to the mother's role than she can handle, the family may have difficulty assuming new roles. In contrast, families who are chaotic have a low degree of control and structure, and few rules. Sometimes there is no family leader and roles are unclear (Case-Smith, 1998; Humphry & Case-Smith, 2001; Lynch & Morley, 1995; Seligman & Darling, 1997).

FAMILY LIFE CYCLE THEORY

Family life cycle theory addresses how families change over time and go through predictable stages, such as coupling, childbearing, having school-age children, having adolescent children, launching, being a postparental family, and dealing with aging. In addition to going through the predictable stages, families may also experience unexpected changes such as divorce, separation by military service, death, etc. While the life cycle theory consists of fairly predictable events, the therapist must realize that each family is unique. The **transitions** from one stage to another are rarely clear-cut and may occur over a number of years. The characteristics and issues at each life stage are variable, and each family moves through the stages at different rates. In addition, the nature of the family structure may mean that different family members are moving through the stages at different times. Also, cultural factors play a major role in how families experience different life cycles. Moving from one stage to the next causes stress and requires the family to adapt. The interim phase between one stage and the next is known as transition. These changes bring about alterations in needs, interest, roles, and responsibilities of family members (Case-Smith, 1998; Gerson, 1995; Humphry & Case-Smith, 2001; Lynch & Morley, 1995; Seligman & Darling, 1997; Winton & Winton, 2000).

Transitions can be some of the most difficult times for families. Turnbull & Turnbull (1997) describe two factors that tend to reduce the amount of stress families feel during transition. First, in all cultures, the roles of the new stage are known. A ritual, such as a graduation or bar mitzvah, might be a way to observe the transition. These ceremonies let the family know that their roles following the event will be changed. Second, the timing of transition is usually expected. For example, children are expected to go to school at the age of five or six years. For a family with a child with disabilities, the transition might be occurring at an unexpected time. A preschooler with disabilities may go to school at age three.

PARENT/CAREGIVER-AND-CHILD RELATIONSHIPS

As stated earlier in this chapter, it is through the family that the children learn about themselves, their values, and relationships. In infancy the functional aspects of the caregiver-child relationship for the parent are bonding, protection, and responsiveness to the infant's needs, teaching, play, and discipline. For the child, the relationship helps develop attachment, affect regulation and sharing, learning, and play (reference). The first step in the development of relationships is attachment.

ATTACHMENT

The development of **attachment,** the emotional connection, or love, between the newborn and his caregiver(s), is an essential occupational task of infancy and early childhood (Rainville, 1999). Attachment has been discussed previously in this text and is reviewed here with the perspective of family issues in disability. Ainsworth (1982) outlined four stages in the development of the infant's attachment to the caregiver:

- Initial attachment: at 2–3 months the infant exhibits undiscriminating social responses.
- Attachment-in-the-making: by 4–6 months the infant begins to discriminate between familiar and unfamiliar persons.
- Clear-cut, or active attachment: by 6–7 months the infant moves toward one primary caregiver, seeking proximity and contact with that caregiver.
- Multiple attachments: after 12 months, the infant attaches to others.

A discussion of attachment also leads to an examination of the other side of this relationship. This other aspect of the relationship is called **bonding** as the infant develops an attachment with the caregiver, and concurrently the adult bonds with the infant. Bonding is characterized by behaviors such as stroking, kissing, cuddling, and prolonged gazing. These behaviors serve two functions: to express affection and to sustain an interaction between the caregiver and the infant. By the time the infant is 1 month old, most parents are attuned with the baby, and are able to interpret her cry and have learned how to comfort her. In other words, there is a "goodness of fit" (discussed in detail later on) between the infant's needs and the reaction of the caregivers. Parents have also recognized the early indicators of the infant's temperament and know how to calm her or how to avoid overstimulation (Ainsworth, 1982; Brazelton & Cramer, 1990; Lowman, 2000).

EMOTIONAL DEVELOPMENT

The psychosocial development of the infant begins with the earliest interactions or emotional connections with his caregivers. According to Greenspan's theory of psychosocial/emotional development in infancy, the first stage is called *self-regulation and interest in the world.* During the first few months, the infant is focused on organizing information about the internal and external world. The job of the parent is to help the infant regulate these influences. Around the second or third month, the infant moves to the stage Greenspan calls *falling in love.* It is during this period that the infant forms strong attachments to the primary caregivers. She responds to the facial expressions and vocalizations of the caregiver with her own smiles and coos. From 3 to 10 months, the infant begins to learn the art of purposeful communication. At this stage, the infant's smile is purposeful; she has learned that if she smiles, the adults will smile back. Around 9–10 months, the infant is developing an organized sense of self and is beginning to realize how to get different reactions to her behavior (Greenspan & Greenspan, 1985).

CAREGIVER-CHILD INTERACTIONS

The quality of the caregiver-child emotional bond is determined by early interactions. At the most basic level, these early interactions provide physical safety, protection from injury, and food. Caregivers who learn the infant's rhythms and cues and respond appropriately to his needs provide a stimulating environment and give the infant a sense of control over the environment. Supportive and nurturing emotional interactions with caregivers help children learn to perceive and respond to emotional cues, to communicate their feelings, and to form a sense of self. As the child learns to regulate behavior and feelings, he can then move to problem solving and changing what is happening in his environment (Brazelton & Greenspan, 2000). An infant whose caregivers are inconsistent in their interactions or rejecting doesn't expect his emotions or actions to lead to a response from the environment and might view himself as unworthy of love (Case-Smith, 1998). Relationships with caregivers that might be characterized as chaotic or unpredictable might impact the development of emotions and lead to emotion-related disorders such as depression, conduct problems, or social withdrawal (Thompson, 2001).

Early interactions between babies and caregivers have been referred to as an *emotional dance,* where the caregiver is "in sync" with the infant's cues and needs. Some characteristics of successfully early interactions are as follows (Brazelton & Cramer, 1990):

- *Synchrony:* The first step is for the adult to adapt (or match) his or her actions to the baby's rhythms.
- *Symmetry:* In a symmetric dialogue with the baby, the caregiver respects the baby's thresholds and changes to fit the baby's capacities for attention, style, and responses.
- *Contingency:* The caregiver responds contingently to the baby's message, therefore developing a "goodness of fit" based on what does and doesn't work.
- *Entrainment:* As the caregiver and baby achieve a synchrony in the dialogue, the adult can anticipate the child's response and add to dialogue.
- *Play:* The "games" observed between a caregiver and baby are built on entrainment and consist of sequences.
- *Autonomy:* The baby's recognition of control leads to a sense of control, growing out of predictable responses from the caregiver.

For example, if the mother smiles, the baby will smile back. The mother will widen her smile, and the baby will brighten to smile again. After repeating this sequence, the baby may coo. Recognizing the change, the mother will coo back at the baby, this time changing the tone of the vocalization by adding a word. The baby will brighten and repeat the new sound. The mother might even add another word to heighten the interaction. Soon the baby will end the sequence by looking away (Brazelton & Cramer, 1990).

As noted earlier, the ICF model discussed families and caregivers as contextual factors in human function (World Health Organization, 2002). When the human in question is an infant, these contextual factors can have a dramatic, lifelong impact on all realms of function.

Goodness of Fit between Caregiver and Infant

Chess and Thomas (1987) describe a "goodness of fit" where the demands and expectations of the caregivers are consistent with the child's temperament, abilities, and other characteristics. Temperament is discussed in Chapter 3. In this context it is the interaction between the temperament of the child and that of the caregiver that is considered. Many caregivers are able to appropriately match their interactions with the needs of the infant. For example, interacting with a child who is hyperactive might be less stressful for active caregivers than for low-activity ones. Some child characteristics that might impact this goodness of fit include children who have hypo- or hyper-responsive reactions to stimuli, or who are autistic. Infants who were born prematurely might have subtle engagement cues such as alerting or brow-raising, and subtle disengagement cues such as facial grimace or gaze aversion.

Some adult characteristics that might impact this goodness of fit include caregivers who are young, have depression, or have substance abuse problems. Formal assessments, such as the Parent and Caregiver Involvement Scale, are available for analyzing **caregiver-child interactions** (Comfort, 1988). Items on this scale include physical involvement, verbal involvement, responsiveness of caregiver to child, playful interaction, control over child's activities, directions, positive statements, and negative statements. However, many therapists prefer to informally observe and assess the quality of caregiver-child interactions. The purpose of this assessment is to understand the caregiver style and suggest ways to help the caregiver match his or her interactions to the child (Case-Smith, 1998).

SIBLING SUBSYSTEM

As stated earlier, the family consists of several subsystems. The **sibling subsystem** consists of the interactions between brothers and sisters. Powell and Gallagher (1993) describe siblings as the first and most intense peer relationships that children experience. Having a brother or sister with a disability has multiple impacts on the sibling system as well as the family. Some siblings benefit from the relationship, others have negative effects, and others report a neutral experience (Turnbull & Turnbull, 1997).

Sibling relationships vary over time, based on the characteristics such as age, gender, temperament, birth order, spacing, number of children in the family, cultural expectations, and family norms. Factors such as the financial resources of the family, parental adjustment, and attitude play a key role in how siblings are affected by a sibling with disabilities. Siblings can also be impacted by factors related to the disability, such as severity of the disability, the need for specialized care, health needs, and behavioral issues (Frank, 1996; Seligman & Darling, 1997). Considerable literature has documented many positive effects that result from the sibling relationship (Frank, 1996; Powell & Gallagher, 1993; Seligman & Darling 1997; Turnbull & Turnbull, 1997). Depending on the dynamics of the family system as a whole, parents can expect that their children may have some of the following experiences or needs related to their sibling with a disability:

- *A need for information:* Siblings tend to have two views of a disability. The first comes from the information received from their parents and professionals. The second is their "private view," which might reflect confusion about the cause of the disability. Information should be provided so that misconception can be replaced by fact (Frank, 1996; Seligman & Darling, 1997).
- *Caretaking responsibilities:* Since the needs of the child with disabilities can absorb a lot of the family's resources, siblings are sometimes forced to assume a parenting role. Excessive caretaking can result in anger or resentment (Seligman & Darling, 1997). On the positive side, helping with a sibling with disabilities can have a positive effect on self-esteem and self-confidence when the sibling feels that she is making a difference (Frank, 1996).
- *Identity concerns:* There is some indication in the literature that siblings sometimes experience a sense of loneliness and isolation (Frank, 1996; Featherstone, 1980). Other literature, however, indicates no difference in self-esteem and self-confidence (Turnbull & Turnbull, 1997).
- *Careers:* A sibling's career decision might be shaped by caring for a sibling with disabilities in that he may choose a helping profession (Seligman & Darling, 1997).

Overall, Meyer and Vadasy (1994) summarize the potentially negative impacts as embarrassment, guilt, isolation, loneliness, loss, resentment, increased responsibility, and pressure to achieve. On the positive side, opportunities include enhanced maturity, improved self-concept, social competence, tolerance, pride, vocational opportunities, advocacy, and loyalty. "Sibshops" are workshops that provide information and support for siblings of children with disabilities.

FAMILIES AT RISK

In the 2002 *State of Children in America* report, the Children's Defense Fund reports that every 11 seconds a child is reported abused or neglected, every 43 seconds a child is born into poverty, and every minute a child is born to a teen mother. *Risk,* in health terms, refers to the possibility of injury, disease, impairment, or death. A **risk factor** is a personal or environmental factor, as defined in the ICF (World Health Organization, 2002), that leaves the individual at risk or susceptible to injury, disease, impairment, or death.

Both biologic and environmental risk factors, discussed in Chapter 7, may impact the family who has an infant with a disease or disability. *Biologic risk factors* are self-evident, given the situation. The child already has a disease or disability, which is a biologic risk factor. The primary problem may lead to other biologic risk factors, such as poor weight gain and malnutrition. *Environmental risk factors* may be compounded in the presence of an infant with disability. The demands of caretaking may compromise the infant's environment. For example, the costs of caring for an infant with a disability are great. Parents living in poverty must focus their energy and resources on the physical aspects of survival and may have limited resources left to attend to the emotional needs of the children (Rainville, 1999). However, the presence of *protective factors* and social system variables may explain why some children and families deal adaptively and ward off difficulties even in the face of multiple potential risk factors (Epps & Jackson, 2000). Some examples of potential risk factors, protective factors, and community supports are given in Table 9–4.

It is important for therapists working with families to be aware of the potential risks to children and families, and the resources available in the community to help reduce these risks. Information is available through the government agencies in the community responsible for early intervention services, social services, and child protective services. By referring parents to available resources, the therapist is supporting the family in their essential occupational function (Rainville, 1999).

TABLE 9–4	Examples of Risk Factors, Protective Factors, and Community Resources		
Risk Factors	**Child**	**Child-Parent Interactions**	**Family**
	Prematurity; low birth weight; perinatal stress	Decreased parent-child interactions	Mental Illness
	Poor sensorimotor development	Insecure attachments	Substance abuse
	Irritable disposition	Parent-child conflicts	Chronic poverty
	Exposure to substance abuse or violence		Violence
Protective Factors	"Easy" temperament	Mother-child attachment	Parental capacity to cope
	Problem-solving skills	Positive interpersonal relationships	Parental self-esteem
	Sociable; socioemotional robustness	Responsive caregiving	Appropriate developmental expectations
	Behavioral adaptiveness	Authoritative parenting/warmth, structure, high expectations	Basic needs met for food, shelter, medical care
	Faith	Emotional availability	Internal family harmony
			Social supports/connections to extended supportive family networks
Community Resources	Well-baby clinics	Mother-Child Interaction Supports	Community health clinics
	Women, infants, and children programs (WIC)	Developmental services	Family service clinics
	Early identification and referral services [IDEA PL105-17: Part C. Early Intervention]	Early intervention	Welfare and social services
		Feeding team	Drug and alcohol recovery programs
	Head Start	"Mommy and Me" classes	Job training and job counseling
	Even Start	Parental Support	Instrumental support for service delivery
	Public school system [IDEA PL105-17: Part B. School Age Services]	Parent support groups	Child care
		Parent education	Transportation
		Parent counseling	Toy loan
		Social Supports	Translator
		Church programs	Community safety
		Library programs	
		Parks and Recreation activities	

Adapted from Epps & Jackson, 2000; Poulsen, 1993.

FAMILIES AND THE "LESS THAN PERFECT" NEWBORN

Staggering obstacles face new parents as they learn that their baby is not completely perfect in health or development. This is a loss not unlike a death as they mourn the imagined "perfect" child and adapt to the actual child. In addition to dealing with this dramatic loss, parents of the "less than perfect" child also lose the freedom to anticipate the future of their baby, themselves, and the family, for there is no clear picture of this baby as a preschooler, adolescent, adult, or parent themselves in the future. As stated by Stern, Bruschweiler-Stern, & Freeland (1999), "The birth of a severely developmentally delayed or handicapped baby is a trauma that virtually stops time in its tracks . . . suddenly your future is unpredictable, and emotionally unimaginable. At the same moment, your past, full of hopes and fantasies of pregnancy, is obliterated and becomes too painful to remember.

Parents are held prisoner in an enduring present" (p. 183).

Parents of these "unexpected" children must become immersed in learning about the baby's problem and learning to see past the impairment so that they can bond with the actual baby. If the announcement of the problem occurs before bonding has begun, this process is clearly much more difficult, and rejection of the infant may occur. It can be an agonizing experience, as the full nature of the problem isn't clear, and no one can tell them how the child will turn out. New parents are often so overwhelmed that they need additional help and support to meet their own needs as well as those of their child.

SUMMARY

As the first view of human function to integrate the family into the performance factors that influence individual function, the ICF (World Health Organization, 2002) reflects a large body of research support about family systems, and the importance of family-centered care. To be an effective advocate for the child and the family, the therapist must understand the pervasive influence of family dynamics, recognize family risk factors, and then take the time to listen to the families. Families need support and education. There will be many points in their child's development when families need, and are ready for, additional information. Physical and occupational therapists are well-placed to provide this support.

Speaking of

Chronic Sorrow

SUSIE RITCHIE, RN, MPH, CPNP
DEVELOPMENTAL SPECIALIST AND PRIMARY CARE PROVIDER

During pregnancy all parents anticipate the delivery of a perfect, healthy baby. Perhaps nothing is more devastating to mothers and fathers than learning their newborn has a condition that will prevent him or her from becoming a fully functioning independent adult.

For nearly 30 years, I have worked with infants and young children who have developmental concerns. Over that time, I have developed a great appreciation for the impact of the first few months, days, and hours after parents are given a diagnosis that will affect their child and their family for life.

It is during that time of initial diagnosis, when the loss of the "wished-for child" is acutely felt, that mothers and fathers begin to grieve (Solnit & Stark, 1961). This grieving is part of a process of coming to terms with what that loss actually means for their child and their family. Some experience "chronic sorrow" that reflects a lifelong sadness (Olshansky, 1962).

I remember being asked to do a developmental assessment on a newborn with a rare genetic syndrome. When I entered the room, this lovely, articulate mother cried and told me, "The one thing I said to my husband during this pregnancy was, 'I know that I can't handle a baby who isn't okay. I just won't be able to care for a child who is retarded or obviously deformed.' Now, here we are." Fortunately, like most, that mother did "handle" her daughter and did it beautifully. Now, 17 years later, this very bright young woman is about to enter college, despite her obvious physical obstacles. While her parents rejoice in her accomplishments, they continue to grieve for the normal life experiences their child has been and will be denied because of her condition.

There is an excellent video produced by WinStar in 1999 entitled *For the Love of Julian*. In this film, narrated by Susan Sarandon, mothers and fathers discuss that time when they learned that their child would not be like other children due to a developmental disability. The emotion displayed by these families, in many cases years after the birth of the infant, is extremely powerful. I would encourage anyone working with children who have special needs to watch such films, listen to parents, and observe family interactions closely. In doing this, we can all come to understand that "acceptance" of a devastating diagnosis may never be completely possible. Recognizing that "acceptance" is a process that lasts for many years, indeed throughout the lifespan of parents and their special child, hopefully allows professionals and families to grow together in positive and productive ways.

REFERENCES

Ainsworth, M. (1982). Attachment retrospect and prospect. In C. M. Parkes & M. Stevenson-Hind (Eds.), *The place of attachment in human behavior.* New York: Basic Books.

American Heritage Dictionary of the English Language (4th ed.). (2000). Boston: Houghton Mifflin.

Barnwell, D. A., & Day, M. (1996). Providing support to diverse families. In P. J. Beckman (Ed.), *Strategies for working with families of young children with disabilities* (pp. 47–68). Baltimore: Brookes.

Beckman, P. J. (1996). Theoretical, philosophical, and empirical bases of effective work with families. In P. J. Beckman (Ed.), *Strategies for working with families of young children with disabilities* (pp. 1–16). Baltimore: Brookes.

Brazelton, T. B., & Greenspan, S. I. (2000). *The irreducible needs of children: What every child must have to grow, learn, and flourish.* Cambridge, MA: Perseus Publishing.

Brazelton, T. B., & Cramer, B. G. (1990). *The earliest relationship: Parents, infants, and the drama of early attachment.* New York: Addison-Wesley.

Case-Smith, J. (1998). Foundations and principles. In J. Case-Smith (Ed.), *Pediatric occupational therapy and early intervention* (pp. 3–25). Boston: Butterworth-Heinemann.

Chess, S., & Thomas, A. (1987). *Know your child.* New York: Basic Books.

Comfort, M. (1988). Assessing parent-child interactions. In D. J. Bailey & R. J. Simeonsson (Eds.), *Family assessment in early intervention* (pp. 65–94). Columbus, OH: Merrill.

Darling, R. B., & Baxter, C. (1996). *Families in focus: Sociological methods in early intervention.* Austin, TX: Pro-Ed.

Epps, S., & Jackson, B. J. (2000). *Empowered families, successful children: Early intervention programs that work.* Washington, DC: American Psychological Association.

Featherstone, H. (1980). *A difference in the family: Living with a disabled children.* New York: Penguin Books.

Frank, N. (1996). Helping families support siblings. In P. J. Beckman (Ed.), *Strategies for working with families of young children with disabilities* (pp. 169–188). Baltimore: Brookes.

Gerson, R. (1995). The family life cycle: Phases, stages, and crises. In R. H. Mikesell, D. D. Lusterman, & S. H. McDaniel (Eds.), *Integrating family therapy: Handbook of family psychology and systems theory* (pp. 91–111). Washington, DC: American Psychological Association.

Greenspan, S., & Greenspan, N. T. (1985). *First feelings: Milestones in the emotional development of your baby and child.* New York: Viking Penguin.

Humphry, R., & Case-Smith, J. (2001). Working with families. In J. Case-Smith (Ed.), *Occupational therapy for children* (4th ed.) (pp. 95–135). St Louis: Mosby, Inc.

Kaplan, H., & Sadock, B. (1998). *Synopsis of psychiatry* (8th ed.). Baltimore: Williams and Wilkins.

Lowman, D. K. (2000). Development of occupational performance components. In J. W. Solomon (Ed.), *Pediatric skills for occupational therapy assistants* (pp. 65–88). St. Louis: Mosby.

Lynch, R. T., & Morley, K. L. (1995). Adaptation to pediatric physical disability within the family system: A conceptual model for counseling families. *The Family Journal: Counseling and Therapy for Couples and Families, 3,* 207–217.

Mattingly, C. F., & Lawlor, M. C. (2003). Disability experience from a family perspective. In E. B. Crepeau, E. S. Cohn, & B. A. Boyt Schell (Eds.), *Willard and Spackman's occupational therapy* (10th ed.) (pp. 43–53). Philadelphia: Lippincott Williams and Wilkins.

McGongiel, M. J., Kaugman, R. K., & Johnson, B. H. (1991). *Guidelines and recommended practices for the individualized family service plan.* Bethesda, MD: Association for the Care of Children's Health.

Meyer, D. J., & Vadasy, P. (1994). *Sibshops: Workshops for siblings of children with special needs.* Baltimore: Brookes.

McGoldrick, M., Heiman, M., & Carter, B. (1993). The changing family life cycle: A perspective on normalcy. In F. Walsh (Ed.), *Normal family process* (2nd ed.) (pp. 405–443). New York: Guilford Press.

Olshansky, S. (1962). Chronic sorrow: A response to having a mentally defective child. *Social Casework, 43,* 190–193.

Peeks, B. (1997). Revolutions in counseling and education: A systems perspective in the schools. In W. M. Walsh & G. R. Williams (Eds.), *School and family therapy: Using systems theory and family therapy in the resolution of school problems* (pp. 5–12). Springfield, IL: Charles C. Thomas.

Poulsen, M. K. (1993). Strategies for building resilience in infants and your children at risk. *Infants and Young Children, 6,* 37–38.

Powell. T. H., & Gallegher, P. A. (1993). *Brothers and sisters—A special part of exceptional families* (2nd ed.). Baltimore: Brookes.

Rainville, E. B. (1999). The special vulnerabilities of children and families. In S. M. Porr & E. B. Rainville (Eds.), *Pediatric therapy: A systems approach* (pp. 61–120). Philadelphia: F. A. Davis.

Rolland, J. S. (1993). Mastering family challenges in serious illness and disability. In F. Walsh (Ed.), *Normal family process* (2nd ed.) (pp. 444–473). New York: Guilford Press.

Seligman, M., & Darling, R. B. (1997). *Ordinary families, special children: A systems approach to childhood disability* (2nd ed.). New York: Guilford Press.

Solnit, A. J., & Stark, M. H. (1961). Mourning and the birth of a defective child. *The Psychoanalytic Study of the Child, 16,* 523–527.

Stern, D. N., Bruschweiler-Stern, N., & Freeland, A. (1999). *The birth of a mother: How the motherhood experience changes you forever.* New York: Basic Books.

Thompson, R. A. (2001). Development in the first years of life. *The Future of Children: Caring for Infants and Toddlers, 11,* 21–33.

Turnbull, A. P., & Turnbull III, H. R. (1997). *Families, professionals, and exceptionality: A special partnership* (3rd ed.). Columbus, OH: Merrill.

Winton, P. J., & Winton, R. E. (2000). Family systems. In J. W. Solomon (Ed.), *Pediatric skills for occupational therapy assistants* (pp. 11–37). St. Louis: Mosby.

World Health Organization (2002). ICF: International Classification of Functioning and Disability. Geneva, Switzerland: World Health Organization.

Development in the Preschool Years

Anne Cronin, PhD, OTR/L, BCP
Associate Professor
Division of Occupational Therapy
West Virginia University
Morgantown, West Virginia

Objectives

Upon completion of this chapter, the reader should be able to

■ Describe the developmental tasks of the preschool child, including these dimensions: motor characteristics, sensory characteristics, global mental characteristics, specific mental characteristics, play, and self-care.

■ Describe the development of tool use and its impact on function.

■ Identify the major power and precision grasp patterns.

■ Describe school readiness, including physical and cognitive/behavioral task performance expectations.

■ Describe asynchronous development and discuss its impact on function.

■ Differentiate typical characteristics of preschool play and discuss the importance of play in the development of functional skill.

■ Describe the contextual factors influencing the preschool child and the influence of these factors on function and disability.

Key Terms

associative play

asynchronous development

bimanual coordination

calibration

constructive play

cooperative play

discriminative touch

dynamic mobility

dynamic postural stability

equilibrium reactions

eye-hand coordination

fantasy play

fine motor control

flow

graphomotor skills

hand preference

haptic perception

in-hand manipulation

learned helplessness

mastery motivation

negativism

nonvolitional behavior

onlooker play

parallel play

perceptual motor skill

play

playfulness

postural stability

power grasp

precision grasp

school readiness

self-efficacy

sensory integration

sensory integration theory

solitary play

stability limits

static postural stability

static visual acuity

visual discrimination

visual pursuits

visual scanning

visual skills

volitional behaviors

INTRODUCTION

In Western cultures, an infant transitions to toddlerhood when he achieves the developmental milestone of walking, typically between 12 and 18 months of age. This is an important transition, because the period of rapid neuromotor development slows and the developmental focus shifts from acquisition of motor control to acquisition of communication and social and behavioral control. As we will see, physiologic and motor control changes will continue at a rapid rate, but the sudden expansion in communication and social skills will eclipse other areas in contributing to increased function. In infancy the emphasis in development was in the areas of structure and function. In the preschool years true interactive participation and activities occur. The personal and environmental contexts become increasingly apparent in their influence on the rate and types of skills acquired.

Increasingly, experience plays a role in development. As stated by Bruce Perry, "The brain does not just automatically develop the capability to love, create, communicate, or think. Experiences—repetitive, consistent, predictable, and nurturing—are required to express the underlying genetic potential of each child. And it is becoming increasingly clear that it is the experiences of early childhood that play a key role in determining the foundational organization and capabilities of the brain" (Perry, 1998, p. 1). In the 2nd through 4th developmental years the child acquires the basic skills needed to function within her social and cultural

environment. These skills, called *developmental milestones,* usually appear in long lists of skills typical within a culture to a specific age group. In children 1–2 years of age the cultural differences are minimal, but they increase as the child matures. In this chapter developmental milestones will be considered, but the focus will be on the development of general functional skills— such as the ability to shift and rotate small objects within the hand—and **dynamic mobility**—the ability to time, anticipate, and change motions while actively moving. Milestones are useful for screening children but do not give the physical and occupational therapist adequate information to determine whether a delay is based on neuromotor or environmental causes.

The experiences of early childhood play a key role in determining the organization of the brain (Perry, 1998; Parham & Mailloux, 2001). In fact, research has shown that the neurologic organization of any brain area is use-dependent, and neurodevelopment is dependent upon experiences during development (Perry et al., 1995; Shore, 1997). The presence or absence of sensory and motor opportunities in the preschool years can have an impact on the child's developing sense of self and his openness to challenges and learning. Consistent, nurturing, and enriched environments are needed for the young child to reach his potential. The prevalence of early-intervention and programs such as Head Start reflect the importance of early support for families with special needs and demands. Perry (1998) remarks, "The child with neglect, chaotic, and terrorizing environments will have significant problems in all domains of functioning" (p. 1). In this chapter we will focus on the typical activities that preschool children participate in, with a special focus on self-care as an emerging skill as well as on play and playfulness.

BODY STRUCTURES AND FUNCTIONS: MOTOR CHARACTERISTICS

In the preschool age group, body structures should all be present, though still maturing. Physical growth remains rapid, with typical preschool children gaining 5–7 pounds a year (Santrock, 1997). Throughout these early years the brain and central nervous system continue to grow. During this time there is an increase in the number and size of nerve endings and an increase in myelination (Santrock, 1997). It is because of this continued brain growth and neural plasticity that there is such an emphasis on early intervention and early identification of developmental differences. This period affords the most productive time for therapists to make lasting changes in motor function.

Throughout the preschool years children gain muscle bulk, coordination, and strength. Walking becomes smoother and more effortless, and the child gains skill in running, jumping, and climbing. The rate and sequence of skill acquisition vary with the child's environment and social situation. Developmental screening tests list milestones like "pedals a tricycle," which assumes exposure and practice with tricycles or bicycles with training wheels (Figure 10–1). The health-care professional needs to understand the qualitative changes in movement during this period in order to isolate motor skill delay from culture and environmental influences. Another component of motor skills is the necessary physical energy to sustain performance of tasks. Typically developing preschool children are characteristically very energetic and prefer active play. Although they have high energy and activity levels, they may have limited endurance to sustain time-consuming tasks without problems of physical fatigue.

Earlier in this text developmental reflexes and reactions were presented. Such motor behaviors are **nonvolitional,** meaning they occur without thought or planning. **Volitional behaviors,** in contrast to reflexes and reactions, are those behaviors that the individual chooses to use to meet a desired goal. Although volitional behaviors are present in the term infant, they are very limited because the infant does not yet have the postural control, perception, or mental functions needed to support complex actions. In the preschool years the nonvolitional behaviors are refined and changed and increasingly interact with volitional behavior.

DEVELOPMENT OF POSTURAL CONTROL

Postural control is the ability to control the body's position in space, to remain erect in spite of changes in the surface being walked on (Payne & Isaacs, 2001). Postural reflexes and reactions developed in infancy support the development of postural control. The ability to walk upright indicates a mastery of the body's muscle system to overcome the influence of gravity. **Postural stability** is the ability to keep the body balanced and aligned. **Static postural stability** is the ability to maintain the preferred posture when the body is still. This would include the ability to remain upright while sitting in a chair or to stand quietly when waiting in line without leaning against a support. In toddlers, static postural stability is brief, but dramatic improvements occur as the child gains muscle bulk and behavioral control. By the age of 5 most children can stand quietly in line for 2–3 minutes and can sit quietly for 5–10 minutes.

In studies of postural stability, *stability* is defined as that point when the center of the body's mass is aligned over its base of support. **Stability limits** are the farthest that the individual can shift her mass off center without altering her base of support. Children with weak or immature nervous systems may be slow to develop static postural stability and have narrow stability limits. Children with Down syndrome provide an example of this, as they often are slow to sit independently, and when they do sit, they topple to the side easily if they attempt to reach for a toy. The difference in the resting tension in their muscles makes it harder for them to acquire motor skills, and an enriched play environment or preschool program like the one shown in Figure 10–2 is recommended.

Although the balance and postural patterns of the preschool child remain immature, children can engage in a wide variety of challenging motor tasks like ballet, swimming, and gymnastics. Throughout the preschool

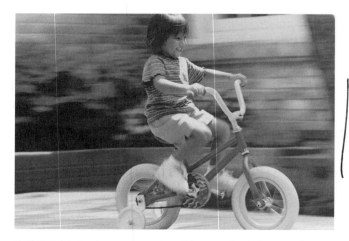

FIGURE 10–1   Large motor play with increasing balance and control for tasks like riding a bicycle emerge during the preschool years. (Image courtesy of PhotoDisc®, Inc.)

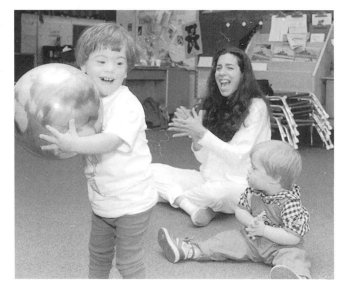

FIGURE 10–2   Larger, more exaggerated movement patterns typify the large motor play of children with Down syndrome.

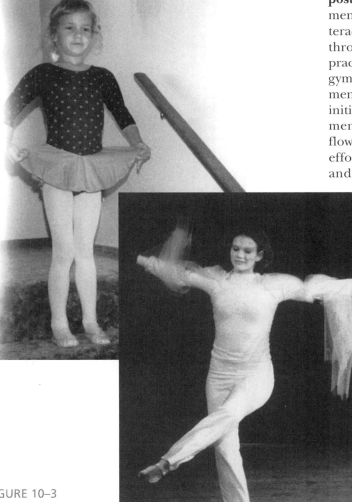

FIGURE 10–3
Movement flow improves in this dancer between the ages of 5 and 16.

years, postural control becomes more adaptive as the child develops the ability to integrate multiple perceptions and gains motor strength and flow. **Flow** is the term used to describe smooth, fluid movements (American Occupational Therapy Association, 2002). While the toddler may have static postural control in many positions, she is likely to also have limited ability to combine mobility and stability patterns functionally for a more active, dynamic form of postural stability. For example, when asked to kick a ball, the toddler will run up to the ball and stop. After stopping and establishing her balance, the toddler can then shift her weight to kick. Flow is likely to be the most noticeable difference between the preschool dancer and the dancer in adolescence. Figure 10–3 shows a 5-year-old dancer next to a picture of the same dancer at age 16. The difference in quality of movement, even in these still photos, is evident.

By about age 5 many children can run fluidly and kick a ball without stopping or compromising their balance. This type of active, adaptive control is **dynamic postural stability,** and it is associated with the development of flow. Dynamic postural control is a complex interaction of muscle strength, perception, and learning through practice. Children gain this skill earlier if it is practiced, as you see in the preschool hockey player or gymnast. Figure 10–4 illustrates some of the improvements in running seen during the preschool years. The initial pattern shown is that of the new walker. The elementary stage shows the older preschooler, in whom flow is emerging and there is more economy of motor effort. Skills in the mature stage, characterized by flow and economy of movement, require practice and are refined into middle childhood.

Equilibrium reactions are complex patterns involving rotational movements along the body axis in order to maintain balance (Shumway-Cook & Woollacott, 2001). These reactions are considered neurologically mature because their presence indicates the integration of earlier primitive and transitional motor patterns. Equilibrium reactions in standing typically emerge between 12 and 21 months of age and are fully mature by age 4. The changes in equilibrium are reflected in the developmental progression of jumping skills. Early jumping mostly involves the legs, and no trunk rotation is observed. As Figure 10–5 shows, in the elementary stage of development common to preschoolers, the upper body has become more active, and trunk rotation is emerging.

Rotational movement around the body axis characterizes equilibrium reactions. Such rotation requires active

Initial

Elementary

Mature

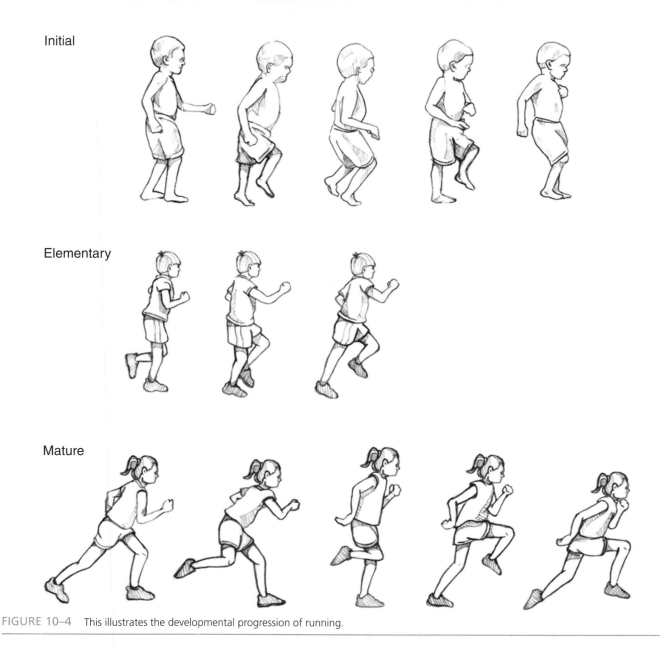

FIGURE 10–4   This illustrates the developmental progression of running.

movement of multiple muscle groups acting together in a smooth, regulated fashion. This smooth rotation movement can occur only when the postural reflexes of infancy have been integrated and a more flexible means of control allows for simultaneous contraction of opposing muscle groups beyond preprogrammed reflex patterns.

Some children are slow to develop this smooth, coordinated control. Children with impairments in motor function, like cerebral palsy or Down syndrome, will have difficulty developing these higher-level skills. Children without obvious motor impairments may still be "clumsy" and slow to refine their equilibrium reactions. In these cases, the limitation is not in developmental milestones but in flow and calibration of

movement. **Calibration** of movement is the judgment of force, speed, and directional control needed when attempting a task (American Occupational Therapy Association, 2002). Difficulties with calibration are evidenced by either too much or too little force being exerted or when the action is performed too quickly. Difficulties with calibration are common when *resting muscular tension* (muscle tone) is outside a typical range. When preschool children try to cuddle with pets, they often hold them either too lightly or too tightly, common errors in calibration (Figure 10–6). Difficulties with calibration are easy to see in broken crayons, spraying juice boxes, and frequent tripping. Calibration errors may also result in unintentionally hurting other children in play.

Initial

Elementary

Mature

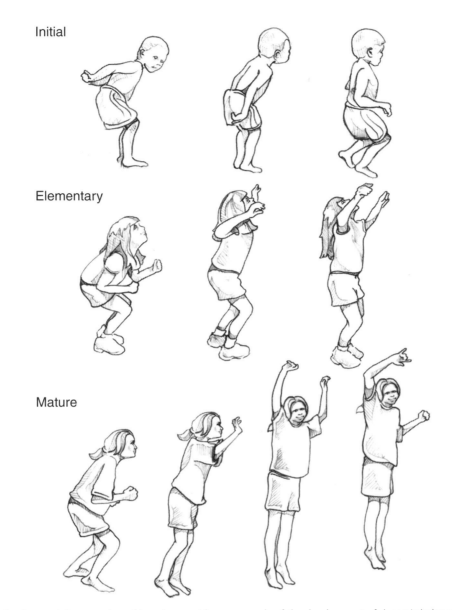

FIGURE 10–5   The developmental progression of jumping provides an example of the development of dynamic balance.

FINE MOTOR DEVELOPMENT

Fine motor development is a significant developmental realm for the preschool child. As mentioned in the discussion of infancy, fine motor development generally refers to those movements produced by the smaller muscles or muscle groups in the body. **Fine motor control,** in this text, includes the coordinated use of the eyes, hands, and muscles of the mouth. While postural control is nonvolitional, fine motor control is largely volitional. The individual must be conscious and self-directed to develop coordination and skill in the small muscle groups. Children with impairments in mental functions often have delayed fine motor skill

development, even in the presence of an intact motor system (Henderson & Pehoski, 1995). It is not uncommon to see a child with profound cognitive impairments who does not develop the ability to hold a spoon or use a pencil even though there is no actual motor impairment limiting him.

From the time that voluntary release is well established (around 15 months), children refine and specialize their grasp patterns based on the characteristics of the object they are grasping. As with other types of motor learning, it is normal to have a lot of variety and experimentation in emerging grasp patterns. There are two major types of grasp that are differentiated (Smith, Weiss, & Lehmkuhl, 1996; Hertling &

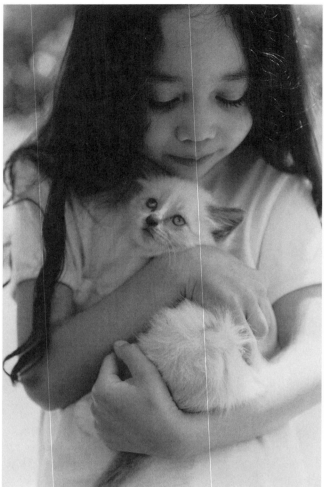

FIGURE 10–6   Calibration includes the ability to hold firmly without squeezing your pet. (Image courtesy of PhotoDisc®, Inc.)

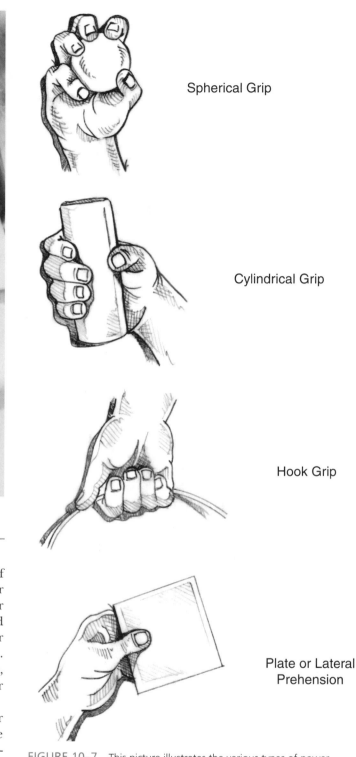

Spherical Grip

Cylindrical Grip

Hook Grip

Plate or Lateral Prehension

FIGURE 10–7   This picture illustrates the various types of power grasps.

Kessler, 1996) according to the position and mobility of the thumb joints. **Power grasp** patterns are used for managing large or heavy objects. Some types of power grasp are *cylindrical grips, spherical grip, hook grip,* and *plate,* or *lateral, prehension* (Figure 10–7). In the power grasp patterns the full strength of the hand is used. These are the patterns used for holding and carrying, and in early toy play. Object size and shape play a major role in the selection of grip patterns.

Precision grasp patterns emerge only slightly later but continue to be refined through adolescence (Henderson & Pehoski, 1995). In spite of their long period of refinement, most forms of precision grasp emerge in the preschool years. Distinctive features of the precision grasp patterns are the unsupported hand and active wrist extension (Shumway-Cook & Woollacott, 2001). Some examples of precision grasp are: "chuck," or *tripod grips, pincer grasp* (the fingertips press against each other), and *lateral prehension* (pad-to-side; key grip) (Figure 10–8). These forms of grasp are refined in the preschool years.

Together with the increase in hand activity and the expansion in types of play the child engages in, there is a change in the physical structure of the hand from the soft, featureless infant hand to a hand with clearly defined arches and muscular areas. It is the development of this hand structure that accommodates the

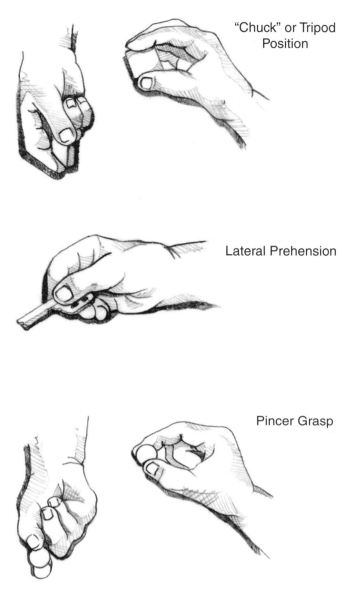

"Chuck" or Tripod Position

Lateral Prehension

Pincer Grasp

FIGURE 10–8   The early developing palmar supinate grasp involves wrist flexion. The later developing grasps show increasing wrist extension and a more distal placement of the pencil.

development of precision grasp and manipulation. Three arches balance stability and mobility in the hand (Figure 10–9). The proximal transverse palmar arch is rigid, but the other two arches, the distal transverse palmar arch and the longitudinal palmar arch, are flexible, and are maintained by activity in the hand's intrinsic muscles (Henderson & Pehoski, 1995).

Failure to play with objects and engage in haptic exploration can lead to inadequate development of the hand muscles and poorly defined palmar arches (Henderson & Pehoski, 1995). Children with limited variety of play are more likely to have difficulty adapting to the tool-use demands of school and to self-care. When there are no cognitive impairments, most preschool children catch up quickly when new tools are introduced. When fine-motor hand tasks are presented in a developmentally appropriate, systematic format, preschool children can develop very fine hand control. Research consistently reports that play and exploration are crucial activities for young children (Perry, 1998; Parham & Fazio, 1997).

SENSORY CHARACTERISTICS

Entering the preschool years, the typical toddler has a fully functional system for receiving sensory information. From infancy, vision is the sensory system that motivates the child to explore the world. Children can see and want to explore things well before they are independently mobile. This is one of the reasons for the popularity of infant walkers. The demanding prewalker now has the ability to move in space and follow up on those enticing visual cues.

With the toddler's ability to move and actively explore the environment, there is a rapid growth in sensory perception, followed by exploration of new motor actions. A controlled, volitional motor act that responds in a dynamic way to sensory perceptions is **perceptual motor skill.** Many of the traditional items on developmental screening tests for this age test specific perceptual motor skills like walking along a line, throwing a ball to a target, and climbing playground equipment. Children with deficits in sensory function or in sensory perception may be able to sit, stand, run, and jump but be unable to manage these perceptual motor tasks. Children with visual impairments are among the most vulnerable and often have delays in development of perceptual motor skills (Gentile, 1997). Children with visual impairments must develop learning strategies to accommodate their limited or absent vision. These children have a unique developmental sequence and should not be assessed on standards developed for the visually intact child.

SENSORY INTEGRATION

The term **sensory integration** is widely used in the neurosciences literature to describe the brain's ability to automatically combine sensory information from a variety of different senses to permit accurate categorization of perceptual information. This neurobiologic process begins in utero and rapidly expands through infancy and the preschool years. It has been the focus of interest and research, and **sensory integration theory** was developed as a tool for therapists. A. Jean Ayres introduced the theory as a frame of reference for therapy interventions in the late 1950s. Since then many other researches have contributed to development of this theory (Parham & Mailloux, 2001), which describes the senses (auditory, vestibular, proprioceptive, tactile,

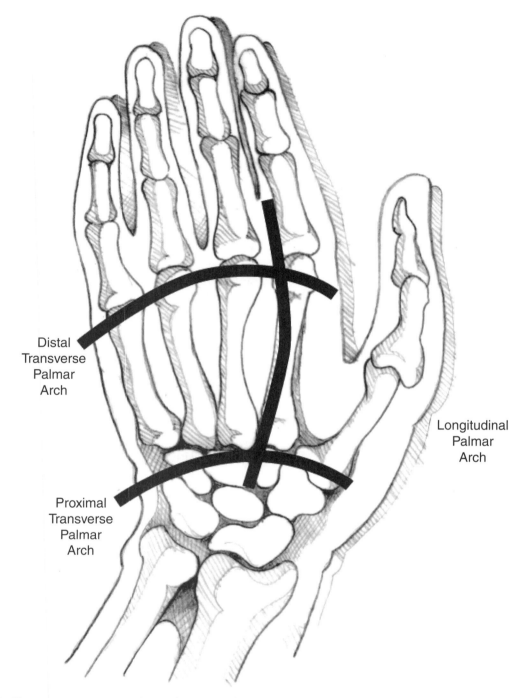

FIGURE 10–9 There are two transverse palmar arches, proximal and distal, and one longitudinal palmar arch.

and visual) as contributing to learning and to the development of important functional skills discussed in this chapter, including regulation of activity level and attention span, eye-hand coordination, visual perception, and many metacognitive functions.

The basic concept of sensory integration theory is that both the global and specific mental functions that allow us to interact and respond in purposeful ways depend on adequate organization of sensory information. Stimuli must be integrated and matched with past experience for accurate information to register, and for the generation of a meaningful response. This is a powerful information-processing network that allows for input from one sensory system to facilitate or inhibit the entire system. This sensory integration process is innate, and it provides an innate drive to seek out new sensory experiences. The innate motivation to move and play that pervades early childhood is believed to be a normal, healthy outcome of sensory integration, which enhances the quality of all developmental processes (Parham & Mailloux, 2001).

This text focuses on typical or "normal" development. At this point it is important to realize that there are individual differences in development, and that there is a continuum of function. In terms of sensory integration, some individuals can integrate sensory information quickly and efficiently, and others need more time or information to come to the same end result. As the discussion proceeds to specific types of sensory function, be aware that an individual may not be equally skilled in using sensory input from all modalities. Children with significant difficulties processing specific sensory modalities may be described as having *sensory integrative dysfunction*. These children often have difficulty acquiring the skills needed to perform well in the school environment.

VISUAL SKILLS

For the purpose of this discussion, the term **visual skills** will be used to describe the ability of the individual to use extraocular muscles to direct the eye. The primary eye movements used in vision are visual pursuits (also called *tracking*) and visual scanning (also called *saccadic eye movements*). **Visual pursuits** are slow, smooth movements, typically used as the gaze follows a moving object. **Visual scanning** involves short, rapid changes of fixation from one point in the visual field to another. Visual scanning is used when searching for something and in reading (Gentile, 2001).

The eye is still immature at birth, and visual skills gradually develop throughout the first 5 years of life (Payne & Isaacs, 2001). The infant has efficient **static visual acuity;** this refers to the ability to discern details when both the person and the target are static. Static visual acuity is useful for reaching and grasping objects, the basic hand skills required in infancy and early in the preschool years. This skill is much used in preschool play activities, as illustrated in Figure 10–10. Static visual acuity is the ability tested in standard eye exams. It is important that visual problems are identified early, because failure to correct this type of problem can hinder the development of eye-hand coordination. **Eye-hand coordination** is the "skillful use of the hand under visual guidance" (Erhardt, 1992, p.13). As eye-hand coordination emerges, the child experiments with hand movements and begins to develop fine hand and eye control.

Visual perception is a "mental function involved in discriminating shape, size, colour, and other ocular stimuli" (World Health Organization, 2002). Children first learn to recognize objects based on their general appearance. This early ability is **visual discrimination,** and it includes the ability to distinguish specific features of an object like shape, size, and color. The visual discrimination of forms precedes the child's ability to copy those forms in drawing tasks. As the preschool child begins to experiment with crayons, he first makes random marks, then can trace and imitate lines he sees someone draw for him. After this, the child can copy simple lines and pictures, and finally he can draw the lines and shapes from memory.

By the age of 4, most children can follow simple instructions and copy patterns for art projects and early writing, as shown in Figure 10–10. This fact illustrates how closely visual and hand skill development are linked. The visually impaired child will be much slower to develop these hand skills, as her perceptions must be based on other discriminative cues, like touch perception.

TOUCH SKILLS

The sense of touch has many different functions in development. The type of touch that warns us of pain or danger is a very diffuse network that causes a protective alerting response. This type of touch is what causes one to startle when tickled from behind with a piece of grass. Light, moving touch is a trigger for this type of protective withdrawal response. Firm touch, as the infant enjoys in swaddling, is a quieting or calming touch. Both of these early touch responses persist throughout life. As the infant gains touch experience, she can begin to identify things as distinct from the more general protective and calming types of touch. This is accomplished by a neurologically newer (more complex) ability to discriminate types of touch. In order for a child to touch things in a manner that encourages the development of perception and memory, her early protective reaction needs to be overridden by discriminative

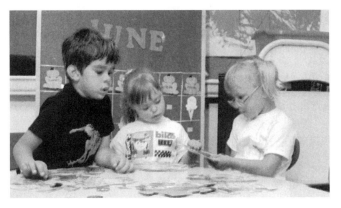

FIGURE 10–10 Prescription lenses can help prevent early delays in eye-hand coordination in preschoolers with visual impairments.

touch perceptions. **Discriminative touch** functions are those aspects of touch that we think about consciously, like how hard, smooth, or curved an object is. Discriminative touch is the type of touch that allows preschool children to learn to use their hands with increased dexterity and acquire tool-use skills. **Haptic perception** is the active memory of touch, texture, shape, temperature, and weight that allows the child to tell you that she has a penny in her hand even when she cannot see the penny.

The information acquired through the combination of haptic perception and visual perception allows for the development of complex, highly refined hand control. When children have difficulty or inefficiency integrating touch information, they often have secondary difficulties in developing fine motor control and self-care skills. A common problem, *tactile defensiveness,* occurs when the child reacts with protective or avoidance responses to what should be nonthreatening touch information. Children with tactile defensiveness may be very selective about the type of clothing they will wear and the type of foods they will eat, and may become very distressed in social situations around other children. Because it leads children to avoid touch and tactile exploration, tactile defensiveness can limit hand skill, self-care, and social skill development.

DEVELOPMENT OF SELF-CARE SKILLS

Even in infancy children are motivated to be active in their care. First holding a bottle and then finger-feeding, the infant participates in self-care. By the preschool years the child is independent in basic mobility but still needs supervision because of poor safety awareness. By 18 months most children feed themselves part of each meal and will wash and dry their own hands, though they are not careful and do not check to see if

dirt remains on the hands. Between 2 and 4 years of age children develop many *activities of daily living (ADLs).* This can be a frustrating time for parents, because the children want to do it themselves but are very inefficient and make many errors.

The order in which children develop self-care skills varies with their culture and experience. Dressing skill often emerges early because it has meaning for the child and is part of the daily routine. Typically in complex skills like dressing the child learns part of a task before attempting the entire skill. Table 10–1 presents a typical sequence of the acquisition of dressing skills for a child growing up in North America.

Children first learn skills that are highly valued by their parents. For children in North America the earliest self-care skills to develop in preschool years are oral hygiene, eating, dressing, and toilet hygiene. In addition to learning to take care of themselves, preschool children imitate and participate in *instrumental activities of daily living (IADLs).* Examples of emerging IADLs in the preschool years are setting the table, picking up toys, washing vegetables, and folding washcloths. In all these tasks the child can actively imitate and participate but will continue to need adult supervision. Preschool children often "practice" IADLs in their play activities, such as by playing house or pushing a toy lawn mower.

Although the sequence of skill acquisition may vary, by the end of the preschool years the child is independent in basic personal care, including toileting, and will be able to function with minimal supervision in the school setting. Some skills may be later to develop because of unusual demands. For example, children with very long or very curly hair may need assistance for several more years to wash, comb, and style their hair. The child's clothing in a cold northern climate may have more layers and more complex fasteners than the clothing typical of warmer climates. Chopsticks are also more complex to manage than western utensils, and in this case finger-feeding may

TABLE 10–1	Typical Sequence of Acquisition of Dressing Skills for Children in North America
Age	**Typical Self-Dressing Sequence**
1 year	Holds out arms and legs, pulls off shoes and socks, pushes arms through sleeves and legs through pants.
2 years	Removes unfastened coat, pulls down pants, finds armholes in T-shirt, and puts on front-buttoning coat/shirt.
3 years	Puts on T-shirt and shoes (may be on wrong foot), puts on socks, manages basic fasteners (zips and unzips, manages large buttons, snaps, buckles), unties and removes shoes, and removes pull-down garment.
4 years	Manages separating zipper, puts on shoes and socks correctly, dresses completely with few errors, consistently finds front and back of garments.

persist later into the preschool years. Self-care independence is a source of pride for the preschool child and a source of embarrassment for the child who has delays in gaining these skills. There is much social pressure in preschool and kindergarten environments to be independent in self-care.

SCHOOL-READINESS SKILLS

One important outcome of successful preschool development is the acquisition of the specific skills needed to be successful in a school environment. **School readiness** is the mastering of prerequisite developmental criteria for success in the school environment. There are no agreed upon criteria for school readiness, but in general a child must be healthy, both physically and emotionally. Children should be largely independent in ADLs and should be able to follow directions. By the age of 5, children should be open to learning and able to communicate with both peers and adults (Kagan, 1999; Kagan, Moore, & Bredekamp, 1995). The specific knowledge and perceptual motor skills needed for school are not universally agreed upon in the education community. Many of the skills that are the focus of the early childhood teacher are also a focus in occupational and physical therapy. Skill areas determined by Coster, et al. (1998) to be relevant to rehabilitation professionals are discussed here.

USING MATERIALS

Using materials requires the ability to use external things to complete a task. This endeavor includes actions like opening and closing a book and using writing utensils. By the age of 5, typically developing children are able to position their bodies and arms to allow them to engage in tabletop activities, although there is some degree of awkward positioning. Typically developing children have the necessary mobility skills to move their bodies through space without difficulty. They walk, bend, and reach for objects; however, they may still need to stop other activities to perform the walking, bending, or reaching task well. By 5 years, the child's bilateral coordination skills are still maturing, and switching hands during a task or failing to use one hand as an assist to stabilize a task are common (Payne & Isaacs, 2001).

Some examples of materials used in elementary school are crayons, pencils, eating utensils, buttons, blocks, and coins. Children between the ages of 2 and 5 learn to manipulate objects in one hand and learn to use one hand as a lead (or dominant) hand while the other hand assists. Tool-use skills are built on vision perception, somatosensory perception, and cognition. The

play of typically developing preschool children includes many types of sensory experiences. For many young children, bathing is a period of recreation and a focal part of the day (Figure 10–11).

Fundamental to efficient tool use is the development of in-hand manipulation. **In-hand manipulation** is "the process of using one hand to adjust an object for more effective object placement, or release; the object remains in that hand and usually does not come in contact with a surface during in-hand manipulation" (Exner, 1992, p. 35). There are three basic types of in-hand manipulation. The first, *translation,* "is a linear movement of the object in the hand from the finger surface to the palm or the palm to the fingers" (Exner, 1992, p. 39). *Shift movements* are the next type of in-hand manipulation. "Shift movements occur at the finger and thumb pads with the alternation of the thumb and finger movement" (Exner, 1992, p. 39–40). *Rotation* is the final type of in-hand manipulation. Rotation involves movements at or near the pads of the fingers that move an object around one or more of its axes.

Exner observed that the skill of in-hand manipulation developed continuously between 18 months and 7 years of age. In her study, all skill types were present in the 7-year-olds, but these children did not have adult proficiency in their use of the skills. In-hand manipulation has received such a focus in this discussion because this type of refined hand skill is needed for the preschool child to become competent in dressing, toileting, independent eating, and a variety of school readiness skills, including scissors use and graphomotor skills.

The hands of an infant are typically chubby with dimples at the joints. Through the preschool years the hands seem to lose their "baby fat" and become increasingly muscular.

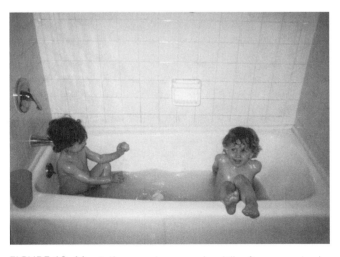

FIGURE 10–11   Self-care and sensory play skills often occur simultaneously in the preschool years.

Graphomotor Skills

Graphomotor skills are the collections of conceptual and perceptual motor skills involved in drawing and writing. Drawing, the art of producing a picture or plan with some implement (pen, pencil), begins to develop first. Writing, the process of forming letters, numbers, and other significant figures, which incorporates language learning as well as sensory and motor skills, develops next. Early in the process of learning to write, children copy the letterforms as they would copy shapes. Prior to the understanding of the alphabet and its role in written language, this letter-copying is more accurately described as drawing. When children with impairments in mental functions learn to write words by memorizing the shape of the word, the children are compensating for difficulty in processing written language by drawing on their graphic skills.

The prehension patterns required for graphomotor tasks are modifications of the three-jaw chuck presented earlier in Figure 10–8. These *tripod grasps*, illustrated in Figure 10–12, emerge during the preschool

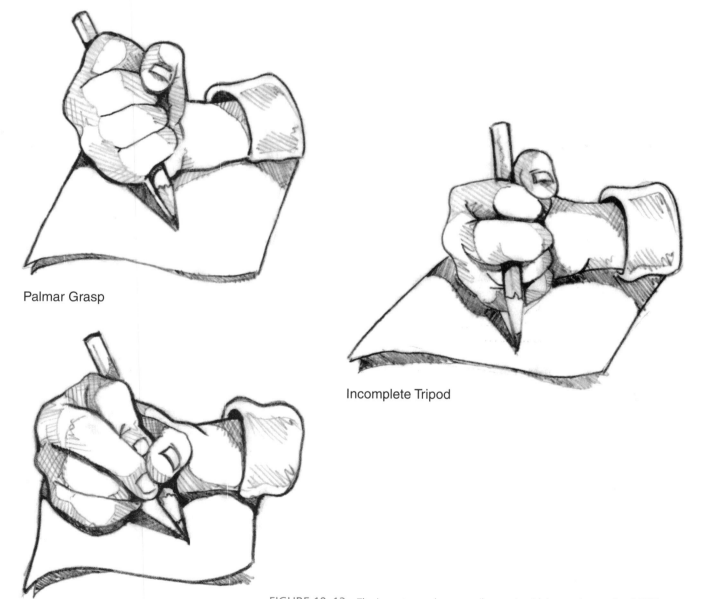

Palmar Grasp

Incomplete Tripod

Tripod Posture

FIGURE 10–12   The immature palmar pencil grasp is widely seen in preschool. With practice in pencil use, the grasp involves more pronation and wrist extension.

years. Unlike the static grasp patterns described earlier, they become dynamic, utilizing in-hand manipulation skills to adjust the tool to meet the demands of the task. This skill will continue to be refined through middle childhood.

The sequence by which children learn graphomotor tasks usually begins with tracing (eyes direct hands to follow visual representation), then imitating (eyes watch and remember another's actions in order to repeat the action), followed by copying (eyes alternate glances between visual representation and own production) (Henderson & Pehoski, 1995). These hand skills are often called "pre-academic" skills in the development literature, because they provide the foundation and tools for later academic learning.

Although there are many technological tools to allow children to compensate for poor graphomotor skill, the combination of visual and haptic perception, kinesthetic awareness, motor control, and memory needed for graphomotor tasks will be needed as well in many other realms of function, including the use of a computer keyboard.

Hand Preference

Early in the preschool years children learn to use the hands in a complementary fashion, with one hand holding or stabilizing materials and the other hand performing the skilled task. The process of using one hand as a lead hand and the other as an assist hand is called **bimanual coordination.** Early in development children frequently switch hands, with either hand taking the lead role in activity. Over the preschool years most children come to consistently prefer one hand as the skilled hand. **Hand preference** is the consistent choice of the same hand for complex skilled tasks. It is established in most children by the age of 4 (Murray, 1995). Hand preference is most typically seen in practiced activities like eating and graphomotor tasks. Although true hand dominance may not develop until age 7, it is in the graphomotor tasks that the lead-assist pattern becomes most highly refined. Failure to develop hand preference can also lead to delayed development of the skilled hand and specific tool grasps associated with writing and drawing.

ATTENTION AND MEMORY

In terms of the ICF classifications of global mental functions, preschool children are competent in consciousness, sleep, and basic orientation and drive functions. The global function of temperament is a personality factor and influences the social and learning style of the preschooler. Intellectual mental functions are developing as the child gains perceptual

motor experience. As noted earlier in this chapter, with the mastery of independent mobility, preschool children become very active and "driven" to explore their sensory environment (Bukatko & Daehler, 2001). Piaget first described patterns of physical or mental action that underlie specific acts of intelligence and correspond to stages of child development. Of the four primary cognitive structures described by Piaget, two fall into the preschool years. These are the sensorimotor period and preoperational period. In the *sensorimotor period* (typically ages 0–2 years), intelligence is demonstrated through motor activity without the use of symbols like written or spoken language. Sensorimotor intelligence is knowledge of the world based on physical interactions and experiences. In the later *preoperational period* (typically 3–6 years) intelligence is demonstrated through the use of symbols, language use matures, and memory and imagination are developed. During this period learning continues to be greatly influenced by experience, and children are *egocentric,* meaning they do not consider the possibility of viewpoints other than their own. Recent studies (Bremner & Bryant, 2001; Bjorklund, 2000; Subbotsky, 2000) have determined that experience and familiarity with the task greatly influence the performance of children on the Piaget experiments. The current belief is that Piaget's theories continue to provide the most important framework for considering cognition in preschool children, but that his theory does not completely reflect the scope of learning and thinking possible in preschool children.

Many cognitive, reasoning, and memory skills have developed in the typical child by the age of 5. These mental functions are needed for the child to perform well in a classroom setting. While there are devices and tools to help compensate for motor and sensory deficits, cognitive deficits are the most limiting in the school setting. For example, attention is one of the most important areas of development in the preschool years and is predictive of school success (Palfrey, 1995). Attention varies with task, social context, and temperament in the preschool years, so there are no general norms for what kind of attention is typical in young children, but Nader (1992, p. 294) reports that "the presence at or before the age of [4 years] of a high degree of activity, lack of ability to sustain attention, and impulsive behavior with little ability to delay gratification is a cluster of behaviors that has been associated with a high risk of school learning problems."

Attention is necessary for learning, and failure to develop adequately in this area may lead to delays in other areas of independent function. Computer games and other applications are increasingly popular with preschool children. Although some games are marketed for the very young child, it is also common for younger siblings to watch a more skilled older sibling, as shown in Figure 10–13, at play.

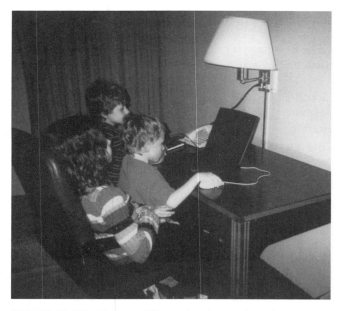

FIGURE 10–13   Younger siblings enjoy the sounds and animation of computer games, as their older sister plays.

Memory development is linked to perceptual experience and language development. The preverbal child exhibits memory in motor learning and demonstrates *rote memory,* mimicking or repeating phrases in a parrot-like fashion without meaning. While memory functions are probably intact in the young child, it takes close observation to assess the competence of short-term and long-term memory, memory span, and retrieval of memory before the child is competent in expressing himself verbally.

FUNCTIONAL COMMUNICATION

The development of language is the single most important functional achievement of the preschool years. Memory and attention are needed for a child to learn and maintain a language system. As noted in Chapter 5, language is a learned code, or system of rules, that makes it possible for us to communicate ideas and express wants and needs. Reading and writing are forms of language, as is speaking. Children with language delays typically also have delays in reading and writing, which are not secondary to difficulties in fine motor control.

TASK BEHAVIOR AND BEHAVIOR REGULATION

School activities require the child to demonstrate an ever increasing array of independent work habits. In the kindergarten classroom there is praise for the child who has the skill to maintain a consistent and effective pace throughout the steps of an assigned task. While distractibility and inconsistent work pacing is normative in

the 5-year-old, delays in acquiring these skills can impact successful classroom function.

Some work habits expected of the primary grades are: remaining in the designated work area, attending to directions, listening in large group activities like storytime, and receiving correction of errors identified by the teacher. Although there is very little regulation of emotional expression in the 2-year-old, emotional regulation is another important requisite for competence in the school environment. Children are expected to accept unexpected changes in routine, to refrain from provoking others, and to use nonaggressive words and actions (Coster et al., 1998).

FOLLOWING SOCIAL CONVENTIONS AND SCHOOL RULES

Social behavior is learned throughout the preschool years. As children gain confidence in walking, the toddler begins to experiment with other forms of personal independence. The preschool years are characterized by growing personal autonomy in social exchanges. Both caregiver and peer relations appear to be necessary for normal socioemotional development (Santrock, 1997). Children who experience much isolation, like immune-suppressed children, may have delays in development secondary to their limited social contact. This is also true of children with mobility limitation, like the child shown in Figure 10–14. Preschool children are very physical and active in their play. Children who cannot keep up on the playground are often left behind.

Early in this developmental period, often around 18 months of age, children begin to exhibit negativism. **Negativism** is an expression of autonomy that includes verbal repetitions of the word "no" and physical resistance in the form of hitting, biting, kicking, and tantrums. The social negativism of this period gives rise to the label "the terrible twos" (Bukatko & Daehler, 2001). In this period a child may say "no" to everything, even things that are liked, in an effort to be in control. This need to be in control also emerges in the areas of self-care. Two- and three-year-olds have basic eating, personal hygiene, and dressing skill, but tend to be slow and make many errors. In addition to "no," the parent of the typical 2-year-old hears "me do it" in self-care tasks. Children who have been very ill or who have a serious activity limitation may appear more passive and dependent than the typical child. In most cases these expressions of autonomy will emerge later when the child is in good health or when the child reaches the motor development level of the typical 2-year-old (Jackson & Vessey, 1996). Negativism usually resolves into more compliant behavior by age 5. Children who remain highly negative are likely to have difficulty in the school setting.

Ambivalence in social situations is common in the young child. This ambivalence occurs when the child

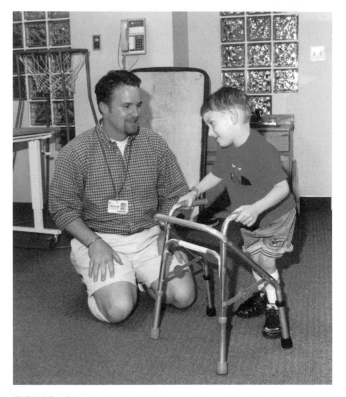

FIGURE 10–14 Preschool children with mobility limitations are likely to have proportionally more social interaction with adults and fewer with peers.

finds something simultaneously attractive and repulsive, as in the case of the child who wants the parent to be present and attending to her every action but cries and withdraws when the parent tries to be active and engage the child socially (Bukatko & Daehler, 2001). This type of behavior, where the child seems to demand attention, then pushes the parent away, is typical as children begin to develop autonomy. As the toddler gains the sense that he can be independent, he also learns that his parents are separate from him. Two- and three-year-olds often dislike being held, but "shadow" their mother, following her everywhere, including to the toilet. At this age children are happiest when free to explore but are within sight of their parents. *Separation anxiety,* mentioned in Chapter 8, is insecurity and emotional distress when removed from someone or something familiar. Separation anxiety and the need to shadow the parent are the reasons that many preschool assessment tools are designed to be given with the parent present. Typically, separation anxiety lessens over time, as does negativism. Children who attend day care and have more experience separating and reuniting with their parents are likely to have little problem starting school. Children who have been primarily in the care of a parent prior to starting school may continue to show some anxiety at separation when they start school. This type of anxiety is normal and resolves over time.

Play

The literature discussing school readiness emphasizes positive adult role models. Incorporating basic social rules like recognizing when they need to ask permission before proceeding, working cooperatively, sharing materials, using acceptable manners, and handling frustration are all skills that make a child "ready to learn" (Kagan, 1999; Kagan, Moore, & Bredekamp, 1995). A key method of learning and practicing these social skills is through play.

Play is "pleasurable activity that is engaged in for its own sake" (Santrock, 1997, p. 240). Play serves many functions for the preschool child. Occupational and physical therapists often focus on the role of play in motor skill acquisition. In addition to providing a practice arena for motor skills, play affords peer interactions, tension release, and advances in cognitive development (Santrock, 1997). Play is a human occupation that occurs at all developmental levels, and play at all ages brings pleasure. The aspect of pleasure is important because pleasure is the basis of the innate drive to repeat the pleasurable activity. This inner drive toward mastery of skills through play is one of the basic premises of *sensory integration theory* (Mailloux & Burke, 1997). Table 10–2 outlines the relationship between play and motor development.

In many ways play contributes to nervous system organization. Play evolves in tandem with the acquisition of developmental skills and becomes increasingly complex. As mentioned, it brings pleasure, as well as a powerful drive to repeat the pleasurable activity (Perry, Hogan, & Marlin, 2000). Children seem programmed with an innate drive for sensorimotor activity and repetition. With repetition comes **mastery motivation,** the "innate drive to find solutions" (Holly & Schuster, 1992, p. 462). Children learn through play and mastery motivation that they have some control over their world and can cause desired change. This belief in their personal power to change things is **self-efficacy.** Self-efficacy is an important school-readiness skill, as it enables the child to be open to challenges and to believe that he can master new skills.

Play is believed to be the primary tool through which the child learns about social and cultural roles and experiments with new skills. **Playfulness** is a characteristic pattern of interaction that includes the tendency to seek opportunities for play, to suspend reality, and to behave with spontaneity (Bundy, 1997). Although some types of play have just been described, play can occur during any activity and can take an infinite variety of forms. Intrinsic drive and motivation are key aspects of playfulness and have been identified in the ICF as global mental functions (World Health Organization, 2002). This aspect of a child's interactions can provide insight into her overall approach to functional behavior.

Early play is reality-based; actions of adults are imitated, and objects are used for their intended purposes.

TABLE 10–2	Interaction between Motor Development and Play		
Motor Behavior	**Approximate Age**	**Developmental Stage**	**Play**
Reflexive/spontaneous rudimentary control	< 1 year	Infancy	Learning self-regulation (peek-a-boo, tactile play)
Mobility and postural control	1–5 years	Preschool	Somatosensory play (large motor, fine motor, music)
Movement calibration and flow	6–10 years	Middle childhood	Socioemotional play (teams, win-lose, turns, sharing)
Skill refinement	11–16 years	Adolescence	Metacognitive play (humor, language, arts, social role-playing)

Mildred Parten (1932) developed a classification of children's play that is still used today. Between about 18 months and 4 years the child learns to be playful in social exchanges and to play independently. This type of play is called **solitary play. Onlooker play** occurs when the child watches other children play, and **parallel play** is common to 2-year-olds, who are very interested in age peers and enjoy their company but have not yet learned to share or play together. Hence, parallel play occurs when children are playing in the same vicinity as one another and are engaged in similar, or parallel, activities. **Associative play,** also common to 2-year-olds, occurs when children enjoy the company of other children but have little organization to their activity. Following one another around in lines, borrowing, and demonstrating toys are examples of associative play. **Cooperative play** "involves social interaction in a group with a sense of group identity" (Santrock, 1997, p. 241) and is more typical of middle childhood and will be discussed in that chapter.

Early **fantasy play** follows, often with the child dressing up or using props and then announcing who (or what) they are. This type of simple fantasy play develops around the same time that expressive language develops. Such fantasy play allows children to mentally experiment with new sensations or roles in a safe environment. It allows children to try out new behaviors for themselves in imagined forms—for example, being the parent, or a monster—allowing for growth in social behavior. Because negative feelings can be expressed in a safe way, fantasy play serves as an important tool for emotional growth. Fantasy also provides a tool to help children organize their "interior language." This role of play is believed to support later academic performance (Holly & Schuster, 1992). Fantasy play typically proceeds through four stages in the preschool years:

- *Reality play:* objects are used in play and are used for their intended purpose.
- *Object fantasy:* objects continue to be used in play but may be used in novel ways. For example, an empty box may be a house, a car, or a bed.

- *Person fantasy:* people's qualities are actively represented. For example, "The car wants a nap," or the traditional "tea party" activity.
- *Announced fantasy:* the child conceives of the game and announces it. Unlike the other types of fantasy play, with announced fantasy the activity is announced and then props are found. (Schuster, 1992)

Fantasy play is a developmental need that contributes to all areas of development. Figure 10–15 demonstrates typical preschool play. There is dress-up and imagination, often inspired by the tools available. Children like the company of others but often spend much of their time doing their own activities near the other children.

Much play at this time is imitative and triggered by both toys and the manner in which the children see those toys used. It is because of these developmental constraints that preschool children are especially vulnerable to the effects of television and movies. The average American child watches about 3–4 hours of television daily. Television can be a powerful influence in developing value systems and shaping behavior. Unfortunately, much of today's television programming is violent. Hundreds of studies of the effects of TV violence on children and teenagers have found that children may (1) become desensitized to violence, (2) accept violence as a way to solve problems, and (3) imitate violence seen on television (AACAP Fact Sheets for Parents, 2003).

Constructive play, the making or building of things, develops between the ages of 3 and 4 and closely parallels the development of manipulation and fine motor skills. This type of play includes puzzles, blocks, playdough, and a variety of art activities. Constructive play allows children to practice emerging fine motor skills and executive functions like planning, sequencing, and error detection. Children who are weak in these areas may avoid this type of play. It is not uncommon for a child to be very active in gross motor type play and avoid fine "constructive" play. Although children without neurologic impairments can catch up when specific skills

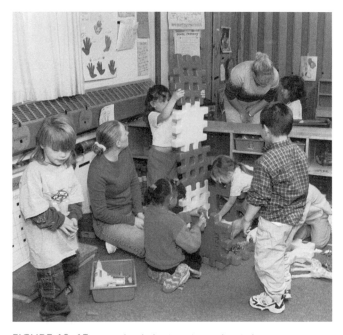

FIGURE 10–15   Preschool play is active and varied.

are required at school, it is best if children are encouraged to engage in a wide range of play activities.

ASYNCHRONOUS DEVELOPMENT

The term **asynchronous development** describes a situation in which the normal developmental progression is highly uneven. This was first described in studies of highly gifted children. Hollingsworth (1942) reported the difficulties of having the "intelligence of an adult and the emotions of a child in a childish body" (p. 282). In gifted children, the gap between the child's intellectual capability and his age-appropriate social and physical skills can lead to frustration and emotional distress. This problem is especially apparent in the preschool years as young children become frustrated when their limited physical capabilities prevent them from acting on their ideas, or from producing the physical products that they imagine.

For example, Jonathan, as a preschooler, was very talented in constructional play and demonstrated extremely precocious spatial perception. His parents accommodated his interests with lots of constructional toys and with art programs for the computer. Jonathan's transition to school at age 5 was very difficult, because kindergarten children are expected to draw a lot. Jonathan drew far better than the typical child but did not have the motor control to draw what he imagined. He tore up his school papers, threw his art materials down, and was very noncompliant. His behavior was baffling to his teachers, because he clearly could draw well. When his parents brought in some of his computer-generated designs, the source of his frustration was more obvious to all.

Children are asynchronous when their development is uneven and out of step with societal norms and their age mates. "Giftedness is asynchronous development in which advanced cognitive abilities and heightened intensity combine to create inner experiences and awareness that are qualitatively different from the norm" (Silverman, 1998). Asynchronous development occurs whenever the physical and cognitive developments are markedly uneven. An example often seen by pediatric therapists is the child with severe motor impairments, like cerebral palsy, and intact abilities to reason. As with Jonathan, these children see and understand what goes on around them but may lack the ability to communicate with others, to explore and experiment, and to act on their ideas. In both the highly gifted child and the child with good cognitive skills and severe motor impairment, the child is at greater risk for developing social and emotional problems. Typically developing children learn self-efficacy through play, as they explore and experiment with the world around them. Children with an asynchronous pattern of development are more likely to feel helpless. Without the motor skills to communicate, the child does not learn routine social exchanges and may be limited to squeals or grunts to get attention. The child knows that this is not normal but knows no options to gain skill in communicating. Megan, a nonverbal 4-year-old with severe athetoid cerebral palsy, has a wide array of eye gestures that her family has learned to read to communicate with her. She does not have any verbal language, and her eye communication system does not work well with outsiders. After her initial attempts at communication failed in the preschool setting, Megan did not try to initiate interaction and was very passive in all the daily classroom activities. Megan learned that she was not effective and could not actively engage others. Megan had learned that she was helpless.

Learned helplessness is a pattern of behavior that occurs when a person is faced with unsolvable problems. Helpless children often interpret failure at a desired task as a lack of ability and tend to give up rather than to try a different strategy (Roedell, 1984). Learned helplessness perpetuates itself: as the child tries less, there is less opportunity for success. So, returning to the example of Jonathan, if he refuses to draw or participate in art activities, over time his skills will fall behind those of the other children and his belief in his inability will be affirmed.

Learned helplessness can occur in any individual, but children with asynchronous patterns of development are at far greater risk of developing this debilitating behavior. Much of what the teachers and therapists of children with asynchronous development do is focus on ways that the children can perform and participate at levels acceptable to them. The early use of powered mobility and augmentative communication devices is advocated so that children like Megan have the chance to move around without the help of others and so that she can communicate complex thoughts.

SUMMARY

The preschool years are a magical time in which rapid social, emotional, and cognitive growth takes place. Children begin to develop unique personalities and can effectively express themselves to others. Play and social relationships play a critical role in preschool development, allowing for exploration, imitation, and practice of basic functional skills. There is more variability in the sequence of skill acquisition in this age group than in infancy, because the new skills acquired require practice and sometimes materials. By the end of the preschool period the child can independently manage basic self-care, follow social conventions, follow directions, and work in a group setting. Successful accomplishment of preschool tasks leaves the child well prepared for the wider environment of school. Children with asynchronous development or some specific impairment may need additional support to be able to function at or near age expectancy.

CASE

1

Brandon

Brandon's mother had HELLP syndrome during pregnancy. HELLP is a rare but serious illness associated with pregnancy. The acronym stands for hemolysis, elevated liver, low platelet. Brandon was born at 33 weeks gestation. He has been diagnosed with failure to thrive, gastroesophageal reflux, and neurologic vision impairment (cortical blindness). Brandon's problems with reflux and some bouts of aspiration pneumonia led to the use of a gastrostomy (G-tube) for nutrition at 5 months. He has been cleared to take foods orally now but consistently refuses to eat foods placed in his mouth.

Brandon is now 3½ years old. He is in the 50th percentile for height and weight. He has the motor patterns typical of children with hypotonia. His mother reports that he is a quiet child who likes to play with toys and sleeps well through the night. Assessment results indicate that Brandon is (1) sitting well, (2) showing rotary transitions, and (3) pulling-to-stand. He is *not* (1) cruising or (2) standing or walking. He is showing pre-standing and walking behaviors. He has a wide variety of grasp patterns, including a fine pincer grasp. His hand skills are most refined when he is in a supportive sitting device like a corner chair. When on the floor or when seated without trunk support he has more difficulty coordinating his hands and his eyes. He prefers to use his side vision in this situation. Brandon has adequate lip closure and tongue control to manage pureed foods. He needs continued support to refine these skills and enhance tongue coordination for the management of additional food textures.

Brandon has no functional communication at this time. Tantrums appear to occur when Brandon doesn't get his way or cannot communicate his needs. Brandon receives special-education preschool services and gets speech therapy three times a week. He receives vision therapy, occupational therapy (OT), and physical therapy (PT) twice a month. The preschool team works collaboratively in their plan for Brandon. His needs are interrelated, and OT and speech work together on oral-motor skills for language and eating. PT focuses on mobility and improving endurance, while both PT and OT work on improved postural control and transitions. The vision therapist consults with all other disciplines to assist with activity adaptations to enhance Brandon's visual processing.

Mobility and communication are the major focus of the intervention process so that Brandon can participate in home, preschool, and peer settings. It is the goal of the family that Brandon will be eating orally and communicating well enough to be able to attend a regular kindergarten classroom. The interdisciplinary team is working to help the family realize this goal by enhancing his access and ability to engage in developmentally appropriate activities.

CASE

2

Trevor

Trevor was born at 41 weeks gestation with no complications. He was a quiet baby and was slow to develop motor control. At 3 months of age he began receiving early-intervention physical and occupational therapy. At 1 year he was diagnosed with cerebral palsy (spastic quadriplegia). Now 2 years old, Trevor has low tone in the postural muscle groups, but high tone in his upper and lower extremities. He is dependent in all mobility and self-care functions.

Assessment results indicate that Trevor (1) is rolling from prone to supine and supine to side, (2) is showing visual attention and reaching for objects, and (3) in supported sitting brings his hands to midline and is able to sit briefly (about 1 minute) without support. He sits with a rounded back and falls backwards with a hip extensor spasm from time to time. He does *not* have (1) protective extension, (2) hip stability in weight bearing, or (3) any locomotor pattern other than rolling. He is showing attempts at weight shift and crawling in prone. When supported in a standing device, he tends to be on his toes.

Trevor is not able to self-feed, nor can he grasp small objects from a tabletop. He can grasp a bottle but shortly drops it. He is alert and interested in persons and things around him. He reaches for toys but is unable to extend his arms fully and often misses his target. He has a raking palmar grasp pattern with his hands and often doesn't like the way things feel. At meals, Trevor avoids all textured food, preferring smooth pureed foods and liquids from a bottle. Trevor needs support with positioning for feeding. He does not have adequate trunk control to sit independently. Emerging skills include taking weight on his legs in a standing position and assuming an all-fours position.

Trevor is able to speak a few words, but they are difficult to understand. He has recently begun to attend the public school special-needs preschool, and the speech therapist has introduced some augmentative communication devices that speak for him. This has made a big difference in his alertness and motivation in all areas. The family is hoping to build on this motivation in motor skill development as well. Trevor receives speech therapy twice a week and OT and PT once a week at school. He is an only child. Both parents are very involved in his well-being but are overwhelmed with the caregiving requirements and expenses. They have been unable to find safe, reliable child-care for Trevor, and therefore seldom do things together (because someone always needs to be home with Trevor).

What kind of goals do you think this family might have?

Speaking of

Chronic Childhood Conditions

ANNE CRONIN, PHD, OTR/L, BCP
PEDIATRIC OCCUPATIONAL THERAPIST

This is part of a transcript of an interview with a mother whose preschool child has cystic fibrosis and diabetes. Understanding typical development is important in understanding how to best support this family. Parents of preschool children with serious health problems are often very isolated from typical support systems.

Has your life changed to accommodate your special child?

Continues

Speaking of Continued

[Laughs]. Do you even need to ask that one? Oh, totally. Completely. One hundred percent. My life isn't anything like it used to be. Well, I don't work. I have a degree in education, but I haven't worked since I had him. And we agreed I'd stay home with him for the first couple of years. But I see no forsee-able way I can go back to work any time soon. Before, I was more active in outside activities. I have no outside activities now. I mean, he is exclusively what I do, and he has so many varied problems; he doesn't have just one. And they all kind of relate, and they all kind of not . . . you know? He's got a lot of medical history. And he's all I do. I mean, literally. I keep the house clean, I get the meals on the table. But because of the asthma, particularly, I have to be real careful with the dust and things like that.

He was sick the minute he was born. I was in labor for three days, then ended up having a caesarian because he was starting to get into trouble. And he ingested meconium. So, from the minute he was born he was sent to the NICU and I didn't hold him until he was a day old, two days old. I went home; he came home days later. At three weeks old, he had his first bowel obstruction. So, he was only home for about ten days before he started getting into trouble. I think we were just numb. Because it was just from day one. We stayed that way. When the pediatrician said, "You know, I think he has cystic fibrosis . . . I want to test for that," I'd never heard of CF. My husband's a registered nurse. He had heard of it in his class. And we just went to the hospital. You're so bombarded with information and things. We really stayed numb until . . . even when he was diagnosed at 17 months with diabetes and he was so terribly sick, and then he developed other obstructions and then I think we got angry. We've had a lot of anger. We had a resident that wouldn't listen to us. And that almost resulted in my son's death. Because we kept telling her, there's something going on, and she kept saying no, it was a reaction elsewhere or something. She lied to us. She told us she had called the endocrinologist, and we talked to the endocrinologist and she didn't know there was a problem going on, which resulted in his second obstruction at that time being much more severe than the first one.

After you got used to the diagnoses, did your perspectives change?

It was something else, because you didn't hear anything good about CF. You heard all the bad stuff. And they told us life expectancy, and you know they told us all this stuff. So that was more stress. Not knowing.

Now, I don't think about it. It's just something else. It's just something I deal with. It's just a part of what I do. I'm the chairman, head, president, whatever of our support group here, and it's just something we do.

How was it for you when it was time to consider preschool?

We didn't do preschool because of the health threat of exposure to more children. When we did start school, I worried about the school schedule, the amount of stress that the teacher has on her, and the fact that he was a real special child and has a lot of special needs. I was concerned about his needs being met in a public school system. I was a public school teacher. I didn't want to put him in a public school. But I went in and talked to the principal, to the teacher, to the secretaries, about learning to do finger sticks, learning to do medicine.

If I were trying to describe what it feels like living with this disease/disability . . . is there something I haven't asked you that you think is important . . . that you would like the world to know about . . . ?

I mean the whole picture, the whole overwhelming picture of his care is very different from the day-to-day. Sometimes I feel so angry I can't think, but it's not at anything in particular. It's like there is a monster living inside this beautiful little boy, and we never know when it is going to all blow up.

REFERENCES

American Academy of Child and Adolescent Psychiatry. (AACAP). (1999). *Fact sheets for parents #13: Children and TV violence.* Retrieved July 17, 2003, from http://www.aacap .org/web/aacap/publications/factsfam/violence.htm.

American Occupational Therapy Association. (AOTA). (2002). Occupational Therapy Practice Framework: Domain and process. *American Journal of Occupational Therapy, 56,* 609–639.

Bjorklund, D. F. (2000). *Children's thinking: Developmental function and individual differences* (3rd ed.).Belmont, CA: Wadsworth/Thomson Learning.

Bremner, A., & Bryant, P. (2001). The effect of spatial cues on infants' responses in the AB task, with and without a hidden object. *Developmental Science, 4,* 408–415.

Bukatko, D., & Daehler, M. W. (2001). *Child development: A thematic approach* (4th ed.). Boston: Houghton Mifflin.

Bundy, A. C. (1997). Play and playfulness: What to look for. In L. D. Parham & L. Fazio (Eds.), *Play in occupational therapy for children* (pp. 52–65). St. Louis: Mosby.

Coster, W., Deeney, T., Haltiwanger, J., & Haley, S. (1998). *The school function assessment.* San Antonio, TX: The Psychological Corporation.

Erhardt, R. P. (1992). Eye-hand coordination. In J. Case-Smith & C. Pehoski (Eds.), *Development of hand skills in the child* (pp. 13–34). Bethesda, MD: The American Occupational Therapy Association.

Exner, C. (1992). In-hand manipulation skills. In J. Case-Smith & C. Pehoski (Eds.), *Development of hand skills in the child* (pp. 35–46). Bethesda, MD: The American Occupational Therapy Association.

Exner, C. (1995). Remediation of hand skill problems in children. In A. Henderson & C. Pehoski (Eds.), *Hand function in the child* (pp. 197–222). St. Louis: Mosby.

Gentile, M. (1997). *Functional visual behavior.* Bethesda, MD: The American Occupational Therapy Association.

Henderson, A., & Pehoski, C. (Eds.). (1995). *Hand function in the child.* St. Louis: Mosby.

Hertling, D., & Kessler, R. M. (1996). *Management of common musculoskeletal disorders: Physical therapy principles and methods* (3rd ed.). Philadelphia: J. B. Lippincott.

Hollingsworth, L. S. (1942). *Children above 180 IQ Stanford-Binet.* Yonkers-on-Hudson, NY: World Book.

Holly, K., & Schuster, C. (1992). Cognitive development during the school-age years. In C. Schuster & S. Ashburn (Eds.), *The process of human development: A holistic life-span approach* (3rd ed.) (pp 444–466). Philadelphia: Lippincott.

Jackson, P., & Vessey, J. (Eds.) (1996). *Primary care of the child with a chronic condition* (2nd ed.). St. Louis: Mosby.

Kagan, S. L. (1999). Cracking the readiness mystique. *Young Children, 54,* 2–3.

Kagan, S. L., Moore, E., & Bredekamp, S. (Eds.). (1995). *Reconsidering children's early development and learning: Toward common views and vocabulary.* Report of the National Education Goals Panel, Goal 1, Technical Planning Group (ED 391 576). Washington, DC: Government Printing Office.

Mailloux, Z., & Burke, J. P. (1997). Play and the sensory integrative approach. In L. D. Parham & L. S. Fazio (Eds.), *Play in occupational therapy for children* (pp. 112–125). St. Louis: Mosby.

Murray, E. (1995). Hand preference and its development. In A. Henderson & C. Pehoski (Eds.), *Hand function in the child: Foundations for remediation* (pp. 154–163). St. Louis: Mosby.

Nader, P. R. (1992). Five years: Entering school. In S. Dixon & M. Stein (Eds.), *Encounters with children: Pediatric behavior and development* (2nd ed.) (pp. 291–302). St. Louis: Mosby.

Palfrey, J. S. (1995). School readiness. In S. Parker & B. Zuckerman (Eds.), *Behavioral and developmental pediatrics* (pp. 261–264). Boston: Little Brown.

Parham, L. D., & Fazio, L. (1997). *Play in occupational therapy for children.* St. Louis: Mosby.

Parham, L. D., & Mailloux, Z. (2001). Sensory Integration. In J. Case-Smith (Ed.), *Occupational therapy for children* (4th ed.) (pp. 329–381). St. Louis: Mosby.

Parten, M. (1932). Social play among preschool children. *Journal of Abnormal and Social Psychology, 27,* 243–269.

Payne, V. G., & Isaacs, L. D. (2001). *Human motor development: A lifespan approach* (5th ed.). Boston: McGraw Hill.

Perry, B. D., Hogan, L., & Marlin, S. J. (2000). *Curiosity, pleasure and play: A neurodevelopmental perspective.* Paper written for HAAEYC Advocate, June 15, 2000, and retrieved April 27, 2002, from www.ChildTrauma.org.

Perry, B. (1998). *Neurodevelopment and early childhood: How exploration and play grow a healthy brain,* Civitas Press. Retrieved October 25, 2002, from http://www.ecmma.org/readings/across.html.

Perry, B. D., Pollard, R., Blakely, T., Baker, W., & Vigilante, D. (1995). Childhood trauma, the neurobiology of adaptation and 'use-dependent' development of the brain: How 'states' become 'traits.' *Infant Mental Health Journal, 16,* 271–291.

Santrock, J. (1997). *Life-span development* (7th ed.). Boston: McGraw-Hill.

Shore, R. (1997). Rethinking the brain: New insights into early development. Summary from Conference: *Brain development in young children: New frontiers for research, policy and practice.* New York: Families and Work Institute.

Shumway-Cook, A., & Woollacott, M. (2001). *Motor control: Theory and practical applications.* Philadelphia: Lippincott, Williams and Wilkins.

Roedell, W. (1984). Vulnerabilities of highly gifted children. *Roeper Review, 6,* No. 3.

Silverman, L. (1998). Through the lens of the giftedness, *Roeper Review, 20,* No. 3.

Smith, L. K., Weiss, E. L., & Lehmkuhl, L. D. (1996). *Brunnstrom's clinical kinesiology* (5th ed.). Philadelphia: F. A. Davis.

Subbotsky, E. (2000). Causal reasoning and behaviour in children and adults in a technologically advanced society: Are we still prepared to believe in magic and animism? In P. Mitchell & K. Riggs (Eds.), *Children's reasoning and the mind* (pp. 327–347). Hove, England: Psychology Press/Taylor & Francis.

World Health Organization. (2002). ICF: International Classification of Functioning and Disability. Geneva, Switzerland: World Health Organization.

CHAPTER 11

Middle Childhood and School

Anne Cronin, PhD, OTR/L, BCP
Associate Professor
Division of Occupational Therapy
West Virginia University
Morgantown, West Virginia

Objectives

Upon completion of this chapter, the reader should be able to

- Describe the developmental tasks of middle childhood, including these dimensions:
  - Body structures and functions
  - Sensorimotor characteristics
  - School tasks and demands
  - Physical tasks
  - Cognitive/behavioral tasks
  - Self-care/self-management skills
  - Play
- Compare the development of thought and executive functions through the context of the child's expanding environment to the process observed in the younger child.
- Describe the role of peer relation and social behavior in middle childhood.
- Discuss common emotional stressors of the middle school years.
- Explain the role of language and literacy skill development on the overall functional performance of the child.
- Describe play and playfulness in the context of middle childhood and skills acquisition.

Key Terms

body schema

coincidence-anticipation (CA) timing

cognitive map

figure-ground perception

inclusion

kinesthetic perception

low vision

motion hypothesis

object play

rapport talk

report talk

self-management skills

social competence

social knowledge

social referencing

spatial awareness

stress

temporal awareness

temporal organization

virtual (electronic) play

INTRODUCTION

Vgotsky (1978) states, "Every function in the child's cultural development appears twice: first, on the social level, and later, on the individual level; first, between people (interpsychological) and then inside the child (intrapsychological). This applies equally to voluntary attention, to logical memory, and to the formation of concepts. All the higher functions originate as actual relationships between individuals" (p. 57). It is in the middle childhood years that social and cultural learning blossoms. Physiologic and motor changes continue throughout this period, but by the age of 6, typically developing children will have the basic sensorimotor skill needed to negotiate the world. School, peer interactions, and a greater awareness of the diversity in the world of people predominate in the experience of middle childhood.

Earlier in this text you have been presented with the historical debate concerning the varying roles of nature and nurture in human development. In infancy and early childhood there is strong support for nature as preeminent. In middle childhood the evidence swings toward the nurture position, with the child's performance contexts emerging as important influences on development. After the age of 5 the basic body functions and structures are intact. Myelination of the brain continues, with the areas of the brain associated with focused attention developing until the end of the middle childhood period (Santrock, 1997). The developmental focus of the school-age child falls into the ICF models of Activities and Participation and Environmental Factors (World Health Organization, 2002).

BODY FUNCTIONS AND STRUCTURES

By the age of 6 the child's general body build and the relationship of height to weight norms are predictive of his adult body proportions (Schuster & Ashburn, 1992). The typical, well-nourished child grows 2–3 inches a year during the ages of 6 to about the age of 11 (Santrock, 1997). During this time body proportions gradually change as the relative size of the head decreases, and increases in skeletal and muscle mass replace "baby fat." During the preschool years the greatest area of growth is the trunk, and the center of gravity is usually at about the mid-thoracic region (near the end of the ribs) when the child is standing. In the years between 6 and 10 most of the growth is in the limbs, and the center of gravity drops farther, to about the level of the umbilicus. This change in proportion is shown in Figure 11–1.

As the center of gravity drops, the child's ability to balance and to maintain balance while running improves. As the center of gravity shifts, the child is better able to balance during activities involving the manipulation of objects, as in sports (Payne & Isaacs, 2002). There has been much research on the refinement of postural control during childhood demonstrating that postural responses grow faster and more reliable over time (Shumway-Cook & Wollacott, 2001). In this age group the large muscles of the body are considerably more developed than the small muscles, and girls are generally about a year ahead of boys in physiologic development (Gallahue & Ozmun, 2002).

In addition to a lowering of their center of gravity, during the middle childhood years children make dramatic increases in muscular strength. The motor skills of stability and alignment when standing or sitting and when moving and interacting with objects in their environment are essential skills for many of the activities that school-age children perform on a daily basis. Children of this age routinely use backpacks to transport their schoolbooks and supplies from home to school. Children without problems with stability or alignment are able to adjust their trunks and center of gravity to accommodate their backpacks as they get on and off the school bus, and walk home. This postural flexibility is illustrated in Figure 11–2.

Several research studies indicate that grip strength increases by between 260% and 393%

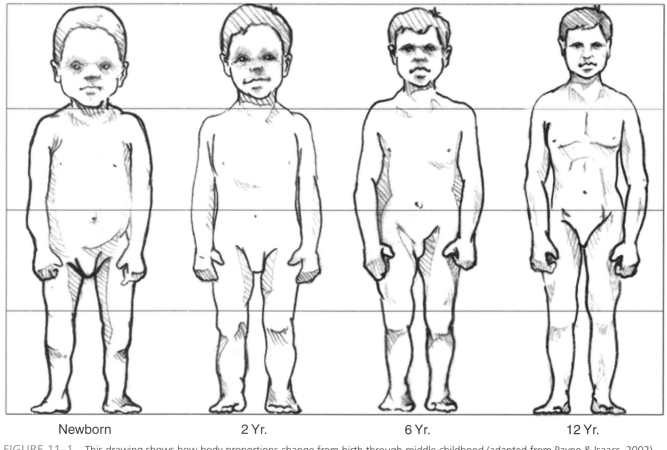

Newborn   2 Yr.   6 Yr.   12 Yr.

FIGURE 11–1   This drawing shows how body proportions change from birth through middle childhood (adapted from Payne & Isaacs, 2002).

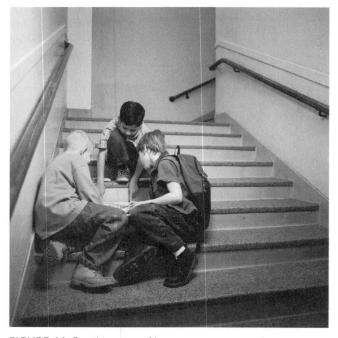

FIGURE 11–2   This group of boys can manage complex postural control, adapt to irregular environmental features, and manage school backpacks. (Image courtesy of PhotoDisc®, Inc.)

between the ages of 7 and 17 (Payne & Isaacs, 2002). In the preschool years children can walk, bend, and reach for objects, but often have to stop other activity to manage this. Now children walk, bend, and reach casually, grabbing an apple as they walk through the kitchen or high-fiving a friend as they pass in the hall. Motor skills continue to develop throughout childhood. In middle childhood there is a dramatic increase in the ability to precisely calibrate movements to the demands of the task.

Physical differences associated with gender begin to become apparent during middle childhood. Throughout life females are less likely than males to develop physical or mental disorders (Santrock, 1999). In studies of brain metabolism, girls have more metabolic activity in the area of emotional expression, and boys have more metabolic activity in the area of physical expression (Gur et al., 1995). Vuontela et al. (2003) report that between the ages of 6 and 13 girls demonstrate greater maturity in the areas of audiospatial and visuospatial working memory. These basic brain functions are important to the developmental demands for this age group and have important impacts on the child's overall development.

SENSORY CHARACTERISTICS

In middle childhood the mechanisms for visual and auditory perception continue to refine. Attention span in middle childhood gradually extends, although at all ages within this group children can attend for hours on tasks that are highly motivating to them. With increasing attention comes increasing perceptual awareness. There is an interrelationship between perceptual development and the increasing calibration of movement seen in the ages 6 through 10. Children with significant sensory deficits at birth consistently show delays in motor coordination in middle childhood, reflecting the link between sensory function and motor skill (Payne & Isaacs, 2002).

In addition to needing intact sensory systems for motor skill development, children need self-directed sensory experience for cognitive and perceptual development. The **motion hypothesis** proposed by Shaffer (1999) is based on a series of studies of kittens that compare variables of active and passive movement on the development of visuospatial skills (Payne & Isaacs, 2002). These studies suggest that self-produced movement is important in the development of depth perception and spatial judgment. While this explanation of perceptual development continues to be contested, it is an important consideration in advocating for early assisted mobility for children with serious motor limitations like cerebral palsy. Although it is common to rely on simple strollers while the child is young, school-age children with no experience of independent mobility may have difficulty learning to control a power wheelchair.

VISUAL DEVELOPMENT

One of the standard screening items for the kindergarten child is a test of visual acuity. *Visual acuity* is the ability to focus the eyes in order to distinguish details in the visual display. Vision is a predominant sensory input system used in the traditional school environment. For this reason visual difficulties are important to identify early. **Low vision** is a term used to describe very limited sight that can interfere with a person's daily routine activities. Children with low vision have a clear pattern of asynchronous development, with normally developing cognitive and intrapersonal development, and delays in all areas that require information from the visual world (Lampert, 1998).

Children with low vision face special challenges in school, where great emphasis is placed on learning through printed material. Severely visually impaired children must rely on ear-hand coordination rather than eye-hand coordination. Ear-hand coordination develops 1–2 years later than eye-hand coordination in typically developing children, accounting for some of the motor delays seen the school setting. In addition, persons who are visually impaired develop compensations in a highly refined sense of touch.

Visual Perception

The following aspects of visual perception mature in middle childhood:

- Perception of size constancy is the ability to recognize that objects maintain a constant size even if their distance from the observer varies. This allows the child to accurately judge the size of objects. This skill typically matures by age 11.
- Perception of figure and ground allows the child to locate and focus on an object embedded in a distracting background, and matures at about 8 years of age.
- Perception of depth is the ability to judge distances and to recognize the three-dimensional nature of objects; it matures at about age 12.
- Perception of movement involves the ability to detect and track a moving object with the eye and matures at about 10 years of age (adapted from Goggin, 2003).
- Although it is widely reported that boys in this age group have better math and visuospatial skills than girls, the gender differences are actually small and may be due to different social and cultural expectations (Santrock, 1999).

Figure-ground perception "is the ability to separate an object of regard from its surroundings" (Gallahue & Ozmun, 2002, p. 259). This skill is refined between the ages of 4 and 13 and is important in many self-care and academic tasks. Visual figure-ground is necessary for completing school worksheets and determining front from back when dressing. Auditory figure-ground is the ability to single out the teacher's voice in a busy classroom, or to hear the ice-cream truck coming down the street while you are watching TV. Because figure-ground perception requires attention, sensory input, and memory, it is poorly developed before middle childhood. Auditory figure-ground becomes functional in typically developing children about the age of 8 (Jackson & Vessey, 1996). For the visually impaired child, auditory figure-ground is the crucial sensory tool needed for interacting with other children in classroom settings. For this reason, visually impaired children are likely to feel isolated and excluded in ordinary classroom activities. In addition, it is common for children with attention deficits to have difficulties with figure-ground perception of all types, especially in distracting environments like the schoolroom.

Kinesthetic Perception

Kinesthetic perception is the interpretation of information regarding the relative position of the body parts to each other, the position of the body in space, and an awareness of the body's movements (Goggin, 2003). Kinesthetic perception, like visual perception, includes many distinct perceptual skills. These include *stereognosis*, the recognition of objects by manipulation, and perception of the extent of limb movements (Shumway-Cook & Woollacott, 2002). To develop proficiency in playing most musical instruments, a high degree of kinesthetic perception is needed. Elementary-school age is when most children are typically introduced to instruments, and many, like the 10-year-old shown in Figure 11–3, become proficient.

It is also kinesthetic awareness that allows for the large increase in skills seen in "ball" sports in this age group. The children can visually fixate on the ball, while being kinesthetically aware of their position and the movements needed.

SPATIAL AWARENESS

By the age of 6 children have developed a **body schema** and have an internalized sense of the space that their body occupies (Gallahue & Ozmun, 2002). The child's body schema combines somatic awareness with experiential memory of movement potential. In other words, the body schema is how the child answers questions like, "Will I fit into that box?" or, "Can I get to the ball before it falls into the water?" The body schema construct does not lend itself easily to research but seems logically related to the motion hypothesis mentioned earlier. As children move and challenge their physical abilities, they gain cognitive information about the

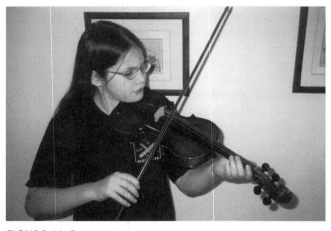

FIGURE 11–3 The violin is a very difficult instrument to play, requiring very discrete hand movements guided entirely by kinesthesia and proprioception.

limits of their body, the body schema. Without the experience of self-controlled movement, this schema is probably slower to develop.

Body schema is the foundation for the understanding of spaces external to the individual. One of the primary strategies taught to parents of children with severe visual impairments is a variety of play activities to enhance the development of body schema. Typical children with poorly developed body schema often appear clumsy in middle childhood but are able to function in routine activities by compensating with their visual skills. Children with low vision do not have a backup system to use in compensation and can become quite fearful and resistive of both movement and large group activities without the support of a well-developed body schema.

Spatial awareness is the understanding of both near and far space around an individual and is assessed by the accuracy in locating items within that space. Spatial awareness in the 6-year-old may be limited to planning how to toss a paper into the wastebasket. By the age of 10, children are not only aware of space in a dynamic manner but are beginning to plan using cognitive maps of the space. **Cognitive maps** are a type of metacognition involving mental manipulations of remembered sensory experiences superimposed on a desired task (Hommel, Gehrke, & Knuf, 2000). More simply, cognitive maps help you remember how to get around in your own house and, in a more complex situation, help you reason where the bathroom might be, based on past experience.

Cognitive mapping emerges in middle childhood and continues to develop through adolescence. It is the conceptual tool that provides the foundation for geometry and the visual analysis of information in charts and graphs (Chown, Booker, & Kaplan, 2001). Cognitive maps are widely used in school and in IADL tasks to improve **temporal organization**, the orderly and logical sequencing of steps and sequences of a task from start to finish.

Children organize their actions into a logical series of steps, and this is a cognitive map that leads them from task initiation, continuing each step of the activity in a logical and effective way until they complete the task. When they initiate an activity like setting the table, school-age children mix logical order with impulse, perhaps putting out the plates before the placemats, observing, and then moving the plates to place the mats under them. With practice, the sequence improves, and the order of task completion increasingly makes sense.

TEMPORAL AWARENESS

Understanding basic time concepts is a component of most elementary curricula. **Temporal awareness** is not about time in the academic sense but rather as it relates to the planning, sequencing, and altering of movements (Gallahue & Ozmun, 2002). These movements may be unique to the body, as in a series of jumping jacks, or they may be planned to coincide with an external stimulus. Temporal awareness is needed for most repetitive motor activities, including bicycling, skipping rope, and playing the piano. Children with difficulty in temporal awareness may appear awkward or clumsy.

In the primary school years there is a gradual improvement in reaction time. *Reaction time* is the time delay between the presentation of a stimulus and the motor response to that stimulus. In the ages between 7 and 10 reaction time is slow and may cause difficulties in both eye-hand and eye-foot coordination (Gallahue & Ozmun, 2002). There is much individual difference in reaction time, and it is a crucial feature that determines success in sports in this age group. In some cases, a slow reaction time may be related to poor temporal awareness.

Coincidence-anticipation (CA) timing is "the ability to initiate and complete a motor pattern with the arrival of a moving object, at a previously set interception point" (Bard, Fleury, & Hay, 1990, p. 283). This complex skill allows the child to play the whole array of sports. Research on CA timing indicates that it improves between the ages of 7 and 18 and then plateaus (Haywood, 1980, 1993).

CA timing is necessary in many activities but is easily illustrated in Figure 11–4, demonstrating normal developmental stages of catching. In the initial development of catching, the child is static, may turn away from the ball, and traps the ball in his arms rather than opening and positioning his hands for the catch. In the mature stage, which is typical of middle childhood, the eyes follow the ball into the hands, the arms adjust to the flight of the ball, and the hands grasp the ball in a well-timed motion. More complex CA timing is seen as children practice ball-related sports like softball, shown in Figure 11–5.

HAND DOMINANCE

As described in Chapter 9, the process of using each hand differently begins in the preschool years. By the time the child enters school, at the age of 5, a consistent hand preference is usually seen. The development of handedness is considered in terms of not only which hand is used but also how consistently the preferred hand is used in a variety of everyday tasks. Patterns of mixed dominance—use of a different hand for specific skilled tasks—are more common than previously documented (Santrock, 1997). It is not unusual for a child to have one preferred hand for eating and writing and a different preferred hand for sports. There appear to be no differences in development of motor skills

between children with right- and left-hand preferences. In a study by Tan (1985), however, children with no hand preference by the age of 4 had significantly poorer motor performance. The development of a dominant "skilled" hand in bimanual patterns allows the child to specialize and develop the refined dexterity needed for writing, keyboarding, and other school demands.

ACTIVITIES AND PARTICIPATION

In the ICF, the category of Activities and Participation includes learning, communication, mobility, self-care, interpersonal relationships, and community life (World Health Organization, 2002). Contemporary views of human intelligence and learning, including that of Piaget, were presented in Chapter 3. While Piaget provided much of the seminal work in understanding cognition in the preschool child, his model of cognition supposes that development is innately driven, and does not account for the influence of peers and social interaction.

Vgotsky (1978) argued against Piaget's theory on the basis that cognitive skills and patterns of thinking are the products of the activities practiced in the social institutions of the culture in which the individual grows up. In this conception, both the history of the society in which a child is reared and the child's personal history influence the way in which that individual will think (Thomas, 1993). In this section we will discuss many skills that are culturally determined as well as self-care, school function, and interpersonal behaviors. Unlike the progression of motor skills presented in earlier chapters, there is wide cultural variation in what type and quality of performance is expected in this regard.

ZONE OF PROXIMAL DEVELOPMENT

Vgotsky believes that children actively construct knowledge to meet sociocultural demands (Santrock, 1999). When analyzing human learning, Vgotsky (1978) described a *zone of proximal development (ZPD)* that relates to emerging skill areas. The ZPD consists of "tasks that are too difficult for the child to master alone, but that can be learned with the guidance and assistance of adults or more-skilled children" (Santrock, 1999, p. 214). The ZPD includes, at its lower end, the skills the child can perform alone, and extends to include the skills the child can accomplish with assistance.

Because learning requires the support and expertise of others, Vgotsky argues that cognitive skills and patterns of thinking are not primarily determined by innate factors but are the products of the activities

Initial

Elementary

Mature

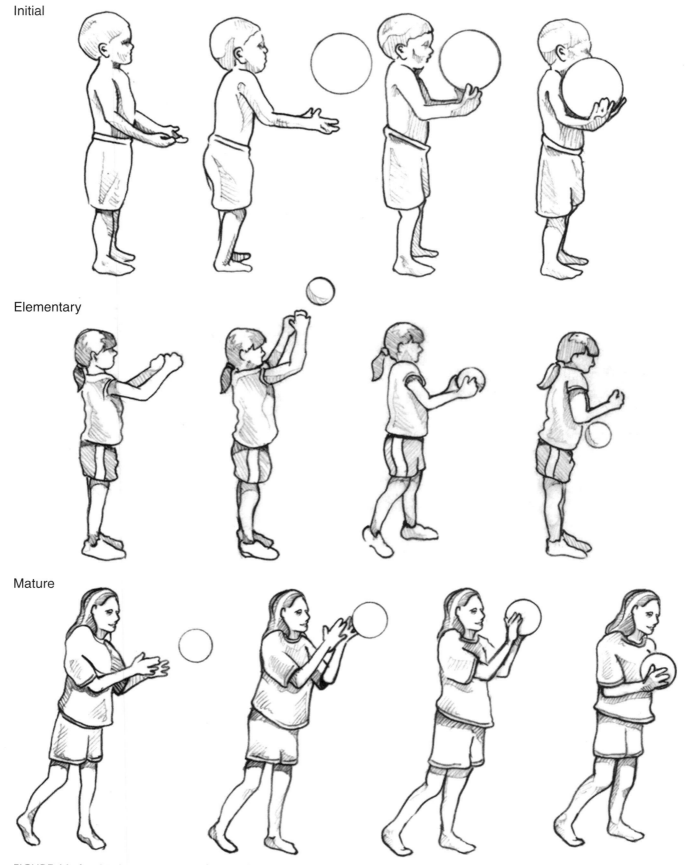

FIGURE 11–4   This drawing re-creates the typical acquisition pattern for learning to catch a ball (adapted from Shumway-Cook & Woollacott, 2001).

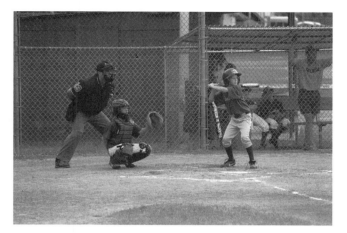

FIGURE 11–5 Softball requires highly developed coincidence-anticipation timing. Prior to achieving this skill level, children play "t-ball" and hit a stationary ball.

practiced in the social institutions of the culture. In this approach, cognitive development is inseparable from the language, culture, and society of the child.

SCHOOL FUNCTION

In middle childhood, one of the most influential social institutions is the child's school environment. For most children the middle childhood years include extended periods of time away from home, in a school setting. While schools are intended to be safe, nurturing environments, they are for many children a place where the child is not seen as positively or treated as gently as in the home environment. Santrock (1999) reports that "evidence is mounting that early schooling proceeds mainly on the basis of negative feedback" (p. 308). At school both the teachers and the student's peers give the child new ideas about himself. Children from low-income and ethnic-minority backgrounds are more likely to have school difficulties than are middle-class counterparts (Mare, 1996; Tozer, Violas, & Senese, 1998).

These difficulties become more complex if a child has a congenital or early-onset condition that results in impairment. This child may not be aware of the impact of the impairment before she attends school with typically developing peers. In the period of 6–10 years of age the child becomes increasingly aware of the social significance of the impairment (Murphy & Crocker, 1987; Rubenfeld & Schwartz, 1996).

Schuster & Ashburn (1992) describe adaptation to physical disability as a process, which during the school years is characterized by both affective awareness and cognitive rebellion. This means that the child is aware of the ways in which he is different and is aware that the condition will persist. It also means that the child developmentally wants to fit in and often responds with

anger, fantasizing normalcy, and refusing to cooperate with interventions (Schuster & Ashburn, 1992). In spite of the great advances in technology and special education, there are many barriers to school function for the child who is different from the norm. Murray and Greenberg (2001) studied 289 fifth- and sixth-grade children to find that "students with disabilities had greater dissatisfaction with their relationships with teachers, poorer bonds with school, and perceived higher school danger than did students without disabilities" (p. 25).

There are some programs, like Special Olympics, that provide support and build avenues for children with special needs to participate in childhood occupations. Unfortunately, these programs are stigmatized as programs for the cognitively impaired, and children without cognitive limits may avoid them for that reason. The ideal of keeping children with disabilities in the mainstream of school life has many benefits but may also leave the child with activity limitation on the sidelines.

Children with very different conditions, like those with particularly high IQ scores (Silverman, 1999; Roedell, 1984), learning disabilities (Pavri & Monda-Amaya, 2001; Vaughn, Elbaum, & Schumm, 1996), cystic fibrosis (D'Auria, Christian, & Richardson, 1997), and spina bifida (Blum, 1983) reported loneliness and a sense of isolation in school during middle childhood. Children who develop asynchronously are likely to need some additional support to function optimally in the school environment.

SCHOOL TASKS AND DEMANDS

Although the focus of public education is to acquire academic skills, children develop many other crucial functional skills in the school environment. As children progress through school there is less teacher direction and a greater demand for independence in their assignments and in managing their time. Although there is much attention focused on the academic portion of the school, school curricula are often very specific on subject areas like mathematics, reading, and science while offering no official curricula goals in school participation. School participation includes interactions in instructional settings, effective organizational strategies, involvement in testing activities, and peer interactions. The goals of typical schools for children in the age range of 6–10 are similar to these:

- Master the basic skills of reading, writing, language development, and mathematics.
- Develop positive relationships with their peers and adults.
- Learn to deal in a mature way with their emotions.

- Explore and pursue interest in the arts and sciences.
- Develop into a physically fit and healthy individual.
- Promote the moral and civic values of their community.
(Briggs Elementary School, 2003)

School is an arena for children to practice emerging metacognitive skills. During middle childhood children learn cognitive monitoring. **Cognitive monitoring** is "the process of taking stock of what you are currently doing, what you will do next, and how effectively the mental activity is unfolding" (Santrock, 1997, p. 278). This is the skill that allows children to persist in school tasks like completing a book report or solving a math problem. Participation in school environments requires a complex interaction of developmental skills. In some cases adequate skill levels are present in isolation, but the combination of demands during the day leads to activity limitation. For occupational and physical therapists working in school environments, effective functional interventions will emphasize improving the child's participation in the school environment in all the areas that have been described.

An assessment tool called the *School Function Assessment (SFA)* (Coster et al., 1998) was designed to measure a child's ability to participate in school. This tool reflects that functional performance is context-specific, and that skills seen in one specific set of circumstances may not be seen in different circumstances. For example, a child may be able to walk well down a long corridor when there is no crowd but may be unable to perform at the same level in a busy corridor or when carrying schoolbooks. In the United States, determination of participation includes type of classroom assignment (regular classroom or special-education classroom) and the following non-classroom school settings: playground, transportation, bathroom/toileting, transitions between areas within the school, and mealtimes. The extent to which the student is able to participate in a given activity can be analyzed in terms of quality of task performance, the types of assistance the child needs to complete the task, and any adaptations to the task that are made to enable the child to be successful (Coster et al., 1998).

SELF-MANAGEMENT SKILLS

Although it is not listed as part of the curriculum, there is a hierarchy of **self-management skills** that is taught in school settings, and expectations increase with the academic level of the child. Some strategies used by teachers to support this type of self-management skill development are to post a daily schedule of classroom activities, establish classroom routines for common tasks like collecting homework, and develop transition activities that prepare students for a change in classroom focus. As students gain skill they are expected to be more independent on both individual and group tasks, including initiating and arranging time to complete the task, pacing task performance, and carrying out task steps in the correct sequence. During the ages from 6 to 10 there are dramatic decreases seen in impulsivity and increases in personal error detection. Although individuals vary greatly in the sequence and timing of self-management skill acquisition, by the age of 11 most children are in self-care, mobility, and social function as illustrated in Table 11–1.

TABLE 11–1	Self-Care Skills in Middle Childhood	
Self-Care	**Mobility**	**Social Function**
Able to eat all types and textures of food.	Able to move effectively between standing and sitting in a variety of situations.	Able to demonstrate comprehension of verbal and written instructions.
Uses eating and drinking utensils well.	Able to get in and out of vehicles, including cars and buses.	Able to convey information to others that is clear in meaning.
Able to effectively brush both teeth and hair.	Able to move at the same speed and distance as the crowd in corridors and out of doors.	Able to work with others to solve problems in ordinary situations.
Able to dress and undress independently and appropriately for the weather.	Able to manage independent mobility on rough and uneven surfaces.	Able to demonstrate basic safety awareness in familiar situations.
Able to manage both personal hygiene and toileting tasks.	Able to manage stairs and ladders within routine environments.	Able to function independently in a variety of familiar community settings without assistance.

SCHOOL ACTIVITY PERFORMANCE

In middle childhood postural control should include the necessary trunk control and balance needed to perform expected occupations. The balance skills expand as sports and other athletic pursuits become more common. In middle childhood individuals may develop specialized skills in dance, gymnastics, martial arts, and team sports.

Schoolchildren are expected to reach to grasp objects that they need when they are on the floor, in the desk, or across a counter in the school cafeteria. In middle childhood bilateral-coordination skills mature, and increased dexterity and improved in-hand manipulation are seen as students shift and adjust their pencils, open condiment packets, and develop skill with musical instruments. These new skills may continue to be conscious but with practice become habits and no longer need cognitive direction.

Many complex bi-manual skills are needed in the school setting. These include carrying both single objects and trays full of objects, opening and closing all types of doors, moving through a line (like a cafeteria serving line) gathering needed objects in a reasonable time, managing a backpack or book bag full of books, and safely carrying fragile objects.

Children in school settings are expected to have a well-developed hand dominance and good finger dexterity. Handwriting is a part of most academic programs, and the expectation that the child has both the motor skills and the strength to write long paragraphs and essays is common in classrooms of 10- and 11-year-old children. Many children now begin to use the computer at the same age that they learn to write, as shown in Figure 11–6. Children can manage the computer mouse and game controllers long before they can type effectively. Although touch typing is not taught in most primary curricula, the tactile kinesthetic awareness needed for effective typing is becoming increasingly important in the school setting.

SCHOOL ACTIVITY PERFORMANCE: COGNITIVE/BEHAVIORAL TASKS

Functional communication is the effective sending and receiving of information. Although most developmental tests include items like "follows one-step commands," by the age of 6 most children are able to follow complex two- and three-step commands with conditions—for example, "Go to your seats and get out your pencils; it is almost time for spelling." Functional communication is a complex interaction of attention, auditory perception, socioemotional maturity, analysis of task, and task sequence.

Tannen (1990) describes gender differences in functional communication. The two types of talk she

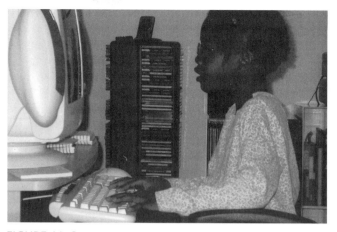

FIGURE 11–6 Children can manage the computer mouse and game controllers long before they can type effectively.

describes, rapport talk and report talk, become apparent in middle childhood (Santrock, 1999). **Rapport talk,** "the language of conversation and a way of connecting and negotiating relationships" (Santrock, 1999, p. 317), is the communication style typical of girls. **Report talk,** which gives information and directives, is the communication style typical of boys. Talk between boys in middle childhood is more likely to be boasting and arguing, with a focus on status and hierarchy between the persons in the group. Talk between girls of this age is more likely to be intimate, with turn-taking and reciprocity. Girls of this age seem to be more interested in being liked by others, while boys are more likely to be competing for position (Santrock, 1999).

MENTAL FUNCTIONS

Attention is a mental function incorporating "concentration with the mental powers upon an object; a close or careful observing or listening" (American Heritage Dictionary, 2000). Attention allows the child to focus as directions are given and to notice the features of tasks so that the task can be stored as memory. Attention is the critical underlying skill for the more involved mental tasks of memory and understanding. It is also critical as school tasks become more complex and more time-consuming to complete.

Cognitive Factors

As children start school, they also begin to compare themselves with their peers and begin to experience stress. **Stress** is "the response of the individual to the circumstances and events (called stressors) that threaten them and tax their coping abilities" (Santrock, 1997, p. 268). It is both the day-to-day experiences and major life events that cause stress. Stress may come from school demands, peer aggression, or family turmoil. Moderate levels of stress are considered to be positive and to enhance learning. Although stress can be a positive influence on development, chronic or high levels of stress lead to a higher risk for illness, depression, and social withdrawal (Kaplan & Sadock, 1998).

For many children, school is the first time they experience achievement pressure. In middle childhood stress can come from outside sources (such as family, friends, or school), but it can also come from the child's own perceptions and expectations. Stresses in the preschool years are most likely to come from events, like injury or divorce. In middle childhood, the child begins to measure himself against others and feel pressure because he perceives himself to be less than he should be. As children get older, the social pressure to fit in creates additional stress. It is during the years of middle childhood that individuals with developmental differences and asynchronous development are likely to have the most difficulty in social situations. In middle childhood, children are susceptible to many types of stress, including stress from parental illness, personal illness, child abuse and neglect, and athletic-performance pressures.

Learned helplessness and underachievement are believed to be the result of prolonged demands on the child that she is unable to meet (Shuster & Ashburn, 1992). Indicators that a child is overly stressed are short-term behavioral changes, including mood swings, acting out, changes in sleep patterns, or bed-wetting. The American Academy of Child and Adolescent Psychiatry (2002) reports that some children experience physical effects to prolonged stress, most typically stomachaches and headaches. In middle childhood children may begin to lie, bully, or defy authority in response to perceived stress (Kidshealth, 2002).

As children begin to read the emotional reactions of other people and use this information to guide their own behavior, they are **social referencing** (Kaplan & Sadock, 1998). This process of comparison provides a coping tool for dealing with ambiguous situations. It is through social referencing that children who are developmentally different speculate on the long-term impact of their impairment or developmental asynchrony.

Related to social referencing is **social knowledge**. Children's ability to understand and interpret peer relationships becomes increasingly important to this age group. Dodge, Murphy, and Buchsbaum (1984) were pioneers in this area of research, describing five steps in acquiring social knowledge:

1. Decoding social cues
2. Interpreting social cues
3. Searching for a response
4. Selecting an optimal response
5. Taking action

Social knowledge is involved in all aspects of peer relations, classroom cooperation, friendships, and aggression. Dodge et al. (2003) have performed 20 years of research on social-knowledge skill as an influence on aggression and friendship behaviors. They found that early peer rejection predicts growth in aggression, especially in boys. The children in Figure 11–7 have compensated for their varying ages to successfully negotiate social referencing and friendship formation.

CARRYING OUT DAILY ROUTINE

By the age of 10, a child's school participation includes carrying out daily routines. Children begin to learn simple routines in early childhood and become increasingly able to organize their time and materials to initiate and complete the task independently. In order to gain these skills in a functional manner that generalizes between situations, children must begin to abstract and generalize ideas and consider new features of the environment and how they might affect performance of a desired task. While many routines can be taught in a rote fashion, they will remain isolated to the conditions

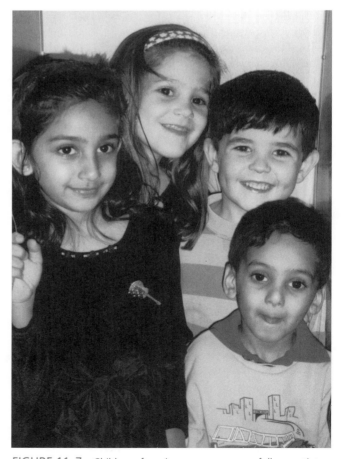

FIGURE 11–7 Children of varying ages can successfully negotiate social referencing and friendship formation.

under which they were taught if the child is not able to manipulate information, integrate new features, and solve problems as they present themselves. These are higher-level mental manipulations that emerge in middle childhood and continue to develop into adulthood.

Many *instrumental activities of daily living (IADLs)* emerge in middle childhood. Most children of this age help with household and classroom chores. They are competent users of the telephone and many kitchen appliances. As children begin to do chores and earn their own money, they learn to manage money, plan, and shop. By the end of this period the typical child can manage money and social interactions to make a purchase and collect the correct change.

PLAY AND PLAYFULNESS

Most adult memories of play are of their middle childhood years. Many of the comic strips and stories in the popular press are of children in this age group—for example, "Calvin and Hobbes," "Peanuts," and "Foxtrot." Play in middle childhood includes the fantasy and constructive play described in Chapter 9, but it also includes sports, nature exploration, and unstructured playground time. It is in the early school years that children come to understand bullies and gender expectations, and learn to cooperate. In middle childhood children have many free-time choices. Common free-play choices identified by McHale, Couter, and Tucker (2001) were specific hobbies, sports, games, outdoor play, television viewing, and reading. In middle childhood gender differences in play become evident, and children will tend to avoid any activity group that is numerically predominated by the opposite gender, regardless of the activity (Sandberg & Meyer-Bahlburg, 1994). It has been consistently observed in North American studies that boys tend to engage more in aggressive rough-and-tumble play and group play with rules. Boys' games often have winners and losers; arguments are often a part of these games (Santrock, 1999). Girls were found to be less physical and engage in smaller group conversations as a form of play. Girls' play was more likely to be parallel and less rule-driven (Moller, Hymel, & Rubin, 1992). Many play activities preferred by school-age children challenge their motor abilities, as seen in the young girl's attempts to master her scooter in Figure 11–8.

There have been many different strategies used to distinguish and conceptualize the great diversity seen in play. In this chapter we will focus on the context of play. During this developmental period, children continue to engage in the types of play learned earlier while adding increasingly more complex play to their repertoire. In contemporary America it is not

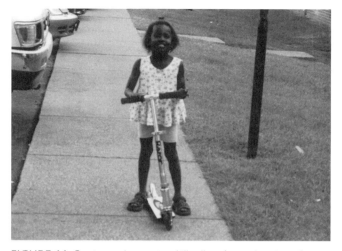

FIGURE 11–8 Increasing motor skills allow for exploration of scooters and other new challenges.

uncommon for 6- and 7-year-old children to become involved in competitive athletics (Gallahue & Ozmun, 2002). There has been much controversy about this current trend in terms of the child's physical and emotional readiness for sports participation. Recent research suggests that poor conditioning, overtraining, and poorly qualified coaches are the major risks in youth sports. The rate of injury, even in traditional contact-collision sports like football, is similar to or lower than that for adults when these conditions are controlled for (Gallahue & Ozmun, 2002).

SOCIAL CONTEXTS

In middle childhood children spend much of their time outside the home in school and other community activities. In addition to interacting in many more environments, as middle childhood progresses children are more likely to be relatively independent in their activities, with less adult direction. Social skills are a collection of isolated and discrete learned behaviors that are modeled on the child's lived experiences. Young children develop skills through imitating others in the home and community setting they spend time in. **Social competence** refers to the smooth, sequential, appropriate use of these skills in a dynamic way across contexts. The development of social competence in multiple environments is a key developmental achievement of middle childhood (Dodge et al., 2003). This is the time of intense peer contexts, including play in "forts," secret hideouts, summer camps, and clubs. During middle childhood, children develop a distinct peer culture in which the rules differ from those common in their interactions with adults. The social skills needed in peer-play contexts will be different from those needed among peers at school and in peer interactions involving teachers, coaches, and counselors who structure activities.

Peer Contexts

In middle childhood some solitary play continues, but play is most typically a peer-group activity (Chandler, 1997). Much of the peer culture in this age group is gender-specific and distinctive. As noted earlier, boys are described as playing in groups, incorporating rough-and-tumble, or aggressive, play that is focused on competition for dominance. Girls tend to play in smaller groups and focus on forming close relationships (Fromberg & Bergen, 1998). In preschool most play is with cultural and socioeconomic peers. In the school-age child, there are greater opportunities to interact with children of different backgrounds.

Ideas of "popularity" emerge first in middle childhood as some children are sought out as associates, while others are shunned (Hubbard & Coie, 1994). Research on popularity suggests that social status is related to an understanding of emotion, the accurate interpretation of facial expression, and the ability to use personalized information about others in social situations. Popular children, Dodge, Murphy, & Buchsbaum (1984) found, are better able to detect the social intentions of their peers than are other children. The ability to make and keep friends is associated with positive social adjustment and classroom performance (Chandler, 1997). One of the most consistently cited concerns of mothers with children having attention deficit hyperactivity disorder is their child's failure to form friendships and his or her exclusion from social activities like birthday parties (Cronin, 1995). Children with learning differences may be "included" in the classroom but actively excluded or marginalized by peers in play (Fromberg & Bergen, 1998).

Children use their peer group to model their social and interpersonal behavior. It is this tendency to model peers in middle childhood that has lent the greatest support for **inclusion** in the school setting. Inclusion in education means that all students in a school, regardless of their strengths or weaknesses in any area, are part of the regular school community. There is evidence to support the theory that children with cognitive impairments and other developmental differences develop more appropriate and positive social interaction when placed with typically developing peers. There has been some evidence that inclusive education practices do result in improved social behavior for many children (Vogler, Koranda, & Romance, 2000), but the bulk of the evidence is quite mixed or openly negative (Slee & Weiner, 2001). Although inclusive education was originally promoted as optimal for all children, there is evidence that children with impairments placed in the regular classroom often have fewer social interactions and a low friendship status in peer groups

(Ridsdale & Thompson, 2002; Brice & Miller, 2000; Cheney, Osher, & Caesar, 2002). This is especially true with children who have compromised ability to perceive nonverbal communication in others, particularly children with hearing impairments, autism, and some types of learning disabilities (Byrnes & Sigafoos, 2001; Mesibov & Shea, 1996; Lloyd, Wilton, & Townsend, 2000).

Children choose friends who share similar characteristics and interests, and they may begin to explore relationships with children who are different through the positive mechanisms of sharing, helping, complimenting, and encouraging. More negative interactions that serve the same purpose are gossiping, directing, teasing, and criticizing. Bullying and victimization are common in middle childhood (Boulton, Trueman, & Flemington, 2002). Peer reports agree that *bullying* includes hitting and pushing, threatening people, and forcing people to do things they don't want to do (Boulton, Trueman, & Flemington, 2002). In this research, "fewer pupils, but still more than half, agreed that 'name calling,' 'telling nasty stories about other people,' and 'taking people's belongings' were types of bullying" (Boulton, Trueman, & Flemington, 2002, p. 353).

During middle childhood, bullying and victimization are typically directed at the child with few friends and little peer support (Pellegrini & Long, 2002). Evidence from groups of children with diverse differences in development and impairment suggest that children who experience differences in development or learning also experience more limited friendships and peer acceptance (Wiener & Schneider, 2002; Dudgeon, Murray, & Greenberg, 2001; Massagli & Ross, 1997). Children may go to great lengths, including refusing special tools like splints or crutches, to keep from standing out or drawing additional attention to themselves. This behavior can be a significant challenge for parents and therapists.

Research on friendships and popularity in average children suggests that unpopular children exhibit behaviors that make them stand out and lead to rejection. Putallaz and Wasserman (1990) attributed the following behaviors to children who had few friends: asking questions that were irrelevant to the group topic; talking about themselves and their problems, feelings, and interests when others were doing something else; introducing new topics abruptly; disagreeing when first joining a group; and not understanding how to disagree positively. Rather than work cooperatively, these unpopular children tended to call the group's attention to themselves, tried to control group activity, and acted to distract the group. In addition, it is common for children with poorly developed peer skills to cry easily and substitute monologues for conversations, interrupting peers (Fromberg & Bergen, 1998).

Adult Contexts

Parents, educators, and other adults influence children's play in many ways. By encouraging specific activities and providing access to "appropriate" peers, parents influence the choices children make. While this has always been true, increasingly television and computer games constitute the leisure time of children in middle childhood (Larson, 2001). These activities are designed and provided to children by adults and are thus included in this section on adult contexts. The social and environmental context influence play. Play for one child may be perceived as work by another. For example, parents who expect excellence in sports may change the category of the activity from the realm of play to that of work.

Because play is important to the development of adult functional behavior, it has been widely adopted as a tool for therapy to assist the child with developmental differences to gain new skills. The careful choice of toys to elicit certain therapy goals is the adult use of object play. **Object play** is the manipulation of objects in an intrinsically motivated activity that is not focused on some externally imposed goal. Therapeutic interventions using object play are among the most widely recommended of strategies in all disciplines working with preschool children. Object play continues to be effective as a skill development tool in middle childhood, but the objects become more sophisticated, often utilizing open-ended constructional tools like art materials and building blocks.

Object play may or may not be adult-directed play. By providing appealing art materials or costumes, the adult may elicit specifically desired play activities. Restricting the availability of some objects, like toy guns or trading cards, is likely to lead to creative object substitutions for an established pattern of object play.

Virtual (electronic) play is intrinsically motivated activity that is chosen as a form of leisure (rather than as a school or learning activity). Television viewing is a type of electronic play that has become one of the primary leisure activities of school-age children (Wright et al., 2001; McHale, Couter, & Tucker, 2001; Sherry, 2001; Charton, et al., 2000). Research on television viewing indicates that it may be associated with increased aggression (Sherry, 2001) and a decrease in other desired behaviors. The Academy for Child and Adolescent Psychiatry states that "time spent watching television takes away from important activities such as reading, school work, playing, exercise, family interaction, and social development" (2002, Facts for Families # 54). Video games, Internet explorations, and computer games have the same effect of limiting alternative play behaviors but have been found to have the same or less of a tendency to inspire aggressive behavior than television (Larson, 2001; McHale, Couter, & Tucker, 2001; Sherry, 2001).

Many types of virtual play are solitary activities, but increasingly, social options are emerging. Many of the handheld game devices can be connected, allowing for multiple players, as shown in Figure 11–9.

Game devices are very common. Children carry them with them to most of their activity environments, including the car, in public transportation, and on playgrounds. Although this trend does not encourage fitness in typical children, assistive technology can interface with these devices and offer children with physical limitations a venue to participate in "normative" play.

There is much concern about the exposure of children to pornography, criminal activity, and exploitation when using the Internet. While caution is urged in both the content and time spent engaged in electronic play, the medium of the Internet in particular has afforded some new and positive opportunities for children's social development. The parameters of Internet play (anonymity, interactivity, and connectivity) provide a nonthreatening format in which to explore roles and personal identity (Maczewski, 2002; Subrahmanyam et al., 2001). Many organizations associated with specific conditions or special interests have Internet sites and Web-based forums. Although research has not caught up with the explosive development in this area, it appears that the Internet may provide an audience of peers with similar experiences and a forum for self-expression and peer support (Jones, Zahl, & Huws, 2001).

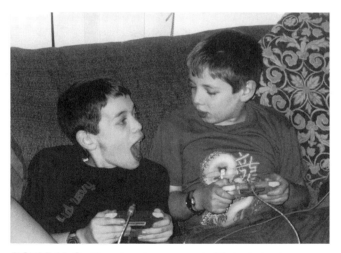

FIGURE 11–9 These boys have connected their electronic game devices and can choose either to compete or to solve puzzles cooperatively.

SUMMARY

The period of middle childhood is characterized by the understanding of one's self and one's culture beyond the home. The greatest developmental demands of this period, often called the *school-age years*, are associated with active participation in the school environment. While this is generally a healthy period, children of this age group are susceptible to stress-related problems, depression, and sports injuries. Children with developmental differences or impairments are at a particular disadvantage because they now learn to measure themselves against their peers rather than by the more lenient adult measure of how far they have come.

As children enter puberty, they have formed ideas about themselves and what their own strengths and weaknesses are that they will carry into adolescence. Through play and school friendships that endure, children learn to negotiate the complex interpersonal world of their community.

Speaking of

School Challenges

HANNAH McMONAGLE
PARENT OF A YOUNG MAN WITH ASPERGER'S SYNDROME

The focus in schools today is that of academics, good grades, and sports. These are the things that my son Gregory does well. Gregory does well in academics, but he has difficulty making friends. When things happen that are out of order or unplanned, or he is losing a game, he will fly into a tantrum and wave his arms and cry very loudly. He will confront any teacher or group of teachers without a qualm. Teachers report that he is uncooperative and confrontational, and often will refuse to participate.

Last year Gregory was tested by many specialists and was diagnosed with Asperger's syndrome. The occupational therapy report showed that he had difficulty with certain tasks in school. His writing is often illegible, and his organization is poor in terms of how the work is set out. He often misses part of the written instructions. My own impression is that he has some form of learning disability and is often unable to get his thoughts on paper in any kind of coordinated fashion.

At his school I requested an IEP [special education support], and the school principal asked why I wanted it, as Gregory had very high standardized test scores. I was very annoyed by this comment and pointed out to her that my concern was that academics was only one part of the education. My concern was the education of the whole child; the schools seem to forget that social skills are a very important part of education.

Gregory sees everything in terms of black and white. Many of the social expressions that we take for granted, Gregory is unable to read. For example, if you tell him to sink or swim, he would interpret this literally. One day I was talking to Gregory and said, "I could have died," and his mouth fell wide open.

He is unable to look people in the eye and will look down and away when he is introduced to someone. In church he is unable to hold hands with anyone other than his brother or myself. If he is upset about something, he will shout loudly no matter where he is. He will not initiate conversation with other kids but will stay on the fringe and might be drawn in after several sessions.

Gregory's grades are good, but will he be able to ever leave home and take care of himself? Will he be able to shop, ask for help, and manage the social expectations of college or a job? What is an education worth if it does not lead him toward a productive adult life? Why should the kids with obvious physical impairments but no difficulty with the social environment at school qualify for special help more easily than Gregory, whose limitations are invisible?

REFERENCES

American Academy of Child and Adolescent Psychiatry. (AACAP) (2002). *Facts for families #54: Children and watching TV*. Retrieved July 2, 2003, from http://www.aacap.org/publications/factsfam/tv.htm.

American Academy of Child and Adolescent Psychiatry. (2002). *Facts for families #66: Helping teenagers with stress*. Retrieved July 2, 2003, from http://www.aacap.org/publications/factsfam/66.htm.

American Heritage® dictionary of the English language (4th ed.). (2000). Boston: Houghton Mifflin.

Bard, C., Fleury, M., & Hay, L. (1990). *Development of eye-hand coordination across the lifespan*. Columbia, SC: University of South Carolina Press.

Blum, R. W. (1983). The adolescent with spina bifida. *Clinical Pediatrics, 22,* 331–335.

Brice, A., & Miller, R. J. (2000). Case studies in inclusion: What works, what doesn't. *Communication Disorders Quarterly, 21,* 237–241.

Briggs Elementary School Home Page (2003). Retrieved July 30, 2003, from http://www.briggs.k12.ca.us/.

Charlton, T., Panting, C., Davie, R., Coles, D., & Whitmarsh, L. (2000). Children's playground behaviour across five years of broadcast television: A naturalistic study in a remote community. *Emotional and Behavioural Difficulties, 5,* 4–12.

Cheney, D., Osher, T., & Caesar, M. (2002). Providing ongoing skill development and support for educators and parents of students with emotional and behavioral disabilities. *Journal of Child and Family Studies, 11,* 79–89.

Chown, E., Booker, L., & Kaplan, S. (2001). Perception, action planning, and cognitive maps. *Behavioral and Brain Sciences, 24,* 882–884.

Coster, W., Deeney, T., Haltiwanger, J., & Haley, S. (1998). *School function assessment: User's manual*. San Antonio, TX: The Psychological Corporation.

Cronin, A. (2001). Psychosocial and emotional domains. In J. Case-Smith (Ed.), *Occupational therapy for children*. St. Louis: Mosby.

D'Auria, J. P., Christian, B. J., & Richardson, L. F. (1997). Through the looking glass: Children's perceptions of growing up with cystic fibrosis. *Canadian Journal of Nursing Research, 29,* 99–112.

Dodge, K., Lansford, J., Burks, V., Bates, J., Pettit, G., Fontaine, R., & Price, J. (2003). Peer rejection and social information-processing factors in the development of aggressive behavior problems in children. *Child Development, 74,* 374–394.

Dodge, K. A., Coie, J. D., Pettit, G. S., & Price, J. M. (1990). Peer status and aggression in boys' groups: Developmental and contextual analyses. *Child Development, 61,* 1289–1309.

Dodge, K. A., Murphy, R. M., & Buchsbaum, K. (1984). The assessment of intention-cue detection skills in children: Implications for developmental psychopathology. *Child Development, 55,* 163–173.

Dudgeon, B. J., Massagli, T. L., & Ross, B.(1997). Educational participation of children with spinal cord injury. *American Journal of Occupational Therapy, 51,* 553–561.

Fromberg, D. P., & Bergen, D. (1998). *Play from birth to twelve and beyond: Contexts, perspectives, and meanings*. New York: Garland Publishing.

Gallahue, D., & Ozmun, J. (2002). *Understanding motor development* (5th ed.). Boston: McGraw-Hill.

Goggin, N. (2003). *KINE 3500 Lecture 4: Perceptual-Motor Development*. Retrieved July 30, 2003, from http://www.coe.unt.edu/goggin/kine3500/350lec4.htm.

Gur, R., Mozely, L., Resnick, S., Karp, J., Alvi, A., Arnold, S., & Gur, R. (1995). Sex differences in regional cerebral glucose metabolism during a resting state. *Science, 267,* 528–531.

Haywood, K. (1980). Coincidence-anticipation accuracy across the lifespan. *Experimental Aging Research, 6,* 451–462.

Haywood, K. (1993). Lifespan motor development (2nd ed.). Champaign, IL: Human Kinetics.

Hommel, B., Gehrke, J., & Knuf, L. (2000). Hierarchical coding in the perception and memory of spatial layouts, *Psychological Research, 64,* 1–10.

Hubbard, J. A., & Coie, J. D. (1994). Emotional correlates of social competence in children's peer relationships. *Merrill Palmer Quarterly, 40,* 1–20.

Kaplan, H., & Sadock, B. (1998). *Kaplan and Sadock's synopsis of psychiatry* (8th ed.). Philadelphia: Williams and Wilkins.

Kidshealth. Retrieved October 28, 2003, from http://www.kidshealth.org/parent/emotions/feelings/stress.html.

Jones, R., Zahl, A., & Huws, J. (2001). First-hand accounts of emotional experiences in autism: A qualitative analysis. *Disability and Society, 16,* 393–401.

Lampert, J. L. (1998). Working with students with visual impairment. In J. Case-Smith (ed.), *Occupational therapy: Making a difference in school system practice* (pp. 37–42). Bethesda, MD: American Occupational Therapy Association.

Larson, R. W. (2001). How U.S. children and adolescents spend time: What it does (and doesn't) tell us about their development. *Current Directions in Psychological Science, 10,* 160–164.

Maczewski, M. (2002). Exploring identities through the Internet: Youth experiences online. *Child and Youth Care Forum, 31,* 111–129.

Mare, R. (1996). *Family structure, social change, school outcomes, and educational inequality*. In A. Booth & J. Dunn (Eds.), *Family-school links*. Hillsdale, NJ: Erlbaum.

McHale, S., Crouter, A., & Tucker, C. (2001). Free-time activities in middle childhood: Links with adjustment in early adolescence. *Child Development, 72,* 1764–1778.

Moller, L., Hymel, S., & Rubin, K. (1992). Sex typing in play and popularity in middle childhood. *Sex Roles, 26,* 331–353.

Murray, C., & Greenberg, M. T. (2001). Relationships with

teachers and bonds with school: Social emotional adjustment correlates for children with and without disabilities. *Psychology in the Schools, 38*, 25–41.

Pavri, S., & Monda-Amaya, L. (2001). Social support in inclusive schools: Student and teacher perspectives. *Exceptional Children, 67*, 391–411.

Payne, V. G., & Isaacs, L. D. (2001). *Human motor development: A lifespan approach* (5th ed.). Boston: McGraw-Hill.

Pellegrini, A. D., & Long, J. D. (2002). A longitudinal study of bullying, dominance, and victimization during the transition from primary school through secondary school. *British Journal of Developmental Psychology, 20*, 259–280.

Putallaz, M., & Wasserman, A. (1990). Children's entry behavior. In S. R. Asher and J. D. Coie (Eds.), *Peer rejection in childhood. Cambridge studies in social and emotional development* (pp. 60–89). Cambridge, UK: Cambridge University Press.

Ridsdale, J., & Thompson, D. (2002). Perceptions of social adjustment of hearing-impaired pupils in an integrated secondary school unit. *Educational Psychology in Practice, 18*, 21–34.

Roedell, W. (1984). Vulnerabilities of highly gifted children. *Roeper Review, 6*, 127–130.

Rubenfeld, P., & Schwartz, A. (1996). Early onset of a disability: Its impact on development and adult outcomes. *Psychosocial Process, 9*, 60–63.

Schuster, C., & Ashburn, S. (1992). *The process of human development: A holistic lifespan approach* (3rd ed.). Philadelphia: J.B. Lippincott.

Sandberg, D., & Meyer-Bahlburg, H. (1994). Variability in middle childhood play behavior: effects of gender, age, and family background. *Archives of Sexual Behavior, 23*, 645–663.

Santrock, J. (1997). *Life-span development* (7th ed.). Boston: McGraw-Hill Publishers.

Shaffer, D. (1999). *Developmental psychology: Childhood and adolescence* (4th ed.). Pacific Grove, CA: Brooks/Cole.

Sherry, J. L. (2001). The effects of violent video games on aggression: A meta-analysis. *Human Communication Research, 27*, 409–431.

Shumway-Cook, A., & Woollacott, M. (2001). *Motor control: Theory and practical applications* (2nd ed.). Philadelphia: Lippincott, Williams and Wilkins.

Silverman, L. K. (1999). The universal experience of being out-of-sync. *Advanced Development.* Special Issue: 1-12.

Subrahmanyam, K., Greenfield, P., Kraut, R., & Gross, E. (2001). The impact of computer use on children's and adolescents' development. *Journal of Applied Developmental Psychology, 22*, 7–30.

Tan, L. E. (1985). Laterality and motor skills in four-year-olds. *Child Development, 56*, 119–124.

Thomas, M. (1993). *Comparing theories of child development* (3rd ed.). Belmont, CA: Wadsworth.

Tozer, S., Violas, P., & Senese, G. (1998). *Social foundations of education.* Burr Ridge, IL: McGraw-Hill.

Vaughn, S., Elbaum, B. E., & Schumm, J. S. (1996). The effects of inclusion on the social functioning of students with learning disabilities. *Journal of Learning Disabilities, 29*, 598–608.

Vuontela, V., Steenari, M., Carlson, S., Koivisto, J., Fjallberg, M., & Aronen, E. (2003). Audiospatial and visuospatial working memory in 6–13-year-old school children. *Learning and Memory, 10*, 74–81.

Vgotsky, L. S. (1978). *Mind in society.* Cambridge, MA: Harvard University Press.

Wiener, J., & Schneider, B. (2002). A multisource exploration of the friendship patterns of children with and without learning disabilities. *Journal of Abnormal Child Psychology, 30*, 127–141.

World Health Organization. (2002). *ICF: International classification of functioning and disability.* Geneva, Switzerland: World Health Organization.

Wright, J. C., Huston, A. C., Vandewater, E. A., Backhands, D., Scantlin, R. M., Kotler, J. A., Caplovitz, A., Lee, J., Hofferth, S., & Finkelstein, J. (2001). American children's use of electronic media in 1997: A national survey. *Journal of Applied Developmental Psychology, 22*, 31–47.

CHAPTER 12

Adolescent Development

Dianne F. Simons, PhD, OTR/L
Assistant Professor
Department of Occupational
Therapy
Virginia Commonwealth University
Richmond, Virginia

Objectives

Upon completion of this chapter, the reader should be able to

▨ Identify the developmental challenges faced by younger and older adolescents.

▨ Discuss the relationship between developmental challenges and engagement in occupation.

▨ Identify types of typical adolescent participation in areas of occupation.

▨ Identify performance skills and performance patterns of typically developing adolescents.

▨ Identify the influence of context in typical adolescent occupational participation.

▨ Recognize the contributions of body functions and body structure to occupational participation in typically developing adolescents.

Key Terms

adaptation skills	model of optimal development	vocational development
biologic challenges	older adolescents	weight training
career	performance skills	work
career literacy	psychological challenges	younger adolescents
educational participation	self-definition	
leisure	sociocultural challenges	

DEFINING THE PERIOD OF "ADOLESCENCE"

The word *adolescence* is derived from the Latin word *adolescere*, which means "to grow in maturity" or "to grow into adulthood" (Kimmel & Weiner, 1995; Kaczmarek & Riva, 1996). Lerner (2001) identifies adolescence as a period of self-examination and emerging identity that spans the second decade, during which the individual changes from "being childlike to adultlike" (p. 4). Adolescence has been described as a phase of life beginning in biology and ending in society (Petersen, 1988). The onset of adolescence is somewhat less problematic than determining its conclusion, but individual differences play a major role in defining entry and exit of this period for specific individuals. Most authors (Kimmel & Weiner, 1995; Steinberg, 1996; Lerner, 2001) recognize the onset of adolescence as marked by the physical and physiologic changes of puberty. This marker is generally agreed upon despite the fact that there can be a range in age of several years between the time that these physiologic changes take place in one individual compared with another. Early development occurs in some young people as early as age 8, but it is not considered abnormal for puberty to occur as late as age 16.

Although the physical and physiologic changes associated with puberty are recognized as the "official" markers of the beginning of adolescence, it is the psychological and social changes that take place in young people that are often the most evident signs of adolescence onset. For some young people, longstanding cultural traditions serve as formal markers of the beginning of the adolescent period. Some religious faiths recognize entry into adolescence with a formal rite of passage. In the eyes of the faith these rites are more accurately viewed as an official acknowledgment of the transition from childhood to the status of being considered a man or a woman. This passage gives young people rights to attend prayer services that are restricted to adult members of the faith.

Young boys of the Jewish faith have their *bar mitzvahs* (Figure 12–1) and young girls their *bat mitzvahs*

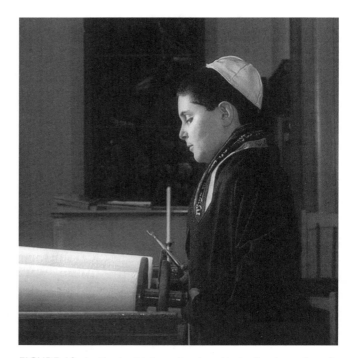

FIGURE 12–1   The Jewish bar mitzvah and bat mitzvah are rites of passage that acknowledge 13-year-olds as adults in the eyes of the synagogue and the Jewish community.

when they turn 13. Lengthy study precedes this formal religious ceremony. The young person often wears symbolic, ceremonial dress to mark the occasion. Festivities and celebration, frequently quite elaborate, resembling a wedding reception, follow the formal religious service. Some Christian denominations have periods of study and religious ceremonies that also typically occur at this age. *Confirmation* recognizes that adolescents have matured to the point of being able to make independent, informed, personal decisions about their faith. This ceremony is an acknowledgment by the church that the adolescent is no longer dependent upon parents to make important decisions for her. She is old enough to make decisions of faith for herself. These religious rituals are some of the few remaining rites of passage in contemporary society that acknowledge that

13-year-olds are regarded differently by society or at least by the members of their faith community.

Specifying the end of adolescence is more problematic due to the lack of a clear marker or indicator of the achievement of adulthood. There is no physical or physiologic change to mark the conclusion of adolescence. The marker of living independently from parents or other adult caregivers is recognized to be predominantly a psychological and social accomplishment. The age when this marker is accomplished varies significantly among individuals. Even at the societal level there are inconsistencies in regard to determining the age of adulthood. A young person can join the military, marry without parental consent, and vote at age 18 but cannot purchase alcohol until age 21.

One of the proposed indicators of attainment of adulthood is economic independence from parents or other adults (Steinberg, 1996). This rite of passage could take place when a young person assumes responsibility for his own financial support by entering the workforce, or by making the necessary arrangements to support himself financially on educational loans or through a combination of work and educational loans. As societies become increasingly complex and technologically developed, the requirement for advanced education and training extends the period of time that is necessary to sufficiently prepare to enter the workforce. As the requirements for higher education and training continue to expand, economic independence occurs later in young people's lives. It has been asserted that the period of adolescence evolved in Western cultures as a direct result of the mandatory education and child labor laws. These laws, which arose in response to the abuses of the Industrial Revolution, brought large groups of young people together for the first time and labeled them as a developmental group (Klein, 1990). The transition from adolescence to adulthood is probably best described as a process that takes into account a number of variables unique to an individual that would include financial support, work, education, and relationship factors.

For the purposes of this chapter we will divide adolescents into two groups: **younger adolescents**, ages 12 to 15 years, and **older adolescents**, ages 16 to 18 years of age. Eighteen has been an age selected by some authors (Wagner, 1996) as the age that most typically corresponds with completion of high school, a physical move away from the family home, and initial entry into the labor force or postsecondary education.

Two key events mark the division between younger and older adolescents: the ability to obtain a driver's license and drive independently without direct adult supervision, and the ability to go to work in the community without restrictions or limitations. This distinction, which roughly divides adolescence into a first half and a second half, is designed to help readers understand the extensive changes that occur during this relatively short, 7–8 year, time period. Texts on human development, by their very nature, discuss generalities and examine trends and patterns of behavior typical of a particular age span. While it is essential to have a general understanding of common characteristics of a particular age group, it is equally important to recognize that individual differences occur at all ages. In adolescence it is the factors related to those individual differences that particularly define the transition from adolescence to adulthood for a particular person.

CONTRIBUTIONS OF RESEARCHERS IN SOCIAL SCIENCES

Early descriptions of adolescent development such as that presented by psychologist G. Stanley Hall (1904) presented adolescence as a period of "storm and stress." Anthropologist Margaret Mead began refuting these ideas fairly soon thereafter when her book, *Coming of Age in Samoa* (Mead, 1928), concluded that storm and stress were culturally conditioned and specific to North America and Europe. Research spanning the last 35–40 years indicates that while some youth do experience a stormy period in response to the challenges of adolescent development, this is not the case for most youth (Laurensen, 1995; Petersen, 1988). Summarizing the results of four decades of research, Weiner (1992) refuted "the mythical notion of normative adolescent turmoil" (p. 8) and reported that approximately 80 percent of adolescents manage this life stage without serious problems. Contemporary scholars are much more focused on developmental variation—diversity—both among people (inter-individual differences) and within persons (intra-individual differences) and emphasize the physical and social context on such variation, including the significant role of culture and history in shaping adolescent development (Lerner, 2001).

DEVELOPMENTAL CHALLENGES

The major developmental challenges can be clustered into biologic challenges, psychological challenges, and sociocultural challenges. All three areas of challenge are intertwined. These three areas coincide with the domains of human function—physical, psychological, and social function—presented in Chapter 1. The **biologic challenges** include accepting the changes in bodily appearance and in physiologic functioning associated with a physically mature body. The **psychological challenges** involve emotional and cognitive changes that result from the ability to think abstractly and hypothetically. These thought capabilities allow adolescents to "know who they are, guess who they may become, and plan what they may do" (Lerner, 2001, p. 12). The psychological changes of adolescence require individuals to deal with their changed biologic self and to develop a new, revised sense of self. The primary developmental challenge in the psychological area is the development of the **self-definition** that guides the selection of roles that they plan to play in society.

Wyn and White (1997) made a particular point of emphasizing that while "growing up" does involve the establishment of an identity, this identity "is not necessarily 'fixed' and may go through significant change in one's life" (p. 54). They argue that identities change throughout life in conjunction with changes of life circumstances, but that adolescence is the first time in an individual's life when identity construction becomes a central developmental process. As adolescents construct their identity, they construct realistic ambitions and reasonable ideals for themselves. This process frequently involves relinquishing wishes for an ideal self, ideal parents, ideal people in authority, ideal educational institutions, and ideal government, and gaining acceptance of people, systems, and themselves as less than perfect.

The psychological challenges of self-definition and future plans blend inextricably with the social and cultural challenges. The **sociocultural challenge**, finding appropriate societal roles that are suitable physically and psychologically, is a crucial developmental task for adaptive functioning. As their social identity develops, adolescents accept certain social, ethical, moral, and legal responsibilities. Experts in adolescent development agree that for a healthy, positive adaptive sense of self to emerge, successful performance in roles that have meaning to the individual and that provide that person with successful experiences is essential (Lerner, 2001).

OPTIMAL DEVELOPMENT

W. G. Wagner (1996), a counseling psychologist, proposed a **model of optimal development** that includes six interacting developmental domains: biologic, cognitive, emotional, social, moral, and vocational. Using an approach that resembles goal setting for therapeutic intervention, Wagner proposed that upon an adolescent's reaching age 18, indicators in each of the domains could be used to measure achievement of optimal development. These indicators, or goals, are applicable to all adolescents. An understanding of optimal development is helpful to occupational and physical therapy students in order to understand the goals of healthy adolescent development. A description of each of Wagner's goals follows:

- *Biologic:* "Adolescents will be alive and healthy, physically mature, and engaged in health-

enhancing behaviors, including proper diet and regular exercise" (p. 364).
- *Cognitive:* "Adolescents will engage in efficient and purposively idiosyncratic thinking of a more hypothetical, multidimensional, future-oriented, and relative nature that is based on prior life experiences, including the completion or near completion of at least 12 years of formal education" (pp. 367–368).
- *Emotional:* "Adolescents will be emotionally aware, feel secure and self-confident, be determined and optimistic about the future, and possess the resilience needed to overcome adversities" (p. 371).
- *Social:* "Adolescents will possess the social skills and maturity needed to engage in cooperative, genuine, and trusting interaction with others, including friends and at least one valued and living intimate, and to recognize and understand the perspective of others, including those of a different age, gender, and culture" (p. 373).
- *Moral:* "Adolescents will have internalized and will follow a personalized set of abstract moral principles that are socially responsive in their integration of the principles of fairness/equity and consideration of the feelings and needs of others, including those of different age, gender, and culture" (p. 377).
- *Vocational:* "Adolescents will be aware of their unique potential, be career literate, have developed employability skills and experienced the fulfillment of productive employment, and have developed a life plan that incorporates a multi-role conceptualization of career and is based on personal preference rather than social biases related to gender, race, or ethnicity" (p. 380).

ADOLESCENT PHYSICAL DEVELOPMENT

The rate of development at puberty is more rapid than at any other time of life except infancy (Carnegie Council on Adolescent Development, 1989). Girls enter the transition to adolescence an average of 1.5 to 2 years earlier than boys do. The timing of onset of physical changes of adolescence is related to a multitude of factors, including heredity and environment. The endocrine system, particularly the influence of gonadotropic (GnRH) hormones that regulate the release of estrogen and testosterone, is particularly important in adolescent development (Gallahue & Ozmun, 2002). The physical changes of adolescence include changes in height, weight, and sexual maturity.

Everyone has experience with the adolescent growth spurt during which 20 percent of adult stature is attained. The growth spurt itself relates to the velocity of the change in height, or the amount of change that occurs in a relatively short period of time. In boys, the peak height velocity is at 14.1 years. The peak height velocity is greater and lasts longer in boys than in girls, in whom it occurs at 12.1 years (Murphy, 1990). In girls 95 percent of adult stature is attained by age 16½ and the remainder by the 18th birthday. In boys 95 percent of stature is attained by age 18, with the last 2 percent occurring by the 20th birthday. This rapid skeletal growth may result in certain variations becoming increasingly evident or even pathologic, such as the case of idiopathic scoliosis. *Idiopathic scoliosis* is a curvature of the spine that manifests itself in the prepubertal years and requires aggressive management during the period of rapid skeletal growth.

Weight gains during adolescence follow patterns similar to those for height but are also greatly affected by environmental factors (Gallahue & Ozmun, 2002). A major societal concern is the onset of obesity at younger and younger ages. The percent of body fat in American adolescents is higher than it was 10 years ago, a fact that is attributable to both an increasingly sedentary lifestyle and changes in diet (Gallahue & Ozmun, 2002). As males pass through adolescence, their proportion of body fat tends to decrease, whereas for females, it tends to increase (Murphy, 1990).

Puberty, driven by changes in the endocrine system, is a period in which changes in secondary sex characteristics appear and the reproductive system reaches maturity. In girls, secondary sex characteristics include the budding of nipples and breasts, followed by pubic-hair growth and growth of genitalia. In males, secondary sex characteristics include the physical growth of the testicles, followed by pubic hair. Later, axillary hair and facial and body hair appear (Gallahue & Ozmun, 2002). The onset of menses is the definitively identified event signifying puberty in females, typically occurring in American females at around 12 years. For males, the highlight of puberty is less obvious but may be considered the first ejaculation of mature sperm, sometime during middle adolescence (Gallahue & Ozmun, 2002).

The most common method of assessing physical maturity in adolescents is known as the *Sex Maturity Rating Scale (SMR)*, developed by Tanner, and otherwise referred to as *Tanner stages.* The SMR is a method of using visual inspection of genitalia or breasts and pubic hair to evaluate stages of pubertal development. Tanner Stage I is considered *preadolescence*, evidenced by absence of pubic hair, flat breasts in females, and absence of pubic hair in males. Tanner Stage II is considered *early adolescence*, and is characterized by sparse pubic hair; small, raised breasts in females, and enlargement of testes with darkening of pubic hair in males. Stages III and IV are considered *middle*

adolescence. Coarsening and curling of pubic hair characterize stage III. In girls Tanner Stage III is characterized by enlargement and raising of the breasts, whereas in males there is an increase in penis size. Stage IV in girls is characterized by the areola and nipple forming a separate contour from the breast and in males by continued growth of the penis. Stage V for both sexes is characterized by adult genitalia.

MOTOR PERFORMANCE SKILLS

The motor skills of a typically developing adolescent continue to be refined as the adolescent ages. **Performance skills** are those motor skills that underlie the ability to physically perform in the environment. The motor skills of stability and alignment when standing or sitting and when moving and interacting with objects in their environment are essential skills for many of the activities those adolescents perform on a daily basis. In order to engage in many of the activities that are valued by adolescents, particularly athletic pursuits, balance is a prerequisite ability. The balance skills evidenced by cheerleading teams, dance teams, and gymnastics teams demonstrate clearly the capabilities of some young people within this age group. Of course, not everyone can balance on one foot while being held aloft in a teammate's hand stretched to full extension, but in general adolescents possess the balance to safely go through their day-to-day activities without difficulty.

Typically developing adolescents are able to balance, stabilize, and position their bodies and arms to allow them to engage in a myriad of tasks from grooming to playing a musical instrument to rollerblading or skateboarding. Reaching and bending are mobility requirements in everyday activities like getting into a car or bus seat or a school desk and for many artistic and athletic activities, such as painting, playing tennis, and turning a page of music while playing an instrument. Routine performance of instrumental activities of daily living (IADLs), like vacuuming, ironing, and cooking, and activities of daily living (ADLs), like showering, self-feeding, hair care and styling, and toilet hygiene, all require bending and reaching for efficient performance of the task. (Both ADLs and IADLs are discussed later.) Typically developing adolescents are expected to have the ability to bend, to flex, and to rotate their trunks without any restrictions or stiffness. By adolescence, a young person's bilateral coordination skills have fully matured. They routinely use two hands or one hand and another body part to accomplish any desired task that requires stabilizing and manipulating objects. They open small makeup containers and the rings of a three-ring binder without problems. Athletic and artistic activities often require excellent bilateral coordination.

Adolescents have the grasp-and-release patterns, the isolated finger movements, and the in-hand manipulation skills to pick up, shift, and adjust their pens or pencils in their hand to take notes in class, to rotate their pencils in their hand to use the eraser end of the pencil, to pull a key out of a pocket or purse and insert it in the ignition, and to put coins into soda machines without difficulty. These actions are a part of the routine, everyday tasks performed by adolescents. Their focus is on the task of taking notes, correcting a mistake to solve a math problem accurately, or starting a car. The underlying motor abilities that they need in order to perform these desired activities never cross their conscious mind once the activity has been mastered. An adolescent learning to drive needs to learn how to insert the key and turn on the engine, but he does not have to think about how to hold the key. Many of the occupations pursued by adolescents require high levels of isolated finger movements. Manipulation skill allows young people to play musical instruments, to do detailed drawings, and to do extremely fine needlework or craft activities.

For adolescents to complete most of the tasks that are part of their day they need smooth, fluid arm and hand movements. *Flow* in the upper extremities is normal and expected in typically developing adolescents. Flow allows them to eat and drink, hit a baseball, throw a discus or shot-put, bowl a bowling ball, cast a fishing line, or play a guitar without a thought about the underlying motor skills required for these highly valued pastimes. Although flow refers to the upper extremities, the same principles hold true for the lower extremities. Adolescents need smooth, fluid leg and foot movements to kick soccer balls or footballs, for example.

Although motor skills continue to develop generally into the 20s, adolescents have learned to precisely *calibrate* their movements. There may be some initial misjudgment when attempting a task for the first time or two, as evidenced by either too much or too little force being exerted or when an action is performed at too quick a speed, but once a typically developing adolescent has been sufficiently familiarized with a task, problems with calibration would not be expected. Adolescents are capable of highly developed calibration, such as that seen in masterfully playing the drums or the violin. They learn the importance of calibration when they learn to drive. Proper braking requires calibration skills, and the skilled use of a clutch and accelerator simultaneously certainly requires the ability to calibrate as well. Table 12–1 gives examples of typical adolescent activities where motor skills are observable.

In infancy and early childhood, characteristics of motor performance are often described in terms of *milestones*, or *skill acquisition*. Nearly all children display the attainment of these skills, such as walking, running, hopping, skipping, throwing, and playing movement-oriented games such as T-ball. Although children differ from an early age in how well they play ball, for example, nearly all children are able to achieve the milestones. However, by adolescence there is a clearly quantitative aspect to motor skill performance manifested by such parameters as strength, speed, power, reaction time, and endurance. Hence the name *performance skills* is often applied to these refined motor patterns. There are differences among individuals on these parameters based on environmental factors, such as training and practice, as well as innate factors, such as gender and body type. Figure 12–2 illustrates a spontaneous game of football. This sport involves complex motor coordination skills as well as much proprioceptive input.

Changes in motor skill performance correlate with physical growth. For example, it is suggested that changes in balance ability occur as the high center of gravity in the child is displaced progressively lower through adolescence. Overall, this tends to coincide with steadily improving static and dynamic balance throughout the adolescent period. The phenomenon of "adolescent awkwardness" has been difficult to document through quantitative study. The current conclusion is that this phenomenon exists in some individuals, mostly males, at the time of peak height velocity. Adolescent awkwardness is a transient phenomenon and tends to affect mostly those boys who were high performers at the onset of their growth spurt (Payne & Isaacs, 1999).

Changes in strength during adolescence have been documented for both abdominal and grip strength. There are definitive gender differences. For males, upper trunk strength increases linearly through adolescence, whereas for females, the rate of change is much less extreme and is characterized by a nearly straight line (Gallahue & Ozmun, 2002). Grip strength in both males and females increases tremendously during adolescence; however, once again, the absolute increases for males are much higher (Payne & Isaacs, 1999).

Changes in strength relate to changes in *body mass index (BMI)*, which is a measure of percent body fat. In adolescence, under the influence of testosterone, boys tend to become leaner, whereas females tend to develop more body fat (Payne & Isaacs, 1999). Therefore, strength differences between the sexes are related to the amount and type of muscle fiber available for contraction. With respect to endurance, males tend to improve steadily up until age 16. Females display a more erratic course, characterized by improvement up until age 14 and then a regression such that the difference between males and females widens considerably through adolescence (Gallahue & Ozmun, 2002). In the case of flexibility, both sexes tend to improve slightly through adolescence, with a dropoff and typically decreasing flexibility beginning at about age 17 (Gallahue & Ozmun, 2002). Of course, all of these differences in physical-performance parameters for both genders are significantly affected by training.

TABLE 12–1	Motor Skills			

Examples of Activities Engaged in by Typically Developing Adolescents During Which Performance Skills Are Observable

Motor Skills	School	Home	Work in Community	Play/Leisure and Social Settings in the Community
Posture—Refers to the stabilizing and aligning of one's body while moving in relation to task objects with which one must deal.				
• Stabilizes	Moving from class to class without the need for support.	Moving around in the shower to wash oneself.	Walking from the counter to the fry station in a fast-food restaurant without stopping.	Running a sprint on the track.
• Aligns	Standing in classroom to give a presentation without needing to lean on a podium.	Standing at the sink to wash dishes without leaning against the counter.	Standing beside a table taking a customer's order.	Standing at the free-throw line to shoot a basket.
• Positions	Arranging one's position in front of one's locker to allow efficient access to the locker.	Standing slightly to the side to allow room for the refrigerator door to open.	Restocking shelves at an effective distance from the objects being removed from the carton and placed on the shelf.	Positioning oneself the proper distance from home plate to allow the bat to cover the plate when swinging the baseball bat.
Mobility—Relates to moving the entire body or a body part in space as necessary when interacting with task objects.				
• Walks	Walking the school corridors between classes.	Walking from one room to another to answer the telephone.	As a hostess, walking in front of customers to show them to their table.	Walking around a shopping mall with friends or family members.
• Reaches	Reaching for papers being passed back by the student sitting at the desk in front of them.	Reaching into the back of a drawer for a "scrunchie" hair tie.	Reaching into the pizza oven to remove a cooked pizza.	Reaching a tennis racquet up for an overhead smash.
• Bends	Bending down to pick up a backpack from the floor.	Bending over to tuck the bedsheets and blanket under the mattress.	Bending over to pick up trash in a volunteer cleanup activity.	Taking a bow after a drama performance.
Coordination—Refers to using more than one body part to interact with task objects in a manner that supports task performance.				
• Coordinates	Opening a soda bottle using both hands.	Brushing hair with one hand while blowing it dry with a hair dryer in the other hand.	Carrying a serving tray of food and drinks.	Clapping for a touchdown, goal, or performance.
• Manipulates	Opening a three-ring binder.	Opening a twist tie on a bread package to make a sandwich.	Using a pen to write down a customer's order on an order form.	Making beaded jewelry or knotted friendship bracelets.
• Flows	Pouring a beaker of solution into a test tube in chemistry.	Applying eyeliner and mascara.	Refilling customers' water and tea glasses.	Playing a violin.

Continues

TABLE 12–1 Motor Skills *Continued*

Strength and Effort—Refers to skills that require generation of muscle force appropriate for effective interaction with task objects.

Motor Skills	School	Home	Work in Community	Play/Leisure and Social Settings in the Community
• Moves	Pulling open a desk drawer to take out supplies.	Pulling a fitted sheet over the mattress when making up a fresh bed.	Pushing a wheelbarrow of mulch to the landscaping bed where it is needed.	Sliding pieces across a game board.
• Transports	Carrying a lunch tray from the lunch line to the table.	Carrying a laundry basket from the bedroom to the laundry room.	Carrying a puppy from the examining table to the scale to be weighed.	Carrying equipment from the gym or field house to the playing field.
• Lifts	Picking up a book from the library shelves.	Passing a shared bowl of food to other people at the dinner table.	Picking up a hammer to begin nailing.	Picking up a "flyer" in a cheerleading formation.
• Calibrates	Writing without putting too much pressure on the pen or pencil.	Cutting food on the dinner plate effectively without scratching the plate.	Pouring the correct amount of batter onto the grill to make pancakes of the right size.	Striking the keys of the piano with the correct amount of pressure, not too lightly, not too heavily.
• Grips	Maintaining a grip on pens and pencils to take notes.	Holding silverware to cut meat and eat.	Gripping the clips on skirt/pants hangers to open them to restock clothing for sale.	Gaining and maintaining grip on the baton that is passed between members of a relay team.

Energy—Refers to sustained effort over the course of task performance.

• Endures	Completing a 7-hour school day without excessive fatigue.	Finishing homework and/or chores without having to stop due to physical fatigue.	Completing a 4-, 6-, or 8-hour shift lifeguarding without undue exhaustion.	Playing an entire field hockey game without an undue number of breaks to rest.
• Paces	Working on in-class assignments with a consistent, steady rhythm.	Not rushing through or "taking forever" to complete homework, chores, meals, or personal hygiene.	Taking the required time to fill orders and check on customers who need refills in the coffee shop.	Pacing one's running speed to compete in a cross-country track event.

ADOLESCENT COGNITIVE DEVELOPMENT

Basic knowledge of development includes an understanding of cognitive development, which was first described in Chapter 3 of this text. Piaget's (1972) stage of *formal operations* is characterized by symbolic thought, mental operations on abstract representations, and hypothetical-deductive reasoning. In addition to abstract thinking, other changes in thinking processes occur during adolescence, such as the development of a more efficient form of thinking that results from an increased speed of information processing (Kail, 1993) and a greater awareness of an increased knowledge base (Keating, 1990).

Emerging cognitive skill areas are in the realm of metacognition. Chapter 3 of this text describes metacognitive monitoring functions as mental activities that let us think about what we are doing before, during, and after we do it. Adolescents are typically very self-aware and are able to detect errors in their work as well as to organize their actions to complete a desired task. Intellectual awareness, the individual's knowledge about personal thoughts and feelings as they influence performance, develops and becomes central to adolescent reasoning processes.

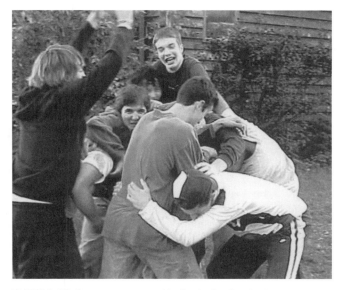

FIGURE 12–2   Contact sports like football reflect both cultural and developmental trends. These young men are demonstrating highly refined movement skills in this rowdy form of social interaction.

PROCESS SKILLS

As ordinary ADL and IADL skills became routine, the adolescent develops elaborate *process skills* to allow the transfer and adaptation of previously learned tasks to new environments. Adolescents use the process skill of knowledge throughout the day as they choose the right tools before initiating the task, and they know what task objects are needed for different activities that compose a part of their day. They also have the knowledge to use the tools and materials that they have chosen for different tasks according to their intended purpose. Although they may occasionally substitute objects, like a washcloth for a toothbrush, or a knife for a fork, they know the purpose of the task objects that they use for various tasks and in most cases use them appropriately and safely.

TEMPORAL ORGANIZATION

Temporal organization pertains to the orderly and logical sequencing of task steps from start to finish. Adolescents initiate tasks and the steps within a task in every activity they undertake within a day. They initiate their ADLs, their homework assignments, and their spontaneous play activities. Once they begin an activity, they continue each step of the activity and sequence the steps in a logical and effective way until they complete the task and terminate the activity. When they initiate an activity like cleaning the car, they generally follow some kind of logical order such as starting with removing the trash and vacuuming the interior, cleaning the windows on the inside, washing the car with soap, wiping down the wheels and tires, and finishing the task with rinsing and drying the vehicle. The order makes sense. They don't start one step, change to another step without finishing the last step, illogically order the steps, or stop prematurely. Typically developing adolescents have an understanding of sequencing and time, and they can hypothesize and plan an activity from start to finish. Adolescent organizations frequently organize car washes to raise money for some group or organization. They understand the scope of the task, and the steps involved. They may stop and play around or flirt by squirting the hose at each other, but they will complete the task.

ADAPTATION

Adaptation skills relate to the ability to anticipate, correct for, and benefit from the consequences of errors that naturally arise during routine task performance. An adolescent, for example, may notice that when he moves a ruler too quickly after drawing an ink line, the ink smears, and he will respond by waiting a minute or so for the ink to dry sufficiently before moving the ruler the next time. He may notice that a page is jutting out beyond the others in his notebook and open the binder to line up the bottom hole of the paper with the appropriate ring of the binder. The need to accommodate one's actions within the workspace by changing their method or the way that they use a tool is a basic way that young people learn from experience. An adolescent may find that attempting to read her social studies textbook is difficult with the radio playing even though she just completed her math homework with no problems with the radio playing. She will adjust to the new situation by getting up and turning off the radio until she gets the social studies chapter read.

A typically developing adolescent benefits when he can anticipate the consequences of not studying, or not practicing, or not taking the necessary time to do a task correctly. Adolescents adapt through experiences with IADL tasks, ADL tasks, educational tasks, work tasks, social participation tasks, leisure tasks, and play tasks. Errors that occur naturally during tasks, as well as the successes that result from doing tasks, become important contributors to adaptation and development. Table 12–2 lists examples of typical activities in which the process skills of adolescents are observable.

ADOLESCENT PSYCHOLOGICAL AND SOCIAL DOMAINS OF DEVELOPMENT

The transition in cognitive development to abstract and hypothetical thinking is accompanied by a greater focus on internal emotional states, and greater awareness of the situational and mental aspects of emotions and the complexity of emotions, such as the ability to experience contrasting emotions simultaneously (Harris, Olthof, & Meerum Terwogt, 1981). Basic knowledge in social development includes recognition

TABLE 12–2	Adolescent Process Skills

Examples of Activities Engaged in by Typically Developing Adolescents During Which Performance Skills Are Observable

Process Skills	School	Home	Work in Community	Play/Leisure and Social Settings in the Community
Energy—Refers to sustained effort over the course of task performance.				
• Paces	Working on in-class assignments with a consistent, steady rhythm.	Not rushing through or "taking forever" to complete homework, chores, meals, or personal hygiene tasks.	Taking the required time to fill orders and check on customers who need refills in the coffee shop.	Pacing one's running speed to compete in a cross-country track event.
• Attends	Paying attention and taking notes during a class lecture in math or science.	Paying attention to family conversations without being distracted by extraneous noise or sights from the TV or radio.	Attending to the safety of the people in the pool rather than to non–job-related activity.	Paying attention to the football play rather than being distracted by the talk from the opposing team.
Knowledge—Refers to the ability to seek and use task-related knowledge.				
• Chooses	Selecting the correct notebooks and textbooks from a locker prior to the next class or series of classes.	Choosing the lawn-mower and edger to mow and trim the lawn.	Choosing four place-mats, napkins, forks, knives, spoons, plates, and glasses to set the table for four people.	Choosing a Frisbee from a closet full of games and sporting goods equipment.
• Uses	Using pens, rulers, compasses, and paper for their intended purposes.	Using a toothbrush and dental floss for their intended purposes.	Using the designated dish sponge to clean the dishes but not using it to clean the floor.	Using a basketball and net to shoot hoops with friends.
• Handles	Supporting a full beaker of solution with two hands to prevent it from spilling or being dropped.	Carrying a dinner plate from the table to the kitchen sink with two hands.	Supporting a pitcher of water with two hands when refilling customers' drinking glasses.	Using two hands and lifting from under the piece when transporting unfired greenware to the kiln to be fired.
• Heeds	Completing an in-class assignment without missing any part of it.	Loading all of the dinner dishes into the dishwasher, filling the soap dispenser, and starting the dishwasher.	Upon seeing a customer leave, going to the table, clearing it, wiping it clean, and resetting it with napkins and silverware.	Continuing to play tennis, alternating between forehand and backhand sides of the court until the conclusion of the game, and continuing play until the set and/or match is concluded.
• Inquires	Asking questions of the teacher only when the information has not been given previously.	Not needing to ask about the washer settings once they have been fully explained.	Asking the supervisor for clarification when a customer asks a question about something that has not been previously explained.	Asking the coach questions only about plays or techniques that have not previously been explained.

Continues

TABLE 12–2	**Adolescent Process Skills** *Continued*			
Process Skills	**School**	**Home**	**Work in Community**	**Play/Leisure and Social Settings in the Community**
Temporal Organization—Refers to beginning, logical ordering, continuation, and completion of the steps and action sequences of a task.				
• Initiates	Starting to work on a test, following directions from the teacher.	Beginning homework without a reminder.	Seeing a customer enter the shop and proceeding to ask if he needs help locating something.	Beginning routine stretches at the beginning of practice without being told.
• Continues	Continuing to complete each step in a biology or chemistry lab without stopping to do something else.	Continuing to vacuum a room completely without being distracted by the surroundings.	Continuing to make and bake pizzas without losing concentration on the task.	Continuing to play basketball despite heckling from spectators.
• Sequences	On a block schedule, attending classes in the correct order for the given day.	Following the steps of a recipe in the order specified by the instructions.	Collecting payment and giving change before filling food order so food does not get cold.	Following Robert's Rules of Order (motion, second, discussion, amendment, vote on the amendment, vote on the motion) to run a club meeting to keep the meeting on task.
• Terminates	Stopping work when the assignment has been completed rather than stopping prematurely or persisting unnecessarily.	Signing off Internet messaging on the computer after spending a reasonable amount of time on-line.	Stopping work on cleaning the tiles around the pool once the full perimeter has been covered.	Leaving a party in progress with sufficient time to return home by set curfew time.
Organizing Space and Objects—Refers to skills for organizing task spaces and task objects.				
• Searches/locates	Locating pen and paper in a full backpack.	Looking for a knife and cutting board in kitchen drawers, for peanut butter in the cabinet, and for jelly and bread in the refrigerator.	Searching for clothing items or shoes in the stockroom to find the size needed by a customer.	Searching the school directory to locate club members' telephone numbers and E-mail addresses.
• Gathers	Collecting pencil, paper, notebook, textbook or computer, ruler, protractor, compass, and calculator for geometry class.	Collecting shirt, pants, underwear, socks, and shoes from closet and drawers.	Picking up items at the end of the register and placing them in grocery bags.	Putting bat, glove, batting gloves, sweatbands, cleats, towel, and uniform in bat bag to take to a softball game.
• Organizes	Setting up supplies and space in art class so water and paint will not be knocked over inadvertently.	Arranging textbooks, notebooks, notebook paper, and snacks on desk in a way that minimizes the likelihood of a spill.	Arranging beverage cups in a portable rack to carry into the stadium to sell.	Setting up easel, canvas, paints, palette, brushes, and stool to prepare to paint a landscape.
• Restores	Shutting down the Internet on the library computer after doing a search in the library.	Putting folded, clean clothes away in closet and drawers.	Returning ketchup and mustard bottles and salt, pepper, and sugar containers to the table after refilling.	Returning helmets, shoulder pads, balls, and protective equipment to the locker room.

Continues

				Play/Leisure and Social Settings in
Process Skills	School	Home	Work in Community	the Community

TABLE 12–2 Adolescent Process Skills *Continued*

Adaptation—Relates to the ability to anticipate, correct for, and benefit by learning from the consequences of errors that arise in the course of task performance.

Process Skills	School	Home	Work in Community	Play/Leisure and Social Settings in the Community
• Navigates	Moving around the cafeteria without bumping into tables and chairs or people.	Moving around the kitchen without bumping into counters or cabinets.	Walking around the store without bumping into clothing displays or clothing racks.	Avoiding getting too close to players from the opposing team when playing soccer.
• Notices/responds	Noticing that an error was not fully erased and finishing the correction process completely.	Noticing that the laundry hamper is full and starting the washing machine.	Blowing the lifeguard whistle upon noticing a young child running around the pool.	Noticing that the pitcher is throwing outside pitches and moving closer to the plate to hit the ball.
• Accommodates	Noticing that the teacher follows the textbook and moving the textbook into closer view.	Realizing that buttoning was off by one hole and unbuttoning and rebuttoning shirt.	Adjusting the umbrella to maintain shade on the lifeguard stand.	Turning down the volume on the car radio upon noticing a detour and slowed traffic.
• Adjusts	Realizing that there is no chalk in the tray and going to a neighboring classroom to get a piece of chalk for the club meeting.	Noticing that the vacuum is not picking up dirt and lint as it should and stopping to change the filter bag.	Upon seeing an empty water glass, fetching the pitcher to refill the glass.	When a trash bag becomes full, going to get a new bag during a community cleanup effort.
• Benefits	Discovering that the teacher's study guide covered most of the test questions and using the next test guide to improve performance.	Separating saturated colors from whites after turning the laundry pink as a result of mixing them.	After leaving a pizza in the oven for too long, setting the timer as an auditory reminder to remove the pizza after 20 minutes.	Sending out meeting reminders before the next meeting after realizing that attendance was low due to a lack of publicity about the meeting time.

of the rise in influence of the peer group in adolescence. Friends are extremely important to teenagers and also benefit them greatly. Adolescents with more intimate friendships are more likely to be described as better adjusted and more socially competent (Wagner, 1996). Ainsworth (1989) described a typology of adolescent friendships ranging from *acquaintances*, with whom an adolescent shares pleasantries on an intermittent basis, to *companions*, with whom they interact regularly and with whom they share common interests, to *intimates*, with whom they form close bonds and whose opinions they respect and whose support they highly value.

Ainsworth (1989) asserted that the romantic relationships that develop during adolescence represent complex interactions of attachment, reproductive, and caregiving systems that develop skills and attitudes that enhance intimacy during engagement and marriage later in life. Although conformity to a peer group has been often cited as a peril of adolescence, research indicates that peer influences in junior and senior high school tend to be positive and to encourage prosocial behavior rather than negative. Positive peer pressure, such as encouraging academic performance to remain eligible for athletic team participation and insistence on the use of a designated driver when a peer has consumed alcoholic beverages, is a benefit of caring friendships (Wagner, 1996).

CONTEXTS FOR ADOLESCENT DEVELOPMENT

Adolescents spend their time in a variety of physical and social contexts, but all or most of these contexts occur within a limited geographic area and social network, except for special occasions. They generally attend school for a good portion of the day when school is in session, so this is an especially influential context. The remainder of their time is spent in their home, neighborhood, and surrounding community—at shopping centers, friends' houses, neighborhood parks, athletic and recreation facilities, theaters, bowling alleys, and restaurants. Unless their school draws from geographic areas with neighborhoods that are diverse, adolescents, particularly younger adolescents, may have a limited view of the world. High schools generally draw from larger geographic areas than do middle schools or junior highs, but even high schools may, because of boundaries, draw from areas with limited ethnic and cultural differences. Socially, adolescents spend time with classmates, teammates, family members, and networks of friends.

MAJOR AREAS OF OCCUPATION

Cross-national research on time use by 2,315 adolescents in 11 European countries and the United States revealed that among those 12–17 years old, boys used 70 percent of their time and girls 74 percent of their time on what the researchers classified as *necessary activities.* Necessary activities included sleeping, body care, eating, going to school, school, homework, chores, and shopping. A large portion of an adolescent's day is devoted to these three major areas of occupation that will be discussed: activities of daily living, instrumental activities of daily living, and education (Alsaker & Flammer, 1999). Other areas of occupation common to this age group will be presented next.

ACTIVITIES OF DAILY LIVING (ADLs) IN ADOLESCENCE

By the age of 12 children have acquired most of the skills for *activities of daily living* that they need to become autonomous. They are responsible for feeding, bathing, grooming, feeding, toileting, and dressing themselves. If parents or caregivers have purchased most of their clothes for them up until this time, there may be a noticeable change in motivation to make their own selections and choices of clothes. With the recent trend of adolescent and adult clothing styles influencing the design of children's clothes, parents may have exercised limits on the styles of clothing that they bought for their children. During adolescence the choice of dress is often one of the first ways that a young person expresses her autonomy from parental control.

Good hygiene skills, such as routine tooth brushing, hair care, daily bathing, and hand washing before meals are generally acquired earlier in childhood. By the time that an individual becomes an adolescent, verbal reminders are not routinely needed unless these habits were not sufficiently established previously. As boys and girls begin to physically mature and body odor becomes an issue, proper hygiene may need reinforcement in the form of verbal reminders until the use of deodorant becomes a habit. As girls experience the first few months of their menstrual periods, instruction in feminine hygiene and the proper disposal of used feminine hygiene products is needed. Once these new hygiene skills have been

established, young adolescents are expected to continue them independently without adult supervision.

Preoccupation with these areas of occupational performance is related to self-esteem. Satisfaction with one's physical appearance and body image is consistently the variable most related to self-esteem (Coleman & Hendry, 1999). Social acceptance by peers, academic achievement, and athletic success also correlate with self-esteem, but appearance has the greatest influence. Adolescents care about how they look. Although girls as a rule tend to develop interests in fashion, hairstyles, and fragrances a little earlier than most boys, boys and girls become interested in their appearance and their physical attractiveness during adolescence. Suburban shopping malls are often known for being frequented by young adolescents who spend hours, especially on the weekends, familiarizing themselves with the latest styles and doing comparison shopping.

Choosing the way one looks from an appearance standpoint is an early expression of experimentation with self-definition. It is not unusual for some adolescents to move through a series of group identities trying different ones on for size to determine if the group is a good match for them personally. It is not uncommon for adolescents to use the style of their hair and their choice of dress to communicate their identification with a particular group, the members of which tend to look and dress in a particular distinctive style. Appearance also contributes to the development of their social identity. Many girls learn to wear makeup as adolescents, as illustrated in Figure 12–3.

Activities of Daily Living (ADLs) in Older Adolescence

Older adolescents have further developed their habits of bathing, toileting, grooming, hygiene, dressing, and feeding. At this point their basic skills for their culture

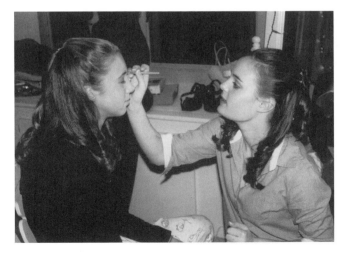

FIGURE 12–3 The grooming task of applying makeup is important to some adolescent girls every day, and even more so on special occasions like school dances.

and environment are acquired and will be retained through adulthood. During the transition to adulthood, these daily tasks are so ingrained in the lives of typically developing adolescents that little to no attention is paid to them unless a problem arises. Because independence in these areas is an essential aspect of adolescents' lives, when circumstances arise that prevent independent functioning in this area, occupational and physical therapy practitioners should respect how important this area of functioning is to young people of this age. Typically developing young people who were gaining autonomy from parents and other adults and who become dependent upon them again as a result of an injury, illness, or a disability need understanding, support, and validation of their discomfort with this situation, because it runs directly contrary to developmental process.

In addition to basic ADL skills, two other ADL activities are worthy of mention. Sleep/rest is recognized as an ADL in the OT Practice Framework (AOTA, 2002). Older adolescents sometimes "push the bar" in regard to getting sufficient sleep and rest. Evening work hours, staying up late at night to finish homework or to study for a test, watching television, playing videogames, surfing the Internet, or communicating with friends via the computer are all reasons for late bedtimes. These late bedtimes coupled with having to get up early the next morning to get ready for school can result in less than optimal levels of sleep for many adolescents. Weekend mornings are often the times to make up for sleep time lost during the week, but school performance may be affected by lack of sufficient sleep. Even typically developing adolescents may need to be reminded of the relationship between sufficient levels of sleep and ability to participate fully in waking occupations.

INSTRUMENTAL ACTIVITIES OF DAILY LIVING (IADLs) IN YOUNGER ADOLESCENCE

Most Americans 12 to 15 years of age live in homes with either one or both parents and other members of their family. However, some may live in other social arrangements, such as with grandparents, in foster care, or in an institutional setting, like a group home or a residential school. Regardless of the setting and social environment of their home or living arrangement, most adolescents have responsibility for some *instrumental activities of daily living (IADL)*. Young adolescents may be responsible for keeping their room neat, making their bed, taking out the trash, cutting the grass, setting the table, washing dishes, doing their own laundry, and helping with the housecleaning. They may vacuum or dust furniture or clean the bathroom. Many adolescents learn to prepare simple cold and hot meals using the microwave, stove, and oven. Adolescents whose parents both work and those who have younger siblings

may be responsible for preparing simple dishes, such as hot dogs, pizza, and macaroni and cheese for their siblings. Adolescents enjoy productive tasks like baking brownies, cookies, cakes, and muffins, and some have experience with making pasta dinners.

Other IADL tasks often performed by adolescents include the care of pets and the care of younger siblings. Care of personal and family pets often begins during childhood and continues into adolescence. Feeding, grooming, and exercising pets, and cleaning pet cages, litter boxes, aquariums, and the like, teach young people to provide the required care and nurturing for another living being. Those 12 to 15 years old are often expected by parents to be old enough to supervise and monitor the safety of their younger siblings. When adolescents perform baby-sitting services for other members of the community and receive pay for their time and effort, it may be viewed as a work activity rather than as an IADL, but within the context of their own home and with family members this activity can be classified as an IADL.

If adolescents take medicine routinely, they are increasingly expected to assume greater responsibility for their own medication management. There is a general relinquishing of responsibility on the part of the parent and assumption of responsibility on the part of the adolescent that takes place over time. Shopping is considered an IADL, but for the most part, the type of shopping that is done by adolescents is more correctly categorized as a leisure activity. Adolescent shopping is nonobligatory and engaged in during discretionary time. There may be some adolescents who have the responsibility of doing the grocery or drugstore shopping for their families, but it is not typically the responsibility of adolescents to perform those tasks unless they have assumed more adultlike roles within the family. As adolescents age, they typically become more involved in IADLs.

Increasing responsibility for IADL tasks allows the adolescent to contribute to the family, fosters self-discipline and self-reliance, and helps adolescents gain the essential living skills that they will need one day to live independently from their parents or guardians. Younger adolescents may just be learning these skills, and the quality of their work may vary substantially based upon their exposure to instruction and the degree of adult supervision or direction. What a younger adolescent considers "clean" or "finished" may vary substantially from an adult's perspective, but with guidance, some direct instruction, and specific performance criteria, IADL performance tends to improve with practice and experience.

Instrumental Activities of Daily Living (IADLs) in Older Adolescence

By the age of 16 most adolescents have acquired the necessary skills to participate in basic home management, meal preparation, and child and pet care activities as a result of participating in these tasks within the context of their home on some kind of a regular basis. Although school, work, and social schedules might interfere with routine performance of keeping bedrooms and bathrooms vacuumed, dusted, and cleaned to their parents' standards, older adolescents have the ability to do these chores when they are required to do them. Keeping older adolescents responsible for completing tasks at home can become a challenge for parents, especially when their adolescent children are increasingly motivated to spend less time with the family and to spend more time with peers.

Some older adolescents strongly support the operation of the household with their daily performance of cooking, cleaning, and supervision of younger siblings. Families with a single head of household and families where both parents work are more likely to place greater demands on their adolescent children to assume responsibility in the home than are those families where one parent assumes most of the responsibility for home management and meal preparation. As adolescents approach the age that they begin contemplating moving out of the family home, they may develop a greater interest in performing tasks that they see as developing the skills necessary for living independently. Even if they have not performed clothing-care and meal-preparation tasks earlier in their lives, they may seek out adult assistance for acquiring these skills in the months or year prior to an anticipated move from the family home.

With the opportunity to earn money at a job, older adolescents often need to learn to manage the money they make. Some adolescents of driving age have responsibility to pay for or contribute to their insurance costs and gasoline and routine maintenance costs for the automobile that they drive. Pay from part-time work is often the impetus to open a checking or savings account for the first time. For many adolescents, learning to budget money is linked to saving money for a large purchase, such as for travel, a car, or college expenses. Once an older adolescent begins to work, she is introduced to income tax. Refund opportunities are another excellent motivator to acquire the skills to complete a simple tax return.

The ability to legally drive a car and having access to an automobile, whether that occurs in the form of a shared family vehicle or one that is provided to the adolescent primarily for his use, changes his life significantly. He begins to explore his community more broadly and learns how to drive to all of the places that interest him. Driving allows adolescents to explore their community in relation to the location of malls, movie theaters, bowling alleys, golf courses, restaurants, and other places of interest in addition to learning the driving routes to school; to church, synagogue, or temple; and to community centers and friends' homes. The ex-

perience of driving a car independently expands the world of an adolescent in new ways. She learns about nearby neighborhoods, counties, and towns that border her community, and she often gains access to a broader and more diverse group of people. This expanded view of the world prepares the adolescent for participation in new contexts.

Regular performance of IADLs contributes to an adolescent's *self-definition,* a term introduced earlier in this chapter. She views herself in the role of a contributor to her family or living unit, and she develops skills that become integrated into her view of herself now and in the future. Success in home management, meal preparation, child and pet care, and budgeting builds confidence in her ability to be the autonomous person that she aspires to become.

EDUCATION IN YOUNGER ADOLESCENCE

Education is one of the most important areas of occupation during both periods of adolescence. Formal **educational participation** includes engagement in academics, nonacademics—such as interactions in lunchrooms and school hallways—and extracurricular activities. Participation in education at the middle and high school level is arguably the most influential performance pattern in the life of most adolescents. During the 9–10 months when school is in session, an adolescent's time is organized around school, transportation, extracurricular activities, and homework schedules. School activities are the most significant contributors to achievement in adolescents.

The cultural expectation in the United States and other developed countries is that all adolescents should be enrolled and attending school until they complete their basic 12 years of education. At ages 12 through 15, students are expected to be attending middle school and their first year of high school. During these years students transition from being in a single classroom with one generalist teacher to having multiple teachers who teach courses in specific subject areas. Students are expected to change rooms and teachers in order to benefit from teachers who have advanced training and specialized knowledge.

Dornbusch, Herman, and Morley (1996) identified school as the major socializing institution outside of the family. They also reported, as did Csikszentmihalyi and Larson (1984), that many adolescents focus more on social and extracurricular achievement during the hours that they spend at their school than they do on academic achievement. A traditional hallmark of social development in adolescence is the emergence of the importance of the peer group. Because young adolescents generally spend 7 hours a day at school and additional time participating in after-school activities and riding on buses to and from school, education and activities associated with attending school occupy a substantial portion of their day.

With each subsequent year of schooling, the expectations of students become greater. They are expected to pay attention in class, to take appropriate notes to help them learn the content, to complete all assigned classwork and homework, to study for tests, and to learn the information identified as essential content of the curriculum. These expectations require organizational skills on the part of the individual student. For most young adolescents this involves organizing their use of time, caring for their supplies and materials, and focusing attention on information that their teachers, parents, and other adults tell them is important to know. Study habits, such as having a designated time and place to do homework each night, are often established while the child is in elementary school. If they have not been established, middle school often serves as the catalyst for the establishment of these study habits as homework becomes more difficult and time-consuming. As expectations and demands increase over the course of middle school, adaptive habit patterns become increasingly important.

During adolescence students become increasingly less dependent upon parents or other adults to assist them, and they gain greater responsibility for their own academic success. They may continue to seek out and ask specifically for adult assistance in particular subject areas or with particular assignments, but in general students become increasingly less dependent on parents or other caregivers to motivate them and oversee their performance. Academic success and accomplishments contribute to feelings of productivity, competence, and self-efficacy, whether those achievements occur in the form of a test or project grade, a teacher selecting one's work to be read aloud or posted in the classroom, or a good report card. Academic success plays an important part in the self-definition process. It is often successes in particular classes that begin the process of defining one's strengths and abilities. By the end of middle school young adolescents are beginning to use their academic experiences to "rule in" and "rule out" possible future interests that may lead to further study and eventually to possible career choices.

Education in Older Adolescence

By the time that they are sophomores in high school, adolescents' level of comfort with the expectations of high school has grown substantially. They have a familiarity with a larger building, and they have learned about the increasing academic demands of high school. They know what behaviors are acceptable in the classroom and what behaviors are not. They know the consequences of studying and preparing for class and tests

and those of insufficient preparation. Study habits are generally well established by this time, but these habits may be challenged, or proven ineffective, as courses become more challenging and more demanding. High school students may be able to continue independently in their preparation for tests, but they may discover that for some courses there are distinct advantages to forming alliances with classmates, such as study buddies or study groups. As students grow older they begin making the connection between their coursework and their future as a college student or a worker.

By the time that they are in their last two years of high school, older adolescents choose the electives that match their interests, skills, and abilities. Teachers can play a significant role in the ruling-in and ruling-out process. Motivated, enthusiastic teachers can spark an interest in a young person through their teaching and nurture that interest with their support and encouragement. Likewise, teachers who lack enthusiasm for their job or the content that they teach can squelch a student's budding interest in an area unless that interest is nurtured outside the classroom.

Learning to Drive

One elective course that is extremely important to most high school students is the course on driver's education. The specific age to obtain a learner's permit varies by state, but it is generally around age 15 to 15½ years. To obtain a driver's license in most states, students must pass a driver's education course approved by the Department of Motor Vehicles. Most high school students take driver's education as a semester-long high school course. Obtaining a driver's license is a major milestone in the life of a teenager. It is also an important milestone in terms of gaining autonomy from parents and other adults who are responsible for transporting younger adolescents to places that they want to go. This independence is a social marker of the transition from young adolescent to older adolescent.

The extracurricular activities sponsored by high schools are generally far more extensive than what is typically offered at the middle-school level. Students can choose to be involved in a variety of clubs, organizations, or groups. Some of these organizations allow the students to enhance the academic experience in an area of study that interests them, like foreign language, performing arts, science, technology, debate, and forensics clubs. Other clubs, like Distributed Education Clubs of America (DECA), Future Business Leaders of America (FBLA), Future Educators of America (FEA), Family Career and Community Leaders (FCCLA), Health Occupations Students of America (HOSA), and Future Farmers of America (FFA), foster involvement in activities related to students' career interests. These activities, which contribute to **career literacy** (discussed further later on), could be considered as extensions of their education. Involvement in other clubs and organizations sponsored by high schools include clubs that are oriented toward community service, such as Key Club, Interact Club, Students Against Drunk Driving (SADD), Students Against Violence Everywhere (SAVE), and Student Organization for Developing Attitudes (SODA).

A large portion of the life of a high school student revolves around his life at school. Satisfaction in this very important area of occupation colors his perception of himself and the world. Typically developing older adolescents recognize the value and the importance of their education to the course, direction, and future of their lives. Although not all students arrive at age 18 or 19 knowing exactly what they want to do in regard to a career choice, their educational process during these 3–4 years of older adolescence plays an important role in helping them formulate an identity that includes further education, work, and career plans.

PLAY AND LEISURE

Play is often associated with children and leisure with adults. It seems logical, then, that adolescents who are in the process of transitioning from children into adults might very well experience both, and they do. **Leisure** is defined as "a nonobligatory activity that is intrinsically motivated and engaged in during discretionary time, that is, time not committed to obligatory occupations such as work, self-care, or sleep" (p. 250). Whether their appeal is more strongly related to their productive, pleasurable, or restorative aspects (Pierce, 2001), play and leisure activities provide adolescents with many opportunities to develop their minds, bodies, and spirits. Throughout adolescence, participation in leisure occupations is a major component of most young people's lives. It is also a major contributor to their identity. Adolescents who participate in high levels of structured extracurricular activities report higher school satisfaction (Gilman, 2001). Passmore (2003), an Australian occupational therapist, found that achievement and social leisure activities positively influenced mental health in adolescents by enhancing competency, global self-worth, and self-efficacy.

Middle school is often a student's first exposure to extracurricular activities sponsored by the school. Academic organizations are a component of many middle-school extracurricular offerings. Clubs like the science or ecology club or foreign language clubs promote learning beyond the classroom and help students further define academic areas of interest. Middle schools offer a number of athletic and other organizational activities. High school generally provides a wider

range of choices of extracurricular activities than middle school, and interests may become more defined as an adolescent matures, but in general there is a fair amount of stability in leisure pursuits during adolescence and into young adulthood (Raymore, Barber, Eccles, & Godbey, 1999). Extracurricular activities, including team sports as illustrated in Figure 12–4, support the development of special interests.

ADOLESCENTS AND SPORTS

During adolescence, individuals tend to diverge in their interests, with some becoming increasingly focused on sedentary activities while others become known as athletes. One particular reason for this change is suggested by Hartner's model of *perceived competence*, which states that individuals who engage in successful sports endeavors are motivated to continue participation. It has been suggested that there is a developmental shift in what children perceive as "success," with the young child gauging success by the game outcome or parental feedback, whereas older children tend to rely on peer comparisons (Payne & Isaacs, 2002). It appears that children participate in sports primarily to have fun, and failure to achieve that goal is a major reason for children and adolescents to discontinue participation in the sport (Payne & Isaacs, 2002). Team sports like basketball, soccer, football, wrestling, baseball, and softball are popular pastimes with adolescents at the middle-school level. These sports become even more challenging and competitive at the high school level.

Athletic achievement is the most publicly recognized and heralded of the domains of achievement (Dornbusch, Herman, & Morley, 1996). Information about athletic accomplishments is spread throughout the school and community. Athletes, especially those

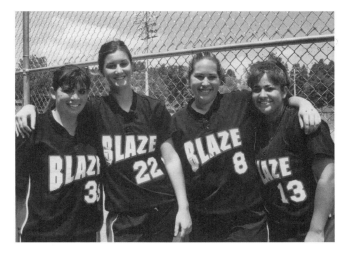

FIGURE 12–4 Team sports allow many adolescents to develop physical abilities and to make close friends.

who excel, become a focus of attention due to their special sport team jackets or dress on game days, having attention focused upon them at pep rallies, on the public address system, and in school and community newspapers. Although research on sports and school in the United Kingdom and the United States (Whitehead, Evans, & Lee, 1997) has shown that adolescents view success in academics as more important than success in athletics, especially as they age, athletics remain a valued leisure pursuit for many adolescents.

There are some common injuries experienced by young athletes. These include physeal or growth-plate injuries, overuse injuries, stress fractures, shoulder impingement syndrome, atraumatic osteolysis of the distal clavicle, Little League elbow, patellofemoral syndrome, Osgood-Schlatter disease, osteochondritis dissecans, and Sever's disease (Patel & Nelson, 2000). One area of major concern for injuries is the increasingly common participation by children and adolescents in weight training. Payne and Isaacs (2002) differentiate between weight training, weight lifting, and power lifting. **Weight training** has been shown to be effective when done in the short term and when supervised by knowledgeable adults. Weight training is a planned regimen of exercise using resistance, typically involving free weights. Weight lifting and power lifting are considered sports that are designed to demonstrate maximum performance. Generally, maximal lifts, full squats, and power lifts are to be avoided in the prepubescent athlete (American Academy of Pediatrics, 1990).

EXPANDED CONTEXTS FOR LEISURE

Leisure activities are influenced by context and access to the necessary space and equipment. For example, access to a golf course and a set of clubs permits adolescents to develop an interest in playing golf. Adolescents who have access to oceans, bays, rivers, lakes, and other bodies of water have another group of leisure activities made available to them. They enjoy boating, canoeing, fishing, and a variety of water sports like water skiing, jet skiing, and duck hunting. Likewise, if they have access to countryside and forests they often grow up enjoying hunting for birds, deer, and other game. Access to hiking and biking trails allows an interest in backpacking, camping, and mountain biking to develop. Young people who live in the country or who have access to rural settings often enjoy spending their leisure time caring for, and showing, cattle or other livestock or riding horses. Leisure activities are also influenced to a great extent by social context. Younger adolescents are especially dependent on parents and other caregivers to transport them to the locations where they can pursue their interests.

Although adolescents are able to make choices for the ways that they want to spend their own leisure, they may have been introduced to particular leisure interests by parents or caregivers who support their participation in that leisure activity. Parents who participated in a particular sport or activity when they were adolescents may coach them. As adolescents age they may to choose to continue participation in these interests, to refine their interest in a particular way, or to spend their time in other ways. Second-generation artists, musicians, and dancers may continue involvement in these arts but choose another medium or genre than the one that they participated in when they were younger children and guided more directly by their parents.

Many adolescents value organized preplanned leisure activities, but a large amount of young people's leisure time is not planned in advance. This use of time usually involves informal play activities that are engaged in spontaneously for the experience of the moment. These include activities like listening to music, hanging out with friends, picking up a book or magazine to read for pleasure or a musical instrument for the sheer enjoyment of playing, watching television, shopping, dining out with friends, going to movies, watching movies on videotape or DVD, playing videogames or computer games, communicating with friends via the Internet, talking on the telephone, riding a bike, taking a walk, or playing spontaneous "pickup" games of basketball, tennis, Frisbee, street hockey, or catch. Most of these activities involve little or no advanced planning and just happen in the moment.

VOCATIONAL AND CAREER DEVELOPMENT

Although we often use the terms *work*, *career*, and *vocation* interchangeably, they represent different aspects of human occupational performance. **Work**, in our context, refers to a trade or other means of livelihood. Work may be a job to earn money while you are in college that has no long-term bearing on your vocational or career goals. A **career** is an organized path pursued by an individual for an extended period. Current researchers have expanded the conceptualization of career to include a variety of work in people's lives including occupational, family, and leisure roles (Richardson, 1993; Merrick, 1995). "Personal competence" and "feelings of mastery" have been identified as important to an adolescent's selection of and commitment to a particular career.

Basic knowledge in this area would include an understanding of the importance of *career literacy* (mentioned earlier in this chapter) at this life stage. Adolescents become career-literate through observation of significant others, media portrayal of careers, and part-time employment or volunteer experience in the community. The

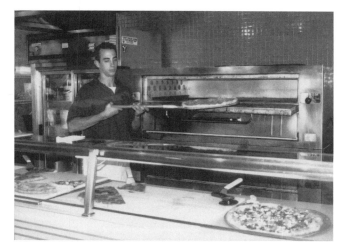

FIGURE 12–5   Many adolescents over 16 work part-time in service related jobs.

term *vocation,* or **vocational development,** refers to the affective aspect, or "calling," associated with finding one's life's work. Participation in part-time employment contributes to development of work attitudes and habits and provides young people with the opportunity to learn about the relationship that exists between the work, remuneration, and work satisfaction (Wagner, 1996). Figure 12–5 shows an adolescent at work. Development of vocational interests starts early in adolescence and continues throughout the whole developmental period.

PAID WORK BY YOUNGER ADOLESCENTS

Generally, young adolescents, 12 and 13 years of age, are considered too young to work. The Fair Labor Standards Act (FLSA) sets 14 years of age as the minimum age for employment and limits the number of hours worked by minors under the age of 16. These minimum-age requirements do not apply to minors who are employed by their parents or guardians, except in very specific areas (e.g., mining, manufacturing). Adolescents who are 14 and 15 years old cannot work more than 3 hours on a school day or 18 hours in a school week. They can, however, work up to 8 hours on a non-school day or 40 hours in a non-school week, which permits them to hold jobs during school vacations and breaks. They are also limited in regard to the times when they are allowed to work (7 A.M. to 7 P.M.), except during the summer months from June 1 through Labor Day, when evening hours are extended to 9 P.M. (U.S. Department of Labor).

The ability to enter the workforce without these kinds of restrictions is one of the markers of the transition from younger adolescence to older adolescence. Every state has its own laws regulating employment of

minors. If the state law and the FLSA overlap, the law, which is more protective of the minor, takes precedence. Some states require employment certificates; other states do not. Some states require certificates for youth under age 18; others require them for employees under age 14 or 16. In some states employment certificates are issued through the schools and in others they are issued through the Labor Department.

Some young adolescents take on responsibilities for which they are paid, such as baby-sitting for young children, doing yard work for neighbors, pet-sitting, delivering newsletters, being paid by community organizations for refereeing athletic activities, or staffing a concession stand. These tend to be occasional jobs rather than regularly scheduled work opportunities. These short-term work opportunities allow young people to make some of their own spending money to purchase things that they want, like compact discs and clothes, or to spend on entertainment. In general, however, younger adolescents in America often do not hold regular jobs, even on a part-time basis.

PAID WORK BY OLDER ADOLESCENTS

The ability to work without limitations, coupled with the societal expectation that older adolescents should begin taking on the responsibility of working at least on a part-time basis during their summer breaks from school, is a key marker of the transition from younger adolescence to older adolescence. The ability to work and the license to drive a car independently at age 16 or 16½ are frequently related. Older adolescents often work to pay for their weekly use of gasoline, automobile maintenance costs, insurance fees, and other expenses related to the automobile that they drive.

For adolescents aged 16 and above, the maximum work hours are generally the same as for adults. There is still a requirement that students cannot work more than 4 hours on a school day unless she is enrolled in the Work Experience Education program at her high school. Those 16 to 18 years old are allowed to work between the hours of 5:00 A.M. and 10:00 P.M. on days preceding a school day and from 5:00 A.M. to 12:30 A.M. on days preceding a non-school day. Students who are involved in Work Experience Education are allowed to work up to 23 hours per week, any portion of which may be during school hours (U.S. Department of Labor). Increased maturity and the flexibility of scheduling make older adolescents more desirable employees than younger adolescents. Some companies make it a policy not to hire young people under age 16. Although the data may be somewhat dated now, Csikszentmihalyi and Larson (1984) found that high school students worked an average of 7.4 hours per week.

Older adolescents may limit their work schedules to weekends during the school year or work only during their summer breaks when school is not in session, but some adolescents balance working regularly in a part-time job with their school schedule. Some adolescents are fortunate enough to find employment in areas in which they have a possible future career interest. They may find work assisting in an engineering office, an accounting firm, a beauty salon, a doctor's or dentist's office, an architectural firm, a service station, or a well-respected restaurant. Work opportunities like these give young people the opportunity to receive mentoring from an engineer, accountant, cosmetologist, manicurist, doctor, nurse, dentist, dental hygienist, architect, interior designer, master mechanic, or chef. These kinds of experiences can have a significant impact on an adolescent's occupational-choice process. The process of considering various work and career paths is one of the most important developmental challenges of this age. Real-world opportunities help young people rule in and rule out possibilities.

VOLUNTEER WORK

Many young people get involved in community service through school- or church-sponsored volunteer activities. They volunteer for jobs such as working in soup kitchens, cleaning up parks and roadways, visiting or making favors for people who are hospitalized, collecting canned goods, staffing collection and distribution sites for families in need, or providing free child-care for parents who are enrolled in English-as-a-second-language classes or who are participating in welfare-to-work programs. Young people donate their time and energies to improve conditions in their local communities, and some young people even travel to impoverished areas of the country or to other countries to do mission work in these areas of need. Schondel and Boehm (2000) identified three motivational factors among adolescent volunteers: *socialization*, the desire to help others and to experience personal growth; *self-actualization*, the need to achieve and to receive affirmation through recognition, admiration, respect, and social approval; and *relatedness*, the need for social contact and desire to engage in prosocial behavior.

SOCIAL PARTICIPATION BY YOUNGER ADOLESCENTS

Social participation is an area of occupation of particular importance to younger adolescents. The importance of peer relationships is a hallmark of adolescence. As mentioned previously, school often serves as the setting where many of these influential relationships are formed and sustained. As children grow into adolescents, their circle of friends increases in size. They make choices of their own friends and are somewhat less restricted by geographic distance as they venture farther into the community on foot, by bicycle, by bus, or by arranging for parents to transport them. Often several neighborhood elementary schools will feed into larger middle schools or junior highs, exposing adolescents to a broader and often more diverse group of students. The structure of a middle-school day, with the changing of classes, the use of lockers, and participation in elective courses, exposes younger adolescents to more people of their age than their single-classroom elementary school structure allowed them previously.

Younger adolescents form close relationships with same-sex peers. They are often quite aware of peers of the opposite sex, and certainly friendships between boys and girls of 13–15 years of age do happen, but closer, more intense, trusting female-female and male-male relationships tend to grow out of the same-sex chums characteristic of school-age children. Overnight "sleepovers" at each other's houses with these close friends are frequent occurrences for boys and girls during middle school. They enjoy just spending time with their friends regardless of what they may do to fill the hours. They may pass the time shooting baskets; looking at photographs, yearbooks, or magazines; listening to music; playing videogames; shooting pool; playing Ping Pong; skateboarding; watching television, videos, or DVDs; or talking and eating, but the time is really time spent developing relationships.

Although some younger adolescents "go out," this usually does not involve dating in the traditional sense. Groups of younger adolescents may arrange to meet at the movies, or a boy and girl may talk on the telephone or hang around together at school. They may even attend a special event together such as a school-sponsored dance, but relationships rarely last more than a few weeks to a few months. Figure 12–6 shows the physical closeness common to adolescent friends.

The majority of the social participation that takes place during younger adolescence occurs in conjunction with other areas of occupation, particularly as a part of nonacademic and extracurricular education and in conjunction with play or leisure activities. Lunchtime in the cafeteria of most middle schools is a major social event. Although the task from the school's perspective is for the students to eat, the task from the students' collective perspective is relax and have fun talking to their friends.

Some younger adolescents view after-school programs as activities that provide structure and supervision of younger children and are too juvenile for them once they have become middle-school students. Some after-school programs recognize this phenomenon and offer "drop-in" programs for middle-school students that promote opportunities for activities that appeal to adolescents to dispel the association with day care. Successful

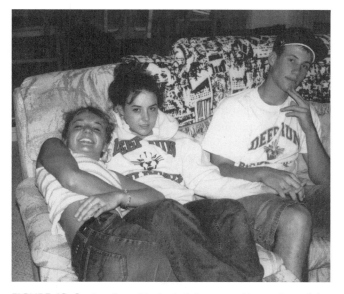

FIGURE 12–6   Comfort with physical closeness with members of the same sex precedes comfort with physical contact with the opposite sex.

after-school programs for younger adolescents offer more opportunity for positive social interaction than children have when returning to homes without adult supervision. Research has demonstrated that after-school programs are successful in reducing the incidence of smoking, drug use, and unsafe sexual practices by providing young people with a safe, structured environment, with caring adults, high expectations for academic attainment and behavior, help with problems, and opportunities to gain the abilities and knowledge they will need as they mature (Kahne & Bailey, 1999; McLaughlin, Irby, & Langman, 1994). Research by Kahne, Nagaoka, Brown, O'Brien, Quinn, & Thiede (2001) indicated that after-school programs provide more attractive affective contexts than students experience during the school day and as such are an important non-school context for adolescent development.

As students become increasingly responsible for their own schoolwork, and as they become more closely connected socially to their peers, they begin looking to their peers for homework assistance rather than asking for help from their parents as they did when they were younger. In recent years, among those young people who have access to technology, new means of communication through electronic mail, instant messaging, chat groups, and cellular telephones have further contributed to enhanced social participation by adolescents after school hours. These technologies allow peer groups of friends to maintain communication even when they are separated from one another physically. Younger adolescents learn quickly from their peer network about how to get connected. Instant messaging is a fascinating new form of communication. It is not unusual for an adolescent to be involved in as many as 10 or more online communications simultaneously.

Communication is usually informal, and short. They often use a shorthand language, such as *brb* for "be right back" or *g2g* for "got to go." Messages are generally devoid of capitalization or punctuation, and accurate spelling is irrelevant. When I responded briefly with a "Hi, Mer" to an instant message that popped on to my screen as I worked at home on my computer one evening, before I even typed the explanation that it was me and not my daughter working at the computer, the reply immediately came back: "this is sooo dr simons!" My capitalization and punctuation gave me away instantly!

FAMILY PARTICIPATION

As the younger adolescent's peer group develops and strengthens, he relies less on the family, but the family still remains an important influence in the lives of younger adolescents. Most adolescents continue to maintain close, warm, accepting relationships with their parents (Grotevant, 1998). Galambos and Ehrenberg (1997) report that optimal adjustment occurs among adolescents whose parents encourage age-appropriate autonomy and maintenance of close ties to the family. Families present a lot of opportunities for social interaction. A variety of dyads, triads, and group interactions occur regularly between parents and their adolescent children, between siblings, and between extended family members and adolescents. All of these interactions provide the younger adolescent with opportunities to develop the skills to get along with other people. Mealtimes, transportation and travel times, visits, vacations, and weekends or weekday evenings at home are typical times for social participation within the family. Many adolescents continue to enjoy going out to eat, going to the movies, or watching television together with their families.

Research on resiliency has shown that the presence of a caring adult is an extremely important asset in the life of a young person. Caring, supportive relationships have been shown to be a protective factor for positive youth development (Tierney & Grossman, 1995; Werner, 1987; Werner & Smith, 1982). As younger adolescents begin to push for greater independence, parents have the challenge of allowing them to experience greater autonomy, but within limits. These boundaries are frequently the source of friction between parents and their adolescent children as the determination of what is considered reasonable and safe is often quite different when viewed from the perspective of an adult than it is from the perspective of a 12–15-year-old adolescent.

COMMUNITY PARTICIPATION

Other opportunities for social participation occur through involvement in activities in the community. Younger adolescents may swim or play football, baseball, soccer, or softball for a community league or competitive travel team in addition to their participation in a school team. They may be active in faith-based youth groups or choirs or groups at the Boys or Girls Club or the YMCA or YWCA. They may be active members of Boy Scout or Girl Scout programs. All of these kinds of activities provide opportunities for social interaction as well as participation in leisure activities. As adolescents become increasingly involved in activities at school and in the community, parents have new opportunities for involvement in activities that support their child's participation.

Parent-child discussions following an adolescent's involvement in an athletic or arts event, and informal conversations that take place while transporting children to rehearsals and practices, are often social interaction times between parents and their adolescent children. Social interactions with peers and with parents and other caring adults provide multiple opportunities for younger adolescents to develop a variety of communication and interaction skills, which in turn contribute to formation of identity. Young people define themselves by the company that they keep. Participation in the social groups that are a part of their lives contributes extensively to their self-definition. They see themselves, and other adolescents see them, as belonging to particular social groups. Discovering appropriate societal roles that are well suited to them physically and psychologically occurs in part because of the social experiences that they have throughout adolescence.

COMMUNICATION AND INTERACTION SKILLS

Adolescents who are developing typically engage in social interaction experiences throughout their days at school, at home, and in the community. Interactions with peers in the hallways of school, on the sidelines of a practice field, or at a party require appropriate physicality. Teens make physical contact when shaking hands or hugging each other upon seeing each other after a time apart. They know when touching is appropriate and when it is not. They use eye gazes to communicate and interact with others. Eye contact communicates interest in the person and the discussion and contributes to sustaining an interaction.

They also learn to use effective gestures to indicate, demonstrate, or add emphasis to their discussion and to coordinate the movement of their body in relation to others. These coordinated physical maneuvers include adjusting the space between themselves and others to demonstrate respect for other people's comfort zones. Adolescents communicate a great deal through body-language postures. Leaning forward and sitting back with crossed arms and legs convey messages of acceptance and interest in the first case and rejection and disinterest in the second. Adolescents generally practice appropriate

physicality first with peers of the same sex and adults like their parents, teachers, and their friends' parents. Gradually they gain confidence in the physical aspects of their communication and interaction and develop a level of comfort interacting with peers of the opposite sex. Pinning a boutonnière on a lapel or a corsage on a date's dress for the first time, as in Figure 12–7, illustrates the challenge of becoming comfortable with the physicality aspects of touch and proximity that occur on a first date.

Healthy communication and relations require that an adolescent focus her speech and behavior on the ongoing social action and contribute to the social process. Adolescents engage in a series of interactions as they walk the halls between classes. They have the ability to change focus to the ongoing social action multiple times as they pass or pause to speak briefly with different friends or groups. An adolescent relates by acknowledging receipt of social messages; giving indications of interest; offering assistance, encouragement, and compliments; displaying concern about other people's feelings; using appropriate humor; and offering ideas, opinions, and suggestions. These actions result in the establishment and maintenance of rapport. The close friendships and dating relationships associated with adolescence provide the perfect opportunity for young people to build and practice these relationship-building and relationship-maintaining skills. Friends help their peers through successes and disappointments, celebrations, and heartbreaks. Table 12–3 presents the adolescent abilities.

As adolescents grow older, dating becomes more common and more frequent. Identification with the role of someone's boyfriend or girlfriend often contributes

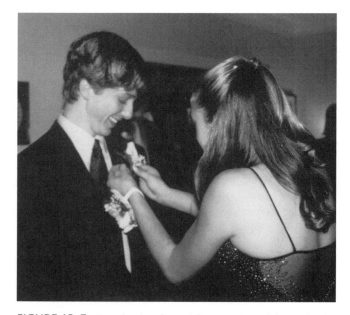

FIGURE 12–7 Experiencing the social conventions of dating for the first time can be awkward initially, until physical contact with the opposite sex becomes more familiar and comfortable.

TABLE 12–3	Adolescent Communication and Interaction Skills			

Examples of Activities Engaged in by Typically Developing Adolescents During Which Performance Skills Are Observable

Communication/ Interaction Skills	School	Home	Work in Community	Play/Leisure and Social Settings in the Community
Physicality—Refers to using the physical body when communicating within an occupation.				
• Contacts	Shaking hands with a buddy in the hall.	Hugging a sibling or parent.	Shaking hands with the employer at a job interview.	Patting a teammate on the shoulder or back after a good play.
• Gazes	Looking at the teacher when asking a question.	Making eye contact with a parent when asking permission to go somewhere or to do something.	Making eye contact with customers when taking orders.	Looking coach or advisor in the eye when being advised, corrected, or reprimanded.
• Gestures	Waving to a friend during a change of classes.	Using a hand motion while talking on the telephone to signal to mother to come closer.	Waving people to keep them moving toward the exit when ushering for a concert.	Using hand and arm motions to show enthusiasm.
• Maneuvers	Moving through the crowded cafeteria to sit next to someone at the lunch table.	Approaching parent to ask about being taken to the mall or to the movies.	Approaching a table to take an order.	Sitting down on the bench next to a teammate to give her words of encouragement.
• Orients	Looking up from work to see someone who called out one's name.	Turning away from the TV and looking at mother when summoned.	Looking up and approaching the counter when a customer steps up to the hotel desk.	Looking at a teammate who indicates that she is passing the ball.
• Postures	Demonstrating open, welcoming body language with peers.	Demonstrating open, receptive body language with parents.	Demonstrating open body language when helping someone locate items in the store.	Demonstrating open, warm, receptive body language with teammates.
Information Exchange—Refers to giving and receiving information within an occupation.				
• Articulates	Speaking clearly enough to be understood by teacher when responding to a question.	Enunciating words to communicate activity choices to parent.	Speaking clearly to ask residents and guests to follow the pool rules.	Speaking clearly to convey ideas about potential club projects.
• Asserts	Asserting refusal to ride in a car with someone who has been drinking.	Asserting an interest in attending a concert or party to parents.	Asserting a desire for a raise to an employer.	Asserting interest in playing a different position with a coach.
• Asks	Asking classmates for clarification on requirements for a homework assignment.	Asking siblings for information on their scheduled activities for the coming week.	Asking supervisor to explain some work procedure, such as how to give credits and refunds or process layaway purchases.	Asking club members to share their past experience in providing community service.

Continues

TABLE 12–3	Adolescent Communication and Interaction Skills *Continued*			
Communication/ Interaction Skills	School	Home	Work in Community	Play/Leisure and Social Settings in the Community
Information Exchange—Refers to giving and receiving information within an occupation.				
• Engages	Starting a conversation with the student sharing the lab bench.	Starting a discussion with a parent about college expenses and financial support.	Starting a discussion about the football game that just concluded while working as a hostess.	Starting a discussion with a new player who was brought up to the varsity level from junior varsity.
• Expresses	Sharing excitement or enthusiasm about a common project.	Expressing love and affection to one's family for their support.	Expressing frustration or anger appropriately to coworker who did not fulfill his responsibilities.	Expressing jubilation or sadness upon winning or losing a championship game.
• Modulates	Lowering voice in the library.	Raising voice to call sibling to the telephone.	Raising voice volume to be heard over the ambient noise of the restaurant.	Talking to friends over the music from the band and the announcer on the PA system.
• Shares	Sharing information about oneself with a classmate.	Sharing information about the day with the family at dinner.	Sharing previous experience and successes on a prior job with one's employer.	Sharing plans for a community service project with a club member who was unable to attend the meeting due to a scheduling conflict.
• Speaks	Answering the teacher's guided discussion questions.	Talking to extended family members by telephone about current involvement in activities.	Talking to people as they enter the pool and sign in, show their membership cards, or pay.	Talking to friends about plans for the weekend to go to the movies and to go to a nearby restaurant for dessert after the show.
• Sustains	Carrying on a conversation with friends at the lunch table.	Taking part in a family discussion about summer vacation possibilities and plans.	Talking with coworkers in the break room about their work experiences.	Reviewing the best parts of the team tournament experience with teammates.
Relations—Refers to maintaining appropriate relationships within an occupation.				
• Collaborates	Working with a classmate on a science or social studies project.	Working together with family members to clean the house or work in the yard.	Working with a partner to restock shelves.	Working as one of an elected group of officers to make plans for club programs and activities.
• Conforms	Showing behavior expected of students when in class.	Adhering to family rules about curfew and using the car.	Meeting the employer's expectations about arriving on time for work in a clean and neat uniform.	Attending all scheduled practices unless excused by the coach.

Continues

TABLE 12–3	Adolescent Communication and Interaction Skills *Continued*			
Communication/ Interaction Skills	School	Home	Work in Community	Play/Leisure and Social Settings in the Community
Relations—Refers to maintaining appropriate relationships within an occupation.				
• Focuses	Following along in the book or on the computer with the lesson of the day.	Actively listening to family members describe the events of their day.	Listening to one's supervisor when instructions are being given.	Listening to coach's instructions to modify a play.
• Relates	Creating rapport with teachers and peers.	Maintaining rapport with family members.	Establishing rapport with coworkers and boss.	Creating rapport with teammates, club members, and friends.
• Respects	Altering behavior or language to show respect for adults and friends.	Adjusting behavior to show respect for parents.	Saying "Please" and "Thank you," "yes, Ma'am," and "No, sir," to convey respect to supervisor, employer, and customers.	Refraining from interrupting while coach is giving a motivational speech to the team.

to a teenager's identity. Teens who have healthy self-esteem and who have accumulated experiences that have built confidence in their own skills and abilities can date a variety of people and not rely on a relationship for a sense of self-worth. Every relationship brings out different aspects of one's personality and interests. Dating a number of different people provides adolescents with opportunities to learn more about themselves and to learn about similarities and differences between themselves and other people. They also learn more about the similarities and differences between families and cultures. Some older adolescents become

involved in more committed relationships. These longer-term dating relationships may mature into committed adult relationships, or the individuals may move on to other relationships. Intimate and sexual behavior is often a part of these dating relationships.

Adolescents who are attracted to other members of the same sex may gain greater acceptance of their sexual orientation as they age and mature. It can be argued that homosexual adolescents live in a culture that is less judgmental than previous eras, but acceptance of homosexuality varies greatly in different areas of the country and the world.

SUMMARY

Adolescence is a time of tremendous growth and change in the life of an individual. With childhood behind them and adulthood in front of them, adolescents have a period of 6–7 years to mature physically, but more importantly to develop psychosocially. The developmental challenges of adolescence are to discover oneself and one's abilities; to arrive at a self-definition, or identity, that incorporates these assets; and to determine the societal roles that are suited to who one is physically and psychologically. The means for accomplishing these developmental challenges is engagement in occupation in context. Adolescents who are developing typically use this period of their lives to participate in a variety of self-defining activities on a daily or routine basis. They participate in a wide range of educational, social, work,

IADL, ADL, play, and leisure experiences that develop their bodies, minds, and spirits. The composite result of these many and varied occupational experiences is personal development. These activities develop adolescents' mental, sensory, and neuromusculoskeletal functions and underlying other physiologic functions. An adolescent's continuously improving occupational performance is evident in the observable motor, process and communication, and interaction performance skills that emerge when she engages in her occupation of choice. Adolescents who are provided with the opportunities to choose and experience a wide array of occupations set in a wide range of naturally occurring contexts will be provided with the conditions to promote optimal development.

Mark

Mark was 15 years and 8 months old when I met him. He was in the first semester of his sophomore year in high school. His parents brought him to the outpatient adolescent substance-abuse treatment program where I worked after he was suspended from school for having marijuana on school grounds. He was an attractive, thin young man who looked somewhat vacant and sad when I introduced myself to him in the lounge. Although he was initially hesitant to talk to me, he relaxed when I suggested that we could take a walk and sit outside while we talked.

During our interview Mark shared with me that his parents were both professional people with very busy work schedules. He also said that he had a sister who was away at an elite state university, majoring in premed. Unlike his "perfect" sister, he had struggled with school for as long as he could remember. He confirmed the report in his chart that he had started drinking beer during the end of seventh grade and that he had been using marijuana on a daily basis for about a year. He told me that he had taken "speed" on two occasions, but that he didn't like the way it made him feel.

Mark told me that he had been shy in elementary and middle school and he had trouble fitting in when he started high school last year. He "wasn't one of the smart kids, or preppie kids, or jocks." He had been asked by some "skaters" to join them after school. He tried to get the hang of skateboarding but "was terrible at it." He said that he had never been very coordinated. His dad tried to get him interested in playing football and baseball when he was younger, but even though he played several years of Little League ball, he was "always the worst player on the team" and finally had chosen to quit.

When things didn't work out for him with the skater crowd, Mark started hanging out with two students who were the ones who introduced him to "smoking weed." Getting high relaxed him and made him feel better about life. He admitted that his schoolwork wasn't good, because in his opinion "it was completely boring." He hated school because every subject that he took required reading. His parents had come to expect poor report cards from him, and their comment was always the same, that they "didn't expect As and Bs. They just didn't want to see Ds and Fs. He should just keep trying to do his best and they would be satisfied."

He told me that when he was younger he used to enjoy collecting and organizing baseball cards and playing videogames, but now he spent most of his free time hanging out with his friends or in his room listening to music and watching TV or DVDs. At home he would frequently fix his own TV dinner in the microwave because he generally got hungry before his parents got home.

His parents gave him an allowance of $25 a week, but his allowance was not tied to any responsibilities around the house. They had never forced him to do chores because they had a cleaning service that came in weekly, and his mom had always done the family's laundry. He had no goals except to get his driver's license in 7 months. He had no idea of what kind of work he might want to do someday, and he had never tried to get involved in any extracurricular activities at the school.

I was concerned about Mark from a developmental standpoint. His cannabis addiction had derailed his development. He was living every day in the present and had no vision of his future. Although he was from a quite affluent family, he tended to see his family as more of a stressor than a resource. He had not had many opportunities to experience success academically, athletically, or socially. His self-definition was very limited and negative. Both of his parents had been involved in their respective careers, leaving him essentially to raise himself. He had not been given responsibility for any IADLs except for preparing his own TV dinners. In school nothing interested him. I questioned whether his problems with reading were a result of a learning disability and whether he had ever been tested. His social life was limited to two friends, and they were a negative influence. He had no defined leisure interests that contributed to his feeling productive or accomplished, or about which he expressed feelings of pleasure or enjoyment.

Continues

Case 1 Continued

Treatment at the outpatient program included individual and group therapy with the substance-abuse counselors and weekly individual and multifamily group counseling with the family therapist. As the OT on the program team, I focus on helping clients explore new interests and restore prior interests, develop the self-confidence to cope with challenges in their lives, and experience success in occupational challenges like preparing a meal or writing a song. In Mark's case, as with other adolescent clients like him, my emphasis was on having him begin the process of redefining himself and thinking about his future.

I helped Mark look at the way that he had been spending his time, to consider whether the activities that he had done regularly contributed to feelings of productivity, pleasure, and restoration, and if not, what replacement activities appealed to him. Organizing a weekly schedule helped him consider how to develop healthy habits that would sustain a life in recovery. Mark particularly enjoyed the outdoor groups that I co-led with one of the support staff on the program's Ropes and Initiatives course. He used his last experience, being belayed on one of the high initiatives, a 30-foot wire suspended 35 feet in the air between two trees, as a metaphor for the challenge of his recovery. I worked with Mark to explore leisure opportunities in the community, and before the 4-week outpatient program was over Mark had signed up for a weekend hiking trip sponsored by the local YMCA.

A significant decision for Mark, and one with which he struggled at length, was the choice about whether to maintain his relationships with his two substance-using "friends" or to break off his relationships with them and work at developing new relationships with people who were supportive of his recovery. Despite testimony from other clients in aftercare telling him about the danger of maintaining relationships with people who continue to use drugs, he felt that he could remain friends without being tempted to use when he was around them.

Through the process of OT and family therapy, and despite Mark's initial resistance, he and his parents were helped to recognize the benefit of being given reasonable responsibilities at home, like doing his own laundry, taking out the trash, and keeping his room and bathroom clean. Mark successfully completed the program and was able to level with his parents about his feelings of inadequacy growing up in a home where the expectations were so high for academic and athletic success. When Mark left the program he stated emphatically that he wanted to stay away from drugs, but he had a hard time accepting that he could never drink alcohol even when he was old enough to do it legally. After attempting to make it on his own without attending aftercare and relapsing on two occasions, Mark admitted that support was essential to his recovery.

I happened to run into Mark at the mall food park about a year after he left the program. The general rule in therapy, to avoid risking a breach of confidentiality, is not to speak to former clients when you happen to cross paths in the community, but in this case Mark approached me. Although still a little shy, he told me that he still had problems with school, but that he was getting help from a tutor and that his grades were getting better. He had gotten his driver's license during the summer, taken a part-time job at a store that sold backpacking and hiking gear to help pay for the cost of his insurance, and had taken several good hiking trips. He smiled sheepishly as he bragged that he had also "gotten pretty good at ironing" his own shirts and pants. Before we said good-bye, he said, "When I was in treatment you made me start thinking about my life. I wasn't really ready to hear everything that you had to say at the time, but now a lot of the things that you talked about keep coming back to me! Thanks!" As therapists, we don't often have the privilege of seeing the long-term effects of our treatment on our client's lives, and not every client benefits from our services. However, when you are fortunate enough to hear a comment like Mark made, it keeps you motivated for a long, long time!

CASE
2

Jeremy

SCOTT DAVIS, PT, MS, OCS
ORTHOPEDIC PHYSICAL THERAPIST

Jeremy was a 13-year-old eighth-grader who was very active in school and community sports. He began playing organized sports at the age of 5 in a community T-ball league and has played baseball ever since. When Jeremy got to middle school he started playing football. The coaches quickly identified him as being a talented athlete. In the fall of his eighth-grade year, the basketball coach asked Jeremy if he was interested in trying out for the basketball team. Despite never having played organized basketball, Jeremy earned a spot on the team and excelled due to his athleticism and quickness. During the last two weeks of the basketball season, Jeremy began complaining of bilateral knee pain. He was no stranger to minor aches and pains from playing sports over the years. Jeremy was a very competitive athlete and did not want to lose playing time, and he certainly did not want the other boys to think that he could not handle the rigors of basketball practice, so he did not initially tell his coach or his parents about the pain. When the pain became persistent and hurting even when he was at rest, he decided to tell his parents.

When Jeremy's mother found out about the pain, she immediately took him to their family doctor, who diagnosed him with "growing pains." With his parent's fear alleviated by the diagnosis, Jeremy continued to play despite the pain. Then, in late winter, after the basketball session was over, his pain began to subside. Despite playing baseball in the spring and summer, he had no further complaint of knee pain. In mid-August during the second week of football practice, Jeremy's pain began to gradually return. By the time the season started in early September, he could hardly run. He complained to his parents that he had pain when he walked down hills and down steps. He also had pain when he tried to sprint or jump. His parents decided that it was time to take him to see a local orthopedic surgeon whom they knew from church.

Dr. Price performed a detailed history that revealed that Jeremy played baseball from April to July, football from August to November, and basketball from November to February. The only time that he was not involved in sports was during the month of March. Dr. Price was quick to recognize that Jeremy was having pain not only during activity but also after exercise, suggesting a more chronic condition. During Dr. Price's observation he noticed no joint swelling or redness and no biomechanical malalignment. Jeremy had good range of motion and normal isometric strength of his quadriceps and hamstrings. Dr. Price did notice that Jeremy had very poor flexibility, particularly of his rectus femoris. The only place that Jeremy was tender was over the tibial tubercles on both knees.

Dr. Price was pretty confident of the diagnosis but decided to order plain radiographs, since Jeremy was still growing and had open epiphyseal plates. The radiographs revealed a slight separation of the epiphysis at both tibial tuberosities, which was a sure sign of Osgood-Schlatter's disease.

Dr. Price explained the diagnosis to Jeremy and his mother. Jeremy's mother still seemed somewhat confused about why he had no pain over the summer. Dr. Price explained that this condition was exacerbated primarily by the jumping and eccentric loading that was common in both basketball and football wide receivers. He also explained that Osgood-Schlatter's disease was very sensitive to the volume of exercise performed, and that Jeremy may have been well within his exercise envelope while playing baseball but exceeded his limits with basketball and football. Dr. Price suggested an evaluation by a physical therapist who specializes in sports-related injuries. He requested that Jeremy be given a home program that would improve his flexibility and increase his eccentric quadriceps strength. Dr. Price told Jeremy's parents that Osgood-Schlatter's disease is a self-limiting condition that if treated conservatively would resolve, but that if he continued excessive activity there was a possibility of avulsing his tibial tubercle.

I had the opportunity to see Jeremy for his physical therapy. I instructed him in proper quadriceps stretching and closed kinetic chain eccentric strengthening exercises. I also discussed the importance of being honest with his parents about when and how much pain he was having. I also

Continues

Case 2 Continued

discussed the importance of recognizing the early signs and symptoms of overuse and how to manage his acute pain by relative rest and ice. I also counseled Jeremy about the importance of adequate rest and suggested that he might want to consider choosing two of the three sports to play. This would give him a chance to recover after each season.

Jeremy was seen a second time two weeks later to evaluate his progress and make sure that he was doing his exercises correctly. At the time of the second visit he was not having any pain and was back to playing football. Jeremy decided that he would stick to baseball and football, which were his two favorite sports, and give up basketball. Since I knew Jeremy's family, I was able to follow his sports career. He was able to play baseball and football without further problems. He excelled in baseball and in his senior year of high school he was offered a chance to play college baseball at a local Division III college.

Speaking of

Those Teen Years

ANDREA EARLE MULLINS, MS, OTR/L
OCCUPATIONAL THERAPIST, GRAFTON SCHOOL

Working with adolescents is something I enjoy immensely. I work with people in all stages of adolescence, from 12- and 13-year-old young adolescents to young adults of 19 and 20. I am an occupational therapist at a private, not-for-profit school and residential treatment program for children and adolescents who have experienced sufficient difficulties functioning in their home or public school environment to justify their placement at our facility.

My experience growing up with a family friend who has a *pervasive developmental disorder* was the driving force behind my interest in this area of practice. I especially remember the challenges he faced during adolescence in developing friendships and participating in social activities. I so wanted to work with young people with these types of challenges that I was willing four years ago to accept a job in this setting in a nontraditional occupational therapy role, as a behavior specialist. My focus in that role was on designing individualized *positive behavior support* programs to help students and staff persons learn techniques that promote adaptive behaviors and improve overall quality of life. A little over a year ago I transitioned into the "traditional" occupational therapy role in this program. I found that my experience as a behavior specialist was completely compatible and highly complementary to my training as an occupational therapist.

The students I work with are diagnosed with a variety of disabilities, including autism, Asperger's disorder, mental retardation, and various psychiatric disorders like bipolar disorder, attention deficit disorder, and major depressive disorder. One of my main roles as an occupational therapist is to help these students engage in the process of forming their own unique identity. I have worked with many teenagers who have missed out on so many important stages of social and self growth. Many of the students with whom I work do not have active family involvement. Many are under custody of the state department of social services. Most of them are extremely limited in their social engagement

Continues

Speaking of Continued

with "typically developing" peers. Although they have disabilities, these adolescents, like all young people, need satisfying social roles for the future.

I engage students in activities that provide them with the opportunities to discover their interests and preferences, and they begin to define their own unique identities. As we do this, an amazing process often unfolds. For example, I worked for over a year with a young woman in her late adolescence. When I first began working with "Sue," she was not able to identify any personal interests other than watching TV. She had lived in foster care and group homes for most of her life and had not been exposed to many basic activities that life has to offer. She had never actively explored her values, interests, and beliefs. People who worked with Sue told me that she was "lazy," "bossy," and "unmotivated." We started to explore her interests and values in a very nonthreatening way. We completed interest checklists and gradually began to explore various choices. When Sue expressed an interest in animals, we began to work with our therapy dog at the end of each session, performing grooming tasks and taking the dog for walks. I always tried to make sessions fun and enjoyable. We discovered that Sue had many interests that she had never previously had the chance to experience or explore. Over the course of the next several months, she began volunteering at a local animal shelter. Since then she has progressed to a level of independence that is allowing her to work toward a career in dog grooming. As she discovered her unique talents and gifts, she began to open up in many ways, expressing an enthusiasm for life that she had never shown before. Her progress has unfolded into all areas of her life. Today she is working on becoming a leader and advocate for other people with disabilities.

REFERENCES

Ainsworth, M. D. S. (1989). Attachments beyond infancy. *American Psychologist, 44,* 709–716.

Alsaker, F. D., & Flammer, A. (1999). *The adolescent experience: European and American adolescents in the 1990s.* Mahwah, NJ: Lawrence Erlbaum Associates.

American Academy of Pediatrics. (1990). Strength training, weight and power lifting, and bodybuilding by children and adolescents. *Pediatrics, 86,* 801–803.

American Occupational Therapy Association. (2002). Occupational therapy practice framework: Domain and process. *American Journal of Occupational Therapy, 56,* 609–639.

Carnegie Council on Adolescent Development. (1989). *Turning points: Preparing American youth for the 21st century.* New York: Carnegie Corporation.

Csikszentmihalyi, M., & Larson, R. (1984). *Being adolescent: Conflict and growth in the teenage years.* New York: Basic Books.

Coleman, J., & Hendry, L. B. (1999). *The nature of adolescence* (3rd ed.). London and New York: Routledge.

Dornbusch, S. M., Herman, M. R., & Morley, J. A. (1996). Domains of adolescent achievement. In G. R. Adams, R. Montemayor, & T. P. Gullotta (Eds.), *Psychosocial development during adolescence.* Thousand Oaks, CA: Sage.

Fisher, A. G. (2001). *Assessment of motor and process skills* (Vol. 1) (User manual). Fort Collins, CO: Three Star Press.

Galambos, N. L., & Ehrenberg, M. F. (1997). The family as health risk and opportunity: A focus on divorce and working families. In J. Schulenberg, J. L. Maggs & K. Hurrelmann (Eds.), *Health risks and developmental transitions during adolescence* (pp. 139–160). Cambridge, UK: Cambridge University Press.

Gallahue, D. L., & Ozmun, J. C. (2002). Understanding motor development. New York: McGraw-Hill.

Gilman, R. (2001). The relationship between life satisfaction, social interest, and frequency of extracurricular activities among adolescent students. *Journal of Youth and Adolescence, 30,* 749–768.

Grotevant, H. (1998). Adolescent development in family contexts. In W. Damon & N. Eisenberg (Eds.), *Handbook of child psychology: Social, emotional, and personality development* (Vol. 3) (pp. 1097–1149). New York: Wiley.

Hall, G. S. (1904). *Adolescence* (Vols. 1 and 2). New York: Appleton.

Harris, P. L., Olthof, T., & Meerum Terwogt, M. (1981). Children's knowledge of emotion. *Journal of Child Psychology and Psychiatry, 22,* 247–261.

Kaczmarek, P. G., & Riva, M. T. (1996). Facilitating adolescent optimal development: Training considerations for counseling psychologists. *The Counseling Psychologist, 24,* 400–432.

Kahne, J., & Bailey, K. (1999). The role of social capital and youth development: The case of "I have a dream" programs. *Educational Evaluation and Policy Analysis, 21,* 321–343.

Kahne, J., Nagaoka, J., Brown, A., O'Brien, J., Quinn, T., & Thiede, K. (2000). School and after-school programs as contexts for youth development: A quantitative and qualitative assessment. In M. Wang & W. Boyd (Eds.), *Improving results for children and families by connecting collaborative services with school reform efforts.* Greenwich, CT: Information Age Publishing.

Kail, R. (1993). Processing time decreases globally at an exponential rate during childhood and adolescence. *Journal of Experimental Child Psychology, 56,* 254–265.

Keating, D. P. (1990). Adolescent thinking. In S. S. Feldman & G. R. Elliott (Eds.), *At the threshold: The developing adolescent* (pp. 54–89). Cambridge, MA: Harvard University Press.

Kimmel, D. C., & Weiner, I. B. (1995). *Adolescence: A developmental transition.* New York: Wiley.

Klein, H. (1990). Adolescence, youth and young adulthood: Rethinking current conceptualizations of the life stage. *Youth and Society, 21,* 446–471.

Laurensen, B. (1995). Conflict and social interaction in adolescent relationships. *Journal of Research on Adolescence, 5,* 55–70.

Lerner, R. M. (2001). *Adolescence: Development, diversity, context, and application.* Upper Saddle River, NJ: Prentice Hall.

Lerner, R. M., & Galambos, N. L. (1998). Adolescent development: Challenges and opportunities for research, programs, and policies. *Annual Review of Psychology, 49,* 413–446.

McLaughlin, M. W., Irby, M. A., & Langman, J. (1994). *Urban sanctuaries: Neighborhood organizations in the lives and futures of inner-city youth.* San Francisco: Jossey-Bass.

Mead, M. (1928). *Coming of age in Samoa: A psychological study of primitive youth for Western civilization.* New York: Morrow.

Merrick, E. N. (1995). Adolescent childbearing as career "choice": Perspective from an ecological context. *Journal of Counseling and Development, 73,* 288–295.

Murphy, J. M. (1990). The Pediatric and Adolescent Athlete. In B. Saunders (Ed.), *Sports physical therapy* (pp. 151–157). East Norwalk, CT: Appleton and Lange.

Passmore, A. (2003). The occupation of leisure: Three typologies and their influence on mental health in adolescence. *OTJR: Occupation, Participation, and Health, 23,* 76–83.

Patel, D. R., & Nelson, T. L. (2000). Sports injuries in adolescents. *Medical Clinics of North America, 84,* 983–1007.

Payne, V. G., & Isaacs, L. D. (1999). *Human motor development: A lifespan approach.* Mountain View, CA: Mayfield Publishing Company.

Petersen, A. C. (1988). Adolescent development. *Annual Review of Psychology, 39,* 583–607.

Pierce, D. E. (2002). *Occupation by design: Building therapeutic power.* Philadelphia: F.A. Davis.

Raymore, L., Barber, B., Eccles, J., & Godbey, G. (1999). Leisure behavior pattern stability during the transition from adolescence to young adulthood. *Journal of Youth and Adolescence, 28,* 79–103.

Richardson, M. S. (1993). Work in people's lives: A location for counseling psychologists. *Journal of Counseling Psychology, 40,* 425–433.

Schondel, C. K., & Boehm, K. E. (2000). Motivational needs of adolescent volunteers. *Adolescence, 35,* 335–344.

Steinberg, L. (1996). *Adolescence* (4th ed.). New York: McGraw-Hill.

Tierney, J. P., & Grossman, J. B. (1995). *Making a difference: An impact study of the big brothers/big sisters.* Philadelphia: Public/Private Ventures.

U.S. Department of Labor. *Youth and labor.* Retrieved June 28, 2003, from http://www.dol.gov/dol/topic/youthlabor/index.htm.

Wagner, W. G. (1996). Optimal development in adolescence: What is it and how can it be encouraged? *The Counseling Psychologist, 24,* 360–399.

Weiner, I. B. (1992). *Psychological disturbance in adolescence.* New York: John Wiley.

Werner, E. B. (1987). Vulnerability and resiliency in children at risk for delinquency: A longitudinal study, birth to young adulthood. In J. D. Burchard & S. N. Burchard (Eds.), *The prevention of delinquent behavior* (pp. 16–43). Newbury Park, CA: Sage.

Werner, E. B., & Smith, R. S. (1982). *Vulnerable but invincible: A study of resilient children.* New York: McGraw-Hill.

Whitehead, J., Evans, N. J., & Lee, M. J. (1997). Relative importance of success in sport and schoolwork. *Perceptual and Motor Skills, 85,* 599–606.

World Health Organization. (2002). *ICF: International classification of functioning and disability.* Geneva, Switzerland: World Health Organization.

Wyn, J., & White, R. (1997). *Rethinking youth.* Thousand Oaks, CA: Sage.

CHAPTER 13

Family and Disablement Issues Throughout Childhood

Susannah Grimm Poe, EdD
Assistant Professor, Department of Pediatrics
WVU School of Medicine
WG Klingberg Center for Child Development
Morgantown, West Virginia

Objectives

Upon completion of this chapter, the reader should be able to

▪ Differentiate developmental disorder from developmental delay.

▪ Discuss the role of crisis in the family life cycle, distinguishing between developmental and situational crises.

▪ Describe the common developmental disorders of autism, Down syndrome, Fragile X syndrome, cerebral palsy, and attention deficit hyperactivity disorder.

▪ Summarize the theory of transformed parenting.

▪ Discuss the ICF construct of Social Participation as it relates to families and children with developmental disabilities.

Key Terms

chronic sorrow
developmental crises
developmental delay
developmental disorder
diagnosis
Down syndrome

dysmorphism
Entrance Process
Fragile X syndrome
hippotherapy
Operating Processes

pervasive developmental disorder
(PDD)
situational crises
Special Olympics
theory of transformed parenting

DEVELOPMENTAL DIFFERENCES AND THE FAMILY

Approximately 17 percent of children in the United States under age 18 have a developmental disability, and about 1.4 million, or 2 percent, of school-age children have such severe developmental problems that they will require lifelong supportive services (Centers for Disease Control, 2003). Caring for these children involves understanding and caring for the family. In some contexts, such as early intervention, the family is identified as the focus of care, while in other settings, like outpatient therapy, the family is the context for care. The introduction to families presented in Chapter 9 provided support for the inclusion of families as a contextual factor in the ICF classification system. In this chapter, we look not only at the caregivers and family, but also at the characteristics of the child and the family and how these influence the performance abilities of the child.

One objective of this chapter is to introduce helping professionals to developmental disabilities that are first diagnosed in childhood. Another objective is to show how that diagnosis can affect the child's family. Because therapists have such a critical role in the rehabilitation of children with developmental disorders, it is necessary that they understand not only their part in helping the child but also the role of the family and the support systems within the community.

PARENTING THE DEVELOPMENTALLY DELAYED CHILD

Few parents plan to have a child with a developmental disability, although most expectant parents worry about whether or not their baby will be healthy. Once the baby is born, and appears to be well, those concerns usually fade. In fact, more than 99 percent of children who are born without disabilities will not subsequently develop severe disabilities (Batshaw, 2001). Some developmental disabilities are obvious at birth and have

immediate impact on the caregivers. In these cases the infant may have dysmorphic features. **Dysmorphism** is an anatomic malformation or abnormality of shape (Merriam-Webster Medical Dictionary, 2002).

Other conditions are present at birth but are not observable until the infant is older. The first indicator that a child may have a developmental problem may occur when milestones are not reached at the expected times. In some children there may be additional indicators that cause concern, including dysmorphic features, escalating behavior problems, coordination or tone problems, difficulties with vision or hearing, repetitive play, and/or lack of interest in socializing with peers.

When parents realize their child is not on the same developmental path as other children his age, they understandably want to know what is causing the delay and what to do to help the child catch up with peers. The first professional they talk with is usually the child's primary-care physician or pediatrician. General pediatricians routinely perform developmental screenings on each child during every well-child visit and can discuss with the parents where the child tests in each domain of development. These domains of development were presented in the context of the ICF classification system in Chapter 1. If questions remain about the child's development, features, or behavior, general pediatricians usually refer the child to professionals specializing in the developmental concerns, including pediatric neurologists, pediatric geneticists, developmental psychologists, developmental pediatricians, occupational therapists, or physical therapists, for further evaluation.

While each of these professionals may be assessing the child for a diagnosis, each may approach the child in a different way, depending on their area of specialty. A pediatric neurologist is concerned with the functioning of the brain, while a geneticist will explore the family history of disorders and determine if blood tests are necessary to detect chromosome abnormalities. A developmental psychologist looks at the level of life-skills and awareness the child has, including social ability and communication style, while a developmental pediatrician will review medical history and order any tests she feels necessary to clarify the child's medical condition. The Occupational Therapy Practice Framework (2002) and the Guide to Physical Therapy Practice (2001), reviewed in Chapter 1, give insight into the roles of these professionals. In many situations, all these professionals work together as a team to provide all the information necessary to establish a clear and accurate diagnosis.

While many parents and professionals are reluctant to label a child with a diagnosis early in life, there is benefit in an early diagnosis for all developmental disabilities. A **diagnosis** is a professional decision, or label, reflecting the supposed nature and cause of the developmental differences presented by the child. The diagnosis may provide an answer for a parent who has been concerned that something is wrong with his child's development. Knowing the diagnosis also can provide parents with the road map they need to begin treatment, and early treatment is important for the success of the child with developmental differences. The earlier help begins for the child, the more progress she can make toward improvement. Additionally, knowing the diagnosis can help the parent find important support and information from others in similar situations.

Developmental delay and developmental disorder are separate but often related labels given children who fail to reach developmental milestones at the expected times. Developmental professionals use the term **developmental delay** to describe a child who is slow in development but who has the potential to catch up. For example, a child born prematurely, without complications, may not initially meet all milestones at the expected time but usually catches up around the age of 2 years. **Developmental disorder**, however, implies a more pervasive and chronic delay and is used as an umbrella term for a variety of diagnoses, including mental retardation, cerebral palsy, and autism. These disorders can impair the physical, cognitive, social, sensory, and communication abilities of the affected child. While children with a developmental disability can continue to make progress in development, most often they do not catch up with typically developing peers (Batshaw, 1997).

Developmental disabilities can originate before, during, or after birth. Often the most severe developmental disorders occur prenatally as the result of maternal infection, substance abuse by the mother, exposure of the fetus to damaging substances in the environment, a genetic or chromosomal disorder, or an unknown reason. At the time of birth, complications such as placenta previa, premature rupture of membranes, labor that does not progress, toxemia, and prematurity may cause oxygen deprivation that can lead to brain damage that at term may result in cerebral palsy and cognitive problems. Traumatic brain injury, lead poisoning, infections, and metabolic disturbances are some of the reasons developmental disabilities may occur after birth.

FAMILY RESPONSES TO DIAGNOSIS OF DEVELOPMENTAL DISABILITY

A *family crisis* is any problem that cannot be resolved with the family's normal or routine problem-solving skills. During the period of crisis, the family may struggle to maintain its normal structure and organization. In the *family life cycle* theory presented in Chapter 9 of this text, family crises are opportunities for change and growth. Crises are a normal part of family life; the family life cycle theory distinguishes two types of crisis. The first type, the **developmental crises**, are those experienced by families that influence the structure and identity of the family, or they may be created by traumatic and unforeseen incidents. The most common stressors identified with developmental issues involve situations where individuals are leaving or entering the family system. A sample of developmental crises may include new marriage/relationship, birth/adoption of a child, children entering school, and children entering adolescence. As frustrating as these stressors might be, they are generally predictable and part of the normal cycle of all families (Case-Smith, 1998; Humphry & Case-Smith, 2001; Winton & Winton, 2000).

Another category of crises, the **situational crises**, encompass the situations in life that come suddenly, without warning. These unexpected circumstances may be distinguished by loss, from loss of an "imagined" child as described in Chapter 9 to the loss of control of the course of one's life. Developmental and situational crises happen to all families, but families within a culture experience similar, predictable developmental crises, whereas the situational crises a given family experiences are unique to that family (Shepard & Mahon, 1996). Having a child with a developmental disability is an example of a situational crisis.

From the literature on family life cycle theory, we know that any family member's situation influences all other family members (Shepard & Mahon, 1996). Having a child with any type of chronic condition is stressful for families, but research indicates that there is no more dysfunction in these "challenged" families than seen in control families (Cadman et al., 1991; Schor, 2003). As health professionals we often label these children as "ill," but families are more likely to view them as "normal" and in good health (Shepard & Mahon, 1996). It is essential that we, as professionals, learn more about these conditions, and consider these children in the context of the family and the community, rather in terms of a child's degree of difference. If we are to be successful in supporting the child, we must work within the perceptions and concerns of the family (Cronin, 2003).

As presented in Chapter 9, the birth of the "less than perfect" infant is a time of extreme distress. Interestingly, later diagnoses acquired in childhood or adolescence are often met with mixed emotions. Following an initial period of heartbreak, some parents express relief. For parents of children with hidden or subtle differences, like attention deficit disorder, the assigning of a diagnosis affirms the parents' difficulty in supporting and managing their child (Cronin, 2003). Developmental differences require the family to adapt to the situation, even when there is no official label for what they are experiencing. These families know that their parenting experience differs from the norm and may feel affirmed in their perceptions by the acquisition of a label.

In most cases the diagnosis of a disorder in a child sends parents on a quest for information. One of the most crucial roles of health professionals is to help parents find and critically evaluate information about treatments for their child. With easy access to Internet search engines, families often get overwhelming, conflicting, and sometimes dangerous information. The health professional should be able to help families sort through this information to provide safe and evidence-based resources for care of their child.

COMMON DEVELOPMENTAL DISABILITIES

The most commonly known developmental disabilities include the autism-spectrum disorders, mental retardation, Down syndrome and other genetic syndromes, cerebral palsy, attention deficit disorders, and learning disabilities. Each of these disabilities can vary from mild to severe, and children can have more than a single diagnosis. While the cause of most developmental disabilities is not known approximately 75 percent of the time, there are predictable developmental disorders that result from chromosomal or metabolic abnormalities or from the use of alcohol by the mother before birth.

Pervasive developmental disorder (PDD) is the name given to the spectrum of disorders that have four characteristics in common: impairments in both verbal and nonverbal communication; stereotypical interests, activities, or behaviors; impairments in social interaction; and a history of developmental delay before age 3. The spectrum of PDD includes several conditions, the most common of which are autistic disorder, pervasive developmental disorder—not otherwise specified, and Asperger's syndrome.

Autistic disorder, or *autism*, as it is commonly called, is diagnosed when the child has moderate to severe problems with socialization and communication, and restricted patterns of behaviors or interests. The child must have also been identified with delays before age 3, with early delay most commonly in the area of communication and/or socialization. Autism can be evident in the 1st or 2nd year of life but is usually diagnosed around age 3. Within the diagnosis of autism come varying levels of disability—for example, one child with autism may have interest in other children and will play near others while another child may prefer to be alone and will withdraw from peers. One child may have enough functional words to ask for what he wants, while another may be completely nonverbal and wait to have her needs met. Some children with autism will be affectionate with familiar people while others pull away from any touch. Almost three fourths of children with autistic disorder are considered to have IQs in the impaired range (Kaplan & Sadock, 1998). The diagnosis of *pervasive developmental disorder—not otherwise specified (PDD-NOS)* indicates that the child either does not fully meet criteria for another autism-spectrum disorder or does not have the degree of impairment described in autistic disorder (Kaplan & Sadock, 1998).

A child with Asperger's syndrome will exhibit difficulties with social relationships, reading nonverbal cues, and understanding the nuances of the environment associated with the other diagnoses on the spectrum; but she does not have the significant delay in language development found in autistic disorder, and she will have a normal to high IQ (Kaplan & Sadock, 1998).

Mental retardation can have unknown etiology or can be linked to a genetic disorder. Mental retardation is used commonly to describe a child who has limited cognitive skills and self-help skills. There are three areas in which criteria must be met for this diagnosis: the person must have an IQ below 70, have the onset of these problems before age 18, and demonstrate difficulty with adaptive functioning. To demonstrate difficulty in adaptive functioning, the child must have delays or differences in at least two of the following areas: communication, self-care, home living, social/interpersonal skills, use of community resources, self-direction, functional academic work, leisure, health, and safety (Batshaw, 1997).

The severity of mental retardation can fall into one of four categories. Children with mild mental retardation generally have an IQ score of 50–70; those with moderately mental retardation, 35–55, and those with severe mental retardation, 20–40. The label of profoundly mentally retarded is applied to a child who has an IQ score below 20 to 25 (Kaplan and Sadock, 1998). Most children with the diagnosis of mental retardation require some support for participation in everyday activities.

Down syndrome is the most common genetic cause of mental retardation. Named for John Langdon Down, who first described the physical features of people with the syndrome in 1866, it occurs in about 1 in 900 births. A *syndrome* is defined by a set of physical characteristics that occur together, and in a child with Down, those characteristics include distinctive facial features, a single crease near the top of the palm, and a large space between the big toe and the first toe. Eyes that slant upward, an epicanthal fold (a fold of skin at the inside corner of each eye), a small nose, a flat nose bridge, and a broad, short neck are some of the expected facial features of a person with Down (Batshaw, 1997).

Fragile X syndrome is another one caused by chromosomal abnormalities that result in mental retardation as a core symptom. The most common form of inherited mental retardation, Fragile X is a sex-linked genetic abnormality in which the mother is the carrier, transmitting the disorder most severely to sons. While it affects approximately 1 in approximately 2,000 to 3,000 births, the incidence of occurrence is 1 in 2,000 to 3,000 males and 1 in every 2,500 females (Batshaw, 1997). Males usually have a moderate to severe intellectual disability, while females usually have less severe intellectual impairment but more emotional difficulties. About 20 percent of people with Fragile X syndrome demonstrate autistic-like behaviors such as limited eye contact, hand flapping, hand biting, language delay, and sensory abnormalities. The physical characteristics that often accompany this syndrome include a long, narrow face; head circumference above the 50th percentile; malformed and/or large ears; strabismus, or lazy eye; hyperextensible joints; a high, arched palate; poor muscle tone; flat feet, and large testicles in males. Behavior problems and developmental delays, particularly in speech, are also common features of Fragile X (Batshaw, 1997). Fragile X is difficult to diagnose in infants, but as the child grows, his physical features become more distinct as behavioral indicators increase.

Fetal alcohol syndrome, described in Chapter 8, is a birth defect that is often not diagnosed until the child is 2–3 years old. *Cerebral palsy (CP)*, also mentioned briefly in Chapter 8, is the most common congenital (present from birth) disorder of childhood, but it is often not diagnosed until the child's motor skills have developed enough to determine dysfunction. It affects muscle tone and coordinated movement and can result in problems with eating, bladder and bowel control, breathing, and learning. There are three types of CP: *spastic*, which causes stiff and difficult movement; *athetoid*, causing involuntary and uncontrolled movement; and *ataxic*, which causes a disturbed sense of balance and depth perception (Batshaw, 1997).

CP affects about 5 in every 2,000 children and about 5 percent of children who are born prematurely (Kids Health for Parents, retrieved July, 17, 2003, from http://www.kidshealth.org/parent/medical/brain/cerebral_palsy.html). It may be possible to identify this condition early, within the 1st year of life, in children born with risk factors present. When a baby is full-term and has none of the risk factors associated with CP, the first sign of the disorder may be a delay in normal developmental milestones but could also include abnormal muscle tone, uncoordinated movements, and persistent infantile reflexes like the Moro reflex. A later diagnosis often indicates a milder delay. CP, like other developmental disorders, cannot be cured, but it can be managed with appropriate intervention, including physical, occupational, and speech therapies.

Attention deficit hyperactivity disorder (ADHD) is a developmental disorder characterized by the inability of the child to stay focused on tasks or activities and by her demonstration of poor motivation, frequent boredom, and lack of understanding of the consequences of her behavior. For many children, hyperactivity and impulsivity accompany this lack of focus. The problems with attention and behavior often cause problems in learning and at home. ADHD is one of the most common of the developmental disorders and occurs in 4–12 out of every 100 children (Kids Health, retrieved July, 17, 2003, from http::/www.kidshealth.org/parent/medical/learning/adhd.html).

LABELING THE DIFFERENT CHILD

Even though most parents want to know the reason for their child's differences, the moment of diagnosis is almost always a memorable and heartbreaking moment in the life of the family. Research reports consistently indicate that this pause in the momentum of the family is almost always painful, sad, and overwhelming (Shepard & Mahon, 1996). Even when a diagnosis is expected, hearing the words said aloud, or seeing them written down, has a finality that challenges denial and begins the process of reconfiguring the status quo.

Parents who learn of a child's disability after what seemed like normal development, as is often the case in autism, find that they are in a dramatically different role than the one they had assumed at the birth of the child. They must learn as much as they can about what the diagnosis means, locate sources of support and education, and juggle the rest of the demands of family life—all while grieving the loss of the idea of the healthy, normal child and "typical" family. The grief doesn't end when the diagnosis is accepted. These feelings of helplessness, isolation, embarrassment, blame, confusion, denial, guilt, anger, and depression, intensely felt at the time of diagnosis, will recur over the years, especially at the times when the child would have experienced major turning points if the disorder were not present (Shepard & Mahon, 1996). Parents who had thought themselves to be accepting of a child's diagnosis often report that sorrow occurs again when the child might have been getting his driver's license, attending the senior prom, or graduating from high school. It often helps parents to learn that the feelings they are experiencing are normal responses to their perceived loss (Johnson, 2000). Hopelessness and despair can be diminished when the parents begin at whatever level of interaction they can manage with their child as the first steps toward regaining control and reorganizing their lives (Johnson, 2000).

THEORY OF TRANSFORMED PARENTING

Seideman and Kleine's (1995) **theory of transformed parenting** offers one interpretation of the stages that families go through after receiving a diagnosis of developmental disability for their child. Their research is based on interviews with parents of children with mental retardation and developmental delay. They use the word *transformed* to indicate the change that occurs from the fundamental character of the pre-diagnosis parenting role into a new form of parenting, one that goes beyond the originally envisioned role. Their first stage, or the **Entrance Process**, occurs when the parents receive the diagnosis and respond to that diagnosis, and is followed by a series of processes that help family members cope with the continuing needs of the child.

THE ENTRANCE PROCESS

The Entrance Process begins with parents sharing their concern about their child with a physician and finding out what the diagnosis is. Parents often describe the moment of diagnosis in detail but can recall nothing else about the visit to the doctor. For many it is a time of turning inward to absorb the impact of the news and to come to an understanding of how different their new reality will be. For some parents, that moment may be short-lived. Learning the name of the enemy, or the diagnosis, begins the battle for those who cope by meeting challenges head-on and deal with stress by mobilizing resources (Seideman & Kleine, 1995).

Other parents need time to accept the diagnosis, to grieve the loss of "normal," and to recreate their lives to include the demands inherent in the diagnosis. Some faced with an unwanted diagnosis will work to deny the reality of it by rejecting any information about their child's condition and by choosing not to go for further evaluation or enroll in treatment programs or become involved with support groups. Most parents in Seideman and Kleine's study (1995) needed some time to understand the truth of the diagnosis and to interpret what it could mean in the life of the child and the family. Accepting the diagnosis often came only when the parent had time to learn and think about the diagnostic information. Initially, these authors found, most parents focused on the day-to-day well-being of the child rather than fully absorbing what the diagnosis meant for the future (Seideman & Kleine, 1995).

Once a diagnosis is given, parents may turn to extended family members and close friends with the news. Some parents reported receiving support from family members, but in some cases the parents actually had to provide the support to others learning the news. By informing extended family and friends, parents begin the task of turning outward and constructing a new reality for the family. Constructing that new reality is an important but ongoing process, as the needs of the child will change over time. Once the family's circle of family and friends are included in the diagnosis, the next outward move includes finding appropriate care and treatment for the child. Parents must find education, socialization, and medical care for their child and, along the way, support services for themselves (Seideman & Kleine, 1995).

ACCOMMODATION

After creating a new framework for the family that includes accommodation to the needs of the child, the family can experience a new sense of normalcy as these routines become ingrained in everyday life. Parents usually construct daily routines to channel their children into the directions that are most desirable (Kellegrew, 1999). Simple daily rituals like bathing and dressing provide children with thousands of opportunities to practice and develop the skills necessary to become independent adults. The more symbolic, like bedtime prayers, transmit the values of the family and the culture.

Parents of children with disabilities also utilize daily routines to teach their child basic skills and, most importantly, to normalize the family experience. Routines provide stability in the face of constant change and can enhance the parent's sense of control in an unpredictable situation (Cronin, 2003). This new normalcy can be tenuous, however, especially for children who have ongoing medical needs. Hospitalization, for example, was described as one of the most demanding times for a family, not only because the child was ill and the hospital stay disrupted normalized routines, but because it served as a reminder that the child was different.

OPERATING PROCESSES

The next stage experienced by parents, called the **Operating Processes** by Seideman and Kleine (1997), includes the tasks of creating a mindset, experiencing chronic sorrow, and adapting by actions. "Creating a mindset" refers to the use of cognitive strategies to deal with everyday problems. "Guarding hope" is also a technique used during this stage; while parents hope for the best outcome possible, they learn to remain cautious as a result of previous disappointments. "Comparing downward," another task described in this stage, refers to the comparisons made by parents when they realize other families and children have more problems than they do and acknowledge that their own child could have been worse than she is. A parent may also employ the technique of "redefining the situation" by considering a philosophic perspective such as "everything happens for a reason," or "God doesn't give people more than they can handle" (Seideman and Kleine, 1997).

Chronic sorrow is a perpetual part of the performance process, according to Seideman and Kleine (1997). Parents experience recurring sorrow when faced over and over again with the child's enduring impairments, especially when they cannot participate in the rites of passage that parents of typically developing children experience: graduation, marriage, and grandchildren. Parents report that one of the most difficult times occurs as the child reaches the age of maturity without functioning independently in society. Another is when parents realize that their dependent child will likely survive them but still require extensive care. Especially as parents age, the demands and needs of a seriously impaired child can present extreme personal and environmental pressures on the parent. In this case the aging parents may be functionally disabled by the supervision and care demands placed on them by their child.

Through chronic sorrow can come good. Some parents show great determination to master the complexities of the disorder and use those abilities to help their child as well as others in a similar situation. Family members of persons with disabilities have been seminal in developing many support groups and community resources.

FAMILY HEALTH AND WELL-BEING

A substantial amount of literature examines the types of stress experienced by families who include a child with a developmental disability. Browne (1998) proposed that these stressors included anxiety about the future, behavior of the child, severity of the diagnosis, and negative attitudes from the community.

Weiss (1991) reported that parents of children with disabilities in her study experienced six major stressors associated with the care of that child. Those stressors included dealing with professional and support services, strains on the family, stigmatization, the child's behavior, concerns regarding the child's future, having insufficient information to care for the child, and the child's need for constant supervision. Weiss found that the age of the child or the parent did not contribute to

this stress, nor did the length of the caregiving, the marital or educational status of the parents, or the perceived adequacy of the family income (Weiss, 1991).

In spite of these increased stressors, families that make persistent and early accommodations in the social and occupational realms differ little from control-group families in their physical and mental health. This continues to be true particularly when their children reach school age and older, even while they continue in the non-normative and demanding role of parenting a child with a disability (Seltzer et al., 2001). One reason for this, these authors suggest, is the advent of mandated educational and social services for children with disabilities, which perhaps takes some of the burden of care from the parents.

While the physical and emotional health of parents of children with developmental disabilities did not differ from that of the control group in the study by Seltzer et al. (2001), the professional careers of those parents did. Research has indicated that the expected life course and well-being of parents whose children were diagnosed with developmental disabilities early in life differ from the life course and well-being of parents whose children initially developed normally (Selzer et al., 2001). These parents of early-diagnosed children learned to make accommodations in their work schedules early based on the needs of their child, and those accommodations had long-lasting effects, resulting in decreased likelihood of paid employment and, for those parents who did work, more work-family strain. These parents also reported fewer social contacts with friends even though they did maintain some social relationships.

Self-efficacy has been identified as an important variable in understanding the relationship between parents' mental health problems and child behavior problems (Hastings & Brown, 2002). The construct of self-efficacy was first described in Chapter 10 as the belief in the individual's personal power to change things. Mothers and fathers of children with autism have high levels of potential mental health problems, anxiety, and depression (Hastings & Brown, 2002). For mothers self-efficacy functions as a mediating variable, while for fathers self-efficacy is not mediating but a moderating variable acting as a protective factor. The researchers contend that self-efficacy plays an important role for both parents in preventing or alleviating mental health problems.

The only groups of parents that did not have physical and emotional health similar to the control group were parents of children diagnosed with severe mental health problems. Parents of children with these diagnoses had the worst physical and mental health outcomes in middle age, even though they had had greater social involvement and had made few accommodations earlier in their family life. Perhaps this was the result of the stigma of their child's diagnosis and the extra demands of caring for and living with a child with a severe mental illness. Or it could be a result of timing—many mental health diagnoses are made later in childhood (Gorman, 2003).

In addition to self-efficacy, the stigma associated with some diagnoses, and the timing of the diagnosis, some researchers have found that the characteristics of the individual child can influence the well-being of the child's parents (Cronin, 2003).

DIFFERENCES BETWEEN PARENTS

Many contextual factors influence how the family copes with the care of a disabled child. In this case the ICF classification model can be applied to the family in reflecting the interrelatedness of context and function (World Health Organization, 2002). Mothers and fathers often adapt to the child's diagnosis in very different ways and at different times, sometimes complicating their relationship as well as the immediate needs of the child. The relationship and degree of cohesiveness between parents is one of the most important factors in the success of the marriage and the care of the child.

Mothers and fathers may experience different types of adaptation to the diagnosis and the needs of the child, complicating the initial adjustment as well as the ongoing care of the child. There are commonalities and differences in the father's and the mother's perception of the parenting role and their individual experiences with the child. Researchers have found differences in the results of their studies looking at the effect of common stressors between parents.

For example, Krauss (1993) found that mothers and fathers report similar levels of parenting-related stress overall, and the effects of that stress were well below those considered to be clinically significant. There were no differences between male and female parents in social isolation, depression, or sense of competence. The types of stressors, however, varied between mothers and fathers. Mothers reported more difficulty in adjusting to the personal aspects of parenting, such as health, role restrictions, and relationship with spouse than did fathers in this study. Krauss (1993) found the most powerful correlates and predictors of stress for both mothers and fathers were the individual characteristics of the parents themselves. Those aspects include their appraisal of the professional's control over their child's development, of the family environment and its adaptability and cohesiveness, and of the helpfulness of social support network. The weight of these factors differed between mothers and fathers, with parenting stress among fathers being more sensitive to the effects on the family environment. Mothers may be less affected by aspects of family function, as mothers are generally the ones creating that environment.

Krauss found that mothers differed from their husbands in the effect of social support on their parenting stress: mothers reported that social support worked better in relieving parental stress than did fathers. Fathers were consistently troubled more than were mothers by various aspects of their relationship with their child, including their attachment and reinforcement. Fathers also reported more stress related to the child's temperament, such as mood and adaptability, than did mothers, and perceived their families as less emotionally cohesive and adaptable.

Roach, Orsmond, and Barratt (1999), in their study of parents of children with Down syndrome, found that parental involvement in child care, parental stress experienced by the partner, and parental employment may influence the stress of parents of young children with Down. They found that fathers who share in the day-to-day aspects of child care may not only ease the mother's child-care burden but may also experience greater perceived competence in their parenting role and experience less perceived difficulty in attachment relationships with their young children.

Dyson (1997) examined fathers' and mothers' experiences with parental stress, family functioning, and social support during the school years of their children with disabilities and found that fathers and mothers are similar in their family experiences involving a child with disabilities. Fathers and mothers of children with disabilities did reveal greater degrees of stress than did the fathers and mothers of children without disabilities. The parental stress that was perceived and experienced by fathers and mothers was related to their own and their spouses' appraisal of the functioning of their family in terms of nurturance, the ability to maintain the family system, and facilitation of personal growth. The parents of children with disabilities also had a disproportionately greater level of stress relating to their children than did families of children without disabilities. Fathers who evaluated their families as emphasizing personal growth and having organized routines experienced less stress. When wives perceived greater family emphasis on personal growth of family members, the fathers had less stress. As mothers experienced and perceived greater social support, a more positive family relationship, a stronger family emphasis on personal growth, and a well-organized family system, they reported less stress, and when their husbands reported the same goals, the mothers also indicated lower stress levels. The researcher concludes that parental stress associated with a child's disability was influenced by family psychological resources (Dyson, 1997).

CHARACTERISTICS OF CHILD

Anderson and Hinojosa's research (1984) described the effect of the child's developmental age on parent-child interaction. The child's ability to interact through loco-motion and play can be rewarding to parents of young children. When the child has a disability that allows few opportunities for this kind of play and interaction, that diminished exchange can affect parent-child relationships. As the child grows, the ability to walk upright has symbolic meaning to parents; it's an important milestone that signals the young child's movement toward separation and individualization. As a result, parents of nonambulatory children with little means of getting needs met besides reliance on their parents may have difficulty in viewing their child as a separate person.

A developing vocabulary is another important milestone for young children. Those children who cannot communicate verbally may become frustrated in their attempts to convey their needs and desires and even their developmentally normal negativity, according to Anderson and Hinojosa (1984). Object manipulation and pretend play, which are important factors in learning coping skills, may not be understood by young children with fine motor problems, learning disabilities, and autism-spectrum disorders.

All in all, these developmental lags change the nature of "normal" parenting. Many parents become over-protective of the child with a disability and do not allow him the independence necessary for normal separation, even when the child is ready, or they transmit their fear to the child, making him afraid of separation. Parents may become too overwhelmed with daily care to set consistent behavioral limits for the child and, as a result, he develops behaviors so demanding that he soon is controlling the home.

SIBLINGS

In all families, the relationship among siblings is among the most important, and complicated, of all human interactions. Regardless of the circumstances, siblings share the bond of family experience from their earliest moments until their last. In childhood, siblings can be a captive audience, available companions, and rivals. They are the measuring sticks by which all achievements are judged. Through sibling relationships, the social, emotional, and psychological development of each child is honed.

While the discovery that a child has a disability has as profound an impact on each member of the family, researchers (Meyer & Vadsay, 1994) have found that the concerns of siblings are often very different from those of parents. These concerns include

- Embarrassment over the sibling's behavior or appearance.
- Fear that they might develop the disability.
- Guilt over not having a disability while a brother or sister does.

- Jealousy or anger over the amount of time the care of the sibling requires.
- Pressure to achieve more in order to make up for the brother or sister's disabilities.
- Worries that they may have caused the disability.
- Concern about the future care of the disabled sibling.

The family environment plays an important role in how the sibling adjusts to the diagnosis of a developmentally delayed brother or sister. The number of children in the family, the kind and severity of the disability, the lifestyle and resources of the family, the way parents adjust to the disability, the age differences among children, the type and quality of community support services, and the coping mechanisms already in place in the family are all part of that environment.

At all ages there can be a gap between what the sibling of a child with disabilities understands on an intellectual level and what she feels on an emotional level. She may understand that her brother or sister did not choose to be disabled, yet still resent him or her for that disability.

Preschool children are usually capable of understanding the differences between themselves and their siblings but accept the special needs as part and parcel of everyday life. Children in elementary school who are venturing out into the company of other children are more aware of the differences between themselves and their disabled sibling than they were when they were younger. They have gained the ability to understand the sibling's disability and his special needs if they are explained in a concrete and clear manner. They may also begin to feel shame or embarrassment as they realize the differences between themselves and their sibling, while also feeling protective toward the sibling. A big concern of children this age is that the sibling's disability is contagious or that something is wrong with them, too. Typically developing siblings may also feel guilty for the negative thoughts or feelings they have about their disabled sibling. To gain their parent's attention, they may try to compensate by becoming overly helpful and well behaved or act in just the opposite manner by being noncompliant and difficult.

The major developmental task of adolescence is breaking away from the family. As the typically developing adolescent's peer group becomes more and more important, she may experience more embarrassment over her developmentally disabled sibling and stop bringing friends into their home. She may also feel conflicted about being able to break away, not only because the sibling cannot expect to become independent but also because she is leaving the sibling behind. Conversely, the well sibling may feel unfairly tied to home because of caretaking responsibilities. Growing awareness will lead the adolescent to consider what the future holds for her sibling with a disability and what role she will play in that future.

At any age the nondisabled child needs to understand what his sibling's disability is and what to expect in the future. He needs to be shown the strengths and weaknesses of his sibling, and realize that the sibling is not completely defined by the disability. He may need help in learning ways to interact with his sibling, not just as a caretaker but through typical peer relations.

In addition to age, the gender, birth order, and the nature of the disability can also have some impact on the relationship between siblings, especially in the realm of caretaking. In families of typically developing children, older siblings often assume some of the care for younger siblings. This role is also evident in families of younger children with disabilities, but the normative caretaking role of the older sibling is magnified. In particular, older sisters of siblings with mental retardation are expected to provide more care to younger brothers and sisters with mental retardation (Lobato, 1990). However, in families where the older child is mentally retarded, for example, the younger children often assume the child-care role for the older disabled sibling; thus the role relationship is transposed. This is particularly true if the sibling with a disability has fewer functional competencies (Stonemen et al., 2003).

Siblings were once thought to be overshadowed and overburdened by the care of the brother or sister with a disability. More recent research, however, indicates that the experience of having a sibling with a disability generally has positive effects on the typically developing child and, as a group, they demonstrate more pro-social behavior, leadership, more empathy and helpfulness, and less self-centeredness than children in families without a disabled child (Faux, 1993). They may also have more sensitivity to others, and a greater sense of closeness to the family (Lobato, 1990; Powell & Gallagher, 1993).

Just as the typically developing sibling experiences stress, the child with a disability has unique stressors that contribute to the family mix. Depending on that child's level of self-awareness, she may experience unhappiness at being different, frustration in not being understood, and anger over not having as many options as the unimpaired siblings.

EXTENDED FAMILY MEMBERS

Relationships with members of the extended family can also have an important effect on the adaptation of the family to a diagnosis of disability, especially the relationship with grandparents. Grandparents can be important providers of routine child care to children with disabilities and as such can greatly impact parental well-being. Grandparents are more likely than any other extended family members to help with the care

of the disabled child, indicating the importance of the parent-child bond (Green, 2001). When they participate in the day-to-day care of the child, that participation helps parents maintain a positive attitude and reduces the physical exhaustion inherent in caring for a child with special needs. Grandparents who are involved with the care of the child and who strive to understand the demands of the diagnosis develop a comfort with the child that normalizes the intergenerational relationship. In addition, when grandparents are involved, it is more likely that other family members will join in the care of the child.

The opposite is true when grandparents do not participate in the care of the child. If the reason for nonparticipation is distance or apprehension, parents often have to broker the relationship between the generations, manage the information to the grandparents and thus become involved in the grandparents' acceptance of and emotional reaction to the grandchild. When the grandparent cannot be involved due to age or disability, parents often feel caught in the middle of the need to care for both their child and their parents. Parents in Green's study (2001) often expressed the need to balance the needs of the two generations and assure family members that they could manage both (Green, 2001).

While grandparenting help had a positive effect on family well-being, sources of support outside the family were not found to have as positive an impact on parental adjustment and were often associated with lower levels of well-being than that obtained with grandparenting suport (Green, 2001).

PARENT-TO-PARENT SUPPORT

When a child is diagnosed with a disability, friends and family members who once provided companionship and support to the parents may no longer be able or willing to act in that capacity, either because they are uncomfortable around the child or because they are grieving for the child and family (Hartman et al., 1992). As a result, parents of newly diagnosed children may lose important support just when they are trying to come to terms with their own grief. In some cases, parents feel they must reverse roles and respond to the sadness of those friends and family members in an attempt to console and comfort them.

Very often the most valued source of new support becomes the parents of other children with disabilities. A consistent finding in the social-support research is the importance of the stress-buffering and health-promoting influences of the informal support offered by other parents in similar situations (Dunst, Trivette, & Deal, 1988). This informal support fosters the parent's acceptance and understanding of the needs of the child and siblings.

These veteran parents understand the stresses of caring for a child with disabilities and can model day-to-day problem solving. They can also guide a parent to the most helpful programs and services available and share the skills they have learned in accessing those systems. The connection that such relationships offer helps parents of newly diagnosed children regain a sense of community.

Parent-to-parent support does not need to be informal to be helpful. Many states provide a more formal source of assistance through *Family Support Networks (FSN)*. A coordinated system run by parents of children with special needs, FSNs provide psychosocial support, peer training, and in some instances financial assistance to other families of children with special needs. Network staff can also help parents of newly diagnosed children identify and collaborate with treatment professionals who could benefit the child.

Members of these support networks can serve as positive role models by sharing their own parenting experiences. According to Hartman et al. (1992), the most significant role modeling provided by parents of children with disabilities occurs when more veteran parents demonstrate enjoyment of their children and pride in their accomplishments. They show, by example, that it is possible for families to survive their grief and live relatively happy and productive lives. With support, most parents of newly diagnosed children begin to see themselves as more capable and feel less dependent on others for answers. They begin to identify their own needs and use newly acquired skills to solve problems (Hartman et al., 1992). Eventually these parents will be the veterans and, as they grow in confidence and abilities, this system of support can provide an opportunity for them to reciprocate by helping other parents. Internet support groups can also provide a sense of community and can be especially important for parents of children with rare disorders who live in rural or isolated areas or who are reluctant to meet others face to face.

RESPITE CARE

Because of the demands of care inherent in some developmental disabilities, parents of children with such disabilities often do not have the child-care options that other parents take for granted. Very often the care of the child requires special training, subtle observation, or great physical reserve. Parents who care for children with these needs don't have the normative amount of downtime other parents may enjoy. Wetherow (2003) likens this situation to the care and attention requirements experienced by parents with a small baby but

without the assurance that over time the child will become more and more self-sufficient. Another consideration is the risk of abuse: children who cannot talk or otherwise express themselves, who have difficulty reading nonverbal cues, or who can't differentiate between acceptable and not acceptable behavior are more vulnerable.

Respite care is service provided by local and federally sponsored programs in which trained providers care for a child with a disability, allowing the parents more time to care for the rest of the family, pursue their own interests, or provide individual or family time with other children. In some cases, respite can be provided by extended family or others familiar enough with the child for the parents to be comfortable leaving the care of the child to another. This much-needed service can be invaluable when the caregiver is well trained and competent, available when needed, and dependable. However, when caregivers are not well trained, dependable, or available when needed, they are of little value to the family. Payment for respite care, like many other child-care situations, is usually minimum wage. As Wetherow (2003) explained, there is an expectation that the respite giver will be engaged, nurturing, and involved, but the reality is that the caregiver is barely "keeping the lid on" while watching television or sitting while the child is sleeping. The term *respite*, he contends, doesn't explain the care that is really needed for the child, which may involve medical support or specific behavioral interventions. Rather, it defines the child as a burden or a source of problems. And the regulations of some funding organizations have requirements that limit the opportunities for a true time-out for the parent by allowing respite care only when the parent is out of the home or the care can be provided only inside the child's house.

HEALTH-CARE PROVIDERS

Hospital and clinic staff members are a critical primary support system for parents of children with disabilities, especially families whose children have severe or multiple medical problems. These professionals are central to the diagnosis and treatment of such children, and they can open doors by making referrals and recommendations for additional interventions. But as critical as the medical information they provide is the effect they can have on the family's well-being through their interest, support, and empathy. The approval or disapproval of these health-care professionals, whether directly conveyed or implied, is felt keenly by parents and dramatically affects their well-being as caretakers (Hartman et al., 1992). Professionals must be sensitive to the impact their words have on the parent and thus the care of the child. By recognizing the validity of all the feelings of the parents and responding empathetically, by linking the family to community and state resources for practical help, and by recognizing the positive efforts made in the care of the child, the medical professional can be most effective in treating the child (Hartman et al., 1992).

This sensitivity is important throughout the experience, both before diagnosis and after. Parents need to hear in plain, honest language when there is a problem or one is expected, and what that problem will mean to the functioning of the child. Parents benefit most when professionals read their cues in how much information the family can manage at a time. Supplemental written information that parents can take with them and digest in a familiar environment also helps them understand and manage the often overwhelming challenge ahead.

EARLY INTERVENTION

One of the first resources for parents of young children with developmental delays is *early intervention*. Designed to be both preventative and ameliorative for children with developmental delay, early-intervention programs are mandated by federal legislation and are available in all states. Parents can refer their children directly for services, or the child's pediatrician or other health-care provider can make the referral. Once the child is enrolled in early intervention, an Individualized Family Service Plan (IFSP) is designed to optimize the child's performance, including a consideration of family needs and goals. Sometimes these early interventions successfully help the child meet milestones appropriately, and services are discontinued. But when the child requires continued intervention, the staff will work with the family to transition the child into the next level of educational support, usually a preschool special-needs program. At age 3 each child with special needs is entitled to a free and appropriate *Individualized Educational Plan (IEP)* for age-appropriate cognitive development as well as the supportive therapies (speech, physical therapy, occupational therapy) important to that child's success. A more in-depth discussion of family-centered care as it pertains to early intervention is in Chapter 9.

SPECIAL EDUCATION

Therapists and teachers in *special-education* programs provide an important service for the child with disabilities through interventions to help the child develop the functional skills necessary for development. While therapists may have the technical skills to provide that service, they must also understand the importance of the

collaboration with the parent to best intervene with the individual child. Successful therapy is a mutually dependent process, with the role of the parent being to explain the nature of the child and the values of the family to the therapist and to help implement the treatments recommended by the therapist.

Both the IFSP and IEP, mentioned previously, require that a therapist examine how the family functions as a system. With the parent-child relationship a critical element, the parents' characteristics, parental stress, role expectations, social support, and the characteristics of the child are all assessed (Humphry, 1989). This examination takes into account the parents' level of education, childhood experiences, cultural influences, role identity, past experiences, and role satisfaction, among other factors. For example, knowing the level of the mother's education can affect how the therapist might teach her to carry out treatment objectives. By understanding what the parents expect of the child and the values of the family, the therapist can emphasize the development of the child's skills that best fit with family expectations.

A child who is making progress can help the parents feel competent, and that competency can increase the overall satisfaction and positive emotional environment of family members. On the other hand, a child who is not making progress or who misbehaves can have the opposite effect: parents may feel ineffective, anxious, or guilty. The therapist who is aware of these effects can encourage closer family relationships by explaining the reason for behaviors of the child that might be discouraging to the parents and help parents learn effective ways of changing negative behaviors. The therapist can also help family members celebrate the progress of their child by pointing out even the subtlest of developmental advances and providing appropriate positive reinforcement to parents (Humphry, 1989). In many respects, the time the therapist spends with parents may be more therapeutic than the time spent in treatment with the child (Anderson & Hinojosa, 1984). Conversely, therapists who are not sensitive to the needs of the whole family, or who have not examined how the family functions as a system, can place demands on families that caregivers cannot meet, thus increasing the feelings of inadequacy.

The setting for special-education services may include instruction in a classroom, in the child's home, in the hospital or other institution, or in another setting, but unless the child's IEP requires another location, the child must be educated in the school he would attend if he did not have a disability. Furthermore, the child must receive the special-education instruction in the *least restrictive environment (LRE)*, and the state must ensure that children with disabilities are educated with unimpaired children to the maximum extent possible. Special classes, separate schooling, or other removal of children from a regular educational environment can occur only if the nature or severity of the disorder is such that the child cannot be educated in regular classes with the help of supplementary aids and services. A more in-depth discussion of the *Individuals with Disabilities Education Act (IDEA)*, which supports special-education services, is in Chapter 20.

SOCIAL PARTICIPATION

The Social Participation dimension of the ICF (WHO, 2002) classifies areas of life in which individuals are involved, or in which they encounter societal opportunities or barriers. *Social participation* means being included in school activities, having access to public transit, and participating in recreation and community activities. Social participation can have positive benefits for children, especially young people with disabilities. The involvement of a child with disabilities in community activities not only provides a normalizing event for the family, but it can increase the child's opportunity for social interaction,

Physical activity can make a contribution to the development of the child's coordination, understanding of rules, and cooperation with others. Many children with special needs will require adaptation to be successful. For example, different sizes and weights of balls may be necessary depending on the strength of the child, or the playing area may need to be shortened to accommodate children with coordination problems. The safety of all children is paramount to a successful outing; leaders should be aware of the safety concerns of each child.

Coaches and other leaders must be trained to understand the physical and attentional limits of the child as well as how she communicates, and consider ways to give each child a specific role in the game that will emphasize her abilities. It is important to give all children a chance to lead others, if possible. When children are unable to compete physically in sports or other recreational events, they may find meaningful occupation in supporting a favorite team as "water boy" (or girl) or as manager. Children and their families are better able to cope and gain skills when they are given meaningful roles and the support to be successful in those roles.

Opportunities for community involvement and recreational opportunities are growing in most areas for children with disabilities. Almost every community has Special Olympics programs, and traditional organizations like Girl and Boy Scouts encourage the participation of children with disabilities. **Special Olympics** is an international organization dedicated to empowering children (and adults) with mental retardation to become more physically fit, respected, and productive

through sports training and competition (Mooar, 2002). To be eligible to participate, a child must be at least 8 years old and be identified by an agency or professional as having one of the following conditions: mental retardation, cognitive delays as measured by formal assessment, or significant learning or vocational problems due to cognitive delays that require or have required specially designed instruction. Children with profound disabilities can participate through specially developed motor-activities training programs (Dykens, Rosner, & Butterbaugh, 1998). Figure 13–1 shows a young woman in a wheelchair playing basketball. In this photo she is on a community basketball court. For the highly motivated wheelchair athlete, there are programs available in larger communities. The area of everyday leisure and recreation is the most limited one for the wheelchair user.

Another recreational and educational program for children with handicaps is hippotherapy. **Hippotherapy** uses the movement of the horse as a tool in treatment by physical therapists, occupational therapists, and

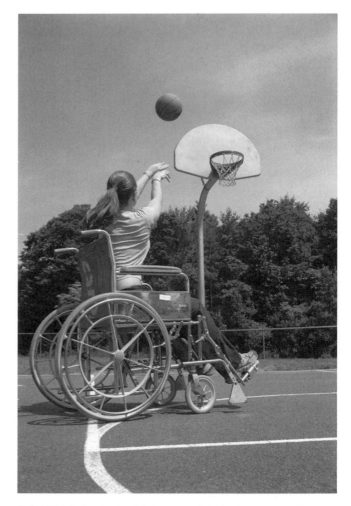

FIGURE 13–1   A wheelchair user participates in a community sports program.

speech-language pathologists in persons with neuro-muscular and developmental dysfunction. In hip-potherapy, the child engages in activities that are both fun and challenging as the therapist modifies the horse's movement and evaluates sensor input. The horse's walk provides sensory input through move-ment, which is variable, rhythmic, and repetitive, and the resulting movements of the rider are similar to the movements of the pelvis while walking (McGibbon et al., 1998). Specific riding skills are not taught in hippotherapy, but the foundation is laid to improve neurologic function and sensory processing.

Aquatic programs, when run by qualified profes-sionals, are another good social resource for children with developmental differences (Hutzler et al., 1998). There are many specialized devices that allow individu-als with severe physical limitations to safely participate in swimming-pool play. Advanced certification is avail-able for health professionals interested in either aquatic therapy or hippotherapy.

SUMMARY

The achievements of a child with developmental diffi-culties are most often different from those expected for the more typically developing child. Just as there is wide variation in what a typically developing child can achieve in adulthood, there is also wide variation in what the child with a developmental disability can attain. In many cases the child's diagnosis and accom-panying deficits can help predict the outcome. For ex-ample, a child with autism who doesn't gain useful speech before age 6 may never have communicative language. Generally, how well the child progresses dur-ing the first 5–7 years of life can predict where she may end up in terms of development, underscoring the importance of early and appropriate interventions (Mathews, 1998).

In addition to the diagnosis, the support of the child's family plays the most important role in the child's outcome. Family characteristics and patterns of interactions can influence not only the child's cognitive abilities but also his social competency and the devel-opment of functional skills. Once the initial impact of the diagnosis is absorbed, the family that accommo-dates the child's disability and normalizes routines is generally most successful.

Speaking of

My Special Gift

CARRIE COBUN
PARENT OF A YOUNG LADY WITH SPECIAL NEEDS

Becoming a mother was a dream I've had since I was a little girl. I couldn't wait to become an adult, get married, and have children. My dreams of the perfect "Gerber" baby were no differ-ent from any other mother's. My dreams were abruptly shattered when my one and only daughter, Amanda Beth, was born 17 years ago . . .

Mandy was different from the very beginning, but like most new mothers, I loved her for just the way she was and refused to believe, initially, that anything could possibly be wrong with her. I had taken excellent care of myself during the pregnancy and had no reason to believe she would not be perfect. I will skip the painful details of being told the news of "brain damage that was severe in na-ture" and "you know she'll never be anything but a baby" and just say that the past 17 years have been a mix of joy, intense grief and sadness, celebrations, and hope.

Mandy was diagnosed as having spastic quadriplegic cerebral palsy when she was approximately 2 years of age. Her type of cerebral palsy involves spastic muscles, involuntary movements, a seizure dis-order, mental retardation, visual impairments, and the inability to communicate using verbal language. Mandy is unable to walk and uses a wheelchair. In addition to all of that, she has had numerous gas-trointestinal problems, which many children do who are unable to walk and move independently.

Continues

Speaking of Continued

She has had numerous surgeries on her bowels as well as a spinal fusion due to a 65 percent curvature of her spine. She always amazes me when she is hospitalized because she endures so much pain and complains much less than adults do!

What have I learned from Mandy? She has never spoken a single word but has taught me more than anyone I know. She has taught me the true meaning of unconditional love. She touches everyone whom she meets and never fails to make those around her smile. When I take her out in the community, whether it's to the mall or Wal-Mart, rarely do we walk by someone who doesn't look upon her with a smile. This is a picture of Mandy and me together (Figure 13–2). She is truly an angel.

Do I have immense challenges that I face each and every day in raising a daughter with special needs? You bet I do! My challenges in raising Mandy are different from those of mothers raising "typically developing" 17-year-olds. Sometimes I envy those mothers who deal with their "normal" teenagers and the problems they deal with; at other times I feel lucky to have Mandy. We are all faced with challenges in life; it's how we deal with them that matters the most.

As Mandy continues to grow into a young adult, the challenges seem to grow with each passing day. I have days where I feel I just can't do it anymore. I feel guilty when I have those feelings, but I realize I am only human. Mandy continues to get heavier, and lifting her is becoming a problem. But the heavier toll is the emotional one that parenting a child with special needs often brings to the primary caregiver. There are days where I feel I am being pulled in a million different directions. *Everyone* seems to want me for something related to Mandy, and Mandy needs 24-hour total care. I do my best to allow her as much independence as possible, but I also understand what she can and can't do.

I have learned many things over the course of the past 17 years from Mandy and those who have cared for her. I have met some of the most wonderful professionals practicing in West Virginia. I have also met some professionals who are in need of intense training in learning how to communicate with parents and their children. I have learned the most from other parents who have children similar to my own. They live the same life as I, and they have been my real teachers.

If I were to offer advice to other parents or professionals caring for children with special needs, I would say this to them: take care of yourself! It took me many years to "let go" of believing that only I could care for Mandy. Over the past several years I have become much better in letting others care for her. In this crazy world in which we live, anything could happen to me. I have to be sure there are others who can care for her as well as I can. With this realization comes another problem: how do parents access quality, affordable care for their children and young adults? This is becoming a major issue for parents across the country. The same problem exists within our elderly population. We expect our children and elderly to receive quality care but pay their caregivers very minimally. Until our state and federal governments make quality respite care a priority on their agendas, it will continue to be difficult to find caregivers for our children.

In summary, my life with Mandy has been filled with joys and challenges. I wouldn't trade Mandy for the world, but I do wish that there were more opportunities for her and for our family to live a more "normalized" life with the supports we need. I still believe that Mandy is a gift to me from God, and I will strive to do my best for her as long as I am able.

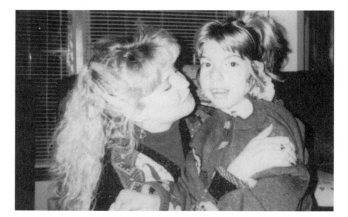

FIGURE 13–2   "Speaking Of" author Carrie Cobun is pictured here with her daughter, Mandy.

REFERENCES

American Occupational Therapy Association. (2002). Occupational Therapy Practice Framework: Domain and process. *The American Journal of Occupational Therapy, 56,* 609–639.

American Physical Therapy Association. (2001). *Guide to physical therapist practice* (2nd ed.). Alexandria, VA: American Physical Therapy Association.

Anderson, J., & Hinojosa, J. (1984). Parents and therapists in a professional partnership. *American Journal of Occupational Therapy, 38,* 452–461.

Batshaw, M. L. (1997). *Children with disabilities* (4th ed.). Baltimore: Brookes.

Batshaw, M. L. (2001). *When your child has a disability: The complete source book of daily and medical care.* Baltimore: Brookes.

Beckman, P. J. (1991). Comparison of mothers' and fathers' perceptions of the effect of young children with and without disabilities. *American Journal on Mental Retardation, 95,* 585–595.

Cadman, D., Rosenbaum, P., Boyle, M., & Offord, D. (1991). Children with chronic illness: Family and parent demographic characteristics and psychosocial adjustment. *Pediatrics, 87,* 884–889.

Case-Smith, J. (1998). Foundations and principles. In J. Case-Smith (Ed.), *Pediatric occupational therapy and early intervention* (pp. 3–25). Boston: Butterworth-Heinemann.

Centers for Disease Control. (2003). *Programs in brief. Developmental disabilities: What is the public health problem?* Retrieved October 3, 2003, from http::/www.cdc.gov/programs/defects8.htm.

Cronin, A. (2003). Mothering a child with hidden impairments. *American Journal of Occupational Therapy* (in press).

Dunst, C., Trivette, C., & Dea, A. (1988). *Enabling and empowering families: Principles and guidelines for practice.* Cambridge, MA: Brookline Books.

Dykens, E., Rosner, B., & Butterbaugh, G. (1998). Exercise and sports in children and adolescents with developmental disabilities: Positive physical and psychosocial effects. *Child and Adolescent Psychiatric Clinics of North America, 7,* 757–771.

Dyson, L. L. (1991). Families of young children with handicaps: Parental stress and family functioning. *American Journal on Mental Retardation, 95,* 623–629.

Dyson, L. L. (1997). Fathers and mothers of school-age children with developmental disabilities: Parental stress, family functioning, and social support. *American Journal on Mental Retardation, 102,* 267–279.

Faux, S. A. (1993). Siblings of children with chronic physical and cognitive disabilities. *Journal of Pediatric Nursing, 8,* 305–317.

Glidden, L. M. (1993). What we do not know about families with children who have developmental disabilities: Questionnaire on resources and stress as a case study. *American Journal on Mental Retardation, 97,* 481–495.

Gorman, J. (2003). Recognizing and addressing the mental health needs of children: A new understanding of treatment options and efficacy. *CNS Spectrum 8,* 249.

Green, A. (2001). Grandma's hands: parental perception of the importance of grandparents as secondary caregivers in families of children with disabilities. *International Journal of Aging and Human Development, 53,* 11–33.

Hastings, R. P., & Brown, T. (2002). Behavior problems of children with autism, parental self-efficacy, and mental health. *American Journal on Mental Retardation, 107,* 222–232.

Hartman, A., Radin, M., & McConnell, B. (1992). Parent-to-parent support: A critical component of health care services for families. *Issues in Comprehensive Pediatric Nursing, 15,* 55–67.

Humphrey, R. (1989). Early intervention and the influence of the occupational therapist on the parent-child relationship. *American Journal of Occupational Therapy, 43,* 738–741.

Humphry, R., & Case-Smith, J. (2001). Working with families. In J. Case-Smith (Ed.), *Occupational therapy for children* (4th ed.) (pp. 95–135). St Louis: Mosby.

Hutzler, Y., Chacham, A., Bergman, U., & Szeinberg, A. (1998). Effects of a movement and swimming program on vital capacity and water orientation skills of children with cerebral palsy, *Developmental Medicine and Child Neurology, 40,* 176–181.

Johnson, B. S. (2000). Mothers' perceptions of parenting children with disabilities. *American Journal of Maternal and Child Nursing, 25,* 127–132.

Kaplan, H., & Sadock, B. (1998). *Synopsis of psychiatry* (8th ed.). Baltimore: Williams and Wilkins.

Kids Health for Parents, Web site sponsored by the Nemours Foundation. Retrieved July 17, 2003, from http://www.kidshealth.org/parent/medical/brain/cerebral_palsy.html.

Kellegrew, D. H. (2000). Constructing daily routines: A qualitative examination of mothers with young children with disabilities. *American Journal of Occupational Therapy, 54,* 252–259.

Krauss, M. W. (1993). Child-related and parenting stress: Similarities and differences between mothers and fathers of children with disabilities. *American Journal of Mental Retardation, 97,* 393–404.

Lobato, D. J. (1990). *Brothers, sisters, and special needs: Information and activities for helping young siblings of children with chronic illness and developmental disabilities.* Baltimore: Brookes.

Mathews, K. (1998). *Developmental delay.* Children's Virtual Hospital. Retrieved October 3, 2003, from http://www.vh.org/pediatric/patient/pediatrics/developmental delay/index.html.

McGibbon, N., Andrade, C., Widener, G., & Cintas, H. (1998). Effect of an equine-movement therapy program on gait, energy expenditure, and motor function in children with spastic cerebral palsy: A pilot study. *Developmental Medicine and Child Neurology, 40,* 754–762.

Merriam-Webster's medical dictionary. Springfield, MA: Merriam-Webster, Inc.

Meyer, D. J., & Vadasy, P. A. (1994). *Sibshops: Workshops for brothers and sisters of children with special needs.* Baltimore: Brookes.

Mooar, P. (2002). Experiences as sports coordinator for the Philadelphia County Special Olympics, *Clinical Orthopedics, 396,* 50–55.

NICHCY. (1998). *Children with disabilities: Understanding sibling issues.* Retrieved October 3, 2003, from http://www.nichcy.org/pubs/newsdig/nd21txt.htm.

NICHCY. (2000). Questions and answers about IDEA. In *News Digest 21 (ND21)* (2nd ed.). Retrieved October 3, 2003, from http://www.nichcy.org/pubs/newsdig/nd21txt.htm.

Powell, T. H., & Gallagher, P. A. (1993). *Brothers and sisters: A special part of exceptional families.* Baltimore: Brookes.

Roach, M., Orsmond, G., & Barratt, M. (1999). Mothers and fathers of children with Down syndrome: Parental stress and involvement in childcare. *American Association on Mental Retardation, 104,* 422–436.

Schor, E. (2003). Family pediatrics: Report of the Task Force on the Family. *Pediatrics, 111,* 1541–1571.

Seideman, R. Y., & Kleine, P. (1995). A theory of transformed parenting: Parenting a child with developmental delay/ mental retardation. *Nursing Research, 44,* 38–44.

Seltzer, M., Floyd, F., Pettem, Y., & Hong, J. (2001). Life course impacts of parenting a child with a disability. *American Journal on Mental Retardation, 106,* 265–286.

Schubert, D. T. (2003). *Sibling needs—Helpful information for parents.* Retrieved October 3, 2003, from http://www.autism.org/sibling/sibneeds.html.

Shepard, M., & Mahon, M. (1996) Chronic conditions and the family. In P. Jackson & J. Vessey (Eds.), *Primary care of the child with a chronic condition* (2nd ed.) (pp. 41–57). St. Louis: Mosby.

Stoneman, Z., Brody, G. H., Davis, K., Crapps, J. M., & Malone, D. M. (2003). Ascribed role relations between children with mental retardation and their younger siblings. *American Journal on Mental Retardation, 95,* 537–550.

The Arc. (2000). *Siblings: Brothers and sisters of people who have mental retardation.* Retrieved October 3, 2003, from http://thearc.org/faqs/sibling.html.

U.S. Department of Education. Office of Civil Rights. *Protecting students with disabilities: Frequently asked questions about Section 504 and the education of children with disabilities.* Retrieved April 2, 2004 from http://www.ed.gov/about/offices/list/ocr/504faqhtml?exp=0.

Weiss, S. (1991). Stressors experienced by family caregivers of children with pervasive developmental disorders. *Child Psychiatry and Human Development, 21,* 203–216.

Wetherow, D. (2003). *Reflections on respite.* Community Works: Retrieved October 3, 2003, from http://www.communityworks.info/articles/respite.htm.

Willoughby, J., & Glidden, L. M. (1995). Fathers helping out: Shared child care and marital satisfaction of parents of children with disabilities. *American Journal of Mental Retardation 99,* 399–406.

Winton, P. J., & Winton, R. E. (2000). Family systems. In J. W. Solomon (Ed.), *Pediatric skills for occupational therapy assistants* (pp. 11–37). St. Louis: Mosby.

World Health Organization. (2002). ICF: International Classification of Functioning and Disability. Geneva, Switzerland: World Health Organization.

CHAPTER

14

Transitions to Adult Life

Steven Wheeler, PhD, OTR/L
Assistant Professor
Division of Occupational Therapy
West Virginia University
Morgantown, West Virginia

with contributions from

Keiba Shaw, PT, EdD
Assistant Professor
University of South Florida
Tampa, Florida

Objectives:

Upon completion of this chapter, the reader should be able to

▇ Understand factors contributing to the attainment of adult status.

▇ Appreciate the manner in which early life experiences impact the transition to adulthood.

▇ Understand theoretical explanations of psychosocial, cognitive, and physical development during the transition to young adulthood.

▇ Identify factors contributing to the decision to leave home.

▇ Understand the transitional process of occupational and vocational choice and the pursuit of related goals.

▇ Recognize the importance of intimacy during the transition to adulthood along with the stages leading up to decisions related to marriage and parenting.

▇ Understand behaviors and experiences that characterize a problematic transition to young adulthood.

Key Terms

adaptive cognition

crystallization stage (of vocational choice)

cycle of violence

experimentation period

fantasy period

Ginzberg, Eli

Holland, John

implementation stage (of vocational choice)

intimacy

isolation

personality types

realistic career exploration

specification stage (of vocational choice)

Super, Donald

tentative period

vocational self-concept

INTRODUCTION

For many adolescents struggling to move beyond the years of turbulence, the idea of adulthood is an exciting one. Adulthood normally represents a time of increased independence, the opportunity to pursue personal goals without the intensity of supervision and structure of previous years. Unfortunately, the transitional years can hardly be considered uneventful and without challenge. Answering the questions "Who am I?" and "Where am I going?" can be difficult during late adolescence, yet establishing a self-concept and personal direction is essential to successful career selection, mate selection, and assumption of community responsibilities.

In fact, the years characterizing the transition to adulthood, normally considered as between the ages of 16 and 24 years, are characterized by dramatic life changes. In addition to being numerous, the changes during the transition to young adulthood are of critical importance given the personal, financial, and social costs associated with unsatisfying careers, unsuccessful marriages, and parenting problems. If problem-solving skills and decision-making ability are influenced by life experience, then the transitioning to adulthood can be conceptualized as a period when major life decisions are made without much life experience upon which to base them.

This chapter will provide an overview of the various issues associated with the transition to young adulthood. Establishing when an individual actually becomes an "adult" is not as clear as one might think, with numerous factors influencing the manner by which one assumes and participates within the roles commonly associated with adulthood. A brief review of psychosocial, cognitive, and physical development during the transitional years will be presented as a means to establish a greater appreciation of the relationship between human development and societal participation. Theoretical ideas on career selection, marriage, and parenting will be discussed with an emphasis on highlighting

factors that contribute to both success and adjustment problems. As in other periods in the life cycle, societal participation as a young adult is highly influenced by the manner in which one has negotiated developmental challenges faced at earlier periods. The coming together of numerous challenges during young adulthood establishes the foundation for the assumption of adult responsibilities.

THE CHALLENGE OF DEFINING THE TRANSITION TO ADULTHOOD

There is no clear formula to determine when one leaves the world of adolescence to become an adult. The human body becomes mature in late adolescence and is at its peak performance from this age through young adulthood. Physical maturity and age are the most commonly considered factors, but even these are variable in Western cultures given the differences in age by which someone is legally allowed to drive a car, vote, consume alcoholic beverages, or get married. Instead of limiting onset of adulthood to a single factor, it is generally agreed that adult status is the integration of chronologic age with cognitive development, physical development, and societal experience. Consideration of the 16-year-old mother, the 24-year-old college student still financially dependent on his parents, and the 20-year-old individual with severe disabilities can help one appreciate the complexity of determining when adolescence ends and adulthood begins. Within the framework of the ICF (World Health Organization, 2002), adulthood is determined primarily by personal and environmental contextual factors.

Defining the transition to adulthood requires an understanding of what actually constitutes adult roles and responsibilities. Magen, Austrian, and Hughes (2002) identified the following developmental tasks as characteristic of the transition to adulthood process:

1. Moving out of the adolescent world while questioning it and one's place in it—a process involving separations, endings, and transformations.
2. Exploring possibilities in the adult world, testing living choices, and consolidating an initial adult identity.
3. Forming a dream with a place in the life structure.
4. Forming a mentor relationship lasting an average of 2–3 years.
5. Choosing an occupation and forming love relationships leading to marriage and family.

Expectations associated with adulthood are heavily influenced by one's culture. In Western culture these expectations typically include leaving high school to pursue higher education or enter the workforce, establishing an independent place of residence away from the family home, establishing relationships that are intimate in nature and that progress toward marriage, and attaining financial independence. As individuals become more independent from their families of origin, societal contextual factors play a larger role in functional performance.

According to Havinghurst (1972), a major difference between adolescence and young adulthood is the removal of preestablished life goals. Up until high school graduation—one of the ultimate achievements of adolescents—many milestones, privileges, and responsibilities were attained by virtue of a significant event, such as a birthday or completion of a school grade. For example, eligibility to obtain a driver's license, participate in various social activities (sports leagues, clubs, etc.), participate in religious activities, and/or vote are bestowed on persons of a particular age. This differs from young adulthood, whereby prestige, privileges, and opportunity become less a reflection of the passage of time and more dependent upon psychomotor skills, emotional strength, and the ability to apply knowledge to situations. In some situations, family connections become more important than actual skills and abilities.

DEMOGRAPHIC TRENDS AND THE TRANSITIONAL YEARS

Despite fluctuations over the past half-century, the number of young adults as a percentage of the American population has remained virtually unchanged from that of 1960 (U.S. Department of Commerce, Bureau of the Census, 1994). However, this does not mean that changes in the demographics of this age group have not occurred. A significant shift has occurred in terms of the racial and ethnic makeup of late adolescents and young adults in the United States. Cultural diversity is on the rise, a trend that is expected

to continue. Growth in the minority populations will be significant, while the white, non-Hispanic segment is expected to show little or no percentage growth (McKenzie, Pinger, & Kotecki, 1999).

The cultural trend in demographics of this population is worthy of consideration in a discussion of how the transition to adulthood is defined. Greater cultural diversity further complicates our defining the stage, given that cultures and societies differ in terms of explaining the appropriate age for leaving school, leaving the home or origin, beginning a full-time job, getting married, and becoming a parent (Shanahan, 2000; Farley, 1996; George, 1993).

PHYSICAL DEVELOPMENT AND HEALTH

The years associated with the transition to adulthood mark a progression toward the attainment of peak physical status and optimal health. Between the ages of 19 and 26 individuals typically reach the optimal speed of reaction time and attain adult growth of the skeletal, respiratory, and cardiovascular systems. An overview of biophysical changes during the transitional years is provided in Table 14–1.

Adolescents and young adults have fewer colds and respiratory problems than children do, and are faced with fewer chronic health problems than can occur at later stages of the life cycle. This age group has benefited considerably from public health efforts to reduce diseases such as polio and measles.

Individuals reach peak maturity in their third decade, at about their early 20s, with functional decline of varying magnitude beginning in subsequent decades (Richardson & Rosenberg, 1989). Decline in physical functioning often is not noticeable, or is easily ignored during young adulthood. Interestingly, the risk of physical inactivity as a young adult was found to be linearly related to low scores received as children on childhood physical fitness tests (Dennison et al., 1988). Also of interest is the fact that athletes who continuously train still experience a decline in physiologic function and competitive performance (Shephard, 1999) consistent with the normal age-related changes taking place over time.

Apparently, being stronger and healthier appears to negatively affect one's belief in the need to practice healthy behaviors. Research has indicated that despite understanding what constitutes healthy behaviors, college students believe that they personally would probably never have a drinking problem or have a heart attack regardless of how much they exercise, smoke, or eat high-cholesterol foods (Weinstein, 1984). Such a tendency to underestimate the personal risks of health-compromising behaviors may help explain why so many young adults develop patterns of poor nutrition, missing

TABLE 14–1 Physical Changes During the Transition to Adulthood

System	Changes
Skeletal system	• Growth essentially complete around 25 years of age. • Vertebral column continues to grow until about age 30.
Neuromuscular system	• Muscular performance at peak performance between 20 and 30 years of age. • Reaction times generally peak just before onset of young adulthood and remain constant until late twenties.
Integumentary system	• After adolescence skin begins to lose moisture, gradually becoming more dry and wrinkled with age. • First signs of gray hair and baldness may appear in young adulthood. • Unwanted hair growth may appear.
Cardiovascular system	• Has established adult size and rhythm by 16 years of age. • Total blood volume of young adult is 70 to 85 ml per kilogram of body weight. • Blood pressure rises slowly from early childhood, and cholesterol levels increase from the age of 21 years.
Respiratory system	• Mature in young adulthood. • Body's ability to use oxygen optimally is more dependent on efficiency of cardiovascular system and needs of skeletal muscle than on maturity of lungs.
Gastrointestinal system	• Digestive tract displays a decrease in the amount of some digestive juices after 30 years of age. • Ptyalin (enzyme used to digest starches) in the saliva decreases after 20 years of age. • Third molars ("wisdom teeth") normally erupt between 20 and 21 years and often need to be removed to prevent irreparable damage to proper occlusion of the jaws.
Genitourinary system	• Total urinary output in 24-hour period ranges between 1,000 and 2,000 ml for the average young adult. • Uterus reaches its maximum weight at about 30 years of age. • Statistically, the optimal period for reproduction in females (in terms of greatest frequency of successful pregnancies) is between 20 and 30 years of age.

Adapted from Ashburn, 1986.

meals, inadequate exercise, poor sleep patterns, and smoking and drinking habits (Santrock, 1999).

Poor personal-lifestyle choices seem common during late adolescence and early adulthood and can have adverse long-term consequences when they impact one's health status. Among the most dangerous and problematic of health-compromising behaviors are risky sexual activities. *Risky sexual behaviors* have been described as those involving multiple sexual partners or high-risk partners, or engaging in unprotected sexual intercourse (Millstein & Moscicki, 1995). Gonorrhea rates have remained high, and rates of acquired immune deficiency syndrome (AIDS) have risen steadily since 1990 despite significant improvements in many areas of public health. Each year in the United States 8 million cases of *sexually transmitted diseases (STDs)* occur in people under age 25 (U.S. Department of Health and Human Services, Public Health Service, 1997).

High-risk sexual activities during the transitional years to adulthood often occur in the context of other health-compromising behaviors such as alcohol and drug abuse (Ericksen & Trocki, 1992). The relationship is such that youth who continue to abuse alcohol and drugs into adulthood also tend to participate in high levels of risky sexual behaviors. The most commonly used and abused psychoactive substance is alcohol, and heavy drinking levels are particularly high during adolescence and young adulthood. In the United States approximately 80 percent of twelfth-grade students report having used alcohol in their lifetimes (Johnston et al., 2000), and nearly half of college students admit drinking heavily (Johnston, O'Malley, & Bachman, 1988).

The actual impact of alcohol and drug use on the eventual transition to adulthood is unclear. For some adolescents, moderate alcohol use appears to be positively related to psychosocial functioning and adjustment to the demands of young adulthood (Labouvie, 1990; Maggs, 1997). For others, however, alcohol use contributes to serious adjustment problems in later life (Hill et al., 2000). During the high school years, those abusing drugs and alcohol demonstrated greater levels of truancy and participated less in recreational and religious activities (Bachman, Johnson, & O'Malley, 1990). College students who drink heavily are more likely to miss classes, sustain physical injuries, and engage in unprotected sex (Johnston, O'Malley, & Bachman, 1990). Further discussion on the dangers of substance abuse and other health-compromising behaviors is provided in the following section, "Applying Theory to Practice." Fortunately, use of alcohol and drugs tends to decrease for the majority as individuals approach their mid-twenties.

Applying Theory to Practice: Hidden Hazard of Peak Physical Performance and Health

Young adults can draw on their physical resources to experience considerable enjoyment and productivity. Social and affective pressures that characterize adolescence and early adulthood tempt individuals to abuse their newly acquired physical and cognitive skills. The fact that they can bounce back from considerable stress and exertion may lead many young adults to push their bodies too far. It is not uncommon for career-oriented individuals to work or study long hours in order to succeed, denying themselves proper nutrition and rest.

The transitional years from adolescence to adulthood mark a period of increased autonomy, affiliation with peers, and risk-taking behavior (Donovan & Jessor, 1985). Alcohol consumption and heavy-drinking episodes (having five or more drinks in a row) tend to be higher during young adulthood than at any other period across the lifespan (Johnson et al., 1998). Estimates of alcohol abuse and dependence prevalence among young adults approximate 16 percent (Grant et al., 1994). Alcohol-use patterns in young adulthood are the product of behaviors often begun during adolescence. The 1999 Mentoring for the Future national survey found that approximately 80 percent of twelfth-graders had used alcohol in their lifetimes (Johnston et al., 2000). Use of cigarettes, marijuana, amphetamines, barbiturates, and hallucinogens is also high in adolescence and young adulthood in comparison to other developmental periods in the life cycle (Merline et al., 2004).

Given these risk statistics and factors, it should be no surprise that the highest percentage of traumatic spinal cord injuries and traumatic brain injuries occurs during late adolescence and young adulthood. Fifty-six percent of traumatic spinal cord injuries occur in persons between 16 and 30 years of age, with the most common age being 19 years (Stover, DeLisa, & Whiteneck, 1995). Statistics on traumatic brain injury indicate a similar occurrence pattern, with those between

the ages of 15 and 24 being at the highest risk. In both conditions, rates of occurrence are higher for males than for females. SCI and TBI also share common causes, with motor vehicle accidents, falls, and violence ranking as the most likely factors. An understanding of the theoretical aspects of and stresses associated with transitioning from adolescence to adulthood is critical for the health professional working with adults with spinal-cord or brain injuries. Negotiating the developmental tasks associated with this developmental stage is particularly difficult in conjunction with the long rehabilitation, recovery, and adjustment process for such injuries. Given that young adulthood emphasizes independent living, financial independence, career development, long-term relationships, and parenting responsibilities, the rehabilitation process with persons with SCI and TBI can be particularly challenging.

What factors influence heavy drinking in late adolescence and young adulthood? It is unlikely that substance abuse during the transition to adulthood can be attributed to a single cause. Research has suggested that youth lacking role models and a productive daily routine are more likely to use and abuse alcohol and drugs, a fact that emphasizes the important roles of institutions such as home, school, and church (Bachman, Johnson, & O'Malley, 1981). As one approaches adulthood, education and relationships become increasingly linked to substance abuse. Findings from a longitudinal study of more than 33,000 individuals from their senior year of high school through their early twenties suggested that

- College students drink more but smoke less than those ending their education at high school.
- Persons engaged or married drink less than single and divorced persons.
- Marijuana use is higher for singles than for married persons.
(Merline et al., 2004)

Stressful life events have also been linked to substance abuse. Evidence suggests that drinking is positively related to stressful life events (Weidner et al., 1998), depression (Sher et al., 1991), and nervousness (Swendsen et al., 2000) during young adulthood and to similar variables during adolescence (Chassin et al., 1996; Hussong & Chassin, 1994). Whether alcohol or drugs are used as a means of psychological coping is subject to individual expectations and influenced by cultural norms. For example, Rutledge and Sher (2001) hypothesize that cultural norms may be more supportive of stress-motivated drinking in men, particularly as they approach their mid-twenties. Fewer gender differences as regards being motivated to drink in an effort to reduce stress have been found among teens coping with problems (Greenberg, Lewis, & Dodd, 1999). The following "Applying Theory to Practice" section provides health professionals with some ideas on how to educate clients attempting to deal with the numerous stresses that characterize the transition to adulthood.

Applying Theory to Practice: Managing Stress During the Transition to Adulthood

The period marking the transition from adolescence to adulthood is marked by a number of major life changes. While unexpected life events such as the breakup of a long-term relationship or illness of a close person can be difficult to cope with, even life changes that are planned, such as a new job, marriage, or moving to a new home, can challenge our ability to cope. Holmes and Rahe (1967) studied the relationship between life events and stress-related health problems. They concluded that an accumulation of significant life events in any one year increases one's vulnerability to stress-related illness. Change disrupts our normal routines and requires that we adjust to new situations, often requiring us to replace old habits and develop new behaviors. In his book, *Free Yourself from Harmful Stress* (1997), clinical psychologist Trevor Powell identifies a number of strategies that an individual can employ to manage change. The health-care professional working with the adolescent or young adult having difficulty managing the numerous changes characteristic of this period may find these ideas helpful. According to Powell, preparing for change involves the following:

- *Develop a positive attitude*: See change as a opportunity and challenge that can make you a stronger and better person.
- *Find out as much as you can*: Having more information about a new situation allows you to be more prepared to deal with the change.
- *Express your own feelings*: Acknowledge fears, and avoid thoughts based on "shoulds," such as "I should be used to this by now."
- *Develop a plan of action*: When dealing with a new situation, look for potential losses and gains. Attempt to maximize gains and minimize losses.
- *Take care of your health*: Eat well and exercise during periods of change.
- *Rally your support network*: Let family and friends know how you feel about the change.
- *Don't take on too much*: Learn how to delegate, and say no to extra commitments.
- *Relax*: Take time away from the situation to allow for emotional repair.

Stress-management skills are critical to a successful transition to young adulthood. The manner in which a particular situation is managed is a reflection of one's interpretation of the event, what it means to the individual, and the person's ability to cope.

SELF-CARE IN THE TRANSITION YEARS

To achieve adult status the individual must have effective strategies for managing ADL and IADL tasks. These tasks may be performed using adaptations and compensations, but the adult is expected to manage the process himself. The AOTA Practice Framework (2002) includes the following self-care activities as integral to independent function: bathing and showering grooming, bowel and bladder management, dressing, eating and feeding, functional mobility, personal device care, personal hygiene and grooming, sexual activity, sleep/rest, and toilet hygiene. By the age of 16 most adolescents have acquired the necessary skills to be independent in all of these areas. In addition, the typical 16-year-old can participate in basic home management, meal preparation, and child- and pet-care activities within the context of their home. In the past many young people were married and beginning their adult life before the age of 20. While most North American teens continue to live with their parents, they possess the IADL skills to support the operation of the household with their daily performance of cooking, cleaning, and supervision of younger siblings.

As discussed in Chapter 12, the adolescent period is characterized by the achievement of many important milestones that prepare the individual to enter young adulthood, which typically occurs upon attainment of relative independence from the parents and a move away from the family home. Although the exact age at which these milestones are reached varies from 18 years of age to the early 20s, certain prerequisite accomplishments are typically achieved. First, as the individual enters young adulthood she is typically independent in IADLs, including clothing care and meal preparation. The ability to earn and manage money has been developed and practiced. The young adult has typically been driving for some time, which has further fostered independence. Finally, upon entrance to young adulthood, the individual has contributed to her self-definition through the increasing ability to make meaningful contributions to her living environment.

CULTURAL DIFFERENCES VERSUS INDIVIDUAL DIFFERENCES

Discussions of cultural influences on development and the process of transitioning to adulthood can be both interesting and controversial. Above all, individual differences among people must be emphasized and stereotyping avoided. Differences appear to exist between cultures, but, even more, tremendous variation in regard to the when, how, and why of the transitional process appears present within cultures. Cultural differences tend to be viewed within the context of a multidimensional phenomenon that encompasses race, gender, and economic resources. For example, while differences have been noted in the timing of marriages and first births between whites and blacks in the United States (Spain & Bianchi, 1996), these differences are greatly diminished when economic factors are controlled for (Oppenheimer et al., 1997). Furthermore, racial and ethnic differences in educational and work choices disappeared when parental education and income, family structure, and aptitude test scores are controlled. Again, while differences may exist across cultures, the extent to which they do is based on a complex array of factors.

UNDERSTANDING TRANSITION TO ADULTHOOD WITHIN LIFE CYCLE

It is difficult to argue with the idea that how we approach the transition to adulthood is heavily influenced by our experiences through life. The *psychosocial stages* of Erik Erikson (1950) are among the most frequently cited to explain how problems during childhood and adolescence can negatively affect our ability to face the many challenges of young adulthood. Clearly, when one thinks of the prerequisites to managing independent living, a career, and long-term **intimacy**, the ability to trust, to be autonomous, to have initiative and industry, and to have established personal identity in regard to sex roles, occupation, politics, and religion must be in place.

The impact of early childhood experiences on one's ability to negotiate the transition from adolescence to young adulthood has received considerable attention from researchers over the years. The theory of the **cycle of violence** is based upon the hypothesis that a childhood history of physical abuse predisposes a person to violence in later years, a notion supported by longitudinal research (Widom & Maxfield, 2001). Figure 14–1 illustrates the cycle of violence. In this cycle, the victim is trapped in a pattern violence where one person in an intimate relationship tries to control the other through force, intimidation, or threats. As the victim feels increasingly isolated, the violence escalates in intensity and frequency.

Studies have found that adverse childhood experiences such as sexual abuse, serious illness of a close person, or major loss events (such as death of close person) can affect one's ability to develop the mature coping skills and emotional strength necessary for successful and satisfying performance of adult roles and responsibilities (Tuulio-Henriksson et al., 2000; Romans et al., 1999).

While our genetic makeup clearly influences who we are, our experiences throughout childhood and adolescence just as clearly contribute to whether or not

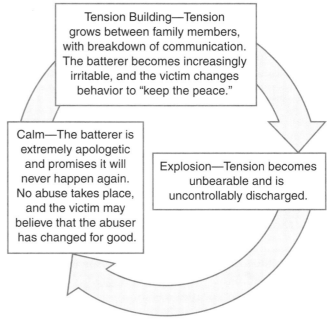

FIGURE 14–1 Cycle of Violence (adapted from Widom & Maxfield, 2001)

we are equipped with the psychosocial, cognitive, and physical skills for prosocial coping and adaptation. When more primitive coping styles persist, the challenge of making life-altering decisions and mastering the inevitable stresses during late adolescence and young adulthood can simply be beyond one's capacity. A number of theories have been developed in an effort to explain the variables contributing to the assumption of adult roles and responsibilities. Those particularly relevant to the transition from adolescence to adulthood will be discussed in the following sections.

THEORETICAL PERSPECTIVES ON TRANSITION TO ADULTHOOD

The number and magnitude of decisions to be made in order to progress to adulthood can create considerable personal confusion and life stress. Among the questions to be successfully answered are

- What are my goals?
- Who am I?
- Whom should I marry?
- Should I have children?
- What kind of career should I pursue?
- What are my priorities?
- What do I value?

As mentioned, Erikson (1950) theorizes that the ability to answer such questions and participate accordingly requires successful negotiation of previous developmental *life tasks.* Those young adults failing to resolve the tasks and conflicts of previous psychosocial stages experience a discrepancy between current life demands and ability to manage. For such individuals, stressful life events, such as loss of a job or a relationship breakup, can trigger a recurrence of previously unresolved task demands and immature coping patterns (Paul, 1992). Persistence or increase in immature coping patterns into adulthood has been associated with the development of psychiatric disturbances (Tuulio-Henriksson et al., 1997).

PSYCHOSOCIAL AND EMOTIONAL DEVELOPMENT

The inability to trust others has an obvious impact on one's ability to establish the level of intimacy and commitment commonly associated with adult relationships. Commitment to another person in a long-term, intimate relationship is virtually impossible for the individual preoccupied with fears of being hurt or rejected. The closer one becomes to another person, the greater the risks of being taken advantage of, having one's personal weaknesses exposed, and failing to meet the expectations of the other. Close relationships always involve an exchange of demands and expectations, some of which are unfortunately difficult and unpleasant (Kiefer, 1988). According to Erikson, persons failing to achieve intimacy in young adulthood experience **isolation**, or the inability to have genuine physical exchanges with others who could offer empathy, understanding, support, encouragement, and insight.

Healthy psychological development permits a greater capacity to manage life stressors in a manner conducive to meeting personal goals. Coping patterns tend to develop away from the neurotic and egocentric patterns of childhood to more pro-social strategies as one enters adulthood. In adulthood there is a trend among both men and women toward greater conscientiousness and self-control, along with an increasing sense of being connected to others in the community. Changes in personality development occurring during the transition from adolescence to adulthood were investigated in a study by Roberts, Caspi, and Moffitt (2001) and are summarized as follows:

- Both men and women become more forceful and decisive.
- Both men and women grow more persistent in work-related efforts.
- Both men and women feel less victimized by life, become less likely to see the world as full of enemies, and become less inclined to hurt other people or seek revenge on those slighting them.

When one develops the psychological and emotional maturity necessary for participation in an intimate relationship, additional levels of maturity and psychological development can be expected. Persons in such relationships have reported an increase in extraversion and self-esteem and a decrease in the traits of shyness and neuroticism (Neyer & Asendorpf, 2001).

COGNITIVE DEVELOPMENT AND ROLE OF EXECUTIVE COGNITIVE FUNCTIONS

Young adulthood is generally considered the period in which an individual approaches his peak of cognitive development and intellectual efficiency. As one moves through the struggles and challenges of adolescence, life experiences accumulate and combine with neurophysiologic changes to establish the foundation for abstract reasoning and mature coping. Much of the behavior exhibited by persons during the transitional years can be explained through an understanding of cognitive development during this period.

The notion of cognitive change beyond adolescence conflicts in some respects with the theory of cognitive development developed by Jean Piaget (1972). According to Piaget, one's highest level of cognitive development is marked by the presence of formal operations and abstract thought attained during adolescence. However, other cognitive theorists suggest that there are considerable differences between adolescent and adult thinking. In adolescence, thinking is more dualistic in nature—acquiring knowledge and differentiating right from wrong. To successfully function in adulthood, the adolescent must give up looking for the absolute truth in favor of the practice of considering a problem in the context by which it is presented (Schaie, 1978). Such a shift in mental activity represents the difference between the requirements during "classroom" activities, where a single answer exists, to managing more complex adult issues such as intimacy and parenting, where a single answer rarely exists.

The ability to think in a manner less constrained by the need to find a single answer has been termed **adaptive cognition**. In an attempt to investigate the presence of such thinking, students were interviewed at the end of each of their four years of college and asked, "What stood out?" during the previous year (Perry, 1981). The students' responses demonstrated a transition from dualistic thinking to more relativistic thought characterized by the ability to "give up" the possibility of a single truth in favor of multiple truths—each relative to the context in which events occur.

Labouvie-Vief (1985) conceptualizes the progression from adolescent to adult thinking as a transition from hypothetical to pragmatic thought. In a sense, such a shift represents a return to the more concrete methods of thinking that characterize childhood.

However, instead of considering such a shift as a regression in thinking, Labouvie-Vief saw the shift as a necessary component to solving real-life problems. As stated previously, managing career, relationships, parenting, and other adult roles requires the ability to accept inconsistencies as part of life, as opposed to hypothetical thinking whereby one seeks to resolve all contradictions.

Theories suggesting significant differences in adolescent and adult thinking are supported by changes in physical brain maturation during the transitional period. *Magnetic resonance imaging (MRI)* studies have discovered that different areas of the brain mature at different rates, a process that continues through adolescence and into adulthood. Of particular interest is the finding that the rate of myelination in the frontal, parietal, and temporal lobes differs in adolescent and adult brains (Thompson et al., 2000). Myelination in the brain implies more mature, efficient connections within the gray matter of the brain and subsequently greater functional capacity. The frontal lobes represent the location of the executive cognitive functions, defined in Chapter 3 as "the mental processes, such as initiation, problem solving, self-awareness, and cognitive flexibility, which organize our thoughts for action" (World Health Organization, 2002). Differences in frontal lobe maturation between adolescents and adults may help explain differences in judgment, degree of impulsivity, coping skills, and problem-solving ability.

MRI studies have also led to hypotheses that adolescents and adults differ in the manner by which emotions are processed within the brain. As adolescents progress toward adulthood, brain activity appears away from the amygdala, a brain center that mediates fear and other "gut reactions" to the frontal lobes (Baird et al., 1999). Such a shift fosters more reasoned perceptions and improved performance in complex emotional situations where considering alternatives and strategies is critical as opposed to acting on instinct.

THE LEAVING-HOME TRANSITION

It is a common occurrence for adolescents to dream of the day when they are "on their own," away from the rules and structure imposed by their parents. Unfortunately, the process of leaving home is not without its share of stressors. Leaving home typically means not only greater financial independence, but also taking greater responsibility for one's actions as well. Both parents and young adults expect that the leaving-home transition will occur around age 18, although notable variation exists in terms of when the process actually occurs (Harley & Mortimer, 1999). Given that taking responsibility for oneself and independent decision making are common markers of adult status, adolescence can be greatly extended in industrialized societies

where successful vocational participation requires many years of education and training.

Although research indicates that the process of leaving home is generally a positive experience (Cohen et al., 2003), difficulties with this transition are predictive of more problematic adjustment into adulthood (O'Connor, Allen, Bell, & Hauser, 1996). A child's leaving home is typically a stressful stage of a family's transition, requiring a redefining of family roles and rituals (Mederer & Hill, 1983). Whether or not the event is a positive one is reflective of the reasons for leaving home and the nature of the dynamics within the family. When leaving home is associated with conflict and discontent within the family, the individual's subsequent adjustment into adulthood is commonly problematic. However, for many families the leaving-home process actually results in a period of increased communication and decreased conflict with parents in comparison to the adolescent years (Cohen et al., 2003).

What are the main reasons for leaving home? The most common reasons are to pursue a job, to attend postsecondary education and training, and to get married or cohabitate. These activities generally represent normal developmental tasks that are consistent with culturally accepted standards of adulthood. Problems with the leaving-home transition are more likely to arise when marred by a history of family disruption and problematic parent-adolescent relationships (O'Connor et al., 1996; Stattin & Magnusson, 1996). Family conflict and less parental monitoring may leave the adolescent without the necessary supports and skills needed for a successful progression to independent living. Research has suggested that persons from divorced families, and particularly from stepfamilies, are more likely than children raised by their biologic parents to leave home at a young age and to do so for negative reasons, such as conflict or friction (Goldscheider & Goldscheider, 1993; McLanahan & Sandefur, 1994). Persons leaving home at younger ages have consistently shown greater risk for adjustment problems in comparison to their peers (White, 1994). Those with substance-abuse problems, lower school achievement, and a history of behavioral difficulties are also at risk for leaving home at earlier ages. When individuals leave home at an early age in an effort to *escape* family turmoil, as opposed to reasons related to education, career, or relationship commitment, they are often unprepared for financial independence and are forced into decisions emphasizing survival over the pursuit of personal goals.

OCCUPATIONAL AND VOCATIONAL CHOICE

Making career choices can be both exciting and frightening. In today's technological society, the transition to adulthood can be difficult for the non–college bound youth who may lack the structure, supports, and opportunities for full societal participation. The importance of decision making related to a career cannot be underestimated given the amount of time people tend to spend at work in adulthood, along with the impact of career on one's self-identity, social networks, and lifestyle. Once again, the adolescent is faced with a major life decision without the extensive life experience upon which to make an informed educated choice. As a result, many who begin college switch from their originally stated majors or leave before completing a degree in the direction of other life options. Furthermore, those beginning in a particular profession may find that the reality of the job differs from established beliefs, resulting in either prolonged dissatisfaction or efforts to switch careers to find one more compatible with their goals.

How do we decide what our career will be? Children often fantasize about "what I will be when I grow up," suggesting that the career-selection process is, at least to some degree, lifelong. However, it is clear that the transitional years from adolescence to adulthood are critical to establishing a suitable work role. As with other developmental milestones that occur throughout life, vocational development and career selection represent the dynamic interaction between the person and the environment. While one's personality obviously plays an important role in career interests, influences such as family support, the presence of role models, educational and training opportunities, and current life circumstances are also considerable. And the changing landscape of career choice and development over the past 25 years has been marked in particular by the changing societal norm of females in the workplace, a subject addressed later in this chapter. Theories looking at the process of vocational choice throughout the lifespan continue to evolve. Among the most common of these are the work of Eli Ginzberg, John Holland, and Donald Super.

GINZBERG'S DEVELOPMENTAL THEORY

Eli Ginzberg's developmental theory (1972; 1988) states that the process of occupational choice follows a developmental progression that begins in childhood and spans into the early adult years. The early and middle childhood years are marked by fantasizing about career options that tend to reflect those professions that are familiar, glamorous, or exciting to the child. It is during this **fantasy period** that a person is likely to express a desire to one day become a teacher, doctor, athlete, or superhero. It typically lasts until approximately age 11 or 12, at which time more realistic thinking about one's eventual career begins.

Decision making within the **tentative period**, according to Ginzberg, is marked by tentative consideration of one's personal skills, capacities, and values. The seemingly endless opportunities that characterized the fantasy period begin to meet the realities of what career one might be suited for. This tentative period is said to begin around the ages of 13 and 14 years and progresses to late adolescence, with an increasing level of awareness of factors that may pose restrictions on available career options. These considerations include economic realities and various potential personal and environmental barriers.

Following the period of **realistic career exploration** during late adolescence, the young adult moves to an **experimentation period** within the chosen career category. Ginzberg views the selection of career category as a process whereby information is collected and various options consistent with one's personality are investigated. Ultimately, **crystallization of vocational choice** occurs whereby a single occupation is selected from within a career category, such as choosing to be a nurse following a period of considering a career in health care.

HOLLAND'S PERSONALITY TYPE THEORY

John Holland's personality type theory (1987) emphasizes the notion of "fit" between one's personality and career selection. Consistent with Ginzberg, Holland indicates that people are attracted to occupations that complement their personalities. The extent to which one is successful and satisfied with her career choice is largely dependent on the strength of this fit. Holland matched six personality traits—investigative, social, realistic, artistic, conventional, and enterprising—to corresponding work environments (Papalia & Olds, 1996). Scientists and detectives, according to Holland's theory, demonstrate an investigative personality; mental health counselors or health-care workers a social personality; and mechanics or plumbers a realistic personality. Artistic personalities would choose a vocation such as writing, music, or art; conventional types would be bankers or lawyers, and enterprising people would have vocations related to sales or managerial positions (Papalia & Olds, 1996). Holland's theory goes on to state that women tend to exhibit more artistic, social, and conventional traits and therefore go into occupations suited to those types. While Holland's theory is most useful, it does not address the fact that many occupations require a combination of skills and traits, nor does it address environmental, social, or cultural influences in the choice of occupation. Additionally, this theory does not address the dynamics that exist between individuals and their environment at work or the development of careers as they age (Papalia & Olds, 1996). Holland's personality types are summarized in Table 14–2.

The idea of matching personality type to career selection has been particularly useful for career and guidance

TABLE 14–2	Holland's Personality Types	
Type	**Personality**	**Occupations of "Fit"**
Investigative	• Highly intelligent, socially indifferent, aloof. • Enjoys working with ideas.	Various scientific occupations.
Enterprising	• Driven by need to dominate others, particularly in regard to personal goal achievement. • Adventurous and persuasive, with strong leadership skills	Sales, politics, various supervisory positions.
Artistic	• Emotionally expressive and prefers individual expression over conformity. • Enjoys working with ideas and materials to express self.	The rarity of occupations that fit this category result in expression through leisure and hobbies. Often forced to choose second or third personality type category for occupational choice.
Conventional	• Values material possessions and social status. • Lower levels of education and prestige than most other personality types. • Preference for more structured tasks.	Secretaries, file clerks, bank tellers.
Social	• Strong preference for interacting with others.	Teaching, social work, counseling professions.
Realistic	• Physically robust, practical, and often non- or anti-intellectual. • Preference for dealing with "real-world" issues over hypothetical.	Construction work, farming, truck driving.

Adapted from Papalia & Olds, 1996.

counselors. Many counselors employ a practice of personality-type assessment as a precursor to assisting adolescents and young adults in making postsecondary education and/or training decisions.

SUPER'S SELF-CONCEPT THEORY

Donald Super's self-concept theory (1957; 1984) views the process of career choice as developmental in nature. The theory postulates that as one moves through childhood, adolescence, and adulthood, vocational decision making becomes clearer and more realistic. Super's theory is unique in its emphasis on the construct of self-concept, meaning ideas about oneself that begin during childhood. The self-concept as it relates to participation in a particular occupation and evolves through adolescence and young adulthood is termed the **vocational self-concept**. The stages that characterize this development are summarized in Table 14–3.

The **crystallization stage** is characteristic of early adolescence, in which only general ideas regarding a career are formulated. In the **specification stage** a more focused development of career ideas and career tracks occurs as the individual moves from early into late adolescence and young adulthood. In their early 20s young adults begin to explore career possibilities through entry-level jobs and/or professional job training, thereby entering

Super's third stage, the **implementation stage**. Establishment and progression of a career begin in the middle 20s, with the individual progressing in his mid-30s up the career ladder. Super's career development theory has been useful in its efforts to explain how individuals across the lifespan make vocational choices, but it has been criticized on the basis that these stages often do not progress in a linear fashion.

ABOUT CAREER-SELECTION THEORIES

Theories such as those of Ginzberg, Holland, and Super serve an important function in that they help us organize ideas and provide explanations about human behavior. Each has made important contributions to our understanding of how individuals pursue and stay satisfied within a particular career. However, as with many theories, criticisms do exist and warrant mention. Santrock (1999) acknowledges that while most people appear to follow a pattern of vocational development, the defined time frames of developmental theories fail to account for exceptions to the rule and individual differences in terms of both timing and sequence. Additionally, pure personality types, as suggested by Holland, are rare given the complexity of individuals.

Table 14–4 shows a comparison of different theories of vocational development. Perhaps the most

TABLE 14–3	Super's Stages of Vocational Self-Concept Development

Stage	Developmental Period	Definition
Crystallization	Adolescence	Consideration occurs of various vocational ideas consistent with one's self-concept.
Specification	Ages 18–21	Ideas about vocational interests become more specified.
Implementation	Ages 21–24	Process of skills training occurs along with experiences needed to pursue chosen career.
Stabilization	Ages 25–35	Individual works within desired profession. May make career changes and return to previous stages.

TABLE 14–4	Theories of Vocational Development Compared

	Theorist		
	Ginzberg (Developmental)	Holland (Personality Type)	Super (Self-Concept)
Childhood developmental period	*Fantasy period,* when career preferences reflect glamorous, exciting careers that bear little relation to eventual career choice.	Early personality development.	Ideas about the self formed (self-concept).
Perspectives on adolescence	*Tentative period,* of evaluating capacities and values during early period. *Realistic exploration* in later period that considers economic and practical realities.	Continued development of personality characteristics that result in one of six personality types. Exploration of careers reflects "fit" between personality type and occupations.	Continued development of vocational self-concept. Growing clarity about the self, and ideas about the self crystallize.
Early adulthood	Experimentation within career category following exploration process.	People attracted to occupations that complement personality. Six basic career-related personality types are investigative, social, realistic, artistic, conventional, and enterprising.	Particular occupations specified between ages 18 and 21. Implementation of career decisions occurs between 21 and 24. Vocational choices stabilize from 25 to 35.

accurate understanding of the career-development process comes from integrating features from each of these theories. It is difficult to argue with the notion that career choice is the culmination of a transitional process beginning in childhood. It is equally likely that one's occupational choice is ultimately influenced by her personality type and self-concept.

Issues and Trends: Female Vocational Choice and Career Development

The past three decades have seen a dramatic rise in the career aspirations of young women, to the point of converging with those of young men. In Western society today, it is expected that women be active participants in the labor force (Crompton, 2003). This view is accompanied by an equal expectancy for women to continue their family responsibilities, placing considerable strain on young women attempting to balance these competing responsibilities. Because women still assume most of the responsibility for childrearing and homemaking, researchers and theorists have become increasingly interested in understanding the factors contributing to career decision making among young women. In general, it has been concluded that by requiring consideration of how to succeed in the multiple roles of parent, partner, and worker, the career decision-making process for women includes a component that differs from that of most men.

What differentiates female career selection from that of men? According to a study commissioned by the American Association of University Women (1991), adolescent women harbored lower hopes for their careers than their male counterparts did and were significantly more likely to state that they lacked the skill or intelligence to attain their desired careers. Farmer (1985) tested a model of career development based on Bandura's (1977) social learning model with a group of high school students and found that background factors contribute significantly to the prediction of career aspiration for both genders. Specifically, women with a high commitment to homemaking were less motivated toward long-term career planning. However, it was noted that for men, high homemaking commitment and high career commitment coexisted.

O'Brien and Fassinger (1993) tested a causal model of career orientation and choice with a group of adolescent women and found contributing factors to include the characteristics of agency, ability, and gender-role attitudes. According to Bakan (1966), *agency* refers to the condition of being a differentiated individual. It is considered to represent the masculine aspects of the personality and is related to the needs for achievement, dominance, and autonomy (Maddi, 1989). O'Brien and Fastinger (1993) found that moderate levels of attachment and healthy individuation between mother and daughter provided an important basis for the daughter's choice of a future career. In addition, women holding more liberal attitudes toward the role of women (i.e., pro-feminist attitudes) in society tended to place greater value on their careers.

McCracken and Weitzman (1997) studied graduate and undergraduate women in an effort to investigate factors contributing to career development and multiple role planning. Their conclusions emphasized the *multiple-role lifestyle* of women and the importance of *self-efficacy* in regard to problem-solving ability to succeeding in career development in the midst of competing family roles. Those appraising themselves as positive problem solvers were considered to be more motivated to approach problems due to the fact that they expected to effectively cope with problem situations. Confidence in problem-solving ability precedes perceived skill in planning for multiple roles. The researchers viewed the process of obtaining and succeeding in the multiple-role lifestyle as a developmental process that required attainment of knowledge about these roles and how to effectively balance them.

ISSUES OF INTIMACY DURING TRANSITION TO ADULTHOOD

Developmental theorists have long emphasized the importance of companionship and intimacy during the transition to adulthood. Erikson (1964) emphasized that the quest to attain intimacy in early adulthood is "a turning point for the better or for worse" (p. 139) with

significant implications for adjustment to adult life. Despite being desired, attaining intimacy poses a considerable challenge for persons using considerable emotional, psychosocial, and physical resources during their adolescent years to achieve personal independence. The challenge of participating in an intimate relationship requires not only that one find a compatible partner, but also that he gives up some of his newfound independence. The individual is redefined within the system of the "couple" and typically must make compromises in personal goals, daily routine, and social relationships to nurture intimacy over time. Associated with intimacy is sexual activity. *Sexual activity* has been identified as an ADL that involves engagement in activities that result in sexual satisfaction (AOTA, 2002). Although physical and occupational therapists are often uncomfortable addressing issues of sexual activity with their clients, it is important to remember that this ADL is highly valued and very much a part of the experience of adulthood.

Is intimacy in young adulthood synonymous with marriage? Not necessarily, although statistics suggest that adults continue to show a strong predilection to marriage. This, despite trends indicating that marriages have become increasingly unstable and that both men and women are marrying later in life than in previous decades. The number of divorced adults in the United States rose from 4.3 million in 1970 to 17.4 million in 1994, increasing at an annual rate of 10 percent (U.S. Department of Health and Human Services (DHHS) (1994). Such staggering statistics appear to have had little effect on people's decision to eventually marry, however, based upon the fact that the proportion of women in the United States that never marry has remained at about 7 percent throughout the twentieth century (Santrock, 1999).

FACTORS CONTRIBUTING TO MATE SELECTION DURING TRANSITION TO ADULTHOOD

Throughout this transition period the young person develops attitudes and values that guide personal relationships. Sexuality, which emerges in adolescence, continues to develop and mature as part of a lifelong process. In their transition to adulthood, most individuals learn to enter into intimate sexual and emotional relationships and understand their own sexual orientation, although they may still experiment.

There is a trend toward increasing acceptance of homosexuality in North America, although this subject continues to be a source of political and societal debate. Psychology and psychiatry have accepted that a variety of sexual orientation is "normative." In the Fourth Edition of the *Diagnostic and Statistical Manual* by the American Psychiatric Association in 1994, only *gender identity disorder* was listed as a disorder related to homosexuality. A diagnosis of this disorder requires that an individual experience a strong and persistent identification with the opposite gender, and a sense of discomfort with his or her own gender. Lesbian, gay, or bisexual orientation without this kind of criteria does not indicate abnormal development. In a survey of over 1,000 high school–based counselors, psychologists, social workers, and nurses, as part of the Healthy Lesbian, Gay and Bisexual Students Project, a majority of the respondents did indicate that lesbian, gay, and bisexual students are at a greater risk than heterosexual students for physical and mental health concerns. These higher risks are associated with social stigmatization (Smith, 2001). Difficulties with peer acceptance, hindered exploration of intimate relationships, and the possibilities of strained or painful family relations often make formation of a positive identity a more difficult process for lesbian, gay, and bisexual young people. Elizur and Mintzer (2001) reported a stage model for same-gender identity formation that includes three steps: self-definition, self-acceptance, and disclosure. Elizur and Ziv (2001) found that family support and acceptance of the gay identity play a significant role in the psychological adjustment of gay individuals.

The progression toward intimacy in Western culture typically follows a defined developmental pattern marked by increasing commitment and redefining of oneself within the context of the relationship. Prearranged marriages are rare, in contrast to some Eastern cultures, necessitating some effort on the part of individuals to find a suitable mate. The prospect of loneliness is unfavorable for most young adults, serving as a motivator to search for a mate and make concessions necessary to foster success within the relationship.

For some people the search for a mate is a long, emotionally exhausting process. For others it is relatively easy. Regardless, the process naturally begins with the availability pool. One's friendships and contacts tend to reflect people with similar interests, education, and goals, as well as comparable social class. From those considered "eligible," initial choice of mate tends to reflect physical appearance and likeable personality in addition to features such as age, height, race, energy level, or social habits (Schuster, 1992). More complex aspects of successful relationships are explored as the couple moves beyond general friendship in the direction of intimacy. Factors such as personal values, religious beliefs, and family goals serve to either maintain or decrease interest in a relationship and are hence critical to the notion of long-term compatibility.

As with other developmental tasks, our preparation for participation in intimate relationships is a culmination of many factors that begin in childhood. One's family of origin plays a key role in not only influencing our values, beliefs, and opinions about intimate relationships, but also in providing approval or disproval about a relationship and a context that either fosters intimacy or serves as a barrier to it. The socialization process leading to adulthood is complex, but given the impact of family on this process, the impact of socialization cannot be underestimated. Family values and beliefs about race, culture, religion, and vocational choice all influence the young person as she explores her expanded social and community environments. Increasingly, diversity is accepted not only in school and in the workplace, but in intimate and marital relationships as well.

Research suggests that family discord contributes to troubled developmental outcomes, although considerably less consensus exists in regard to the extent of this impact (Shanahan, 2000). The absence of stable role models, low parental investment, weakened emotional bonds with their children, and heightened family stresses are among the factors hypothesized to negatively impact the transition to adulthood and ultimately one's beliefs about and reasons for seeking intimacy. Some research has suggested that parental divorce and a lack of economic resources are particularly detrimental to a child's development into young adulthood (Roth & Brooks-Gunn, 2003). In general, however, the magnitude of the relationship between negative childhood experiences, such as poverty and divorce, and negative outcomes in late adolescence and adulthood has been small, pointing to the diversity of families and individuals (Shanahan & Mortimer, 1996; Mayer, 1997). As emphasized by Shanahan (2000), many parents and nonparental adults serve as positive role models and provide nurturing relationships despite adverse family events or conditions.

The impact of culture and social class is discussed in Chapter 4. Culture tends to dictate the manner in which a partner is chosen and the roles of participating individuals as a relationship develops (Schuster, 1992). The same can be said for social class, although to a lesser degree and with greater variation. Research suggests that socioeconomic status and gender influence mate selection, career and lifestyle expectations, and awareness of future life role choices and conflicts (Segal et al., 2001). Persons from lower socioeconomic families are more likely to marry in their teens and early 20s and more likely to have marriage with pregnancy than are upper-class individuals (Saxton, 1990). Middle-class individuals are more likely to marry in their early to mid 20s, often during or immediately after career training (Schuster, 1992). It should be emphasized that these broad categorizations of social class are intended to be representative of trends and not to stereotype individuals. As is generally the case, individual differences and varying environments greatly impact the effect of social class on the mate-selection process.

STEPS LEADING TO MARRIAGE

As discussed previously, while not all long-term, intimate relationships lead to marriage, the vast majority of them do. Our culture greatly influences the steps leading to marriage—a progression that typically involves dating, courtship, and engagement. Most people in Western culture date many people before marriage. The steps leading to marriage and the functions of each as outlined by Schuster (1992) are shown in Table 14–5.

No sharp time line exists between dating and courtship, and the process is bound to repeat itself for the majority who fail to find their future marriage partner on the first try. A couple's engagement typically marks the point at which wedding planning begins and others view the couple as a single unit. Engagement provides added security to a relationship but, given the influence on one's self-concept and the need for personal sacrifices in the spirit of common objectives, it can be a time for increased tension and conflict within the relationship.

CHARACTERISTICS OF UNSUCCESSFUL MARRIAGES

It has long been believed that for any marriage to be successful, certain prerequisites are essential (Masters & Johnson, 1975). Compatibility of interests, values, goals, energy, intellectual skills, and lifestyles serves as the foundation for the shared life experience of marriage. However, as in any relationship, problems will inevitably occur. Skills in negotiation and communication, along with compassion, empathy, and commitment to the relationship, are necessary to meet challenges to the relationship. An extensive body of research has suggested that psychopathology and emotional immaturity negatively impact one's ability to participate in a long-term relationship and ultimately experience marital satisfaction and stability. Particular characteristics that contribute to marital failure include

- Feelings of powerlessness (Begin, Sabourin, Lussier, & Wright, 1997)
- Passive-aggression (Slavik, Carlson, & Sperry, 1998)
- Neuroticism (Karney & Bradbury, 1997)
- Suspicion (Craig & Olson, 1995)
- Chemical abuse (Leonard & Jacob, 1998)
- Depression (Cohen & Bradbury, 1997)
- Borderline pathologies (Paris & Braverman, 1995)
- Hostility, defensiveness, and aggression (Heyman, O'Leary, & Jouriles, 1995)

The divorce rate in the United States hovers around 50 percent. Interestingly, despite knowing that so many marriages fail, adolescents and young adults continue to have high expectations of marital happiness. Research has indicated that college students have a tendency to unrealistically romanticize marriage (Larson, 1988). Such a tendency to romanticize marriage may contribute to a couple's lack of preparation and subsequent difficulty meeting the inevitable challenges that lie ahead.

Is everyone unprepared and unrealistic about marriage during the transition to adulthood? Perhaps to

TABLE 14–5	Functions of Steps Leading to Marriage
Stage	**Functions**
Dating	• Allows an individual to learn about himself or herself.
	• Allows an individual to identify persons compatible with own goals, values, and personality.
	• Offers opportunity to develop personal interests.
	• Provides leisure-time activities.
	• Enhances the status of the individuals involved in dating.
	• Lays the groundwork for the next stage of the progression toward marriage.
Courtship	• Serves as period where at least one member of couple is considering marriage.
	• Period where values, religious beliefs, family relationships, and long-term goals are considered prior to decision on engagement.
Engagement	• Strengthens the relationship.
	• Redefines one's social world through the union of two families.
	• Serves as preparation for married life.
	• Period of in-depth assessment of compatibility between partners.

some degree everyone is, given that one cannot truly understand the challenges of marriage prior to experiencing it. Preparation for marriage is, however, enhanced by healthy family attitudes about marriage. Embree and DeWit (1997) note that marital role expectations are rooted in family patterns beginning in childhood. These authors report that analysis indicates that "personal consumption of alcohol and the experience of sexual abuse during childhood are the best direct predictors of level of satisfaction with the current relationship, with higher alcohol consumption and experience of sexual abuse related to lower satisfaction" (Embree & DeWit, 1997, p. 42).

DECIDING NOT TO GET MARRIED

Not all people choose to get married, a preference that can be difficult to admit in a marriage-oriented society. The conscious decision to remain single can be rooted in positive factors, such as the desire to channel one's energies into career development, or negative factors, such as personal insecurities and fear of emotional intimacy. While the phrase "it is better to have loved and lost, than to have never loved at all" is somewhat commonplace, many fear that becoming intimate and committing to another person is a risky venture that leaves one vulnerable to eventual agony and rejection. Victims of incest or abuse during childhood may develop an intense hatred of the opposite gender (Schuster, 1992). Such a deep hatred is incompatible with the notion of a gentle, loving, and caring relationship.

As stated earlier in this chapter, finding a compatible mate can be a difficult process. For some, remaining single is preferable to accepting "just anyone." For others, staying single means preserving personal freedom without the perceived responsibilities and commitments associated with marriage and parenting. Limiting oneself to a single relationship can be, for such individuals, a personally stifling and unpleasant experience.

Cohabitating without formal marriage is relatively common in Western society. For same-sex couples wanting to share intimacy and reside together, cohabitation is particularly common. Same-sex marriages are not legally recognized in much of the United States. However, gay and lesbian groups continue to advocate for equal recognition and rights, including legalization of same-sex marriage. A 2003 U.S. Supreme Court decision that sodomy laws were unconstitutional was viewed as a major victory by same-sex couples in their quest toward greater societal acceptance. Groups in support of same-sex relationships express the hope that this landmark legal decision will put an end to some kinds of discrimination based on marital status and sexual

orientation (Alternative to Marriage Project, 2003). Canada, Belgium, and the Netherlands currently recognize same-sex marriages (Lotozo & Lubrano, 2003).

PARENTHOOD AND THE DECISION TO HAVE CHILDREN

Changing trends in career planning and marriage have had a direct impact on societal views about parenting. Individuals who are childless are less prone to societal criticisms than in the past generations. Remaining childless is also easier because of advances in birth control. In 1950, 78 percent of all American couples were having children, in contrast to 72 percent by 1996 (U.S. Bureau of the Census, 1996). For those couples deciding to have children, the trend is toward having fewer of them. The average number of children per couple was 3.1 in 1950 but only 2.1 by 1996, representing a downward trend expected to continue. Accompanying these trends are the tendency toward less maternal investment in a child's development (due to increasing focus on career development), a greater investment by males in fathering, and an increased use of institutional care to supplement parental care (Santrock, 1999).

Parenting remains central to what most consider the essential functions of the family within society. Paul (1992) identified the functions of the family to include

- Sexual relations
- Economic cooperation and protection
- Legitimate procreation
- Socialization of offspring
- Enculturalization of citizens
- Social control

Clearly, the decision of whether or not to have children is a major one, with a rippling effect at the level of the individual, the child, and society in general. For many couples, the decision to become parents is part of a well-coordinated plan that considers such factors as educational attainment, personal values, biologic and medical conditions, and the couple's readiness to incorporate parenting roles into their current routine. For others, pregnancy with the prospect of parenting is an unplanned and surprising discovery. In either case, the anticipation is both exciting and stressful and results in a degree of life change that can be difficult to predict. As with other developmental tasks during the transition to young adulthood, romantic illusions about parenting are common and can contribute to unhappiness when they conflict with the reality of parenting. Common myths about parenting include

- The birth of a child will save a failing marriage.
- Children will take care of parents in old age.
- Parents can expect respect and obedience from their children.

TABLE 14–6	Advantages and Disadvantages of Parenting as Reported by Parents

Advantages of Parenting

- Experiencing the stimulation and fun that children add to life.
- Giving and receiving warmth and affection.
- Being accepted as a responsible and mature member of the community.
- Having someone to carry on after one's own death.
- Experiencing new growth and learning opportunities that add meaning to life.
- Gaining a sense of accomplishment and creativity from helping children grow.
- Having offspring who help the parents work or add their own income to the family's resources.

Adapted from Michaels, 1988.

Disadvantages of Parenting

- Loss of freedom, being tied down.
- Financial strain.
- Worries over children's health, safety, well-being.
- Risks of bringing children into a world plagued by crime, war, and pollution.
- Fear that the children will turn out badly, through no fault of one's own.

■ Having a child gives the parents another chance to achieve what they should have achieved in life.

■ Mothers are naturally better parents than fathers.

■ Having a child means that the parents will always have someone who loves them and is their best friend.

■ If parents learn the right techniques, they can mold their children into what they want.

■ Parenting is an instinct and requires no training. (Okun & Rappaport, 1980)

One's views about parenting are a representation of learning and socialization. As such, most parents acknowledge that they find themselves acting or speaking in ways reminiscent of their own parents. Passing on methods of parenting from one generation to the next gives some structure to a complex process for which formal education is generally unavailable. Unfortunately, both desirable and undesirable parenting practices become ultimately perpetuated (Santrock, 1999).

Despite its many challenges, the process of giving birth and becoming parents is a powerful source of adult development. Parents typically report both advantages and disadvantages of being parents, many of which are listed in Table 14–6, based on a study by Michaels (1988).

Today many couples opt to delay parenting until they are "more established." For such persons, tasks such as completing an education and attaining career stability are viewed as prerequisites to meeting the financial obligations of parenting. However, research suggests that the postponing of having children appears to reduce the likelihood of ever becoming a parent. A study by Campbell (1985) found that two thirds of childless couples do not have children because of prolonged postponement. The other third of childless couples made their decision about parenting prior to marriage (Veevers, 1980).

SUMMARY

A successful transition from adolescence to adulthood is marked by the ability to make repeated, major life-altering decisions without the life experiences necessary for complex problem solving. A consistent theme throughout the transition to adulthood is the tendency to view oneself as immune from the risks of unsuccessful careers, failed marriages, career dissatisfaction, and serious health consequences. As a result, the process is generally a challenging one. In today's society, career changes, failed marriages, and parenting crises are common. However, for most, the stage of adulthood is ultimately reached and the experiences of the past become the basis by which future decisions are made in a more informed manner.

The manner by which one approaches and manages the tasks of young adulthood are largely influenced by the experiences of childhood and adolescence. Such experiences combine with genetic factors to make up our unique human characteristics and capacity to participate in satisfying careers, intimate relationships, and community activities. Negative experiences in early life can leave one without the confidence necessary for managing dramatic life changes and assuming adult roles.

Cultural expectations also influence the transition to adulthood. However, many societal norms have been challenged in recent years. Greater numbers of women are putting careers ahead of marriage and parenting. People with disabilities continue to seek greater accessibility to career options, racial minorities continue to fight for equal rights and opportunities, and gay and lesbian groups continue to pressure the legal system to gain greater acceptance for same-sex relationships. As these societal issues unfold, the process of defining when one actually becomes "an adult" is likely to be further redefined and the processes that contribute to a successful transition to this developmental stage better understood.

Speaking of

Labels

COLLEEN ANDERSON
PARENT OF A YOUNG MAN WITH AUTISM AND DEVELOPMENTAL DELAY

When Kenny was a baby, getting a diagnosis that explained why he was developing differently seemed very important to me. When I was told he had cerebral palsy, I thought, "Now I know what I'm dealing with." Then, years later, a doctor did an MRI and found no brain damage, so Kenny could no longer have the diagnosis of cerebral palsy but was diagnosed with autism and developmental delay. The school district checked his IQ and said he was profoundly mentally impaired, all because they had no way to test a child who was nonverbal. The labels changed, but it was all still my Kenny.

Kenny is 22 now. He walks with a walker and communicates with gestures and one or two words and phrases, and on occasion you will even get sentences out of him. Kenny's personality and humor shine through all the labels. Kenny may have major impairments, but he still perceives himself as a young adult ready for the challenges of new people and places. He was unhappy in the rush and crush of the large local high school, and was homeschooled all of those years. Although he qualified for school-based services until the age of 21, at 18 he announced that he was "all done," and we started the next phase of his life.

Kenny has been a volunteer worker at the local Center for Excellence in Disabilities since he finished school. At "work" Kenny met many new people and challenges. His ability to communicate increased more in the first few months than it had for years in special education, because now he had a real need to communicate. He learns more in the real setting than in some "pretend" setting. Since then he has continued to gain skills that no one ever expected a "profoundly impaired" person to gain.

In many ways Kenny is a very typical 22-year-old. He has a job, loves to spend time with young women, teases and flirts, and fights with his mother. Kenny is also Uncle Kenny, a role that has become a central focus of his life. As a parent, I would like to encourage student therapists to look for the person behind the label, and to offer support with community transitions so that more people like Kenny can find a productive niche when they have finished school. Remember, labels are not the person.

REFERENCES

Alternative to Marriage Project. (2003). *Affirmation of family diversity.* Retrieved October 6, 2003, from http://www.unmarried.org/family.html.

American Association of University Women. (1991, January). *Shortchanging girls, shortchanging America.* Washington, DC, American Association of University Women.

American Occupational Therapy Association. (2002). Occupational Therapy Practice Framework: Domain and process. *The American Journal of Occupational Therapy*, 56, 609–639.

Bachman, J., Johnston, L., & O'Malley, P. (1990). Explaining the recent decline in cocaine use among young adults:

Further evidence that perceived risks and disapproval lead to reduced drug use. *Journal of Health and Social Behavior, 31,* 173–184.

Bachman, J. G., Johnston, L. D., & O'Malley, P. M. (1988). Explaining recent increases in students' marijuana use: Impacts of perceived risks. *American Journal of Public Health, 88(6),* 887–893.

Bachman, J. G., Johnston, L. D., & O'Malley, P. M. (1981). *Monitoring the future: Questionnaire responses from the nation's high school seniors, 1980.* Ann Arbor, MI: Institute for Social Research.

Baird, A., Gruber, S., Fein, D., Maas, L., Steingard, R., Renshaw, P., Cohen, B., & Yurgelun-Todd, D. (1999). Functional magnetic resonance imaging of facial affect recognition in children and adolescents. *Journal of the American Academy of Child and Adolescent Psychiatry, 38(2),* 195–199.

Bakan, D. (1966). *The duality of human existence.* Chicago: Rand McNally.

Bandura, A. (1977). Self-efficacy: Toward a unifying theory of behavioral change. *Psychological Review, 84,* 191–215.

Campbell, E. (1985). *The childless marriage: An exploratory study of couples who do not want children.* New York: Tavistock.

Chassin, L., Curran, P., Hussong, A., & Colder, C. (1996). The relation of parent alcoholism to adolescent substance use: A longitudinal follow-up study. *Journal of Abnormal Psychology, 105,* 70–80.

Cohen, P., Kasen, S., Chen, H., Hartmark, C., & Gordon, K. (2003). Variations in patterns of developmental transitions in the emerging adulthood period. *Developmental Psychology, 39(4),* 657–669.

Crompton, R. (2002). Employment, flexible working and the family. *British Journal of Sociology, 53(4),* 537–558.

Dennison, B. A., Straus, J. H., Melits, E. D., & Charney, E. (1988). Childhood physical fitness tests: Predictor of adult physical activity levels? *Pediatrics, 82(3),* 324–330.

Donovan, J., & Jessor, R. (1985). Structure of problem behavior in adolescence and young adulthood. *Journal of Consulting and Clinical Psychology, 53,* 890–904.

Elizur, Y., & Mintzer, A. (2001). A framework for the formation of gay male identity: Processes associated with adult attachment style and support from family and friends. *Archives of Sexual Behavior. 30(2),* 143–167.

Elizur, Y., & Ziv, M. (2001). Family support and acceptance, gay male identity formation, and psychological adjustment: A path model. *Family Process. 40(2),* 125–144.

Embree, B., & DeWit, M. (1997). Family background characteristics and relationship satisfaction in a native community in Canada. *Social Biology, 44(1–2),* 42–54.

Ericksen, K., & Trocki, K. (1992). Behavioral risk factors for sexually transmitted diseases in American households. *Social Science and Medicine, 34,* 843–853.

Erikson, E. (1950). *Childhood and society.* New York: Winston.

Erikson, E. (1964). *Identity, Youth, and Crisis.* New York: Norton.

Farley, R. (1996). *The new American reality.* New York: Russell Sage Foundation.

Farmer, H. S. (1985). Model of career and achievement motivation for women and men. *Journal of Counseling Psychology, 32,* 363–390.

George, L. (1993). Sociological perspectives on life transitions. *Annual Review of Sociology, 19,* 353–373.

Ginzberg, E. (1972). Toward a theory of occupational choice. *Vocational Guidance Quarterly, 20,* 169–176.

Ginzberg, E. (1988). *Young people at risk: Is prevention possible?* Boulder, CO: Westview Press.

Goldscheider, F., & Goldscheider, C. (1993). *Leaving home before marriage: Ethnicity, familism, and generational relationships.* Madison, WI: University of Wisconsin Press.

Grant, B., Harford, T., Dawson, D., Chou, P., Dufour, M., & Pickering, R. (1994) Prevalence of DSM-IV alcohol abuse and dependence: United States. *Alcohol Health Research World, 18,* 243–248.

Greenberg, J., Lewis, S., & Dodd, D. (1999). Overlapping addictions and self-esteem among college men and women. *Addictive Behavior, 24(4),* 565–571.

Harley, C., & Mortimer, J. (1999). Markers of transition to adulthood, socioeconomic status of origin, and trajectories of health. *Annals of the New York Academy of Science, 896,* 367–369.

Havinghurst, R. (1972). *Developmental tasks and education.* New York: McKay.

Holland, J. (1987). Current status of Holland's theory of careers: Another perspective. *Career Development Quarterly, 36,* 24–30.

Holmes, T., & Rahe, R. (1967). The social readjustment scale. *Journal of Psychosomatic Research, 11,* 213–218.

Hussong, A., & Chassin, L. (1994). The stress-negative affect model of adolescent substance use: Disaggregating negative affect. *Journal of Studies on Alcohol, 55,* 707–718.

Johnston, L., O'Malley, P., & Bachman, J. (1995). *National survey results on drug use from the Monitoring the Future Study, 1975–1994.* Washington, DC: U.S. Government Printing Office.

Johnston, L., O'Malley, P., & Bachman, J. (1998). *National survey results on drug use from the Monitoring the Future Study, 1975–1997.* Washington, DC: U.S. Government Printing Office.

Johnston, L., O'Malley, P., & Bachman, J. (2000). *Monitoring the future: National results on adolescent drug use: Overview of key findings, 1999.* Bethesda, MD: National Institute on Drug Abuse, Department of Health and Human Services.

Kiefer, C. (1988). *The mantle of maturity: A history of ideas about character development.* Albany, NY: State University of New York Press.

Krein, S., & Beller, A. (1988). Educational attainment of children from single-parent families: Differences by exposure to gender and race. *Demography, 25,* 221–234.

Labouvie, E. (1990). Personality and alcohol and marijuana use: Patterns of convergence in young adulthood. *International Journal of Addiction, 25,* 237–252.

Labouvie-Vief, G. (1985). Intelligence and cognition. In J. Birren & K. Schaie (Eds.), *Handbook on the psychology of aging* (2nd ed.). New York: Van Nostrand Reinhold.

Larson, J. (1988). The marriage quiz: College students' beliefs in selected myths about marriage. *Family Relations, 37,* 3–11.

Lotozo, E., & Lubrano, A. (2003). Same-sex marriages may be halted at the border. *Philadelphia Inquirer,* June 19, 2003.

Maddi, S. R. (1989). *Personality theories: A comparative analysis.* Homewood, IL: Dorsey.

Magen, R., Austrian, S., & Hughes, C. (2002). Adulthood. In: S. Austrian (Ed.), *Developmental theories through the life cycle* (pp.181–263). New York: Columbia University Press.

Maggs, J. (1997). Alcohol use and binge drinking as goal-directed action during the transition to post secondary education. In J. Schulenberg, J. Maggs, & K. Hurrelman (Eds.), *Health risks and developmental transitions during adolescence* (pp. 345–371). New York: Cambridge University Press.

Masters, W., & Johnson, V. (1975). *The pleasure bond: A new look at sexuality and commitment.* Boston: Little, Brown.

Mayer, S. E. (1997). *What money can't buy: Family income and children's life chances.* Cambridge, MA: Harvard University Press.

McCracken, R. S., & Weitzman, L. M. (1997). Relationship and personal agency, problem solving appraisal, and traditionality of career choice to women's attitudes toward multiple role planning. *Journal of Counseling Psychology, 44(2),* 149–159.

McKenzie, J., Pinger, R., & Kotecki, J. (1999). *An introduction to community health* (3rd ed.). Sudbury, MA: Jones and Bartlett.

McLanahan, S., & Sandefur, G. (1994). *Growing up with a single parent: What helps, what hurts.* Cambridge, MA: Harvard University Press.

Mederer, H., & Hill, R. (1983). Clinical transitions over the family life span: Theory and research. In H. McCubbin, M. Sussman, & J. Patterson (Eds.), *Social stress and the family: Advances and developments in family stress theory and research* (pp. 39–60). New York: Haworth Press.

Merline, A. C., O'Malley, P. M., Schulenberg, J. E., Bachman, J. G., & Johnston, L. D. (2004). Substance abuse among adults 35 years of age? Prevalence, adulthood predictors, and impact of adolescent substance use. *American Journal of Public Health, 94(1),* 96–102.

Michaels, Gerald Y. (1988). Motivational factors in the decision and timing of pregnancy. In Gerald Y. Michaels & Wendy A. Goldberg (Eds.), *Transition to parenthood: Current theory and research* (pp. 23–61). New York: Cambridge University Press.

Millstein, S., & Moscicki, A. (1995). Sexually transmitted disease in female adolescents: Effects of psychosocial factors and high risk behaviors. *Journal of Adolescent Health, 17,* 83–90.

Neyer, F., & Adendorpf, J. (2001). Personality-relationship transaction in young adulthood. *Journal of Personality and Social Psychology, 81(6),* 1190–1204.

O'Brien, K., & Fastinger, R. (1993). A causal model of the career orientation and career choice of adolescent women. *Journal of Counseling Psychology, 40(4),* 456–469.

O'Connell, L., Betz, M., & Kurth, S. (1989). Plans for balancing work and family life: Do women pursuing nontraditional and traditional occupations differ? *Sex Roles, 20(1–2),* 35–45.

O'Connor, T., Allen, J., Bell, K., & Hauser, S. (1996). Adolescent-parent relationships and leaving home in young adulthood. In J. Graber & J. Dubas (Eds.), *New directions for child development: Vol. 71, Leaving home: Understanding the transition to adulthood* (pp. 39–52). San Francisco: Jossey-Bass.

Okun, B., & Rappaport, L. (1980). *Working with families: An introduction to family therapy.* North Scituate, MA: Duxbury Press.

Oppenheimer, V., Kalmijn, M., & Lim, N. (1997). Men's career development and marriage timing during a period of rising inequality. *Demography, 34,* 311–330.

Papalia, D., & Olds, S. (1996). *A child's world: Infancy through adolescence* (7th ed.). New York: McGraw-Hill.

Paul, C. (1992). Psychosocial development during early adult years. In C. Shaw-Schuster & S. Smith-Ashburn (Eds.), *The process of human development: A holistic lifespan approach* (pp. 600–619). Philadelphia: J.B. Lippincott.

Perry, W. (1981). Cognitive and ethical growth: The making of meaning. In Arthur W. Chickering and Associates (Ed.), *The modern American college* (pp. 76–116). San Francisco: Jossey-Bass.

Piaget, J. (1972). Intellectual evolution from adolescence to adulthood. *Human Development, 15(1),* 1.

Powell, T. (1997). *Free yourself from harmful stress.* Westmount, PQ, Canada: The Reader's Digest Association.

Richardson, P. A., & Rosenberg, B. S. (1989). The effects of age on physiological and psychological responses to a training and detraining program in females. In A. C. Ostrow (Ed.), *Aging and motor behavior* (pp. 159–172). Indianapolis: Benchmark Press.

Roberts, B., Caspi, A., Moffitt, T. (2001). The kids are alright: Growth and stability in personality development from adolescence to adulthood. *Journal of Personality and Social Psychology, 81(4),* 670–683.

Roth, J., & Brooks-Gunn, J. (2003). Youth development programs: Risk, prevention and policy. *Journal of Adolescent Health, 32(3),* 170–182.

Romans, S., Martin, J., Morris, E., & Herbison, G. (1999). Psychological defense in women who report childhood sexual abuse: A community study. *American Journal of Psychiatry, 156,* 1080–1085.

Rutledge, P., & Sher, K. (2001). Heavy drinking from freshman year into early young adulthood: The roles of stress, tension-reduction drinking motives, gender and personality. *Journal of Studies on Alcohol, 62,* 457–466.

Santrock, J. (1999). *Life span development.* Boston: McGraw-Hill College.

Saxton, L. (1990). *The individual, marriage, and the family* (7th ed.). Belmont, CA: Wadsworth.

Schaie, K. (1978). Toward a stage theory of adult cognitive development. *Aging and Human Development, 8,* 129–138.

Schuster, C. (1992). Initiating a family unit. In C. Shaw-Schuster & S. Smith-Ashburn (Eds.), *The process of human development: A holistic life-span approach* (pp. 624–644). Philadelphia: J.B. Lippincott.

Segal, H., DeMeis, D., Wood, G., Smith, H. (2001). Assessing future possible selves by gender and socioeconomic status using the anticipated life history measure. *Journal of Personality, 69(1)*, 57–87.

Shanahan, M. (2000). Pathways to adulthood in changing societies: Variability and mechanisms in life course perspective. *Annual Review of Sociology, 26*, 667–692.

Shanahan, M., & Mortimer, J. T. (1996). Understanding the adverse consequences of psychosocial stressors. *Advances in Group Process, 13*, 189–209.

Shephard, R. (1999). Age and physical work capacity. *Experimental Aging Research, 25(4)*, 331–343.

Sher, K., Walitzer, K., Wood, P., & Brent, E. (1991). Characteristics of children of alcoholics: Putative risk factors, substance use and abuse, and psychopathology. *Journal of Abnormal Psychology, 100*, 427–448.

Spain, D., & Bianchi, S. (1996). *Balancing act: Motherhood, marriage and employment among American women.* New York: The Russell Sage Foundation.

Stattin, H., & Magnusson, C. (1996). Leaving home at an early age among females. In J. Graber & J. Dubas (Eds.), *New directions in child development: Vol. 71, Leaving home: Understanding the transition to adulthood* (pp. 53–70). San Francisco: Jossey-Bass.

Stover, S., DeLisa, I., & Whiteneck, G. (1995). *Spinal cord injury: Clinical outcomes from the model systems.* Gaithersburg, MD: Aspen Publications.

Super, D. (1957). *The psychology of careers.* New York: Harper and Row.

Super, D. (1984). Career and life development. In D. Brown & L. Brooks (Eds.), *Career choice and development.* San Francisco: Jossey-Bass.

Swendsen, J., Tennen, H., Carney, M., Affleck, G., Willard, A., & Hromi, A. (2000). Mood and alcohol consumption: An experience sampling test of the self-medication hypothesis. *Journal of Abnormal Psychology, 109*, 198–204.

Thompson, P., Giedd, J., Woods, R., MacDonald, D., Evans, A., & Toga, A. (2000). Growth patterns in the developing brain detected by using continuum mechanical tensor maps. *Nature, 404 (6774)*, 190–193.

Tuulio-Henriksson, A., Poikolainen, K., Aalto-Setala, T., Marttunen, M., & Lonnqvist, J. (2000). Life events and increase in immature defense style during transition to adulthood. *Nordic Journal of Psychiatry, 54(6)*, 417–421.

Tuulio-Henriksson, A., Poikolainen, K., Aalto-Setala, T., & Lonnqvist, J. (1997). Psychological defense style in late adolescence and late adulthood. *Journal of the American Academy of Child and Adolescent Psychiatry, 36*, 33–37.

U.S. Department of Commerce, Bureau of the Census, Current Population Reports, Series P-25. (1994). *Population estimates and projections.* Washington, DC: U.S. Government Printing Office.

Veevers, J. (1980). *Childless by choice.* Toronto: Butterworth.

Weidner, G., Kohlman, C., Dotzauer, E., & Burns, L. (1996). The effects of academic stress on health behaviors in young adults. *Anxiety, Coping, and Depression, 9*, 123–133.

Weinstein, N. (1984). Reducing unrealistic optimism about illness susceptibility. *Health Psychology, 3*, 431–457.

White, L. (1994). Coresidence and leaving home: Young adults and their parents. *Annual Review of Sociology, 20*, 81–102.

Widom, C., & Maxfield, M. (2001). An update on the "cycle of violence." *National Institute of Justice Research in brief,* February, Washington, DC: U.S. Department of Justice.

World Health Organization. (2002). *ICF: International Classification of Functioning and Disability.* Geneva, Switzerland: World Health Organization.

Adulthood

Keiba Shaw, EdD, PT
Assistant Professor
University of South Florida
Tampa, Florida

with contributions from

Anne Cronin, PhD, OTR/L, BCP
Associate Professor
Division of Occupational Therapy
West Virginia University
Morgantown, West Virginia

Objectives

Upon completion of this chapter, the reader should be able to

▪ Identify the landmarks that comprise early, middle, and late adulthood.

▪ Describe the physiologic differences between middle and late adulthood.

▪ Identify motor and sensory characteristics of middle and late adulthood.

▪ Identify cognitive characteristics of middle and late adulthood.

▪ Recognize the role of stress and coping abilities throughout adulthood.

▪ Identify socioeconomic factors and their influence on occupational performance in adulthood.

▪ Recognize the importance of work, leisure, and self-care activities in adulthood.

Key Terms

adaptive coping	functional performance	productivity
apoptosis	Hayflick limit	retirement stage
cognitive appraisal theory	health management	sandwich generation
consolidation stage	implicit memory	sarcopenia
crystallized intelligence	late adulthood	skeletal maturity
deceleration stage	maintenance stage	Type A personality
denervation	middle adulthood	Type C personality
differentiation	palliative coping	Type D personality
establishment stage	physiologic age	working memory
explicit memory	presbycusis	young adulthood
fluid intelligence	presbyopia	

INTRODUCTION

The term *adulthood* spans the spectrum from what society designates as the beginning of maturity at the age of 18 to the end of life. In examining adulthood, it is useful to differentiate between what is considered "early" adulthood versus "middle" and "late" adulthood as there are changes and challenges unique to each era of the individual's life. Using the ICF framework, the age of an individual is a *contextual factor* called a Personal Factor, which has a pervasive influence on health and functional performance (World Health Organization, 2002).

The ages between 20 and 40 years are generally considered **young adulthood,** an age where optimal physical functioning and intellectual reasoning prevail, major decisions regarding significant relationships and career choices are often contemplated and made, and a keen sense of identity prevails (Papalia, Cameron, & Feldman, 1996; Cech & Martin, 2002). According to Papalia et al., in **middle adulthood** (ages 40–65), normal age-related changes in physical functioning begin to occur, a more sophisticated level of thinking is adopted, and changes begin to occur within the family system. Additionally, middle adults may begin to experience their mortality and begin to have a sense of panic that they have not met their lifelong goals. Inclusive in **late adulthood** are the years 65 and older. In this age group physical functioning may be a concern, as normal age-related changes taking place in physiology are possibly compounded by chronic illness and disease. In addition, psychosocial issues may become increasingly paramount as the nuclear family may not be intact and one must contend with the loss of close friends and loved ones. Individuals in this age category tend to ponder their life accomplishments, move into retirement, and devote more time to leisure activities.

PHYSIOLOGIC CHANGES IN ADULTHOOD

Physiologic age is defined as a "person's ability to adapt to the environment in normal life situations or life crises" (Richardson & Rosenberg, 1989, p. 159, in Ostrow). While this may be true, there is a general decline in physiologic functioning as one ages chronologically. In the ICF categories of Body Structures and Functions, there are typical, age-related changes that will be presented in this chapter. As a result of access to improved advances in medicine and in preventative health care (Cassel, 2001), individuals today can expect to live well into old age, barring any physical trauma or illness. According to the National Vital Statistics Reports, in 2000 the average life expectancy for a baby born in the United States was 74.1 years for males and 79.5 years for females (Minino & Smith, 2001). Longer life expectancy will lead to a greater percentage of people experiencing the normal age-related physiologic changes in the musculoskeletal system that occurs as one progresses from young through middle adulthood and finally into late adulthood.

BONE

The bony skeleton provides structural protection of the internal organs and central nervous system. In addition, it serves as a basis for muscle and ligamentous attachments while also accounting for 14 percent of adult weight and approximately 98 percent of adult height

(Cech & Martin, 2002). The structural integrity of bone is determined prior to birth, with full maturity and manifestation of its strength and weakness presenting itself during growth and aging (Seeman, 2002). The dynamic nature of bone is evident in its ability to model and remodel throughout an individual's lifespan. **Skeletal maturity** is often reached by young adulthood and is illustrated by the attainment of maximal, or peak, bone mass between the ages of 25 and 35 (Cech & Martin, 2002). During middle adulthood, bone loss will begin to exceed bone formation due to the process of remodeling, whereby osteoblasts and osteoclasts work together to produce new bone (Seeman, 2002). As remodeling takes place, a small degree of bone loss is to be expected. Bone loss appears to be mediated by gender. For women, bone loss accelerates after menopause as a result of decreasing levels of estrogen within the body (Seeman, 2002).

Figure 15–1 illustrates the changes in bony tissue resulting from aging. Bone loss that exceeds that of "normal" aging is called *osteoporosis*. Before menopause, it has been estimated that women lose approximately 1 percent of bone mass per year and men approximately .5 percent (Guccione, 2000). Research examining the vertebral bodies in men and women has shown that men in their early 20s to 30s, on average, have a 20–30 percent higher peak bone mass and strength than women of the same age (Payne & Issacs, 1999).

CARTILAGE

Cartilage, a type of connective tissue, is derived from primordial mesenchymal cells and when fully developed is capable of withstanding mechanical stress and compressive loads. The function of cartilage is manifold, including the ability to act as a shock absorber, provide a surface for the sliding and rolling between joints, as well as play an essential role in the foundation for bone growth and development (Cech & Martin, 2002).

When cartilage undergoes a mechanical load or compressive force, fluid and nutrients are pushed out. Conversely, as the cartilage is unloaded, fluid and nutrients flow back into the matrix. This process is essential for adequate lubrication and nutrition of the cartilage. With aging, this process is disrupted and often results in dehydration, poor nutrition, and increased degradation of weight-bearing surfaces (Cech & Martin, 2002; Boughie, 2001).

As individuals age, there is a decrease in glycosaminoglycan and chondroitin, components that make up the extracellular matrix, thereby contributing to it becoming brittle and hard (Boughie, 2001; Cech & Martin, 2002). Changes in the structure of the surface of cartilage appear to begin in the adolescent years, with a change in the normal "bluish" appearance of the cartilage as it turns to an opaque yellow (Loeser, 2000; Boughie, 2001). There is a thinning of cartilage with age, particularly articular cartilage, which has been shown to crack, fray, and shred by the age of 30 (Boughie, 2001; Bottomley & Lewis, 2003). It has been suggested in the literature that there is approximately a 30 percent reduction in cell density between the ages of 30 and 100 years noted in hip articular cartilage (Loeser, 2000). Crystal formation and calcification has been suggested to occur within aging cartilage. These changes contribute to the increase in friction with joint

Normal

Osteoporosis

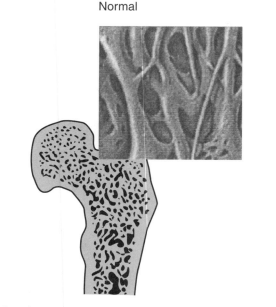
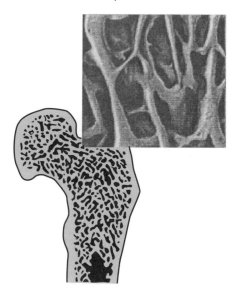

FIGURE 15–1   *Changes in Bone Structure with Osteoporosis*

movement and are contributors to the development of the degenerative condition of osteoarthritis.

LEAN MUSCLE MASS

Several alterations in musculoskeletal physiology begin to occur as young adults move into middle adulthood and then late adulthood. It is well accepted that most adults are strongest physically during their second and third decades. A peak in muscle strength will normally occur as individuals reach their 30s, and they will experience no decline in strength until after their 50s (Payne & Isaacs, 1999). While this may be true, it has been found that the ability to build and maintain muscle mass begins to wane as early as the second decade of life (Nuland, 1999). During this time lean body mass and bone density begin to decrease, with an acceleration occurring in the early 30s (Nuland, 1999). In a study conducted by Kyle et al. (2001) total body mass, lean body tissue, fat mass, and skeletal muscle were examined in 190 men and women age 64–94. The results indicated that fat mass was higher in individuals of age 70–79 than in those of age 60–69 or 80 and older.

Muscle Atrophy

Protein synthesis, while at its peak in the early years, begins to decline with age, thereby diminishing the ability of muscle mass to be synthesized. This age-related decline in muscle mass and thereby muscle strength is referred to as **sarcopenia** (Kyle et al., 2001; Bales & Ritchie, 2002). In individuals younger than 35 years, the protein synthesis rate has been shown to be better than in individuals who were older than 60 years. The prevalence for protein synthesis was also found to be 13–24 percent in persons under 70 years of age and greater than 50 percent in persons over the age of 80 (Welle et al., 1993). Skeletal muscle mass and function decline slowly between the ages of 25 and 70 (Nourhashémi et al., 2001).

Between the ages of 50 and 70 it is estimated that approximately 30 percent of muscle strength will be lost (Nuland, 1999). Studies have found that moderate decreases in strength occur after the age of 50, with the rate increasing up to 15 percent per decade to the age of 70 and increasing to 30 percent thereafter (Payne & Isaac, 1999). In examining the quadriceps femoris using *magnetic resonance imaging (MRI)* in young and old inactive individuals, Trappe, Lindquist and Carrithers (2001) found that the mean cross-sectional area of the quadriceps femoris was significantly decreased in the older men and women, more so than in the young men and women. In a group of individuals ranging in age from 20 to 60 years old, differences in strength of the knee extensor muscles were assessed when performing

isokinetic concentric contractions. The result of this study indicated that there was a decrease in knee extensor strength in both men and women, beginning in the 4th and 3rd decades respectively (Melzer, Benjuya, & Kaplanski, 2000).

Muscle Force

Muscle force production in the young adult remains static, with a slight decline experienced in the middle years of 40–65 (Shepard, 1999). As individuals age, the ability for their skeletal muscles to generate force decreases (Williams, Higgins, & Lewek, 2002). In a study conducted by Pearson, Young, and Macaluso (2002), a comparison of explosive muscle power and isometric strength in the lower extremities of elite master weight lifters and healthy, inactive men of similar age (40–87 years) was conducted. The results indicated a decline in both strength and power in both groups of men with increasing age. Newton, Häkkinen, and Häkkinen (2002) examined the effects of a 10-week periodized resistance-training program on force/power production and muscle strength in young (30–35 years) and older (61–64 years) men. These authors found that the older group of men, like their younger counterparts, have the ability to achieve and increase muscle strength and power output. In a review of the literature, Fiatarone and Evans (1993) reported studies that indicated a decline in muscle force production with age that closely parallels the diminished muscle mass and muscle strength.

These age-related decreases in strength are attributed to several factors. One such factor is a decline in the total number of skeletal muscle fibers according to size, and type (Kirkendall & Garrett, 1998; Bemben 1998; Larsson, Li, & Frontera, 1997). With age there is a reduction in Type II (fast-twitch) fibers while Type I fibers remain relatively stable (Fiatarone & Evans, 1993; Payne & Isaacs, 1999). Other factors thought to contribute to the decline in strength include a reduction in the number of muscle motor units and a reduction in the function of the cardiovascular system. The latter results in the reduction of glycoproteins being transported to the muscles. The ability of the body to repair nerve damage with age might lead to an increase in the loss of muscle mass and therefore reduce function more in older individuals than in those that are younger and experiencing the same loss of the same amount of motor neurons (Welle, 2002).

Age-related changes in neuromuscular innervation and the ability to activate existing muscle may also lead to a decrease in muscular strength in the older adult. It has been suggested that muscle weakness may be secondary to a decrease in central nervous system drive and thereby a decrease in the ability to voluntarily contract a muscle (Thompson, 2000). Kirkendall & Garrett

(1998) reviewed the literature on aging, training, and skeletal muscle and found that electromyography studies have shown that there are age-related decreases in the number of active motor units and an increase in size in low-threshold motor units (Shumway-Cook & Woollacott, 2001). As a normal process, motor unit connections at the neuromuscular junction regularly are disrupted and then reconnected via the process of denervation, axonal sprouting, and reinnervation of the muscle (Thompson, 2000). **Denervation** is to "deprive (an organ or body part) of a nerve supply, as by surgically removing or cutting a nerve or by blocking a nerve connection with drugs" (American Heritage, 2000, retrieved July 21, 2003, from http://dictionary.reference.com/search?q=denervation). This occurrence is demonstrated by the denervation of Type II fibers and subsequent reinnervation by collateral sprouting and expansion of axons, predominantly by Type I fibers (Kirkendall & Garrett, 1998). Another study, this one examining the effects of a six-month resistance-training regimen in both middle-aged (39–44) and older (67–75) men and women, found, among other results, an increase in mean fiber areas of Type I fibers in the older women and an increase in Type IIa fiber area in middle-aged and older women. Additionally, "maximal strength gains were accompanied by significant increases in the voluntary neural activation of the agonist muscles in all subject groups with significant reductions taking place during the initial training phases in elderly women in the antagonist coactivation" (Häkkinen, Kraemer, Newton, & Allen, 2002, p. 61). This finding would lend support to the idea that neural adaptation may play a role in the development of power and strength in middle-aged and older men and women. In a review of animal studies examining age-related changes in the neuromuscular system, it was found that changes in the architecture of neuromuscular innervation involved a reduction in the amount of neurotransmitter released into the synaptic junction and in changes in motor unit size (Balice-Gordon, 1997).

CELL DYNAMICS

In humans, the ability of cells to divide and replicate is limited to some genetically predetermined amount referred to as the **Hayflick limit,** which is approximately 50 replications for an individual human cell (Hayflick, 1974). As reported by Kirkland (2002), studies have found that, proportionally, the ability of cells to reproduce is decreased as one begins to age.

Differentiation, which allows cells to become specialized, is at its peak in younger individuals but begins to decline in the aging adult. This ability to differentiate is partially responsible for the increase in adipose tissue in the older adult. The ability for individual fat

cells to store lipids declines between middle and old age (Kirkland et al., 2002; Kirkland & Dobson, 1997).

Apoptosis is the "disintegration of cells into membrane-bound particles that are then eliminated by phagocytosis or by shedding" (American Heritage, 2000, retrieved July 21, 2003, from http://dictionary.reference.com/search?q=apoptosis). Apoptosis, then, is actually a process of waste removal. It is not readily accomplished in late adulthood. To observe the process of apoptosis in action, go to the Web site http://www.alz.uci.edu/Cellculture1.html for a short movie of the process. In studies, tissue samples from cells no longer capable of dividing have been taken from older adults and observed in a laboratory setting. These cells were shown not to undergo apoptosis, thereby indicating that waste materials may accumulate within the older adult (Kirkland, 2002).

It is apparent that the progressive decline in muscular strength that individuals experience as they age is attributed to diverse biologic processes occurring within the human system. While these changes in the physiology of the aging body are inevitable, it is possible to offset the effects of aging with increased physical activity and exercise.

MIDDLE ADULTHOOD

The period of middle adulthood, ages 40 to 65 years, is one in which the physiologic effects of aging are beginning to manifest. These physiologic changes are compounded by the sedentary lifestyles often adopted during this time. Many middle-aged adults do not exercise, and they make physical activity secondary to competing time demands from other areas of their life, such as work and family (Paplia et al., 1996).

Energy requirements for the aging adult begin to decline after age 40 (Strauss & Blaustein, 1997). In the middle-aged adult, caloric intake is usually not decreased enough to meet the new, lower energy requirements of daily life. This and the normal age-related changes that occur are primarily responsible for the gain in weight seen during this period. In a 20-year longitudinal study of nine 1972 Olympic silver medalist oarsmen, peak power, metabolic responses, heart rate, blood lactate levels, and percent body fat were examined, with results indicating an increase in body fat from 12.3 percent to 15.6 percent in 1992 (Hagerman, Fielding, Fiatarone, Gault, Kirkendall, Ragg, & Evans, 1996). Hagerman et al. (1996) also found that within a 10-year period (1972–1982) the most significant changes in these athletes were seen in percent body fat, which increased from 12.3 percent to 16.3 percent, and in decreases in absolute and relative peak oxygen consumption. Other studies have found that by age 35 aerobic capacity begins a steady decline, gradually accelerating once athletes reach their mid-40s and increasing even more rapidly after age 60 (Anderson, 2002).

SENSORY CHANGES WITH AGING

The changes that occur in the sensory system are gradual and usually begin in the middle of the second decade, becoming more noticeable after the age of 50 (Papalia et al., 1996). The nervous system in conjunction with the sensory system (vision, touch, taste, smell, hearing) is the primary method by which information is gathered, interpreted, and integrated. The nervous system and the sensory system both decline in efficiency in aging.

Vision

Visual perception and depth perception were described in Chapters 10 and 11 of this text. Visual perception skills continue to increase in the 20s and 30s and remain unchanged throughout middle adulthood (Shumway-Cook & Woollacott, 2001). Normal age-related changes begin approximately at the age of 40, with a decrease in near vision happening in everyone (Bonder & Wagner, 2001). Normal age-related changes that take place within the eye involve both external and internal structures. Externally, the eye consists of the orbital cavity, the extrinsic ocular muscles, the eyelids, the conjunctiva, and the lacrimal apparatus. Changes occurring in these areas include increased wrinkling and loss of elastic and orbital adipose tissue, and decrease in tear secretion. Additionally, an inward turning (entropion) or an outward turning (extropian) of the eyelid may occur in individuals as they age. Internally, the eye consists of the sclera, cornea, choroids, ciliary body, iris, pupil, lens, and retina. Changes occurring within these structures include a decrease in the number of cells in the cornea, as well as decreased sensitivity and reduced corneal reflex (Payne & Isaacs, 1999).

Changes in vision occurring with age include decreased lens transparency, decrease in the amount of light contacting the eye, and a decrease in the number of macular neurons by approximately half from the ages of 20 to 80 years old. In a review of literature, Patten and Craik (2000) report that individuals between the ages of 40 and 50 will need some form of visual correction. The process of *accommodation*, whereby an image is focused on the retina, is impaired with aging secondary to deterioration of ciliary muscle action. Ciliary movement is necessary for changing the curvature of the lens. Because of this decline in muscle action, a condition known as **presbyopia** will ensue (Figure 15–2).

Additional impediments to the process of accommodation will occur because of decreased elasticity, increase in size and production of new cells that increase the density of the lens, and the accumulation of degenerated cells within other internal structures of the eye, such as the iris, cornea, and lens capsule. This, in turn, will result in an increased sensitivity to light and glare. The development of *cataracts,* a condition where the lens of the eye becomes opaque, will add to the decrease in light sensitivity.

Hearing

Presbycusis, an age-related impairment that initially causes an inability to hear high-pitched sounds, begins to manifest prior to the age of 25 (Papalia et al., 1996). Hearing is usually optimal in the adult at age 20, with deterioration occurring because of changes in the appendages of the external auditory canal and the *tragi,* which are hairs on the lateral external auditory canal. With age the tragi tend to become larger and more coarse (Meyerhoff, 2002). These changes are seen to occur during young adulthood, beginning in the third decade (Cech & Martin, 2002). The elongation of the tragi will contribute to the buildup of the waxy material, cerumen, within the ear, causing impaction and diminished hearing known as *conductive hearing loss.*

Changes in the inner ear will usually not be seen until the individuals approach their 4th decade. Included in these changes is the degeneration of auditory, vestibular, and supporting hair cells (Meyerhoff, 2002). Sensorineural hearing loss affects the individual's sensitivity to sound, speech comprehension, and maintenance of equilibrium (Bonder & Wagner, 2001). It is estimated that hearing loss producing functional impairment is present in approximately 25 percent of those at the end range of what is considered *middle adulthood,* or the beginning of the "young-old" (Nusbaum, 1999).

The constant exposure to loud noises, such as those encountered by people working in factories or living in industrial cities, may contribute to the loss of hearing during young adulthood. In addressing hearing loss, the best strategy is to prevent damage that may be sustained in these high-volume areas by wearing protective devices such as earplugs or shields.

Olfaction and Taste

The senses of olfaction and taste are intimately linked and serve a common purpose that is related to our perception regarding the different flavors of food (Cech & Martin, 2002; Bonder & Wagner, 2001; Bromley, 2000). The presence of approximately 9,000 taste buds allows individuals to perceive the flavor of food, but as many as 80 percent of these taste buds will atrophy and

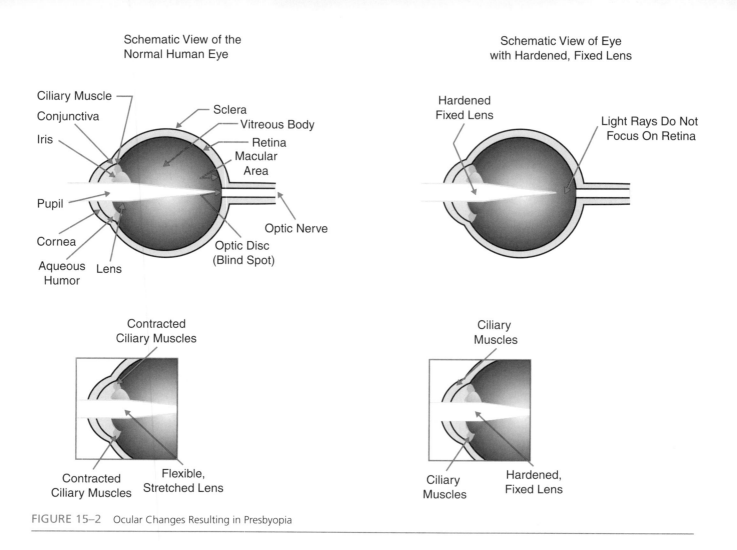

Schematic View of the
Normal Human Eye

Ciliary Muscle
Conjunctiva
Iris
Sclera
Vitreous Body
Retina
Macular
Area
Pupil
Cornea
Optic Nerve
Optic Disc
(Blind Spot)
Aqueous Lens
Humor

Schematic View of Eye
with Hardened, Fixed Lens

Hardened
Fixed Lens
Light Rays Do Not
Focus On Retina

Contracted
Ciliary Muscles

Ciliary
Muscles

Contracted
Ciliary Muscles
Flexible,
Stretched Lens

Ciliary
Muscles
Hardened,
Fixed Lens

FIGURE 15–2   Ocular Changes Resulting in Presbyopia

become impaired with normal aging (Bromley, 2000). In healthy adults, taste cell loss is described as modest, with changes in taste perception, detection, and recognition of type of taste declining. This progressive decline will accelerate in the adult who has chronic medical conditions and who is on a variety of medications (Ritchie, 2002; Bromley, 2000).

The olfactory system originates in the superior aspect of each nasal cavity, with the sense of smell depending upon proper functioning of the cranial nerve I (olfactory nerve) and portions of cranial nerve V (trigeminal nerve). The olfactory nerve and ophthalmic and maxillary divisions of the trigeminal nerve mediate quality of odor detection and somatosensory nuances, respectively (Bromley, 2000). The nose and olfactory system has been shown to deteriorate with age in middle adulthood. The ability to identify odors has also been shown to decline as one ages, in both males and females (Nusbaum 1999). While the decrease in olfactory function occurs with advancing age, women tend to retain olfactory function more than men at any age (Bromley, 2000). This decline in olfaction in conjunction with age-related changes in taste buds may

lead to a decrease in enjoyment of food, thereby resulting in either overeating or malnourishment (Ritchie, 2002; Bromley, 2000; Nusbaum, 1999).

Touch, Pain, and Temperature

In comparison to younger adults, older adults have a reduced absolute sensitivity to vibratory stimuli (Craig & Rollman, 1999) and pain. A noted decline in vibratory sense begins to occur approximately by the age of 50 (Cech & Martin, 2002). Gibson & Helme (2001) have summarized studies that have looked at the aging adults' responses to different stimuli, including noxious heat, electrical stimulation, mechanical pressure or distension, and pinprick, and have concluded that as individuals age there is an increase in thermal pain threshold. The loss of sensitivity to pain stimuli begins to occur approximately at the age of 50. Interestingly, this happens in conjunction with a decreasing ability to tolerate pain (Papalia et al., 1996). In one study, middle-aged and older adults rated pain stimuli lower in intensity than did younger adults (Harkins, Price, & Martelli, 1986; Cech & Martin, 2002).

A decrease in dermal thickness, with the skin at the fingertips becoming less sensitive, occurs during middle adulthood and may affect function and quality of life if an individual is visually impaired (Papalia et al., 1996). A decrease in elasticity and collagen production, thermal sensitivity and pressure, and light touch are also seen with age (Cech & Martin, 2002; Craig & Rollman, 1999).

The ability to adjust to changing temperatures is compromised within aging individuals as the hypothalamus is altered. This compromise may predispose the aging individual to hypothermia or heat stroke. Pacini's and Meissner's corpuscles, the skin receptors responsible for the sensation of pressure and light touch, show a decline in number with aging (potentially 90 percent), with significant increases in thresholds after age 40 (Cech & Martin, 2002).

COGNITION AND MEMORY

In a normal healthy adult, full brain weight is attained by age 30, with individuals experiencing a progressive decline in brain weight as they age. Beginning in middle age, a total of 15 percent of brain weight and volume is lost throughout the lifespan (Cech & Martin, 2002). By 80 years old, individuals will have lost approximately 6–7 percent of their brain mass, with approximately 10 percent loss occurring by age 90 (Uylings & De Brabander, 2002; Bottomley & Lewis, 2003).

Degeneration of nerve cell number and composition occurs with aging, with the total number of cells within the nervous system declining throughout adulthood (Uylings & De Brabander, 2002). The protein beta-amyloid, in conjunction with decaying dendrites and axons, forms amyloid plaques within remaining neuronal cells with aging (Uylings & De Brabander, 2002). In normal brains, neurofibrillary tangles are found in small numbers (Aiken, 1998). The cerebellum may lose up to 25 percent of its cells and synaptic connections, and nerve conduction velocities begin to slow down, thereby affecting balance and fine motor coordination (Bottomley & Lewis, 2003; Papalia et al., 1996). Many central nervous system reflexes and actions controlled by the autonomic nervous system become slow and weak as individuals age (Perlmutter & Hall, 1992).

With normal aging, a larger reduction in the volume in the prefrontal cortex is seen than in the inferior and superior temporal cortex when viewed by MRI (Uylings & Brabander, 2002). The limbic system, specifically the hippocampus, shows a 30 percent decrease in neurons beginning after the age of 30 (Cech & Martin, 2002). It should not come as a surprise that individuals begin to worry that the things by which they define themselves—such as the ability to think, perceive, speak, express creativity, remember, learn, and perform—might begin to wane with age. Interestingly enough, the normal changes that are occurring in the brain and nervous system with age are generally not enough to affect the overall function of the individual in a negative way except through disease states. The ability of the brain and nervous system to replace or adapt to the loss of neurons through plasticity, and the ability to sprout additional dendrites, may serve to compensate for the changes that are taking place. In reality, the areas of the brain that are responsible for sustaining crucial functions remain steady and show minimal changes with age (Cech & Martin, 2002). Cognitive decline is recognized as one of the factors leading to disability in older individuals (Nourhashémi et al., 2002).

Intelligence

Intelligence was introduced in Chapter 3 of this text as the capacity to acquire and supply knowledge. *Fluid* and *crystallized* are two terms used by psychologists to define aspects of intelligence in adulthood. **Fluid intelligence** is the ability to process novel information (Stevens-Long & Commons, 1992); in other words, it is "the ability to apply mental powers to situations that require little or no previous knowledge" (Papalia et al., p. 216). This form of intelligence is more dependent upon the functioning of the neurologic system, and it peaks in young adulthood, approximately by the age of 20, and then progressively declines with age (Cech & Martin, 2002).

Crystallized intelligence, on the other hand, is the ability to apply knowledge gained over time and by experience and uses judgment to aid in deciding how to respond to given situations (Papalia, 1996; Perlmutter & Hall, 1992). This form of intelligence often improves throughout middle age and older adulthood as it incorporates a lifetime of experience, thought, and decision making (Cech & Martin, 2002). Crystallized intelligence is popularly tested via examination of an individual's vocabulary skills, knowledge of facts and figures, and mathematical expertise (Whitbourne, 1996).

It is widely believed that as individuals age their intellectual abilities decline. Although this may be true in some aspects, the pattern of intelligence decline may render this belief false. Some researchers have noted that up to ages 55 to 65, the improvement seen in crystallized intelligence approximately equals the decline in fluid intelligence. In fact, verbal ability has been shown to improve with age (Papalia et al., 1996). Given that the majority of important decision-making positions are held by adults from 50 to 70 years old, the age-related changes that may be occurring with the aging process are often offset by the knowledge and wisdom gained from broader experiences of older individuals; in other words, in real-life decision contexts, these experiences may serve to compensate for the decline in fluid intelligence. (Stevens-Long & Commons, 1992).

Memory

Memories define ideas and beliefs that individuals have relating to their past, which influence thought processes in the present. *Implicit* and *explicit memory* are terms used to describe memory. **Implicit memory,** also known as *procedural memory,* incorporates skills that are practiced and automatic and that primarily involve cognitive or motor components (Perlmutter & Hall, 1992). A good example of this form of memory is demonstrated by the ability to type, play an instrument, or ride a bike almost as efficiently as one did as a younger adult. Memorization of anatomic attachments is an example of *declarative,* or *explicit,* memory. **Explicit memory** contains knowledge about the world and facts and figures that can be detailed verbally (Aiken, 1998). It is dependent upon the medial temporal lobe and hippocampus and allows for abstract thought (Cech & Martin, 2002). As stated previously, the decline in declarative memory may be due to normal age-related changes taking place within the hippocampus itself.

The degree of memory deficit is dependent upon a variety of factors, such as health and level of physical activity and exercise. In a pilot study assessing memory and physical activity in older adults, being more physically active was associated with better performance on a word-list memory task. In addition, the investigators measured exercise self-efficacy and found that higher scores on exercise self-efficacy were significantly correlated with performance on a word-list memory task (Rebok & Plude, 2001). Memory is also dependent on whether the material to be remembered is relevant to the individual's life and the amount of emotional impact that the event or events have on her life.

There is a decline in **working memory** (where past events are associated with present events) in individuals as they age. This decline is due to the fact that information must not only be retained but also manipulated in some way to be retrieved. It has been shown that new information for the older individual can be acquired and recovered, but the new information is forgotten more quickly, and the speed at which the information is processed slows (Luszcz & Bryan, 1999). With aging there is memory loss on some levels secondary to neuroanatomic changes in the brain and the influence of personal factors related to the importance and significance of the information to be retained.

OCCUPATIONAL PERFORMANCE IN ADULTHOOD

Occupation is the "ordinary and familiar things that people do every day" (Christiansen, Clark, Kielhofner, & Rogers, 1995, p. 1015). Human occupations have been studied in terms of the form (observable aspects),

function (intent or use), and meaning (personal significance) (Larson, Wood, & Clark, 2003). Occupations, and these distinct features of them, are important to both individuals and families in adulthood. The term **functional performance** describes the ability of an individual to participate in activities, tasks, and roles during daily occupations (Christiansen & Baum, 1997). The four primary forms of occupation in adulthood are work, play, leisure, and self-care. Each of these areas will be addressed as it relates to adult development.

WORK AND PRODUCTIVITY

Work is any activity that is required for subsistence and perceived competence within a society (Christiansen & Baum, 1997). *Productivity* is a broader term that includes "those activities and tasks which are done to enable the person to provide support to the self, family, and society through the production of goods and services" (Canadian Association of Occupational Therapists, 1995, p. 141). Work and productivity take various forms throughout the lifespan. It is typically in adulthood that work is commonly associated with vocational choice and career. Work can give meaning to our lives, help us define our position in society, serve as an outlet for creativity, be a source of social stimulation, and provide us with an activity that we find fulfilling (Stevens-Long & Commons, 1992).

The two classic theories in the psychological literature that attempt to explain how people choose a vocation and establish a career were presented in Chapter 14. John Holland's theory (1985) incorporates the influence of personality, and Donald Super's theory (1985) proposes that career choice and development occur in stages.

CAREER DEVELOPMENT

As discussed in Chapter 14, Super (1985) proposed eight stages of career exploration and development that span puberty on through to adulthood. The crystallization, specification, and implementation stages are generally associated with adolescence and early adulthood. Establishment and progression of a career begin in the middle 20s, with the individual progressing in his mid-30s up the career ladder. These developments are indicative of Super's fourth and fifth stages, the **establishment stage** and the **consolidation stage.** The sixth stage, known as the **maintenance stage,** generally begins in the mid-40s and is distinguished by the maintenance of prestige, authority, and responsibility. Those in their late 50s who are beginning to distance themselves emotionally and physically define the **deceleration stage.** Super's last stage is aptly termed the retirement stage, as individuals at age 65 make an official break from their careers and move into leisure and recreation (Papalia et al., 1996). As more people choose nontraditional life paths, or make major career changes in middle adulthood, Super's theory becomes less useful.

By the time some individuals reach their mid-40s, the constant drive to excel and achieve has begun to take its toll. Work stressors in combination with everyday life stressors often will contribute to middle-aged adults experiencing burnout and depression while on the job. This is especially true for women, who are often juggling a career and work. There has been a steady increase in the number of women who are participating in the workforce (Bromberger & Matthews, 1994). In fact, women make up approximately half of the labor force in the United States (Kenney, 2000). In a study assessing differences in sources of stress, personality traits, and symptoms of health problems in women of varying ages who work, it was found that young women between the ages of 18 and 29 reported more work-related stressors, daily hassles, financial difficulties, and health problems related to physical and emotional symptoms, along with less healthy personality traits, than middle-aged and older women (Kenney, 2000). These findings were attributed to difficulties in balancing family demands with low-paying jobs that were also unrewarding.

In this same study, middle-aged women, 30 to 45, were found to have significantly more stressors than young or older women. These women reported having more daily hassles and overall stressors than younger and older women that may be attributed to the struggle to maintain and juggle multiple responsibilities as a parent, spouse, employee, student, and caretaker of aging parents (Kenney, 2000). Oftentimes women in the workforce feel that they are not getting the love and the physical and emotional support they require from their partners (Kenney, 2000). Yet a study conducted by Bromberger and Matthews (1994) found that women who work were more psychologically stable—in other words, less depressed—than those who did not. The influence of life stressors should not be underestimated, as it may be that, for women who report low life stress, gainful and meaningful employment may be advantageous, but for women who experience high life stress, the positive effects of employment may be repressed (Bromberger & Matthews, 1994).

OCCUPATIONAL COMPETENCE

For the adult, occupation is an aspect of role performance, and there is an ongoing interaction between the person's expected participation and performance in daily activities, her personal characteristics, and the environmental context (World Health Organization,

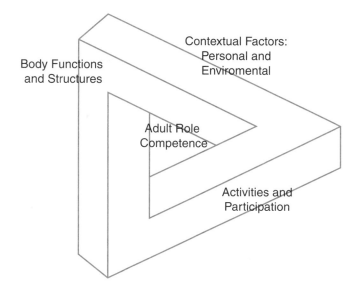

FIGURE 15–3 Occupational Role Performance as Influenced by ICF Domains

2002). Christiansen and Baum (1997) describe this as a continuous dynamic system that requires individual negotiation to be an optimally competent adult. This interaction is illustrated in Figure 15–3. Occupational development during adulthood is driven by the desire for creative participation and the need to maintain role competence.

Work, education, and social participation are all aspects of occupational competence in adulthood. Although the proportion of time devoted to each varies greatly by stage of adult development and individual environmental demands, these three domains of occupation remain a major focal area for adults.

PLAY AND LEISURE

Although normally associated with childhood, play continues to be a feature of adult life. *Play* was described in Chapter 10 as "pleasurable activity that is engaged in for its own sake" (Santrock, 1997, p. 240). The construct of *playfulness*, also introduced in Chapter 10, is equally applicable to adults. Both play and leisure can be considered in the context of specific activities, and in the context of the experience itself. This is important because the determination of any given activity as play or work is based on the interests and values of the person engaged in the activity.

Stevens-Long and Commons (1992) describe *leisure* as "an economically optional activity" (p. 371). This differentiates leisure from play and playfulness, since the latter can exist in a place of employment. Leisure can occur only when the individual has time not devoted to work, self-care, or family demands. This point is important to consider, because although leisure positively influences the quality of life, it is not an option for persons from challenging environmental contexts or with few socioeconomic resources.

Leisure activities are important in maintaining quality of life in adulthood. Engagement in leisure-time exercise was associated with lower risk of consuming a high-fat diet, being overweight, and feeling stressed (Boutelle et al., 2000). Freysinger (1995), based on interviews with 54 middle-aged men, categorized leisure as either self-oriented or other-oriented. She explains, "Through these two types of leisure, adults try to balance social expectations and individual needs, and in doing so adapt to the developmental concerns and issues of middle adulthood" (Freysinger, 1995, p. 71). Leisure can be seen as *agency,* an outlet from the roles of work and family, and as *affiliation,* a way of sharing oneself with others.

Through affiliation, some middle-aged individuals will find pleasure in sharing activities or spending time with family or friends. For individuals who seek this form of leisure activity, leisure is a way of gaining or maintaining closeness with family and friends. In some instances, affiliation with family serves as a way to interact and share in the development of one's children. This is done by serving as a positive role model for learning for the children. In some ways, leisure appears to parallel changes that occur in the family life cycle. Between the ages of 30 and 44, leisure activities tend to be centered on the home and family (Perlmutter & Hall, 1992). After the age of 45, when children are becoming more independent, the focus of leisure activities may expand to reflect this freedom from responsibility (Perlmutter & Hall, 1992).

Having time for oneself and experiencing a sense of autonomy and separation can allow middle-aged individuals to develop parts of themselves and explore and discover new aspects of themselves. Leisure in this form allows middle-aged adults self-expression, feelings of competency, and accomplishment based on mastery of challenging endeavors (Freysinger, 1995). Choosing an activity and gaining mastery over it leads to a sense of pride in oneself, which is important for this age group, as self-esteem may be decreasing as a result of sustained stress.

SELF-CARE

Adult self-care demands are the most extensive of those at any point in the lifespan. In addition to competence in the ADL and IADL tasks described earlier in this text, adults need skill in home management, community mobility, financial management, health management and maintenance, meal preparation and cleanup,

safety precautions and emergency responses, shopping, childrearing, and care of others. Adults who have postponed having children until their 30s and 40s, such as the father pictured in Figure 15–4, have the care-giving demands of both the young parent and the middle-age person with failing parents.

Although self-care and process skills have been refining since childhood, the adult is expected to have effective process skills, including knowledge of the task and the tools for that task. The adult should be able to choose the right tools before initiating the task without hesitation. The tool may be a computer, a forklift, or a pencil sharpener, depending on the task and the challenges offered by it. Occupationally competent adults know what task objects are needed for different activities that make up the day. They have the knowledge to use the tools and materials that they have chosen for different tasks according to their intended purpose in a safe manner.

Adults are more independent in their work and self-care activities than are children or adolescents, and they are expected to be goal-directed in all activities and to see them through to completion. Adults typically complete familiar tasks without asking questions and are aware of the need to seek information when a task exceeds their skill level. Although there is no predetermined age of the developmental stage when the individual first meets these complex IADL demands, by middle adulthood complex skills are needed in

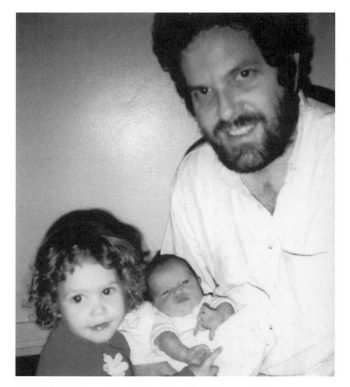

FIGURE 15–4   A Man in His 40s with His Young Children

home management and health management and maintenance.

HOME MANAGEMENT

The AOTA Practice Framework (American Occupational Therapy Association, 2002) describes *home establishment and management* as "obtaining and maintaining personal and household possessions (e.g., home, yard, garden, appliances, vehicles), including maintenance and repairing personal possessions (clothing and household items) and knowing how to seek help or whom to contact" (p. 620). Rowles (2003) describes home as a "place of possession and ownership" and a "place of safety and security" (p. 115). "Home is a repository of the items we have accumulated that catalog our history and define who we are. . . . Little wonder that, for many people, to abandon one's home is, in a quite real sense, to contemplate a severance from self" (Rowles, 2003, p. 116).

Homelessness in adulthood is reflective of demands that exceed the resources of the individual. Homelessness is a pervasive social problem in North America (National Coalition for the Homeless, 2003). In the year 2000 it was estimated that approximately 1 percent of the U.S. population experiences homelessness each year (Urban Institute, 2000). This homeless population, with its self-care needs, has recently been a focus of occupational therapy research and intervention planning (Finlayson, Baker, Rodman, & Herzberg, 2002; Tryssenaar, Jones, & Lee, 1999).

HEALTH MANAGEMENT

Health management and maintenance include "developing, managing, and maintaining routines for health and wellness promotion, such as physical fitness, nutrition, decreasing health risk behaviors, and medication routines" (American Occupational Therapy Association, 2002, p. 620). Given the nature of the responsibilities faced by middle-aged adults, the ability to cope positively with stressful situations is an important aspect of health management. Psychological stress is thought to temporarily increase blood levels of *homocysteine,* a chemical associated with the development of heart disease (Stoney, 1999; Henderson, 1999). Additionally, it has been found that the age onset for hypertension was found to be associated with family stressors (Wickrama, Lorenz, Wallace, Peiris, Conger, & Elder, 2001). When perceived stress and coping resources were examined as predictors of life satisfaction amongst three age groups, it was found that the youngest adults (18–40) experienced the highest levels of stress as compared to the older age groups, 41–65 years and 66 years and older (Hamarat et al., 2001). In

addition, older adults experienced highest satisfaction with life. This is in accordance with other research that has found no significant differences in coping resources among middle-aged (45–64), young-old (65–74), and oldest-old (75 and older) age groups, indicating a more positive life outlook than originally considered (Hamarat, Thompson, Steele, Matheny, & Simons, 2002).

Cognitive appraisal theory, introduced by Lazarus & Folkman (1984), defines psychological stress as a "particular relationship between the person and the environment that is appraised by the person as taxing or exceeding his or her resources and endangering his or her well-being" (p. 11). These authors also identify two forms of coping that are frequently used by individuals of all ages. This model is illustrated in Figure 15–5. The first—*problem-focused*, or **adaptive, coping**—focuses on the problem by attempting to solve the problem, master the situation, or expand resources to deal with the situation. It is primarily used as a coping mechanism when individuals feel that they have a realistic chance to effect change. Changing careers or quitting a stressful job in midlife are good examples of problem-focused coping in the middle-aged adult.

The second form of coping is *emotion-focused*, or **palliative, coping.** With this form of coping the main objective is to feel better through the management of the emotional response to a stressful situation in order to free oneself of the psychological or physical impact (Lazarus & Folkman, 1984; Papalia et al., 1996). People tend to use emotion-focused coping when they feel that they can do nothing to change a stressful condition (Lazarus & Folkman, 1984). The use of substances such as alcohol and cigarettes as a distraction from marital problems arising from difficulties balancing work and family is a good example of emotion-focused coping in individuals who are in middle age.

The coping strategies individuals tend to use are dependent upon the stressful situation(s) in which they find themselves. In alignment with the cognitive appraisal model, individuals will first do a primary appraisal of the situation and ask key questions like, "How threatening is this problem to me? What is the possibility that this event will make me appear incompetent to others? How challenging is this situation?" Once this determination is made, individuals will then go on to do a secondary appraisal, evaluating what, if anything, can be done to overcome, prevent harm from, or improve the situation. It is in the second appraisal that individuals will decide what coping options will best fit the situation (Rodney, 2000; Sarafino, 1998; Lazarus & Folkman, 1984). It is not uncommon for individuals to use a combination of coping styles to deal with stressful situations.

It is evident that the stressors encountered in middle adulthood can have a negative effect not only

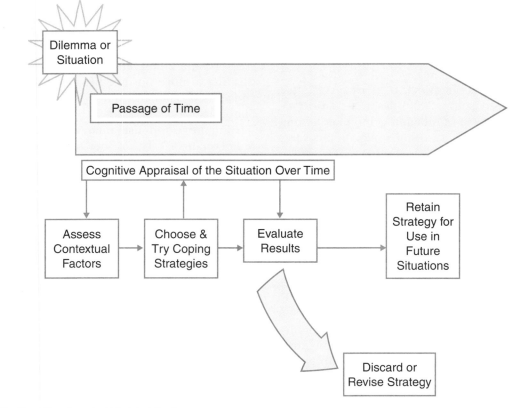

FIGURE 15–5   Cognitive Appraisal Model of Coping

on the health of these individuals, but on the relationships that they have with significant others, such as spouses, children, and colleagues at work. Finding positive and effective coping strategies is especially important and salient for this group of individuals.

CARDIOVASCULAR DISEASE AND CANCER IN YOUNG AND MIDDLE ADULTHOOD

The inability to maintain a healthy lifestyle is of major concern for individuals across the lifespan, but especially for individuals who are in the young and middle-aged categories. In the United States there is an increasing trend toward obesity at a younger age (Kantrowitz, 2001). In a survey conducted by *Newsweek,* 48 percent of middle-aged individuals, often referred to as "baby boomers," ranked getting enough exercise as one of the hardest things to incorporate into their lifestyle, followed by the inability to stop using tobacco or cigarettes at 21 percent (Kantrowitz, 2001). In assessing their own health, individuals in middle age are most concerned about cardiovascular disease and cancer (Kantrowitz, 2001). These concerns are well founded, as scientific literature continues to show relationships between the incidence of heart disease and cancer and the behavioral risk factors for this age group.

Age-related changes occurring in the cardiovascular system are characterized by increased thickness in vascular structures, vascular stiffness, ventricle-wall thickness, altered regulation of vascular tone, and decreased cardiovascular reserve (McLaughlin, 2001). These normal changes in combination with a sedentary lifestyle, poor dietary intake, and other risk factors may contribute to the development of cardiovascular disease.

Cardiovascular disease continues to be one of the leading causes of mortality in both men and women, with the increase in the likelihood of mortality occurring in women after the onset of menopause and in men after the age of 35 (Sawatzky & Naimark, 2002; Kantrowitz, 2001). The lifetime risk of developing *coronary heart disease (CHD)* at age 40, according to the Framingham Heart Study (Lloyd-Jones, Larson, Beiser, & Levy, 1999), is 1 in 2 for men and 1 in 3 for women (Weidner, 2000). In longitudinal studies of Harvard and Pennsylvania alumni, a mild increase in blood pressure in male students ages 15–29 was associated with an increased morbidity and mortality from cardiovascular disease 50 years later (McCarron, Smith, Okasha, and McEwen, 2000), indicating that early life factors can determine disease risk later in life. McCarron et al. (2000) traced a group of University of Glasglow male students with a mean age of 20.5 years who participated in a longitudinal study from 1948 to 1968 and found that systolic and diastolic blood pressure were associated with an increased risk of CHD and cardiovascular disease mortality. Other studies have found an increase in mortality rates as a result of cardiovascular disease in individuals with hypertension in middle age (McCarron et al., 2000).

Cardiovascular Disease and Personality

Type A personality, originally described by Friedman and Rosenman, is characterized by "(1) an intense sustained drive to achieve self-selected but usually poorly defined goals, (2) profound inclination and eagerness to compete, (3) persistent desire for recognition and advancement, (4) continuous involvement in multiple and diverse functions constantly subject to time restrictions (deadlines), (5) habitual propensity to accelerate the rate of execution of many physical and mental functions, and (6) extraordinary mental and physical alertness" (1959, p. 1286). Type A individuals have a faster rate of development of CHD and its complications. This concept has been widely researched and generally accepted (Miller, Smith, Turner, Guijarro, & Hallet, 1996; Smith, 1994). In contrast, at least one study does not support this notion of the Type A personality and its influence on CHD. Case et al. (1985), in a study comparing personality types and the course of CHD in 516 patients 2 weeks after myocardial infarction, did not find a relationship between Type A behavior and CHD progression. Subsequent investigations further complicated this issue. A study by O'Connor et al. (1995) suggested that decreased levels of HDL cholesterol account for the increased risk of nonfatal myocardial infarction in persons with the Type A personality.

More recently, in 1996 Denollet's et al. introduced the **Type D personality** as a strong CHD risk factor. The D stands for a "distressed" personality type—one that has a tendency to experience negative emotions and to inhibit self-expression (Denollet, 2000; Denollet & Van Heck, 2001). Patients with CHD and a Type D personality have a fourfold risk of death compared with non–Type D patients (Denollet, 1998). The precise role of personality types in producing or preventing CHD is unclear. Recent evidence suggests that Type D has displaced Type A as the dominant personality risk factor for this disease.

CANCER

The term *cancer* relates to a multitude of diseases involving uncontrolled growth and spread of abnormal cells that invade healthy normal tissue and may result in death. The occurrence of cancer increases with age, with the onset of most cases beginning in middle age (American Cancer Society, 2004). Four out of 10

Americans develop cancer at some point in their lives (Kantrowitz, 2001). As baby boomers age in the United States, it is predicted that they will face a higher incidence of cancer by the year 2011 (Henderson, 1999). According to the American Cancer Society (2004), approximately 77 percent of cancers are diagnosed in individuals age 55 and older.

Approximately 215,990 new cases of invasive breast cancer will be diagnosed in women in the year 2004, with approximately 40,110 of those women expected to die in the same year (American Cancer Society, 2004). New cases of prostate cancer in the United States were estimated at 230,110 during 2004, with an estimated 29,900 men dying in the same year, making it the second leading cause among cancer-related deaths in men (American Cancer Society, 2004). Like the women in the *Newsweek* survey, approximately 52 percent of middle-aged men were concerned about developing prostrate cancer at some point in their lives (Kantrowitz, 2001). The risk for developing prostate cancer is approximately 1 in 10, with the risk rising significantly after the age of 50. There is, however, some good news in that the deaths among both white and black men from prostate cancer are declining overall (American Cancer Society, 2004), although the rates of death in black men are still twice as high as those for white men (American Cancer Society, 2004). Risk factors for prostate cancer include being over 55 years old, family history of cancer, exposure to heavy metals, African-American race, sedentary lifestyle, and smoking (American Cancer Society, 2004).

Cancer and Personality

It is believed that the reason people with Type A and Type D personalities are at higher risk for heart attack is that their anger and hostility put a burden on their cardiovascular system. **Type C personalities,** on the other hand, have been shown to be at a greater risk for cancer (Temoshok & Dreher, 1992; Temoshok, 2000; Price, 2001). Type C personalities are described as "cooperative and compliant" with authorities but unexpressive and unassertive of their own negative emotions (Denollet, 1998). In this case the belief is that unexpressed negative emotions weaken the immune system. The studies describing the Type C personality are limited and have methodological limitations. Some researchers report that rather than a distinct cancer personality type, there is evidence for cancer being related to depression, and depression could account for the relationship between hopelessness and cancer (Linkins & Comstock, 1990; Zonderman, Costa, & McCrae, 1989). In contrast with coronary-prone Type As and cancer-prone Type Cs, Type Bs are healthy, with a decreased risk for heart disease and cancer. These personality types are compared in Table 15–1.

TABLE 15–1	Proposed Personality Influences on Health		
Type A	**Type B**	**Type C**	**Type D**
Expresses negative emotion.	Consciously controls anger; expresses positive emotions.	Suppresses all emotions.	Suppresses all emotions, especially negative ones.
Cynical.	Optimistic.	Affect is repressed.	Negative.
Self-centered.	Capable of meeting own needs and responding to others' needs.	Self-sacrificing, denying own needs.	Variable.
Anxious.	Relaxed.	Variable.	Anxious.
Has few interests outside work.	Has many interests.	Puts interests of others over own.	Puts interests of others over own.
In control.	Self-supportive.	Helpless.	Variable.
Competitive and active.	Enthusiastic and active.	Fatigued and depressed.	Fatigued and depressed.

ENVIRONMENTAL CONTEXTS

Environmental factors are contextual influences on function that are extrinsic or external to the person (World Health Organization, 2002). Families provide both social and cultural contexts for adult function. Stevens-Long & Commons (1992) note that "the middle generation acts as the load-bearing wall. Middle-aged people take responsibility for the stability of the structure and the welfare of both the younger and older generations" (p. 342).

DIVORCE

For both men and women the divorce rate increased significantly in the 1980s and has mainly remained steady since then (Kreider & Fields, 2002; Choi, 1996). Among young adults age 20–24, 82 percent of men and 67 percent of women had never married; for individuals age 30–34 years, 29 percent of men and 19 percent of women had never married, with a major difference occurring in the 40–49-year-old group, which showed only 12 percent of men and 9 percent of women who had never married (Kreider & Fields, 2002; Choi, 1996). These percentages are significant in that they quantitatively show the potential for additional stressors in this age cohort as a result of attempting to balance marriage, work, and daily life hassles. Of those individuals who have recently married, over 80 percent are men and women between 15 and 44 years old, and most work full time and have children or stepchildren (Kreider & Fields, 2002). From 1971 to 1991 women between the ages of 35 and 45 years were more likely to remain single, and women who were married and worked part or full time doubled (Choi, 1996). The sense of liberation some women gain from divorce may be offset by their struggle to maintain a healthy lifestyle and achieve financial freedom in spite of their emergence into or continuation within the labor arena (Choi, 1996), again giving credence to the struggle that women who work have in maintaining balance in their lives.

THE "SANDWICH GENERATION"

The term **sandwich generation** was coined to describe the role of middle-aged adults who are sandwiched between older and younger cohorts in the population (Figure 15–6). Additionally, this term serves to describe the middle-aged adults who are concurrently serving in roles of both parent to their own children and adult child of a parent (Ward & Spitze, 1998).

These individuals in middle adulthood are often faced with many challenges and responsibilities, including caring for teenaged children and elderly parents at a time when they are facing their own impending retirement, health issues, and mortality (Mikulinger & Florian, 1995). In other words, middle-aged adults are often faced with caring for others while facing their own midlife crisis (Mikulinger & Florian, 1995; Boland-Hamill, 1994). The challenge of assuming the role of caretaker of one's children, spouse, and aging parent in addition to facing one's own life crisis can take a toll on marriage and relationships between caretaker and children and caretaker and parents. It has often been thought that those who are sandwiched between

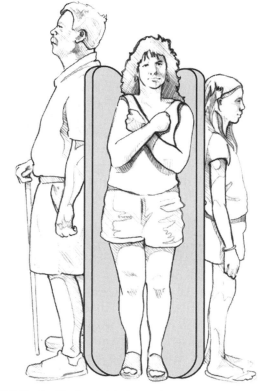

FIGURE 15–6 The Sandwich Generation

younger and older generations would be faced with increased burdens and stress (Ward & Spitze, 1998; Boland-Hamill, 1994). Problems or concerns that surface within the family unit may be an additional source of stress and strain, resulting in dissatisfaction in marital roles as one or both spouses feel neglected and or unfairly burdened (Ward & Spitze, 1998). In a study conducted by Ward and Spitze (1998), those in the sandwich generation, who were primarily in their 40s and 50s, gave support to their children and parents but received little support in return. In this same study, the occurrence of individuals who were providing assistance to a child and a parent was lower than expected. For 50 percent of respondents, the most common scenario for middle-aged adults in their 50s was providing assistance to their child rather than their own parent (Ward & Spitze, 1998).

Women, who are often described within the sociological and psychological literature as "kin keepers," often demonstrate stronger family bonds and are most involved in providing care for their family members (Ward & Spitze, 1998). Women often are credited with having extensive support networks that serve to shield them from stressors related to their roles as caretakers, but it follows suit that these same networks may be in and of themselves a source of strain for these women (Ward & Spitze, 1998; Boland-Hamill, 1994). For both

men and women, being in the sandwich generation is associated with increasing rates of depression, anxiety, substance abuse, suicide, and declining health, in addition to being a time of financial burden and increasing stress from demands on their time from work and family members (Samuels, 1997).

Midlife Crisis

Midlife is often a time of change and experience of losses, illness, and retirement and involves the overall responsibilities associated with being the sandwich generation. As previously mentioned, middle-aged adults are often caretakers of their own children, aging parents, and in some instances grandchildren (Samuels, 1997). Middle age is often characterized as a period of crisis, as the aging adult faces a series of lifestyle changes and demands. Stevens-Long & Commons (1992) review the literature on midlife crisis and report a low point in expression of marital satisfaction, high rates of alcoholism, and a heightened awareness of aging.

Boland-Hamill (1994) assessed parent and adolescent communication in sandwich-generation families and found that a father's midlife development corresponded with his ability to communicate effectively with his adolescent children. In this study the middle-aged father who was experiencing midlife conflicts and concerns about his own aging and accomplishments reported withdrawing inwardly and pulling away from his children, often projecting negative feelings he harbored for himself onto his children (Boland-Hamill, 1994). This was not found to be true for middle-aged mothers, who tended to put the feelings of others at the forefront. Boland-Hamill (1994) did find that the quality of communication between mother and child was disrupted when the mother invested the majority of her energy into caring for aging family members.

Women during this time are experiencing numerous physical, emotional, and social changes as well as varying losses related to the onset of menopause and the loss of their youthful appearance (Banister, 2000). In an ethnographic study, Banister (2000) interviewed women ranging in age from 40 to 53 years and found that midlife is a difficult and confusing time for women. In this study, women often related a sense of decreased self-esteem as a result of physiologic changes associated with menopause, sexuality, and physical attractiveness. The investigator (Banister, 2000) noted that in Western cultures, unlike Native American cultures, midlife transitions are not acknowledged or honored by ritual and are not seen in a positive light.

It is clear that midlife can be a time of challenges for both men and women, but there is research available that supports the notion that midlife crisis is not as commonplace as one might think (Stevens-Long & Commons, 1992). The MacArthur Foundation Research Network on Successful Midlife Development sponsored research that examined the prevalence of midlife events in respondents of ages 28 to 78 years. It was found that people who thought they were experiencing midlife crisis were really experiencing "stressful life events," and those who were truly experiencing a midlife crisis attributed this feeling to the reality of aging and the passage of time (Lang, 2001).

During this time of change, individuals in middle adulthood may take the opportunity to reevaluate their lives and all they have accomplished (or not accomplished) up until this point. They may take midlife as an opportunity to move forward on projects or experiences they have put aside, or they may use this time to renew past goals (Stevens-Long & Commons, 1992). Midlife need not be a time of negativity and distress. It can be translated into a period of growth and renewal and be looked at as a period of maturation and growth mentally, emotionally, and physically.

IMPENDING RETIREMENT

Older workers are more likely to retire than younger workers due to the attainment of financial resources that make retirement attractive and to the societal norm that retirement is expected at a predetermined age (Adams, Prescher, Beehr, & Lepisto, 2002). In our society today a vast number of individuals may go into retirement and remain there for up to 30 years or more (Drentea, 2002). For the middle-aged and older adult, retirement may be welcomed as a time for relaxation, recreation, leisure, and escape from work-related stress, or it might be anticipated with an impending sense of trepidation. As a result, examining the attachments or the amount of self-identity invested in the work role may be warranted.

Work-role attachment is defined as the "degree to which individuals' commitment to their work-role influences their desire to remain a member of the workforce" (Adams et al., 2002, p. 126). According to this theory, workers who have a high degree of job involvement value their role within their particular job; workers who strongly identify with their company are characterized as committed to their organizations, whereas workers who have a high degree of professional attachment value their role as an active member in a particular profession (Adams et al., 2002; Carter & Cook, 1995). Some individuals find their work role alienating, which causes them to look toward retirement as a time of enjoyment or being empowered, whereas other individuals have anxiety about reaching retirement age (Drentea, 2002).

Adams et al. (2002), using work-role attachment theory, found that work-role attachment variables such as job involvement, organizational commitment, and career commitment served as predictors of intention to retire in a sample of men and women ranging in age from 45 to 77 years. In their study, a negative relationship was found between high job involvement and intention to retire, in that some workers felt other roles, such as those involving leisure and family, were exerting a pressure to retire. In other words, those with high job involvement who stay at work longer may experience time conflict with other roles (Adams et al., 2002). The study also found that those who were committed to the organization were less likely to retire and that those who had a high commitment to their profession did not report lower retirement intentions. The lack of retirement in high-career-commitment individuals may be due to the trend in middle and older adulthood to plan to maintain some level of employment after reaching retirement age (Adams et al., 2002).

In a study performed by Drentea (2002) examining retirement versus employment and mental health, it was found that retirees had a lower sense of control, lower levels of anxiety, less distress, and higher levels of positive affect than those who worked full time. This would indicate that retirement has more of a positive effect on psychological well-being than being involved full time in the workforce. Perhaps retirees are experiencing a sense of autonomy and freedom that those who continue to work do not.

SUMMARY

The years from young adulthood into middle adulthood are complex and characterized by changes occurring in many facets of the individuals' life. These transformations occur as part of a normal developmental process that brings change in the physiology, motor, and sensory systems. Transformation also extends into the many roles assumed by the individual during these years. As demonstrated in this chapter, navigation through the various transformations can be difficult for young or middle-aged adults, but these transformations can also be seen as opportunities to discover or rediscover oneself through exercise, sport, and leisure activities.

ANN CHESTER, PhD
HEALTH SCIENCES EDUCATION PROFESSIONAL, DAUGHTER, WIFE, AND MOTHER

Speaking of

Adulthood: The High Points and Challenges

Christmas vacation? That's when you "work so much you look forward to going back to the office to rest up." When people ask me how my Christmas holidays were this year, I could say they are just a reflection of my life: *complex*. For my family of five, the week of Christmas was decorating, shopping, cooking, wrapping, sending off packages of gifts, and more wrapping. But, turns out, getting ready for Christmas was the easy part. I have always looked forward to the time after Christmas to relax and catch up. Not this year. This year, without thinking about what we were doing, my husband, Jim, and I gave our 16-year-old daughter a room makeover. That translates to spending two solid days buying supplies, taping the edges, and painting trim and walls all over again (even though we just did this 2 years ago). That's the "benefit" of having a daughter interested in interior design who has been inspired by a number of design shows on TV. She chose some unlikely color combination that you'd swear wouldn't work in a room with cedar walls and ceiling. Kelly green on one plaster wall with a window, sky blue on the other plaster wall with the door, and yellow trim on the window. After the painting was finished, we hung her very own photos of flowers (she's so talented) and a couple of neat posters in nice frames. We even put a picture light underneath one big poster over her window to accent it. I must say, the girl has a different eye from mine, but it all worked. When we were done, Jim and I were exhausted, but we love facilitating our kids' achievements: isn't that what being a foundation for your kids is all about?

After one evening of relaxation, Jim and I got the bright idea of paying some attention to ourselves in an effort to enjoy life longer as healthy, fit, and energetic adults. This meant turning our unused basement recreation room into a workout room, with recumbent bike, weight machine, step-and-free weight space, and the essential couch to sit on to contemplate working out. Taking the lead from our artistic daughter, we painted the room cornflower blue, maize, and cranberry. What a job that was . . . still is. It isn't completely done. We had only a day to spend on it. It looks a lot better, though, than it did before. Just getting rid of the holes in the wall and scuff marks from boys playing Ping-Pong and throwing footballs—and occasionally one another—up against and through the Sheetrock. A day for ourselves, that's not too extravagant, is it?

Then we went to my parents' home for New Year's. My parents are both 81 years old and in pretty good health. My sister and her two teenagers joined us from Tennessee. What was supposed to be a relaxing few days playing bridge with our elderly parents turned into a marathon home-moving affair. This involved moving our even more elderly (92) unmarried and childless aunt from independent living to assisted living. This couldn't have been done by my parents, because we're talking a major mess and heavy lifting. Ohhh, myyyy!! It couldn't have been done by the children: they just wouldn't have known how to do what we did. We had a day and a half to move many years of accumulated possessions from a three-room apartment to a single room—quarters less than half the size. My sister and I and my husband and all five of our wonderful children pitched in. Yep, my aunt is now in "assisted living" and happy. She can't find anything, but, then, she couldn't remember where she put stuff before we moved it, so that's not much different. In the move from the old apartment, we found food in the strangest places. We found gallons of gin, bourbon, scotch, white wine from 19??, and tiny little bottles from airlines from who knows what year (people must give the elderly liquor, because I know she didn't buy it. She couldn't carry a cup of coffee, much less a gallon of liquor). We found bills in even stranger places. We found 5,000 pipe cleaners bent up to make cat toys all over the floor. We found inches of dust and kitty litter and coffee spills from one end of the apartment to the other. But we did it! She's moved. She was smiling when we left—till she can't find her favorite coffee cup.

I'm exhausted and mentally overwhelmed with the thought of aging at the moment. My aunt is 43 years older than I am. I came back home from "vacation" and exercised in my newly painted beautiful basement workout space to try to make sure I can continue to live life the way I want to. If I can make it through these years of being responsible for myself (which is hard enough) with a full-time job, plus my children and my parents' generation—I hope to be climbing mountains when I'm 92!

Life in the Middle

TRACY J. HOUGH, COTA/L, BSBA
OCCUPATIONAL THERAPY ASSISTANT AND STUDENT IN MOT PROGRAM

In my post-college adult years I had many typical experiences, including moving, setting up a household, learning to balance my family demands, and keeping space in my life to play.

Now as I look at the young adult students around me I can still remember the enthusiasm and idealistic expectations from that time. Enthusiasm, however, is not necessarily limited to youth; in the middle years, enthusiasm merged with the experiences of life can create an exciting environment; it affords you the opportunity to continue the quest for satisfaction while tempering the limitations of idealistic expectations.

Prior to my work experience and re-education as a certified occupational therapy assistant, I spent my early years in a corporate environment as a manufacturer representative for three different companies over an 18-year span. The life and work experiences there provided me with many of the life skills necessary to succeed in many work environments, including OT, and now also carry over to my education while enrolled as an MOT student. Much of what you learn and develop early on in your professional career transfers to new opportunities, perhaps in a different format, but the skills, qualities, and characteristics remain. These skills—maturity, work ethic, focus, determination—all transition well into career changes.

Each year, I lecture to a graduating OTA class on marketing yourself in an OT environment. What I tell these new grads, many of whom have life experiences, is to use those life experiences and these skills, as skills that translate into OT. Interpersonal skills, time management skills, organizational skills, teamwork, persistence, determination—the "soft skills" learned in life's roles—are skills that carry you through and separate the ordinary OT from the exemplary OT.

The enthusiam gained from entering a new work environment, as a midlife career change, provides the spark so often needed for the middle-aged worker. The so-called burnout can be avoided because the environment and the job-specific "hard skills" are new but the unrealistic expectation of the work environment is tempered.

In my experience, when reentering the workforce at 40 with a new career, I was able to bring a renewed zest for work through my new career and combine it with my life knowledge and experience. I entered the workforce armed with much enthusiasm, eager to practice my new craft. On the other hand, I, from many years of work experience, was able to understand that change does not happen immediately. I also was able to understand that not everything that I would do as a COTA would save the world. That concept and belief was for the youth, the inexperienced. That concept, however, is vital to the young adult because it is part of their development. Idealism is something that fades with maturity but is also something that should never be forgotten. It is the remembrance of that idealism that continues to fire the soul each day, why you continue to persevere. Maturity does not eradicate idealism entirely, but tempers it, channels it, and makes it a memory of how you would like things to be.

REFERENCES

Adams, G. A., Prescher, J., Beehr, T. A., & Lepisto, L. (2002). Applying work-role attachment theory to retirement decision-making. *International Journal of Aging and Human Development, 54,* 125–137.

Aiken, L. R. (1998). *Human development in adulthood.* New York: Plenum Press.

American Cancer Society. (2004). Facts and figures 2004. Retrieved June 10, 2004, from http://www.cancer.org/downloads/STT/CAFF_finalPWsecured.pdf.

American Occupational Therapy Association (AOTA). (2002). Occupational Therapy Practice Framework: domain and process. *The American Journal of Occupational Therapy, 56:* 609–639.

Balice-Gordon, R. J. (1997). Age-related changes in neuromuscular innervation. *Muscle and Nerve, S5,* S83–S87.

Bemben, M. G. (1998). Age-related alteration in muscular endurance. *Sports Medicine, 25(4),* 259.

Blanchard, E. M. (2000). Women's midlife confusion: "Why am I feeling this way?" *Issues in Mental Health Nursing, 21,* 745–764.

Blanchard, F., Jahnke, H., & Camp, C. (1995). Age differences in problem-solving style. *Psychology and Aging, 10,* 173–180.

Boland-Hamill, S. (1994). Parent-adolescent communication in sandwich generation families. *Journal of Adolescent Research, 9,* 458–482.

Bonder, B. R., & Wagner, M. B. (2001). *Functional performance in older adults* (2nd ed). Philadelphia: F.A. Davis.

Bottomley, J. M., & Lewis, C. B. (2003). *Geriatric rehabilitation: A clinical approach* (2nd ed.). Upper Saddle River, NJ: Prentice Hall.

Boughie, J. D., & Morgenthal, A. P. (2001). *The aging body: Conservative management of common neuromusculoskeletal conditions.* New York: McGraw-Hill.

Boutelle, K. N., Murray, D. M., Jeffery, R. W., Hennrikus, D. J., & Lando, H. A. (2000). Associations between exercise and health behaviors in a community sample of working adults. *Preventative Medicine, 30,* 217–224.

Bromberger, J. T., & Matthews, K. A. (1994). Employment status and depressive symptoms in middle-aged women: A longitudinal investigation. *American Journal of Public Health, 84,* 202–206.

Bromley, S. M. (2000). Smell and taste disorders: A primary care approach. *American Family Physician, 61,* 427–436, 438.

Canadian Association of Occupational Therapists. (1995). *Guidelines for the client-centered practice of occupational therapy.* Toronto, Canada: Canadian Association of Occupational Therapists.

Case, R. B., Heller, S., Case, N. B., & Arthur, J. M. (1985). Type A behavior and survival after acute myocardial infarction. *New England Journal of Medicine, 312,* 737–741.

Cech, D. J., & Martin, S. (2002). *Functional movement development across the lifespan* (2nd ed.). Philadelphia: W.B. Saunders.

Choi, N. G. (1996). Changes in the living arrangements, work patterns, and economic status of middle-aged single women: 1971–1991. *Affilia, 11,* 164–178.

Christiansen, C., & Baum, C. (Eds.) (1997). *Occupational therapy: Enabling function and well-being* (2nd ed.). Thorofare, NJ: Slack.

Craig, J. C., & Rollman, G. B. (1999). Somesthesis. *Annual Review Psychology, 50,* 305–331.

Denollet, J. (1998). Personality and coronary heart disease: The type-D scale-16 (DS16). *Annals of Behavioral Medicine, 20,* 209–215.

Denollet, J. (2000). Type D personality. A potential risk factor refined. *Journal of Psychosomatic Research, 49,* 255–266.

Denollet, J., Sys, S. U., Stroobant, N., Rombouts, H., Gillebert, T. C., & Brutsaert, D. L. (1996). Personality as independent predictor of long-term mortality in patients with coronary heart disease. *Lancet, 347,* 417–421.

Denollet, J., & Van Heck, G. L. (2001). Psychological risk factors in heart disease: What Type D personality is (not) about. *Journal of Psychosomatic Research, 51,* 465–468.

Drentea, P. (2002). Retirement and mental health. *Journal of Aging and Health, 14,* 167–194.

Fiatarone, M. A., & Evans, W. J. (1993). The etiology and reversibility of muscle dysfunction in the aged. *Journals of Gerontology, 48,* 77–83.

Finlayson, M., Baker, M., Rodman, L., & Herzberg, G. (2002). The process and outcomes of a multimethod needs assessment at a homeless shelter. *American Journal of Occupational Therapy, 56,* 313–321.

Folkman, S., Lazarus, R. S., Pimley, S., & Novacek, J. (1987). Age differences in stress and coping processes. *Psychology and Aging, 2,* 171–184.

Freysinger, V. J. (1995). The dialectics of leisure and development for women and men in midlife: An interpretive study. *Journal of Leisure Research, 27,* 61–84.

Friedman, M., & Rosenman, R. H. (1959). Association of specific overt behavior pattern with blood and cardiovascular findings. *Journal of the American Medical Association, 169,* 1286–1295.

Gibson, S. J., & Helme, R. D. (2001). Age-related differences in pain perception and report. *Clinics in Geriatric Medicine, 17,* 433–456.

Guccione, A. A. (2000). *Geriatric physical therapy* (2nd ed.). St. Louis: Mosby-Year Book.

Hagerman, R. C., Fielding, R. S., Fiatarone, M. A., Gault, J. A., Kirkendall, D. J., Ragg, K. K., & Evans, W. J. (1996). A 20-yr longitudinal study of Olympic oarsmen. *Medicine & Science in Sports & Exercise, 28(9),* 1150–1156.

Hamarat, E., Thompson, D., Steele, D., Matheny, K., & Simons, C. (2002). Age differences in coping resources and satisfaction with life among middle-aged, young-old, and oldest-old adults. *Journal of Genetic Psychology, 163,* 360–367.

Hamarat, E., Thompson, D., Zabrucky, K. M., Steele, D., & Matheny, K. B. (2001). Perceived stress and coping resource availability as predictors of life satisfaction in young, middle-aged, and older adults. *Experimental Aging Research, 27,* 181–196.

Harkins, S. W., Price, D. D., & Martelli, M. (1986). Effects of age on pain perception: Thermonociception. *Journal of Gerontology, 41,* 58–63.

Hayflick, L. (1974). The strategy of senescence. *The Gerontologist, 14,* 37–45.

Holland, J. (1985). *Professional manual for the self-directed search.* Odessa, FL: Psychological Assessment Resources.

Kantrowitz, B. (2001). Health for life. *Newsweek, 138(11),* 4–11.

Kenney, J. W. (2000). Women's 'inner-balance': A comparison of stressors, personality traits and health problems by age groups. *Journal of Advanced Nursing, 31,* 639–650.

Kirkendall, D. T., & Garrett, W. E. (1998). The effects of aging and training on skeletal muscle. *American Journal of Sports Medicine, 26,* 598–602.

Kirkland, J. L. (2002). The biology of senescence: potential for prevention of disease. *Clinics in Geriatric Medicine, 18,* 383–405.

Kirkland, J. L., & Dobson, D. E. (1997). Preadipocyte function and aging: Links between age-related changes in cell dynamics and altered fat tissue function. *Journal of the American Geriatric Society, 45,* 959–967.

Kirkland, J. L., Tchkonia, T., Pirtskhalava, T., Han, J., & Karagiannides, I. (2002). Adipogenesis and aging: Does aging make fat go MAD? *Experimental Gerontology, 37,* 757–767.

Kreider, B. M., & Fields, J. M. (2002). Number, timing, and duration of marriages and divorces: Fall 1996. *Current Population Reports U.S. Census Bureau,* 70–80.

Kyle, U. G., Genton, L., Hans, D., Karsegard, V. L., Michel, J. P., Slosman, D. O., & Pichard C. (2001). Total body mass, fat mass, fat-free mass, and skeletal muscle in older people: Cross-sectional differences in 60-year-old persons. *Journal of American Geriatric Society, 49,* 1633–1640.

Larson, E., Wood, W., & Clark, F. (2003). Occupational science: Building the science and practice of occupation through an academic discipline. In E. Crepeau, E. Cohn, & B. Schell (Eds.), *Willard and Spackman's occupational therapy* (10th ed.) (pp. 15–25). Philadelphia: Lippincott, Williams and Wilkins.

Larsson, L. (1998). The age-related motor disability: Underlying mechanisms in skeletal muscle at the motor unit, cellular and molecular level. *Acta Physiologica Scandinavica, 163,* S27–29.

Larsson, L, Li, X., & Frontera, W. R. (1997). Effects of aging on shortening velocity and myosin isoform composition in single human skeletal muscle cells. *Cell Physiology, 272,* C638–C649.

Lazarus, R. S., & Folkman, S. (1984). *Stress, appraisal, and coping.* New York: Springer.

Linkins, R. W., & Comstock, G. W. (1990). Depressed mood and development of cancer. *American Journal of Epidemiology, 132,* 962–972.

Lloyd-Jones, D. M., Larson, M. G., Beiser, A., & Levy, D. (1999). Lifetime risk of developing coronary heart disease. *Lancet, 353,* 89–92.

Loeser, R. F. (2000). Aging and the etiopathogenesis and treatment of osteoarthritis. *Rheumatic Diseases Clinics of North America, 26,* 547–567.

Luszcz, M. A., & Bryan, J. (1999). Toward understanding age-related memory loss in late adulthood. *Gerontology, 45,* 2–9.

McCarron, P., Davey Smith, G., Okasha, M., & McEwen, J. (2000). Blood pressure in young adulthood and mortality from cardiovascular disease. *Lancet, 355,* 1430–1431.

McLaughlin, M. A. (2001). State-of-the-art prevention and management of cardiac disease. *Geriatrics, 56,* 45–49.

Melzer, I., Benjuya, N., & Kaplanski, J. (2000). Age-related changes in muscle strength and fatigue. *Isokinetics and Exercise Science, 8,* 73–83.

Mikulinger, M., & Florian, V. (1995). Stress, coping, and fear of personal death: The case of middle-aged men facing early job retirement. *Death Studies, 19,* 413–431.

Miller, T. Q., Smith, T. W., Turner, C. W., Guijarro, M. L., & Hallet, A. J. (1996). A meta-analytic review of research on hostility and physical health. *Psychological Bulletin, 119,* 322–348.

Minino, A. M., & Smith, B. L. (2001). Deaths: Preliminary data for 2000. *National Vital Statistics Reports, 49(12),* 1–40.

National Coalition for the Homeless (2003) Home Page. Retrieved August 1, 2003, from http://www.nationalhomeless.org/index.html.

Neumann, D. A. (2000). Arthrokinesiologic considerations in the aged adult. In A. A. Guccione (Ed.), *Geriatric physical therapy* (2nd ed.) (pp. 56–77). St. Louis: Mosby-Year Book.

Newton, R. U., Häkkinen, K., Häkkinen, A. (2002). Mixed-methods resistance training increases power and strength of young and older men. *Medicine and Science in Sports and Exercise, 34,* 1367–1375.

Nourhashémi, F., Andrieu, S., Gillette-Guyonnet, S., Reynish, E., Albarède, J. L., Grandjean, H., & Vellas, B. (2002). Is there a relationship between fat-free soft tissue mass and low cognitive function? Results from a study of 7,105 women. *Journal of the American Geriatric Society, 50,* 1796–1801.

Nuland, S. B. (1999). Pumping iron. *American Scholar, 68,* 121–124.

Nusbaum, N. J. (1999). Aging and sensory senescence. *Southern Medical Journal, 92,* 267–275.

O'Connor, N. J., Manson, J. E., O'Connor, G. T., & Buring, J. E. (1995). Psychosocial risk factors and nonfatal myocardial infarction. *Circulation, 92,* 1458–1464.

Papalia, D. E., Camp, C. J., & Feldman, R. D. (1996). *Adult development and aging*. New York: McGraw-Hill.

Patten, C., & Craik, R. L. (2000). Sensimotor changes and adaptation in the older adult. In Guccione, A. A. (Ed.), *Geriatric physical therapy* (2nd ed.) (pp. 78–112). St. Louis: Mosby-Year Book.

Pearson, S. J., Young, A., & Macaluso, A. (2002). Muscle function in elite master weightlifters. *Medicine and Science in Sports and Exercise, 34,* 1199–1206.

Perlmutter, M., & Hall, E. (1992). *Adult development and aging* (2nd ed.). New York: John Wiley and Sons.

Price, M. A., Tennant, C. C., Smith, R. C., Butow, P. N., Kennedy, S. J., Kossoff, M. B., & Dunn, S. M. (2001). The role of psychosocial factors in the development of breast carcinoma: Part I. The cancer-prone personality. *Cancer, 91,* 679–685.

Rebok, G., & Plude, D. J. (2001). Relation of physical activity to memory functioning in older adults: The memory workout program. *Educational Gerontology, 27,* 241–259.

Richardson, P. A., & Rosenberg, B. S. (1989). The effects of age on physiological and psychological responses to a training and detraining program in females. In A. C. Ostrow (Ed.), *Aging and motor behavior* (pp. 159–172). Indianapolis, IN: Benchmark Press.

Ritchie, C. S. (2002). Oral health, taste, and olfaction. *Clinics in Geriatric Medicine 18,* 709–717.

Rodney, V. (2000). Nurse stress associated with aggression in people with dementia: Its relationship to hardiness, cognitive appraisal and coping. *Journal of Advanced Nursing, 31,* 172–181.

Samuels, S. C. (1997). Midlife crisis: Helping patients cope with stress, anxiety, and depression. *Geriatrics, 52,* 55–63.

Santrock, J. (1997). *Life-span development* (7th ed.). Boston: McGraw-Hill.

Sarafino, E. P. (1998). *Health psychology: Biopsychosocial interactions* (3rd ed.). New York: John Wiley and Sons.

Sawatzky, J. V., & Naimark, B. J. (2002). Physical activity and cardiovascular health in aging women: A health-promotion perspective. *Journal of Aging and Physical Activity, 10,* 396–412.

Seeman, E. (2002). Pathogenesis of bone fragility in women and men. *Lancet, 359,* 1841–1850.

Shepard, R. J. (1999). Age and physical work capacity. *Experimental Aging Research, 25,* 331–344.

Shumway-Cook, A., & Woollacott, M. (2001) *Motor control: Theory and practical applications* (2nd ed.). Philadelphia: Lippincott, Williams and Wilkins.

Smith, T. W. (1994). Concepts and methods on the study of anger, hostility and health. In A. W. Siegman & T. W. Smith (Eds.), *Anger, hostility and the heart* (pp. 23–42). Hillsdale, NJ: Erlbaum.

Stevens-Long, J., & Commons, M. (1992). *Adult life* (4th ed.). Mountainview, CA: Mayfield.

Stoney, C. M. (1999). Plasma homocysteine levels increase in women during psychological stress. *Life Sciences 64,* 2359–2365.

Strauss, E., & Blaustein, A. (1997). Keeping in shape: Exercise fundamentals for the midlife patient. *Geriatrics, 52,* 62–72.

Super, D. E. (1985). Coming of age in Middletown: Careers in the making. *American Psychologist, 40,* 405–414.

Temoshok, L., & Dreher, H. (1992). *The Type C connection: The behavioral links to cancer and your health*. New York: Random House.

Temoshok, L. R. (2000). Complex coping patterns and their role in adaptation and neuroimmunomodulation. Theory, methodology, and research. *Annals of the New York Academy of Science, 917,* 446–455.

Thompson, L. V. (2000). Physiological changes associated with aging. In A. A. Guccione (Ed.), *Geriatric physical therapy* (pp. 28–55). St. Louis: Mosby-Year Book.

Trappe, T. A., Lindquist, D. M., & Carrithers, J. A. (2001). Muscle-specific atrophy of the quadriceps femoris with aging. *Journal of Applied Physiology, 90,* 2070–2074.

Tryssenaar, J., Jones, E., & Lee, D. (1999). Occupational performance needs of a shelter population. *Canadian Journal of Occupational Therapy, 66,* 188–195.

Urban Institute. (2000). *A new look at homelessness in America*. Washington, DC: Urban Institute.

Uylings, H. B. M., & de Brabander, J. M. (2002). Neuronal changes in normal human aging and Alzheimer's disease. *Brain and Cognition, 49,* 268–276.

Ward, R. A., & Spitze, G. (1998). Sandwiched marriages: The implications of child and parent relations for marital quality in midlife. *Social Forces, 77,* 647–667.

Weidner, G. (2000). Why do men get more heart disease than women? An international perspective. *Men's Heart Disease, 48,* 291–294.

Welle, S. (2002). Cellular and molecular basis of age-related sarcopenia. *Canadian Journal of Applied Physiology, 27,* 19–41.

Welle, S., Thornton, C., Jozefowicz, R., & Statt, M. (1993). Myofibrillar protein synthesis in young and old men. *Endocrinology and Metabolism, 264,* E693–E698.

Wickrama, K.A.S., Lorentz, F. O., Wallace, L. E., Peiris, L., Conger, R. D., & Elder, G. H. (2001). Family influence on physical health during the middle years: The case of onset of hypertension. *Journal of Marriage and Family, 63,* 527–539.

Williams, G. N., Higgins, M. J., & Lewek, M. D. (2002). Aging skeletal muscle: Physiologic changes and the effects of training. *Physical Therapy, 82,* 62–68.

World Health Organization. (2002). *ICF: International classification of functioning and disability*. Geneva, Switzerland: World Health Organization.

Zonderman, A. B., Costa, P. T., & McCrae, R. R. (1989). Depression as a risk for cancer morbidity and mortality in a nationally representative sample. *Journal of the American Medical Association, 262,* 1191–1195.

Aging

Pamela Reynolds, PT, EdD
Associate Professor
Gannon University
Erie, Pennsylvania

with contributions from

Anne Cronin, PhD, OTR/L, BCP
Associate Professor
Division of Occupational Therapy
West Virginia University
Morgantown, West Virginia

Objectives

Upon completion of this chapter, the reader should be able to

▓ Identify demographic characteristics of the aging population.

▓ Understand the three main components of successful aging.

▓ Recognize normal and usual physiologic and cognitive characteristics of aging, including changes in memory, learning, intelligence, cardiovascular, pulmonary, musculoskeletal, neurologic, and integumentary systems.

▓ Describe the psychosocial characteristics of aging, including education and socioeconomic factors, family roles, social support networks, leisure activities, work, retirement, and community roles.

▓ Identify the predictors and the supportive evidence for successful aging.

Key Terms

age-associated memory impairment
  (AAMI)
benign senescent forgetfulness (BSF)
cataracts
fear of falling (FOF)
Fick equation

glaucoma
kyphosis
lordosis
macular degeneration
metabolic equivalent unit (MET)
osteopenia

presbyastasis
selective attention
successful aging
vigilance

INTRODUCTION

The aging process is universal, irreversible, and progressively cumulative throughout the lifespan. Every physiologic function will decline with the passage of time. However, the rate at which physiologic functions diminish is highly variable, as is the quality of life that parallels them. Because the effects of disuse or inactivity mimic aging, it is often difficult to assess the difference between the effects of aging and disuse.

The 2000 U.S. Census (U.S. Census Bureau, 2001) found the median age of the population to be at its highest level ever. In 1990 the median age was 32.9 years old, and it rose to 35.3 by 2000. It is expected to peak at 38.7 in 2035, then decrease slightly to 38.1 by 2050. The aging baby boomers, who were born after World War II between 1946 and 1964, are driving this upward rise in median age. They currently represent 30 percent of the population. The population between the ages of 45 and 54 grew by 49 percent, and the number of people over the age of 85 expanded by 38 percent, between 1990 and 2000. Figure 16–1 illustrates the percent change in population by age groups in that decade.

However, the fastest-growing segment of the population is those over the age of 85. Figure 16–2 displays

the projected percent distribution and growth of the older population by age between 1990 and 2050. In 1995 it was estimated that 3.6 million people were age 85 and over; by 2050 it is projected that this number could increase to 18.2 million. Although numerically small, the population age 100 and older is also expected to expand considerably. In 1995 the centenarian population was estimated at 54,000. It is projected to grow to 214,000 by 2020 and to 800,000 by the year 2050 (U.S. Census Bureau, 2001).

Although age-related changes do not necessarily have to be associated with disease processes, the incidence of chronic disease does increase with age. Concurrently, disability in older persons and the need for assistance also increases with age. Twenty-three percent of persons age 45 to 54 reported some form of disability, but only 4 percent needed personal assistance for it. Among those over 80 years old, 74 percent noted some form of disability, and 58 percent reported a severe disability, with 35 percent requiring assistance. Figure 16–3 depicts the increasing incidence and severity of disability as a factor of age (U.S. Census Bureau, 2001).

There is a high correlation between increasing age, decreasing physical activity, and increasing disability. The classic study completed by Saltin et al. (1968)

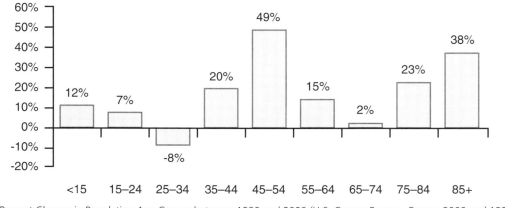

FIGURE 16–1 Percent Change in Population Age Groups between 1990 and 2000 (U.S. Census Bureau, Census 2000 and 1990 census)

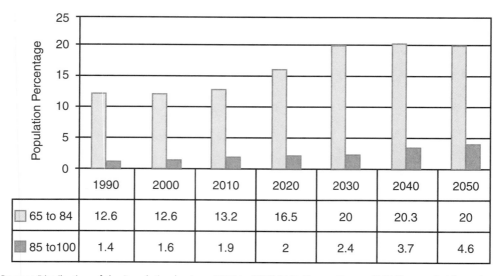

FIGURE 16–2   Percent Distribution of the Population by Age: 1990 to 2050 (U.S. Census Bureau [1996], compiled from data in Current Population Reports: Population Projections of the United States by Age, Sex, Race, and Hispanic Origin: 1995 to 2050)

demonstrated that inactivity and disuse could mimic the physiologic changes that are observed with aging. Smith and Gilligan report that "disuse accounts for about half the functional decline that occurs between the ages of 30 and 70, and aging causes the other half" (Smith & Gilligan, 1983, p. 91).

In 1980 Fries proposed his controversial *compression of morbidity* theory. He noted that although human life expectancy has increased greatly in the past century, maximum lifespan has not increased proportionately. Currently, the years that a person is ill are heavily concentrated in old age. Fries (1980) proposed that if the onset of morbidity and disability could be postponed, or compressed into the last few years of the lifespan, then quality of life would improve and the need for medical care would be reduced. The primary opponents of his theory at the time believed that research funds would be better utilized in finding cures for illness than in the questionable success of preventing or postponing disease and chronic illness.

In 1987 Rowe and Kahn proposed a distinction between usual and successful aging, both characterized as nonpathologic states. Their purpose was to distinguish between two groups of non-diseased older persons. *Usual-aging* individuals were defined as those having normal age-related alterations in physical and cognitive function, such as increases in blood pressure and blood glucose and modest memory impairment. These individuals are considered nonpathologic but at high risk for development of chronic disease(s). In contrast, **successful-aging** individuals were considered low-risk and high-functioning. These assumptions spurred research on the criteria and determinants of successful aging and identification of more appropriate interventions for "normal" elderly. The MacArthur Foundation Research Network on Successful Aging supported much of the subsequent research for these propositions. In 1997 Rowe and Kahn proposed a conceptual framework for successful aging and offered some pathways and interventions that lead to

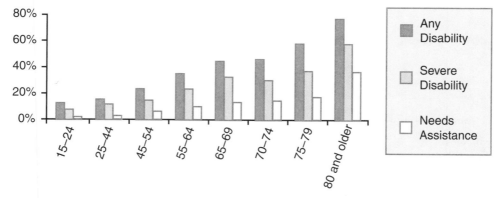

FIGURE 16–3   Disability Occurrence by Age and Severity: 1997

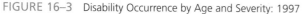

successful old age. The objective of this chapter is to examine the physical, cognitive, and psychosocial characteristics of usual and normal aging. Descriptions of normal aging are presented in this chapter, and factors that predict successful aging are summarized at the end of this chapter.

SUCCESSFUL AGING

There is a growing body of literature that refutes traditionally held views that as a person ages, increased risk of disease and disability is inevitable and part of the intrinsic aging process. Many of the usual characteristics associated with aging are due to lifestyle, environmental, and other factors, which may increase with age but are not age-dependent. In a recent human-twins study, Finch and Tanzi (1997) demonstrated that twins reared apart share less than 35 percent inheritability of lifespan. Environment and lifestyle accounted for the rest of this 65 percent observed variance.

The MacArthur Foundation Research Network on Successful Aging conducted a longitudinal study of older individuals to identify the physical, psychological, social, and biomedical characteristics that were predictive for maintaining high function later in life. Initially the study included 1,189 subjects who were between 70 and 79 years old. After 2 to 2½ years 1,115 subjects were reevaluated, achieving a 91 percent follow-up rate. Pre- and post-study data sets included detailed assessments of physical and cognitive performance, health status, social and psychological characteristics, and blood and urine samples. Several research reports have been published from the results of this study (Albert et al., 1995; Rowe & Kahn, 1997; Unger et al, 1999).

Based on the cumulative outcomes of the MacArthur Foundation studies, Rowe and Kahn (1997) define three components of successful aging as (1) low probability of disease and disease-related disability, (2) high cognitive and physical functional capacity, and (3) active engagement with life. Figure 16–4 displays the interdependent relationship among the components, each of which has subparts.

Low probability of disease not only denotes the absence of disease but also recognizes the absence, presence, or severity of risk factors. Physical and cognitive function indicates an individual's potential for activity and implies what a person can do. Active engagement may take many forms. The two forms of most interest here are interpersonal relations and productive activity. Interpersonal relationships involve communication and interaction with others, exchange of information, emotional support, and direct assistance. An activity is considered productive if it holds societal value, whether or not the individual receives any monetary remuneration (Rowe & Kahn, 1997).

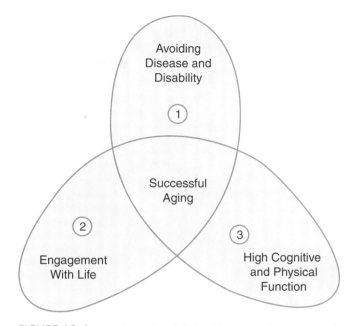

FIGURE 16–4 Interdependent Relationship among Components of Successful Aging. (Reprinted with permission from J. W. Rowe & R. L. Kahn, Successful aging, *The Gerontologist, 37(4)*, 434, 1977, copyright © The Gerontological Society of America)

PHYSIOLOGIC CHARACTERISTICS OF AGING

Movement is essential for activities of daily living, as well as work, educational, and leisure activities. Age-related changes in movement function require an appreciation and understanding of the biologic modifications of aging. As noted earlier in this text, the coordinated support of the musculoskeletal, neuromuscular, cardiovascular, and pulmonary systems in conjunction with the specific metabolic processes are all necessary for functional movement. Although the body's biologic system has a large capacity and functional margins of performance, these functional margins diminish with age. The rate of decline is extremely variable. Inactivity accounts for about half of the functional decline that occurs between age 30 and 70; age-associated changes are ascribed to the other half (Smith & Gilligan, 1983). Exercise training and physical activity can delay and even reverse some of the effects of disuse and aging (Blair & Wei, 2000; Katzel et al., 1995; Thompson, 2000).

Table 16–1 summarizes the age-related physiologic attributes, their functional significance, and effects of exercise training on that attribute (Bottomley & Lewis, 2002b; Bottomley & Lewis, 2002c; Patten & Craik, 2000; Reynolds, 1991; Thompson, 2000).

Common pathologies observed with increasing frequency among the elderly that can accelerate the aging process and increase the rate of functional decline are listed in Table 16–2 by body systems.

TABLE 16–1	Age-Related Physiologic Attribute, Functional Significance, and Effect of Exercise on Change	
Age-Related Change	**Functional Significance**	**Effect of Exercise and Activity**
	Cardiovascular and Pulmonary System	
Decreases of 2–4 bpm resting heart rate.	Decreased cardiac output—if not accompanied by increase in stroke volume.	Does not seem to have any effect.
Decreased cardiac heart muscle and heart volume.	Decreased cardiac output by 25–30%. Decreased maximum stroke volume.	Delays and diminishes decline.
Decreased elasticity of blood vessels.	Increased peripheral resistance. Increased blood pressure. Increased cardiac afterload.	Slows decline and improves cardiovascular proficiency.
Increased systolic blood pressure (10–40 mm Hg). Increased diastolic blood pressure (5–10 mm Hg).	Increased risk of hypertension, AMI, and CVA.	Upon initial onset, elderly persons show a greater decrease in hypertension with exercise training.
Decreased capillary/muscle fiber ratio.	Decreased blood flow to muscle beds and related connective tissue. Delayed healing process.	Delays and diminishes decline. Ratio can actually increase with exercise training.
Decrease of 40–50% vital capacity. Increase of 30–50% residual capacity.	Increased lung compliance. Decreased elastic recoil of lungs. SOB (shortness of breath).	Exercise training may delay or limit these changes. However, in the absence of disease, these changes are compensated for by the respiratory system's large reserve capacity.
Decreased size and number of mitochondria.	Decreased potential to produce energy required for any muscular and/or physiologic work.	Increased volume and size but not number, which contributes to meeting need for increased metabolic energy production.
Decrease of 20–30% functional work capacity (VO$_{2MAX}$/MET level) young-old (55–75) old-old (>75)	Decline in ability to perform ADLs and IADLs. average 5–7 METs average 2.5 METs	Exercise training slows decrease of work capacity and aids in maintaining functional skills and ability to participate in recreational activities.
	Musculoskeletal System	
Decreased bone mineral content.	*Women:* Decrease of 0.75–1%/yr. beginning at age 30–35. Decrease of 2–3%/yr. from menopause to 5 years after menopause. ≈ 30% on bone mineral loss by age 70. *Men:* Decrease of 0.4%/yr. beginning at age 50. Usually not a problem until age 80. Increased risk of bone fracture, especially vertebral, hip, and wrist fractures.	Exercise is beneficial in decreasing the amount of bone mineral loss, and resistive exercises have been shown to increase bone mineral density in some instances.
Increased stiffness of connective tissue surrounding joints.	Decreased flexibility 20–30%. Decreased joint stability and mobility.	Improved flexibility and mobility.
Decreased cartilage water content.	Decreased nutritional fluid exchange in cartilage, leading to increased degenerative joint changes. Loss of height in spine and increased risk of vertebral compression fractures and kyphosis.	Provides increased nutritional fluid exchange for cartilage. Spinal extension exercises can decrease risk of vertebral compression fractures and may help to prevent deformity.

Continues

Age-Related Change	Functional Significance	Effect of Exercise and Activity
Neuromuscular System		
Decrease of 25–40% muscle mass.	Decreased lower extremity musculature > upper extremity. Decreased distal musculature > proximal. Type II (FT) > Type I (SO). Loss of strength and endurance.	Increased strength and endurance. Muscle hypertrophy occurs with resistive exercise training, but is unlikely with only aerobic exercise training.
Decrease of 10–15% nerve conduction velocity.	Changes in threshold for action potential. Increased refractory period. Widening of the synaptic cleft. Functional denervation.	Exercise training increases the proficiency of motor unit recruitment for movement. Neural factors are responsible for initial increases in strength with resistive training.
Decreased "psychomotor speed."	Decreased reaction time. Loss of balance and coordination. Increased risk of falls.	Exercise delays decline and preserves functional reaction time for activities such as crossing a street.
Metabolic		
Decrease of 15% basal metabolic rate.	Decreased physical activity. Loss in muscle mass accounts for age-associated decrease in BMR. Fewer calories are required to supply energy, but nutritional requirements are unchanged.	Slows decline of BMR. Exercise training with adequate intensity will decrease accumulation of internal fat deposits.
Decreased lean body mass.	Diminished strength leads to compromise of ability to perform ADLs/IADLs; increased chance of falls.	Resistive exercise training can increase muscle mass; strengthening muscle of LE has been shown to decrease fall risks.
Increased fat mass.	Increased risk for chronic disorder (atherosclerosis, hypercholesterolemia, hypertension).	Aerobic exercise with adequate intensity can decrease fat mass.
Decreased glucose tolerance and insulin responsiveness.	Increased incidence of non-insulin-dependent diabetes mellitus (NIDDM).	Aerobic exercise improves glucose tolerance and prevents the onset of NIDDM.
Decrease of 30–50% renal function.	Slower clearing of metabolic waste products. Increased risk of drug toxicity and electrolyte imbalance.	Exercise can improve clearing of metabolic waste products.
Decreased total body water.	May present increased risk when exercising.	Adequate hydration is necessary during exercise; however, exercise has not been shown to alter age-related decreases in total body water content.

| TABLE 16–2 | Common Pathologies Observed with Increasing Frequency in the Elderly |

System	Pathologies
Cardiovascular	Coronary artery disease; hypertension; valvular heart disease; left ventricular dysfunction and failure; congestive heart failure; dysrhythmias; aortic stenosis and aneurysms; peripheral vascular disease
Pulmonary	Chronic obstructive and restrictive pulmonary disease; pulmonary edema; asthma; pneumonia
Musculoskeletal	Osteoporosis; degenerative joint disease/arthritis; degenerative disk disease; thoracic kyphosis; Paget's disease, polymyalgia rheumatica; hip, wrist, and vertebral compression fractures
Metabolic/endocrine	Diabetes; hypercholesterolemia; obesity; kidney failure
Peripheral and central nervous system	Cerebral vascular accident; peripheral neuropathies, Parkinson's disease; dementia; Alzheimer's disease
Sensory: Eye	Presbyopia; cataracts; glaucoma; macular degeneration
Sensory: Ear	Presbycusis
Sensory: Vestibular	Presbyastasis, disequilibrium

CARDIOVASCULAR AND PULMONARY SYSTEMS

As a person ages, the cardiovascular and pulmonary systems undergo normal physiologic adaptations. Cardiovascular health risks were introduced in Chapter 15 of this text. In older adults there is tremendous physiologic variation among persons of the same chronologic age. Decreased cardiac output, stroke volume, and maximum heart rate, together with increased systolic and diastolic blood pressure, generally represent the age-related cardiovascular changes. In the absence of disease, age-related declines in the cardiovascular system function will be affected earlier than the slower, progressive aging changes in the pulmonary system. Unlike the cardiovascular system, the pulmonary system has a large functional reserve capacity that can more easily compensate for the physiologic and structural changes in the lungs (American College of Sports Medicine, 2000; Cohen, 1999a; Cohen, 1999b).

Movement requires the coordinated function of heart and lungs as well as pulmonary and peripheral circulation to transport the oxygen and nutrients required to support muscular contraction and functions of other metabolically active tissues. The muscle must have the ability to extract these elements from the vascular and interstitial tissues, and the capability to metabolically generate the energy needed to execute movement. The vascular system must not only deliver oxygen and nutrients to metabolically active tissues, but also be able to remove and dispose of carbon dioxide and metabolic waste products of physical activity. Thus, the muscular component of movement requires the support of the cardiovascular and pulmonary systems. Limitations in either of these systems can affect the function of the others such that heart disease can cause both abnormal breathing and gas exchange response, and primary pulmonary disease can cause abnormal cardiac responses (Peel, 1996).

The relationship between cardiopulmonary function and an individual's maximum performance level or functional capacity is expressed by the **Fick equation:** $VO_{2max} = CO \times a\text{-}\bar{v} O_2$ difference. VO_{2max} is the maximum volume of oxygen the body can utilize; CO is cardiac output, or the product of heart rate and stroke volume; and $a\text{-}\bar{v} O_2$ is the arteriovenous difference, or the measure of the body's ability to extract and utilize oxygen. Cardiac output is referred to as the *central component* of this equation, or the *deliver component.* Arteriovenous difference is referred to as the *peripheral* or *utilization component* (McArdle, Katch, & Katch, 1996).

Maximum oxygen consumption (VO_{2max}) is the maximum energy the body can generate through aerobic processes and represents the functional capacity of the cardiovascular system. It is a measure of the total amount of oxygen that an individual can utilize when doing physical working or exercising from initiation to exhaustion. It is also defined as aerobic, or functional, work capacity and relates to physical endurance. VO_{2max} is considered an overall index of aerobic physical fitness (Cohen, 1999a). For any activity, a person uses only a percentage of her functional capacity. The more vigorous the activity is, the greater the percentage of functional capacity required.

Aerobic, or functional, capacity is greatly affected by age and disease-related processes. Thus, persons having a lower functional capacity will be limited in their ability to perform *activities of daily living (ADLs).* The measure of functional capacity is often expressed as a **metabolic equivalent unit (MET).** One MET is equal to approximately the body's utilization of 3.5 ml O_2 per kilogram of body weight per minute (ml O_2/kg/min). One MET is the average energy cost of just resting. Walking 2 miles per hour requires 2.5 METs. If a person's maximum functional capacity is only 5 METs, that person will have to use 50 percent of his functional capacity just to walk at this pace.

Heart rate and stroke volume are the primary determinants of cardiac output (CO). Cardiac output increases linearly as a function of oxygen consumption during exercise. Heart rate is a major determinant of cardiac output, especially during moderate to maximal exercise. Cardiac output decreases with age, while resting heart rate remains unchanged. Increased stiffness of the ventricular walls due to connective tissue changes and the gradual loss of the contractility strength of the heart contribute to decreased cardiac output. There is also a slight hypertrophy of the left ventricular wall associated with aging (Cerny & Burton, 2001).

The two most prevalent cardiovascular diseases associated with age are hypertension and coronary artery disease. In a longitudinal study, Hagberg (1987) reported that persons free from hypertension and coronary artery disease demonstrated no decreased cardiac output at rest and 5 percent per decade decline in age-related maximum cardiac output, which is consistent with the 5 percent per decade decrease in maximum heart rate. In other words, this suggests that maximum stroke volume is unchanged and that heart function is not compromised in these persons. The comparison group in this study with identified cardiovascular disease had noticeable decreases in resting cardiac output and twice the rate of decline in maximum cardiac output. The implication is that in the absence of hypertension and coronary artery disease, cardiac function can for the most part be preserved in persons who are physically active.

Arteriovenous difference ($a\text{-}\bar{v} O_2$) refers to the ability of the muscles to extract and metabolically utilize oxygen. It is a measure of the difference between the oxygen in the arterial blood entering the muscle beds and the oxygen that remains in the venous blood leaving the muscles. Utilization of the oxygen by the mitochondria to produce the energy for muscle contraction is a complex process also involving oxidative enzymes. The more effectively the mitochondria can extract and use oxygen, the greater the contribution to VO_{2max} and aerobic physical fitness. There is an age-related decrease in the size and number of mitochondria and a decrease in oxidative enzyme activity. The muscle-fiber-to-capillary ratio and total hemoglobin also decrease and contribute to age-related reduction in the arteriovenous oxygen difference (Cerny & Burton, 2001; Cohen, 1999a; McArdle, Katch, & Katch, 1996). However, with exercise training, aging muscle appears to be able to increase both its oxidative capacity and mitochondria volume (Orlander et al., 1978) and capillary-to-muscle-fiber ratio (Larsson, 1982).

Increasing vascular stiffness due to loss of blood-vessel elasticity and increase in arterial wall thickness increase peripheral resistance. In part this contributes to age-related increases in blood pressure. The rise in systolic pressure is generally greater than the rise in diastolic pressure. Higher total peripheral resistance limits the forward movement of the blood into the aorta and through the vascular tree. Consequently, with increased peripheral resistance, the heart attempts to work harder to perfuse the body, and over time, less blood is able to exit the heart, with each beat contributing to chronic increases in afterload that leads to left ventricular hypertrophy and a stretching (and therefore weakening) of the heart muscle (Cerny & Burton, 2001; Cohen, 1999a).

The pulmonary system has a large ventilatory reserve capacity that can compensate for the structural and physiologic effects of aging. However, in the absence of disease, declines in pulmonary system are not noticeable until the individual reaches 60, 70, or even 80 years of age. There is decreased mobility of the bony thorax, with less efficient resting position of the muscles of respiration that alter lung performance. Loss of the alveoli-capillary interface and increased alveolar size secondary to destruction of the walls of individual alveoli are the major forms of lung deterioration found with aging. Lung compliance, or the ability of the lungs to expand, increases with age, as noted by the increasing size of alveoli; and at the same time, elastic recoil of the lungs decreases. Both of these changes lead to increased air trapping and loss of oxygen exchange in the compromised alveolar structures. As a result of these changes, residual volume increases because of increased air trapping within the alveoli and concurrent decreases in vital capacity (Cohen, 1999b). However, secondary to the large functional reserve in the pulmonary system and in the absence of disease, these changes usually do not have a noticeable effect on function until the 8th decade.

BODY COMPOSITION

The progressive increase in body fat accompanied by a decrease in lean body mass beginning about age 30 was discussed in Chapter 15. With less lean muscle mass, there is less metabolically active tissue, contributing to a decline both in the basal metabolic rate and in energy requirements, as reflected in the decline of VO_{2max}. These body changes also increase the older person's risk for chronic disorders such as decreased glucose tolerance, non-insulin-dependent diabetes (Type II), hypercholesterolemia, atherosclerosis, and hypertension (Thompson, 2000). Many of these conditions can be moderated or even reversed with exercise (Blair, 1993).

Total body water content also decreases with age, which is exhibited intracellularly as either dehydration of the cell or a decrease in cell mass when hydration is adequate. Dehydration is a frequent problem in the elderly, especially during exercise. Electrolyte imbalances associated with dehydration are also common with aging (Bottomley & Lewis, 2002).

Degeneration of the articular joint surfaces leads to osteoarthritis and progressive demineralization of bones, resulting in **osteopenia** and osteoporosis, which are the primary earmarks of an aging skeletal system. Osteoarthritis and degenerative joint disease are characterized by atrophy and degeneration of the articular cartilage and hypertrophy of the subchondral bone and joint capsule. In addition to the deleterious effect of aging on joint surfaces, age-related changes in ligaments, tendons, and other connective tissues are characterized by decreased mobility and flexibility.

In Chapter 15, hyaline cartilage, which covers the articular surfaces of most joints, was described. This type of cartilage has no neural or vascular supply and is about 70–80 percent water. Hyaline cartilage depends on the intra-articular fluid content and joint movement for nutritional exchange and for its ability to withstand compressive stresses without structural damage. With aging, water content in the joint decreases, and there is loss of the normal viscosity in the synovial fluid. If range of motion is lost, nutritional exchange to portions of the articular cartilage is also reduced; this leaves the joint vulnerable to developing degenerative changes, especially in the weight-bearing joints (Moncur, 2000).

Collagen is an insoluble fibrous protein found in connective tissue such as tendons, bones, ligaments, and cartilage. Increased *cross-linking* of collagen fibers is seen with aging. It can also be caused by inactivity. The result of cross-linking is that the fibers no longer glide easily with respect to each other, contributing to decreased mobility of these tissues and increased stiffness in the movement of joint structures. In the older person, collagen is less movable and responds more slowly to stretching, but with time it does stretch (Lewis & Kellems, 2002). Older adults are able to demonstrate increases in flexibility with exercise programs emphasizing stretching. These results may be enhanced by modification such as adding weights (Swank et al., 2003). Strengthening the musculature around the joint will also decrease the effect of mechanical stresses surrounding the joint (Lewis & Kellems, 2002).

Osteoporosis is another major manifestation of the aging skeletal system. It affects 15–20 million people, primarily women, and is responsible for thousands of injuries and deaths per year. Osteoporosis occurs when there is an imbalance between bone resorption and bone formation. This process was described in greater detail in Chapter 15. Pathologic fractures of the vertebra, wrist, and hip represent the most common exacerbations of the disease.

Physical inactivity is only one of the many factors contributing to pathogenesis of osteoporosis. During normal activity or exercise, there are three forces acting on the bone: gravity, weight bearing, and the pulling forces of the muscle on the bone. Bone loss occurs when physical levels and weight bearing are decreased. Physical activity increases remineralization of the bone tissue in persons who exercise (Guccione, 2000).

Common changes in aging posture include forward head position, slight **kyphosis,** and changes in lumbar **lordosis** (Guccione, 2000). The intervertebral disks contribute to 20–30 percent of the total height of the spinal column. The water content in the nucleus pulposus of the center of the disk ranges from 70 percent to 90 percent. This water content diminishes with age, and as a result, the height of the disk decreases, which accounts partially for the loss of stature with age (Moncur, 2000). There is a high degree of variability with posture in the thoracic spine and rounding of the shoulders. The normal lumbar lordosis becomes either flatter or more accentuated. Recurring anterior vertebral compression fractures of the thoracic spine lead to wedging and increased kyphosis.

Promoting good postural alignment is important in the treatment and prevention of spinal deformities, especially those that come from or lead to vertebral compression fractures. In a now classic study, Sinaki and Mikkelsen (1984) grouped postmenopausal women who had incurred at least one vertebral compression fracture into one of three back-exercise protocol groups: flexion only, flexion and extension, and extension only. In a two-year follow-up study the incidence of vertebral compression fracture recurrence was 89 percent in the flexion exercise group; 56 percent in the flexion-extension group; and 16 percent in the extension group.

Sinaki et al. (2002), in their latest research study, found that even without hormone replacement, exercises to strengthen back extensor muscles could provide significant protection against spinal fractures in women at risk for osteoporosis and that this benefit lasts for several years. The study involved 50 healthy postmenopausal women, ages 58–75. Twenty-seven performed back-extension strengthening exercises for 2 years, while the other 23 served as the control group. There was no difference in the bone mineral density between the two groups at the end of the 2-year exercise period. However, at the end of 10 years, members of the control group were 2.7 times more likely to have vertebral compression than the back-extension exercise group ($p = 0.0004$). The exercise group also retained a significant advantage in back strength, such that even 8 years after the study ended, its members had less bone density loss than did those in the control group.

NEUROMUSCULAR SYSTEM

Muscle atrophy through the loss of lean muscle mass is among the most notable physical changes that occur with aging. Concurrent with this change is an increase in body fat and connective tissue. Functionally this may limit flexibility and mobility and increase the frequency of soft tissue injuries. Coordination of muscle contractions for functional movements is mediated through peripheral and central nervous systems. There are changes at the neuromuscular junction with aging, and nerve impulse transmission slows.

Gait activities are mediated through the neuromuscular system. Numerous changes in gait occur with aging. They include mild rigidity and less body motion proximally than distally. Automatic movements such as arm swing decrease in amplitude and speed. The base of support or stride becomes wider to improve stability, and step length becomes smaller. More time is spent in the double-support stance with decreased swing-to-stance ratio. Many of these gait changes, including a slower pace, are adaptations that provide an increased sense of safety during walking activities (Lewis & Kellems, 2002).

In the aging nervous system, neurons are smaller and fewer. Nerve conduction velocities decrease concurrently with decreases in neurotransmitters and a widening of the synaptic cleft at the neuromuscular junction (Gutmann & Hanzlikova, 1976). Atrophy of the muscles results from a decrease in both the size and the number of muscle fibers. The most characteristic morphologic change is the decrease in Type II fast-twitch fiber areas that parallels functional decline at the same age. Type I slow-twitch fiber areas remain unchanged or slightly increased. Decreases in mitochondria and oxidative enzyme volumes also contribute to declines in strength.

The functional result of all of these neuromuscular changes is the generalized weakness, impaired mobility and balance, and poor endurance that characterize age-related disability and are associated with frailty. Clinical studies correlate physical frailty with falls, fractures, impaired ability to perform activities of daily living, and loss of independence.

However, strength-training programs are effective in increasing Type I and Type II muscle fiber areas (Larsson, 1982). For significant gains in strength and muscle hypertrophy in elderly persons, a longer resistive-training program is required than for younger persons. Frontera et al. (1988) demonstrated that a vigorous 12-week strength-training program can lead to muscle hypertrophy due to an increase in the size of Type I and Type II muscle fibers. This hypertrophy was not evident until toward the end of the 12-week period. Nonetheless, these results demonstrate that the capacity for increasing muscle mass is retained into old age and that the strength gains are in part due to hypertrophy.

Fiatarone et al. (1994) conducted a randomized controlled trial comparing progressive exercise resistance training for nonexercisers with 100 frail nursing home residents over a 10-week period. The mean age of 63 women and 37 men enrolled in the study was 87.1 ± 0.6 years; 94 percent of the participants completed the study. The training regimen consisted of high-intensity progressive resistive training of hip and knee extensors three days a week for 10 weeks. These muscle groups were selected because of their importance in daily functional activities. At the conclusion of the study, muscle strength increased 113 ± 8 percent in participants who underwent exercise training as compared to 3 ± 9 percent of nonexercisers; gait velocity increased by 11.8 ± 3.8 percent, and stair-climbing power improved by 28.4 ± 6.6 percent versus 1.0 ± 3.8 percent (gait velocity) and 3.6 ± 6.7 percent (stair-climbing power) for nonexercisers. The researchers concluded that low muscle mass and muscle weakness were strongly associated with impaired mobility in frail elderly people and that this association is independent of the effects of chronic disease, dementia, depression, and other age-related characteristics of advanced age. The ability of the aging muscle system to respond to progressive resistive training is preserved. Consequently, correction of disuse can be accompanied by significant enhancement in levels of functional mobility and overall activity (Fiatarone et al., 1994).

INTEGUMENTARY SYSTEM

There are undeniable changes in the skin as it ages. The epidermis thins and flattens, making it more susceptible to shearing stresses, which can lead to blisters and skin tears. The dermis also atrophies and has diminished vascularity. There is a loss of collagen and elastin fibers. Loss of tissue support for the remaining capillaries results in an increased tendency to bruise (senile purpura). Lentigos (flat pigmented age spots) increase with exposure to the sun. The number and size of oil and sweat glands decreases, resulting in less sweat production. Older skin does not stay as moist or as well lubricated as younger skin (Bottomley & Lewis, 2002c). These changes are illustrated in Figure 16–5.

CENTRAL NERVOUS SYSTEM

Although the normal aging process results in changes in the brain and components of the central nervous system, there are no significant associated neurologic impairments or deficits that can be attributed completely to the aging process. The most notable age-related functional changes in the central nervous system include slowing down and deterioration in the quality of movement and changes in the cognitive and sensory systems (Bottomley & Lewis, 2002a; Patten & Craik, 2000). Changes in the motor unit were discussed in the previous section.

There is a linear decline in the size and weight of the brain as an individual grows older. The age-related declines in cerebral blood flow, oxygen need, and glucose utilization by the brain are not significant enough to account for the extent of brain atrophy that accompanies aging. Until recently, the progressive loss of cortical neurons with aging was an accepted premise. However, newer neuroanatomic techniques have

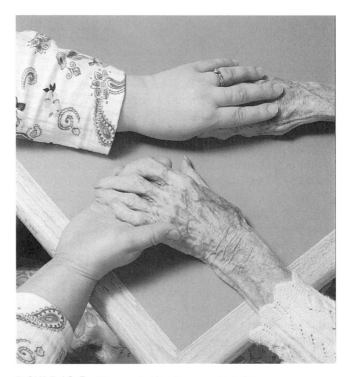

FIGURE 16–5 Changes in Skin Common to Aging

demonstrated across species that cortical neuron loss is not a manifestation of normal aging. The normal changes that do occur with age do not result in significant neurologic impairment and fail to demonstrate any associated neurologic deficit that can be completely attributed to aging.

The aging brain remains plastic in that individuals can purposely continue to gain or retain complex skills. As mature adults, aging persons may have reached their biologic capacity for brain growth, but they can continue to channel their resources or energies into valued skills and activity competence (Hogstel, 2001).

Neuronal loss is a factor in dementing processes (Bottomley & Lewis, 2002a; Patten & Craik, 2000). Decreased gyral thickness and increased size of the ventricles are the two most prominent structural changes. Decreased gyral thickness occurs in the gray or white matter or both. It is not found throughout the cerebral cortex but is limited to certain regions. A progressive increase in the size of the ventricles accompanies the decreased brain weight. It is gradual up to the 7th decade; then there is a marked increase in the 8th and 9th decade (Bottomley & Lewis, 2002a; Patten & Craik, 2000).

There is significant neuronal loss from subcortical regions of the brain such as the thalamus, forebrain, and hippocampus. Acting through a variety of neurotransmitters, these areas of the brain project to and serve as modulators of higher cortical function. Furthermore, subcortical systems are significant sources of neurotransmitters such as dopamine, serotonin, and acetylcholine. Hence, any significant loss of neurons in subcortical areas can lead to depletion of neurotransmitters. Functionally these losses translate into diminishing ability to modulate activity and thus movement.

Another age-related change across species is the loss of Purkinje fibers from the cerebellum. These CNS structures have an important role in regulating various and multiple aspects of movement, including control of posture and balance, locomotion, movement sequencing, repetitive and alternating movements, and smooth eye movements (Patten & Craik, 2000).

It is now evident that much of the loss of brain mass occurs in the myelinated structures of white matter. Not only does the volume of myelin decrease, but also the integrity of it is impaired. Myelin is important for the rapid, accurate, and effective transmission of neural signals. In context, the compromise of the myelinated structures accounts for slowing of psychomotor speed, increased processing time required for complex information, and transmission of motor responses via the corticospinal and peripheral neural pathways (Patten & Craik, 2000).

Early work of Spirduso (1980) suggested that exercise can affect the rate of change in the aging nervous system. She related physical fitness to *psychomotor speed*, or "the speed with which an individual can perform a task which involves reacting motorically to an environmental stimulus" (Spirduso, 1980, p. 851). The reaction time and movements of the more physically fit group of aged persons were faster than those of the sedentary young group. She hypothesized that those who have maintained a high level of physical activity and training are better able to cope with daily environmental hazards such as walking, crossing the street, or driving a car.

SENSORY SYSTEMS

Before the age of 50 most adults have some noticeable declines in sensory system function (Papalia et al., 1996). These changes result in a higher sensory threshold and a decrease in sensory acuity (Hogstel, 2001). Most sensory changes occur gradually, and the individual adapts to these changes with little impact on daily function. By later adulthood many people will self-limit sensory challenges (like driving a car at night) and have adapted their work spaces for valued occupations.

Visual System

Presbyopia, the most common visual problem among older adults, was presented in Chapter 15. This condition results in the physiologic loss of accommodation, or ability to focus on near objects. Photoreceptors in the retina and their related projections to the thalamus and visual cortex exhibit an age-related loss of up to half the cells that process information. The size of the pupil decreases with age (Hogstel, 2001). The smaller pupil size results in a need for brighter lighting for reading and other close tasks. Color discrimination is impacted by age-related changes in the lens of the eye. The lens becomes more opaque (Castor & Carter, 1995) and yellow (Kee, 1990), resulting in increased sensitivity to glare and difficulty discriminating blue-green and violet colors. Pupillary responses diminish or are even absent. Glare and sudden changes in light are problems for the older adult (Patten & Craik, 2000). Tear secretion decreases by up to 40 percent in older individuals (Bottomley & Lewis, 2002a).

The most common visual disorders in older individuals are cataracts, glaucoma, and macular degeneration. **Cataracts** are developmental or degenerative opacity of the lens, causing obstruction and scattering of light to the retina. The scattered light causes images to be blurred, and visual acuity is reduced. Removal of the cataract lens and intraocular lens implant is the therapy of choice. For those who are not candidates for lens implants, contact lenses or cataract glasses are options (Bottomley & Lewis, 2002a).

Glaucoma is one of the leading causes of blindness in persons over the age of 35, yet 95–98 percent of blindness due to glaucoma is preventable. Vision loss from glaucoma is caused by damage to the optic nerve. This nerve acts like an electric cable with over a million wires and is responsible for carrying the images we see to the brain. Increased intraocular pressure is a risk factor for glaucoma. There are two types. *Open-angle* is the most common and has an insidious onset. It is usually painless and asymptomatic until major damage and visual loss occurs. Fluid normally flowing from the intraocular cavity out of the eye through a canal is either decreased or blocked. Medication is usually given to enlarge the canal; sometimes surgery is required. Regular screening examinations are a vital preventative measure. The second type of glaucoma is *acute closed-angle.* Onset is usually sudden and very painful. Increased size of the lens mechanically obstructs flow of intraocular fluid by displacing the lens forward against the iris and cornea, occluding any fluid flow. Intraocular pressure builds up very quickly. Topical eye drops can control the disease, but often surgical intervention is required (Bottomley & Lewis, 2002a).

Macular degeneration is the third major source of visual disability and is more serious than cataracts or glaucoma because it is currently the least treatable. Due to small hemorrhages in the macular area, the individual sees gray shadows in the center of her visual field. However, she can see the outer borders better. This condition significantly limits activity participation and the use of electronic media like the television or a computer (Bottomley & Lewis, 2002a).

Auditory System

Presbycusis, described in Chapter 15, is an inner-ear age-related decline in auditory acuity and the most common cause of hearing loss in adults. The incidence of hearing loss is 50–60 percent in persons 71–80 years of age. Hearing loss is the third most prevalent chronic condition found in community-dwelling older adults; only arthritis and hypertension occur more frequently. It is characterized by a slow, bilateral, symmetrical, progressive high-frequency sensorineural hearing loss that includes poor speech discrimination. Older persons may report no difficulty because the loss is very gradual or because they are very sensitive about admitting the loss. Most typical of aging is a selective high-frequency hearing loss rather than a generalized loss in hearing acuity (Hogsdell, 2001). Presbycusis was once thought to be part of normal aging but now is seen as having a large genetic component (Hills, 2002).

Vestibular System

Complaints of balance problems and dizziness are common in older persons. When no other pathologies are noted, **presbyastasis** is the term used to describe this disequilibrium. Studies indicate that there is a 20 percent reduction in the hair cells of saccule and utricle that sense linear acceleration and a 40 percent decline in the hair cells of the semicircular canals, which monitor angular acceleration of the head. Other factors may contribute to age-related disequilibrium, including vestibular pathology, changes in other sensory systems, and changes in the motor system. Distinguishing presbyastasis from other pathologies and impairments may lead to a more successful treatment outcome (Hills, 2002).

Presbyastasis can lead to individuals' developing a **fear of falling (FOF).** The prevalence of FOF is reported to be between 29 percent and 92 percent among older adults and is associated with poorer health status and functional decline. FOF etiology is multifactorial and affected minimally by physical, psychological, or functional influences. Recommended interventions for FOF include education, environmental safety considerations, discussion of risk-taking behaviors, assertiveness training, and improving physical fitness (Legters, 2002).

Olfactory and Gustatory Systems

The chemical senses of taste and smell become less acute with age, and saliva flow decreases. *Hyposmia* is the decreased sensitivity to smell that occurs in the olfactory system. *Hypogeuia* is the decreased sensitivity to taste that occurs in the gustatory system. Both are reported as age-dependent changes. Decreased perception of both taste and smell may make food less appealing and lead to poor nutrition. It may also place an older person at risk for failing to recognize (1) food that may be spoiled or (2) toxic gases such as cooking or heating fuels, since he cannot detect these warning cues. To compensate for these dampened senses, food choices should highlight appearance and texture for their appeal, and the social aspect of mealtime should be emphasized. Condiments other than salt should be used liberally to augment flavor. Older persons, and their families and friends, should develop a habit of checking pilot lights and stored foods for safety hazards (Hills, 2002).

COGNITIVE CHARACTERISTICS OF AGING

Earlier in this chapter physiologic changes in brain weight and circulation were discussed. In spite of these measurable changes, there is no evidence that normal aging leads to poor cognitive function or mental disorders. Changes in cognition that impact function do begin to appear in later life. In the area of global mental functions, the aged person is likely to experience differences in orientation functions and learning. Difficulties with orientation to time sometimes occur as well. These difficulties seem to be related to the dramatic lifestyle changes associated with aging.

A capacity for cognitive reserve has been demonstrated in the older adult. Although a younger person's ability and efficacy for learning remains higher, older adults' ability to learn and improve their cognitive performances continues (Stevens-Long & Commons, 1992). The changes in learning, related to crystallized and fluid intelligence, are discussed in Chapter 15. Older persons often demonstrate diminished performance in timed learning tasks, in learning that is novel (or in novel environments), and in understanding new methods or situations (Chop & Robnett, 1999). For example, as electronic communication methods like E-mail and cell phones become normative in society, many older persons feel left behind and overwhelmed by the novelty of the communication context.

It is in the realm of the ICF "specific mental functions" that functional change is common and normative.

There are documented aging effects in the areas of attention, memory, psychomotor functions, and perceptual functions (Chop & Robnett, 1999; Hogstel, 2002). Each of these specific mental functions will be reviewed briefly here. Table 16–3 summarizes the effects of aging on specific mental functions.

ATTENTION

Attention, first discussed in Chapter 3, emerges in infancy. There are many specialized types of attention that develop in humans. Children can be distracted from tasks easily by sensory information, like sounds or movement. By adolescence, **selective attention,** the ability to subconsciously screen out extraneous information while focusing on important cues, is well developed. It is selective attention that allows you to sit in a lecture hall with 100 other students and maintain your focus on the instructor. It is also what allows you to function in busy places, like parties. For example, at a party, in spite of the hubbub of voices, you can focus on

TABLE 16–3	Effects of Aging on Specific Mental Functions	
Specific Mental Function	**Functional Changes associated with Aging**	**Retained Functional Abilities**
Attention	• Divided-attention tasks	• Sustained attention to task
Memory	• Short-term and working memory • Newly learned materials	• Long-term memory • Procedural information • Overlearned information
Psychomotor	• Reaction time and speed of performance • Unfamiliar and difficult tasks • Oculomotor skill (including visual tracking)	• Verbal abilities and performance • Familiar and/or easy tasks • Routine habits
Emotional		• No changes in this area
Perceptual	• Difficulty with figure-ground perception	• Changes related to specific areas of sensory loss
Executive functions	• Abstract reasoning • Mental flexibility	• Decision making • Planning and carrying out plans • Deciding which behaviors are appropriate under what circumstances
Mental functions of language and calculation		• No changes in this area
Mental functions of sequencing and coordinating complex, purposeful movements		• Changes related to specific areas of motor and psychomotor loss

Adapted from Chop & Robnett, 1999.

the voice of the person you're holding a conversation with. And although it may seem that you've filtered everything else out, if someone mentions your name in another conversation, you immediately pick it up. Selective attention "is an essential aspect of perception, information processing, and everyday behavior. In many situations, people engage in divided attention, or the allocation of attentional resources to two simultaneous sources of stimulation" (Hogsdel, 2002, p. 88). An example of this would be checking your E-mail while talking on the phone. On divided-attention tasks, the performance of the older adult decreases, with a more rapid decline after age 70 (Kline & Scialfa, 1997).

Vigilance is "the ability to maintain attention on a task for a sustained period" (Hogsdel, 2002, p. 87). This skill is used when a person must remain highly focused on a task for a long period of time, like driving on winding mountain roads or doing assembly-line work. Performance on vigilance tasks decreases with age and does not seem to be changed by practice to support the skill (Kausler, 1991). The impairments in function in the older adult are greatest when the task is rapidly paced or lengthy, or when the individuals must hold information in memory (Kausler, 1991).

MEMORY PROCESSES

Memory changes associated with aging have been extensively studied (Hogsdel, 2001). It is important to be aware that memory is a dynamic process. *Registration* refers to the point where the sensory input is received. If the older person has a hearing loss or a visual impairment, the memory process may be interrupted at this point. *Encoding* is the mental process of assigning meaning to the sensory input and is characterized by active rehearsal of the information. It is in the area of encoding that many older persons begin to lose efficiency (Hogsdel, 2001). *Retrieval* is the process of locating, and producing for use, encoded information. When information is not efficiently encoded, it becomes difficult to retrieve. The memory loss associated with normal aging is greatest when there is a time pressure (limiting time for both encoding and retrieval) and when the situation is novel (more difficult to encode) (Hogsdel, 2001; Bottomley & Lewis, 2002b; Riley, 2001; Schunk, 2001).

Age-associated memory impairment (AAMI) is a recently defined clinical state. It involves complaints of memory impairment with everyday activities and is a very modest loss of memory function in healthy persons aged 50 and older. In contrast, **benign senescent forgetfulness (BSF)** is a term associated with healthy individuals who experience brief transitory episodes of cognitive decline. It is attributed more to inattentiveness and distractions than to the actual aging process. BSF is not severe enough to interfere with daily activities.

Again, bear in mind also that actual memory loss is a classic sign of dementia or other brain-based syndromes. In addition, complaints of memory loss that are not, in fact, actual memory loss are indicative of a depression disorder. Presentation of depression in the elderly is sometimes misdiagnosed as dementia. It is important for complaints of memory impairments to be thoroughly investigated (Bottomley & Lewis, 2002b; Riley, 2001).

PSYCHOMOTOR FUNCTIONS

Reaction time, coordination of complex movements, and use of feedback to adjust movements dynamically all slow with normal aging (Shumway-Cook & Woollacott, 2001). This fact is illustrated in the 30–70 percent decrease in reaching speed between the ages of 50 and 90 years (Williams, 1990). A study by Pohl, Winstein, and Fisher (1996) demonstrated decreases in movement flow and fluidity with aging. This study showed that older adults had significantly more movement adjustments in coordinated reaching than young adults did.

In addition to large motor changes in movement flow, older adults have decreased abilities to manipulate small objects. Cole, Rotella, and Harper (1999) report that the time required to manipulate small objects increases by as much as 40 percent by 70 years of age. This decrease in speed, precision, and flow of movements can have a profound functional impact on performance of ADLs and IADLs by late adulthood.

PERCEPTUAL FUNCTIONS

It is believed that the common changes in perceptual function in aging are secondary to changes in the sensory systems, interfering with accurate sensory registration, difficulties with divided attention, and difficulties encoding information in the working memory (Hogsdel, 2002). Although the older adult may demonstrate increased difficulties with figure-ground perception and spatial awareness, these limitations reflect the interrelationships between attention, memory, and perception.

EXECUTIVE FUNCTIONS

Executive functions, first described in Chapter 3, include "abstract reasoning, inductive and deductive reasoning, and cognitive flexibility to devise alternative solutions to a problem" (Chop & Robnett, 1999, p. 122). Although there are age-related declines in executive functions, these do not occur until after age 70 in healthy adults (Chop & Robnett, 1999).

PSYCHOSOCIAL CHANGES ASSOCIATED WITH AGING

Aging in America reflects a series of "cultural age deadlines" (Settersten & Hagestad, 1996a; 1996b). These are culturally embedded perceptions that deadlines (or time lines) exist to be "on target" with family, work, and educational achievement. When a person confronts these deadlines, it can result in either a sense of satisfaction or a sense of depression. For the older adult in American culture, there has been a focus on retirement and the end of the work career (Stevens-Long & Commons, 1992). Leisure is expected to expand and increase as retirement age is reached, and maintaining independence in personal self-care remains a valued goal in later life.

Later adulthood is typically a period of personality stability and persistence of lifelong belief patterns. Persons who are self-confident in middle adulthood are likely to remain self-confident, and persons who were inflexible earlier in life are likely to retain this trait as well. The concept of *self-efficacy,* discussed earlier in this text, is a person's conviction that he can organize and implement effective strategies to deal with any potential situation that may be novel or unpredictable and/or have stressful components. Studies by McAuley et al. (1999) on physical activity and self-efficacy suggest that continuous participation in activities, regardless of physical fitness improvements, contributes substantially to enhancing self-efficacy. A weaker sense of self-efficacy has been associated with slower gait speed, fear of falling, and general decline in physical and social function. In contrast, self-efficacy has been found to be a positive predictor for adherence to exercise regimens for persons participating in health-promotion programs or recovering from conditions associated with aging, and in survival rates for persons with chronic diseases. Thus, self-efficacy can be an important factor in maintaining functional performance into later life.

EDUCATION AND SOCIOECONOMIC FACTORS

According to the 2000 census, the level of American education keeps climbing; currently 80 percent of Americans have finished high school or had higher education. The number of middle-aged adults, ages 55–74, who have attained bachelor degrees or higher has risen. Consequently, the educational level of the older age groups, 75 and up, will continue to grow. Educational level is a well-established predictor of continual productive behavior, whether the productive activity is paid or not (Herzog et al., 1989).

Turrell et al. (2002) investigated whether and to what extent socioeconomic mobility over the life course affected cognitive function in later life. Life-course research has demonstrated that adult disease is influenced by socioeconomic mobility. This study found that socioeconomic conditions across all stages of the life course seem to make particular contributions to cognitive function in late middle age. The results indicate that each factor of socioeconomic position—childhood, education, and income—makes independent contributions to levels of cognitive functioning in adulthood. Individuals who began their lives in a socioeconomically disadvantaged position and then attained high education and/or income perform better on every test than their less upwardly mobile counterparts. Although childhood status is important, it is not the sole determinant of cognitive function in later life (Turrell et al., 2002).

FAMILY LIFE AND SOCIAL SUPPORT NETWORKS

Studies consistently show that marriage is most satisfactory in later life (Stevens-Long & Commons, 1992). Older persons report greater satisfaction in their marriages and believe their marriages to be more equitable than their middle-aged counterparts do. Studies of marital satisfaction across the family life cycle note a dramatic improvement in couple relations at or near the point when the last child leaves the home (Bahr & Peterson, 1989). For healthy elderly people this is a time for relationship renewal and increasing shared leisure (Figure 16–6).

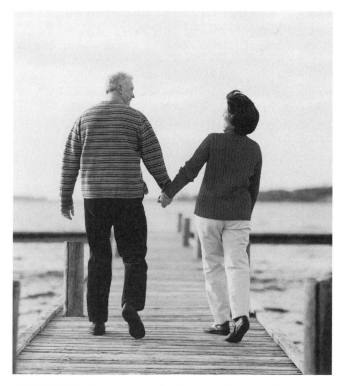

FIGURE 16–6 Sharing leisure time is enjoyed by many older couples. (Image courtesy of PhotoDisc®, Inc.)

American elders continue to have frequent contact with their children and families. However, there is a lot of variability in the amount of contact elderly persons have with their family in spite of ethnic influences and gender-specific roles in caring for aging family members. Daughters tend to have more contact with their aging parents than do sons. Widows have more contact with their children than do their married peers. Married children tend to have less frequent contact with their parents than do unmarried children (Guccione, 2000).

Healthy elders are found to provide both financial and emotional support to their children. With increasing longevity, the amount of time spent being a grandparent has increased, and the roles of grandparents have changed. With so many women entering the workforce outside the home, many grandparents find themselves taking on significant child-care responsibilities. Many grandparents watch their grandchildren mature from infancy to adulthood, and experience having great-grandchildren (Binstock & George, 1996; Guccione, 2000).

When an elderly person becomes sick, she is usually cared for by her spouse. If the spouse is unable or unavailable, caregiving usually falls to a daughter or daughter-in-law. However, with smaller families and fewer children nowadays, and more women entering the workforce, there are fewer women available to care for aging elders. Many middle-aged women find themselves in competing caregiving roles between their children and parents. Research has not demonstrated the role of men in caring for elderly parents. Elderly people who live with their families become part of a multigenerational family and grow old with their children (Guccione, 2000).

Unger et al. (1999) examined the association between social network characteristics and physical functioning according to gender, income, and baseline health function. Social support and social networks have demonstrated protective health benefits in the elderly population, including lower risk of mortality, cardiovascular disease, cancer mortality, and functional decline. Access to information about health and utilization of health services, encouragement of healthy behaviors, provision of concrete aid and emotional support to facilitate coping with life stress, and enhancement of feelings of self-esteem and control may be factors in these outcomes.

One of the findings in the Unger et al. (1999) study was that social support and social networks had a stronger effect on the functional status of men than of women. Women in generally are more skilled at social networking to provide appropriate support at pertinent times. In contrast, men are more reluctant to ask for support. The study also demonstrated a stronger protective effect of social ties for those with lower baseline physical function. Thus, social ties are most important for elderly people with more limited physical abilities. Those with higher incomes appear to be able to remain integrated with a social network, most likely because they are able to afford the transportation and costs of activities.

WIDOWHOOD

Aging carries with it an increasing number of personal losses. One of the significant areas of loss associated with this age group is the loss of a spouse. The grief and bereavement process is difficult not only for the older person but also for their extended family and their friends. In our society death and grief are uncomfortable topics, and the grieving period is supposed to last only a short time (Chop & Robnett, 1999). The feelings of loss, isolation, and extreme sadness can persist for years. When an elderly person is the caregiver for a dying spouse, the emotional situation is extremely complex. With a wide array of reactions, including anger, denial, and poor attention to their own health needs, the caregivers are often in need of both physical and emotional support. Figure 16–7 reflects the importance that memories play for the healthy widowed partner.

Rehabilitative professionals are often interacting with persons at points in the bereavement process. It is important to be aware that disruptions in functional performance in many areas—including cognition, memory, orientation, sleep, and leisure—often are part of the bereavement process (Royal College of Psychiatrists, 2003). Following the death of a loved one, periods of depression are also common.

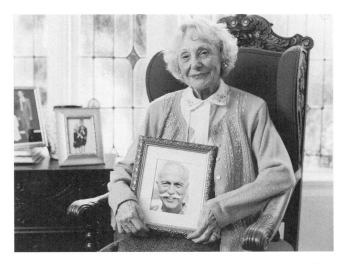

FIGURE 16–7 Memories of the deceased spouse hold comfort for his widow. (Image courtesy of PhotoDisc®, Inc.)

DEPRESSION

Depression is one of the most widespread causes of activity limitation experienced by the elderly (Hogstel, 2002). Although the high incidence of depression in the elderly is commonly attributed to the series of losses and health problems of this age group, recent studies have added new dimensions to our understanding. Depression in the elderly tends to manifest with more ideational symptoms, which are related to thoughts, ideas, and guilt. In addition, older people tend to have anxiety and depression together, rather than depression alone (Ahmed & Takeshita, 1996).

Depression is under-identified in the elderly because their increase in health problems allows for some symptoms of depression to be overlooked. For example, the prevalence of low blood pressure increases with aging. The correlation of depression with low blood pressure also increases as time passes, particularly among men. A study by Barrett-Connor and Palinkas (1994) indicated that "men with low blood pressure scored significantly higher on both the emotional and physical items of a depression test" (p. 447). These same individuals also scored higher on measures of pessimism, sadness, loss of appetite, weight loss, and preoccupation with health than did people with normal blood pressure. This makes low blood pressure a risk factor for the development of depression. Changes in the brain, including neurotransmitter and receptor changes and dementia, increase the risk of depression (Hogsdel, 2002). Figure 16–8 reflects the prevalence of isolation and depression in the aged.

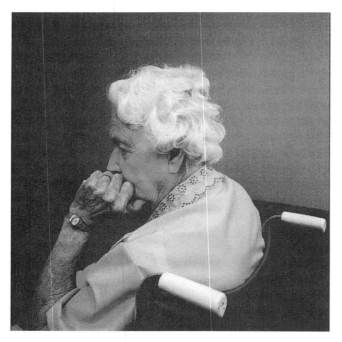

FIGURE 16–8   Depression is a serious functional impairment in the elderly.

Persons with depression have marked activity limitations and diminished functional capacity (Williams, 2002). The apathy, loss of pleasure in daily activities, and fatigue are personal factors that can limit typical activities and participation. Williams (2002) remarks, "For the physically ill elderly person with depression, this loss of functional capacity becomes even more problematic. The deconditioning effects of age and illness combine with depression to result in even more perceived effort required for minor everyday tasks" (p. 166). Unfortunately, many families and health-care providers do not recognize depression in older persons, and it therefore remains untreated.

AREAS OF OCCUPATION

With healthy aging, the individual will remain independent in all of the ADLs discussed in earlier chapters. While changes in balance, reaction time, and endurance are common, simple accommodations to the change in personal skill are all that is needed for continued performance of bathing, showering, dressing, eating, functional mobility, personal hygiene, sexual activity, and sleep. Unlike ADLs, there are some changes in IADLs in the older adult. IADLs are defined as "activities that are oriented toward interacting with the environment and that are often complex" (American Occupational Therapy Association, 2002, p. 620). IADLs may be completed by the individual or delegated to another. The older adult may be more likely than younger persons to delegate tasks like community mobility, home management, and shopping.

EDUCATION

Many older adults continue to choose to participate in learning environments. Learning may be independent study on some topic of interest, it can be associated with a community group, or it may be a structured student-teacher relationship. With the increased leisure some elders experience, it is not uncommon for them to develop long-suppressed interests in skills as diverse as oil painting, learning to play a musical instrument, and golfing. Because of the increasing need for basic computer skills, and the widespread use of E-mail and the Internet for family communications, computer classes have become popular with the elderly.

WORK AND RETIREMENT

According to the *2002 American Perceptions on Aging in the 21st Century* report, 19 percent of persons surveyed age 65 and older are not retired at all. This report also identified a new retirement pattern—simultaneously retired and working persons accounted for 23 percent of the respondents. Increased participation rates of women in the labor force have been the most significant trend in the past 40 years (Sterns, Junkins, & Bayer, 2001). The number of paid hours of work per week is relatively steady for persons 25–54 years old. Beginnings at age 55, the average number of paid working hours of the older adult is markedly lower (Herzog et al., 1989). Currently work and retirement are not mutually exclusive categories. Retirement appears to be a process, not "an event." Those reporting that they are completely retired and not working at all totals only 58 percent (National Council on the Aging, 2002).

Factors influencing the retirement experience include whether the retirement is voluntary or forced. Personal-satisfaction factors linked to retirement include health, income, attitudes, and preparedness for retirement. Voluntary retirees demonstrated higher occupational status, income, health, and life satisfaction than involuntary retirees, who in contrast exhibited signs of poor adaptation. In spite of the 1986 amendments to the Age Discrimination Act that eliminated mandatory retirement policies for most occupations, health and pre-retirement attitudes remained the most significant predictors of retirement satisfaction (Sterns, Junkins, & Bayer, 2001; Kimmel, Price, & Walker, 1978).

Retirement creates many life changes for individuals, which usually include more free time and less income. There are multiple pathways from work to retirement. Mutchler et al. (1999) studied the different exit patterns of a sample of 2,226 white and black men aged 55–74. Over a 28-month period, the patterns of continuous work, continuous nonwork, crisp exits, and blurred exits were studied. A crisp transition is a clear-cut, nonreversed, single exit from the workforce. Gradual but repeated exits and reentries into and out of the workforce over months or years characterized a blurred-exit pattern. Crisp and blurred transitions varied according to age, financial resources, and health status. Crisp transitions are more likely to occur at an age younger than 65. Persons with the poorest of health usually demonstrated a crisp exit. Individuals with limited financial resources and individuals with less than average good health were more likely to have blurred transitions. There is much complexity to the process of retiring, and it can no longer be seen as a single transition (Sterns, Junkins, & Bayer, 2001).

It is obvious that healthier retirees transition more easily into retirement and have higher life satisfaction than unhealthy persons. Recent evidence suggests that married men in moderate to poor health have a lower than expected attachment to work if they have a working wife. Currently there are rising rates of labor force activity among married women; and in the absence of improved health, older men are leaving the workforce at higher rates and making little attempt to reenter it (Mutchler et al., 1999).

Although loss of money in retirement can be a significant stressor, what seems more important is the adequacy of the older person's available income (Sterns, Junkins, & Bayer, 2001). Some researchers suggest that tomorrow's retirees will be at least as well off as their parents. However, with the economic difficulties that began in 2000, the combination of social security and pension income may be viewed as inadequate to support a desired retirement lifestyle. If retirement is less affordable, labor force attachment may become stronger, at least among those older workers in good health (Mutchler et al., 1997).

While late adulthood is typically viewed as a period of retirement from paid work, many elders continue to work in some capacity. The literature has established that an active lifestyle contributes to psychological well-being among older, noninstitutionalized adults (Searle, 1991). Both remunerative employment and volunteer activities help link the older person to his community. For persons in this developmental period, work provides opportunities to pursue and meet personal goals and challenges. Volunteer work also serves to enhance a sense of community and improve quality of life (Chop & Robnett, 1999).

Herzog et al. (1989) provided a comprehensive list of nonpaid productive activities, including maintenance of one home and possessions, volunteer work, housework, child-care, informal assistance to relatives and friends, and care provided to impaired others. Utilizing this expanded definition of productive activities, age differences in productive contributions both paid and unpaid were examined. This study found that older Americans participate in many unpaid activities at levels comparable to younger and middle-aged Americans. In a subsequent study, Herzog and Morgan (1992) confirmed that at all ages, women were found to have at least the same or greater productive time, although more of their productive time was unpaid.

Full-time work is generally calculated on a 40-hour workweek for 52 weeks, or approximately 2,080 work hours per year. Hours of paid work begin to drop sharply after age 55 (Herzog et al., 1989). When all forms of productive activity are combined, 39 percent of those at age 60 reported at least 1,500 hours of productive activity in the preceding year, 41 percent reported 500 to 1,499 hours, and 18 percent reported 1 to 499 hours. Volunteer work hours in organizations peak between the ages of 35 and 55, with informal help to friends and relatives peaking at ages 55 to 64 and remaining significant till age 75 and beyond. The amount of work done by older men and women is substantial (Rowe & Kahn, 1997).

Unpaid productive activities, including formal volunteer work, informal helping of others, housework, and home maintenance, demonstrate much less decrease with age. Many older persons are willing to stay engaged in productive ways. These activities are useful and productive such that if the older person were not providing them, these services would have to be purchased in the market. Thus, older persons should be recognized for the contributions that they are making to society by helping each other and members of the younger generation (Herzog & Morgan, 1992).

PLAY AND LEISURE

There is a positive correlation between increased participation in recreational activities and higher psychological well-being, or more successful aging (DeCarlo, 1974). Ragheb and Griffith (1982) and Russell's research (1987) have clearly shown a positive relationship between contentment with leisure activities and life satisfaction among older adults. Leisure is a statement of identity, about who we are. When an individual has lost or is in danger of losing a valued leisure pursuit, that person also risks losing an important part of herself. Leisure is especially important to the older adult because many of them no longer have their primary identity that came from their work. Leisure is often linked to life satisfaction for men and women with and without functional impairments. Social interaction and friendship are vital to some leisure activities, whereas for other activities solitude is essential. There is no age at which individuals give up involvement in leisure activities (Bundy, 2001).

Little is known about how disabilities affect leisure activities. Many people who experience arthritis, stroke, or another age-related disability will likely decrease their participation in leisure pursuits and lament their loss (Bundy, 2001). In one notable study (Zimmer, Hickey, & Searle, 1997), it was observed that approximately 40 percent of older adults who had arthritis replaced some activities with others; approximately 48 percent quit and were much less likely to add new activity (about 7 percent) or to continue with former activities (about 5 percent). However, it was also noted that those with strong social structures were more likely to continue or replace activities. Thus, leisure activities have important implications for successful aging by providing an opportunity to remain engaged in social and productive activities.

SUMMARY

Multidimensional factors contribute to an individual's healthy and successful aging. Rowe and Kahn (1997) frame three critical domains for successful aging: (1) avoiding disease and disability, (2) maintaining high physical and cognitive function, and (3) remaining engaged in social and productive activities. There is a growing body of literature to support the predictors of success in these domains. Evidence is rapidly growing that many characteristics of so-called usual aging are due to lifestyle. Other factors may be age-related and certainly increase with age but are not caused by the aging process.

Multiple studies presented in this chapter demonstrate that active and fit individuals are at much lower risk for morbidity, mortality, and loss of function when compared with sedentary and unfit individuals. Table 16–4 summarizes the results of studies investigating the relationship of physical activity or physical fitness to selected chronic diseases or conditions from 1963 to 1993.

High physical performance was predicted by both socioeconomic performance and health-status characteristics. There is an increased likelihood of decline in physical performance for older individuals who have a lower income, higher body mass index, higher blood pressure, and lower initial cognitive performance (Albert et al., 1995). Moderate and/or strenuous leisure activity and emotional support from family and friends are predictors of maintenance of physical function. Spirduso and Cronin (2001) examined the effects of exercise intensity on quality of life and independent living in older adults. The most consistent outcomes were that long-term physical activity was related to postponed disability and independent living in the oldest of old subjects, even though there was no evidence that the level of exercise intensity influenced these results. Thus, it appears that moderate levels of exercise, such as leisurely walking, have comparable advantages to more strenuous exercise (Rowe & Kahn, 1997).

Education, strenuous activities in and around the home, peak pulmonary flow rate, and self-efficacy have been identified as direct predictors for change or maintenance of cognitive function (Albert et al., 1995; Rowe & Kahn, 1997). Cognitive ability was evaluated utilizing neuropsychological tests of language, nonverbal memory, verbal memory, conceptualization, and visuospatial abilities. Together these four variables explained 40 percent of the variance in cognitive test performance (Albert et al., 1995).

Education was the strongest predictor, with greater years of school increasing the probability of maintaining high cognitive functioning. The second highest predictor was pulmonary peak flow rate. Other studies have also noted that pulmonary function is a correlate

TABLE 16–4	Summary of Results of Studies Investigating Relationship of Physical Activity or Physical Fitness to Selected Chronic Diseases or Conditions, 1963–1993

Disease or Condition	Number of Studies	Trends Across Activity or Fitness Categories and Strength of Evidence
All-causes mortality	> 10	↓↓↓
Coronary artery disease	> 10	↓↓↓
Hypertension	5–10	↓↓
Obesity	> 10	↓↓
Stroke	5–10	↓
Peripheral vascular disease	< 5	→
Cancer		
colon	> 10	↓↓
rectum	> 10	→
stomach	< 5	→
breast	< 5	↓
prostate	5–10	↓
lung	< 5	↓
pancreas	< 5	→
Non-insulin-dependent diabetes	< 5	↓↓
Osteoarthritis	< 5	→
Osteoporosis	5–10	↓↓
Functional capability	5–10	↓↓

→ = no apparent difference in disease rates across activity or fitness categories.
↓ = some evidence of reduced disease rates across activity or fitness categories.
↓↓ = good evidence of reduced disease rates across activity or fitness categories, control of some potential, good methods, and some evidence of biologic mechanisms.
↓↓↓ = evidence of reduced disease rates across activity or fitness categories, good control of some potential, excellent methods, and extensive evidence of biologic mechanisms; relationship is considered causal.

of cognitive and physical function and a predictor of cardiovascular mortality (Cook et al., 1989).

The amount of strenuous physical activity at and around one's home was surprisingly found to be the third strongest important predictor for maintenance of cognitive function. These data suggest that exercise can potentially improve or maintain central nervous system performance and even memory function (Albert et al., 1995; Rowe & Kahn, 1997). Perceived self-efficacy was found to be the fourth predictive variable for maintaining high cognitive function (Albert et al., 1995; McAuley et al., 1999).

Emerging predictors of productive activity and maintenance of social engagement include functional capacity, education, and self-efficacy. Both men and women functioning at high cognitive and physical levels are three times as likely to be engaged in some form of paid work and more than twice as likely to be involved with volunteer work than those of

comparable age but lower levels of cognitive and physical functioning. An individual's educational level is a well-recognized predictor of continued productive activity, both paid and unpaid (Albert et al., 1995). Continuous participation in activities, regardless of physical fitness improvements, contributes substantially to enhancing self-efficacy (McAuley et al., 1999).

The process of aging begins with birth. It is universal, irreversible, highly variable, and not strongly correlated with chronologic age. Aging undeniably has a sociological impact and challenges the health-care delivery system in both the near and distant future. Many factors can affect the rate and progression of aging, including physiologic, cognitive, and psychosocial attributes. Efforts at understanding healthy aging, lessening risk factors for chronic diseases, and engaging in health-promotion practices offer hope for a better quality of life and successful aging.

JANE PERTKO, PT, GCS
GERIATRIC PHYSICAL THERAPIST WORKING IN HOME HEALTH

CASE

1

Helen

Helen is 78 years of age and was referred to a home health agency for nursing and rehabilitation care. She sustained a left hip fracture 2 weeks ago after falling in her daughter's home. She underwent an open-reduction internal fixation of her left hip the day of the fall. Initial orders were for partial weight bearing (PWB); however, following surgery, she was very confused and agitated, which made compliance with the weight-bearing status difficult. On the 3rd postoperative day, Helen developed a sudden onset of left-sided weakness and slurred speech, which was diagnosed as a possible cerebrovascular accident. She has had some clearing of these symptoms, but she continues to have problems with short-term memory, balance, and safety issues. She also has periods of incontinence. Helen's medical history is significant for hypertension and possible transient ischemic attacks.

While hospitalized, Helen received physical, occupational, and speech therapy. Upon discharge she was able to ambulate 30 feet $\times$ 2 with a walker and moderate assistance (one person) for balance and walker placement. Due to inability to maintain partial weight bearing, gait was changed to weight bearing as tolerated. Transfers required minimal to moderate assistance (one person). ADLs required setup and verbal cues plus minimal assistance for upper-body bathing and dressing, and moderate assistance for lower-body bathing and dressing. Helen's mild confusion contributed to her inability to independently sequence bathing and dressing activities. She was independent in combing her hair, with setup. With time and setup, Helen could feed herself independently but was easily distracted. Speech therapy was discontinued at the time of discharge from the hospital. Although on a bladder-training program, Helen was still having episodes of incontinence and required prompting to go to the bathroom.

The rehabilitation team recommended that Helen's care be continued at a local SNF (skilled nursing facility) for more intensive skilled therapy; however, the daughter refused to investigate this option. "I want to take her to my house. She needs to be with my dad and with her family. Once she is back in familiar surroundings, she won't be so confused. That will make all the difference. I won't put my parents in a nursing home!"

Helen's daughter, Peggy, is 48 years old. She is married and has two children, ages 18 and 20. Her son is a senior in high school, and her daughter is away at college. Peggy has two older siblings—a sister and a brother. Her sister has a serious heart condition and is unable to assist in the care of her parents. Peggy's brother lives in California and is an executive with an investment firm. His business requires frequent traveling, often out of the country. He is divorced and is unable to provide physical assistance with the care of his parents, although he has offered financial support.

Helen and her husband Sam have been living in the same home for over 50 years. It is 10 miles from Peggy. Peggy has been the primary support system for her parents, providing transportation to the grocery store once a week, to all the doctor visits, and to Peggy's sister's home for visits. As many of Helen and Sam's friends are no longer in the area (having either relocated or died), Peggy tries to bring her parents to her home once a week for dinner with her family. It was during this last visit that her mother slipped on a throw rug near the kitchen sink and fell on the ceramic tiled floor, sustaining a hip fracture.

If you question Peggy, you find that both of her parents have been in declining health for the past 4 years. Sam is 82 years old and has severe congestive heart failure. He is very short of breath and deconditioned and has had frequent hospitalizations. Each episode "takes a little more out of him." Sam currently uses a walker for ambulation. Except for outings with his daughter, he is essentially homebound. He quit driving 5 years ago. Helen has also become increasingly frail during the past year and has had several "mini-strokes." These have left her with some balance deficits and mild confusion. Helen tends to want to hold on to furniture or touch the wall when walking in the house. She requires hand-held assistance when walking outside. Prior to this hospitalization, Helen was independent in her ADLs and could prepare light meals, with time. Peggy had arranged for

Continues

CASE
1

Helen *Continued*

Meals on Wheels to come in during the week, and Peggy prepared weekend meals herself. Helen has had several "close calls" in terms of loss of balance but until the fall at Peggy's home had never sustained any serious injuries. Peggy and her husband assist her parents with paying bills and other financial matters.

Peggy's parents are extremely close and, in spite of their recent medical problems, were able to function in their home, with Peggy's assistance. Peggy's immediate family is supportive of Peggy's commitment to her parents. Her husband and children assist as they are able; however, their schedules are fairly busy. Both Peggy and her husband have full-time jobs: she is a legal secretary, and her husband is a professor at the local university. Her son is involved in sports and other extracurricular activities and works part-time at a local sporting goods store. Her daughter is home only for summers and school holidays.

The past year has been particularly trying for Peggy's family. Her husband has tried to talk to her about "making some kind of arrangement for her folks," but Peggy would not discuss it. "Mother and Daddy have always told me that they wanted to stay in their own home, and I must see to it that they can. They are too old to adjust to a new environment—I'm afraid that it will kill them both."

Peggy has converted her den into a room for her parents. It is close to the first-floor bathroom. There are no bedrooms on the first floor, and neither Helen nor Sam can negotiate a full flight of stairs at this time. Peggy was able to take a week off from work when Helen was discharged from the hospital but has since had to return to work. Mary was hired as a "sitter" for Peggy's parents while Peggy worked. She provides assistance, supervision, and light-meal preparation. A CNA from the agency comes in five mornings per week to assist Helen with her personal care, but this will be decreased to three times a week. Peggy and her husband provide full care on the weekends. Helen still has episodes of incontinence and "pleasant confusion." The incontinence is a problem that troubles the entire family. "Mother has always been so neat and clean about herself. This is upsetting for all of us to see her this way. It doesn't seem to be getting any better."

PT and OT goals have been to increase Helen's safety awareness, improve her balance, and increase independence in ambulation, and to help with transfers, home management skills, and ADLs. Helen's plan of care has been certified for 9 weeks.

Helen is now able to get in and out of chairs with only SBA (stand-by assist) but occasionally loses her balance and falls back into the chair. She is ambulating 75 feet with a walker, SBA, and verbal cues for walker placement and safety. She tends to walk too fast at times. She has fallen three times since being home—always at night and when she tries to get out of bed on her own. She has not had any serious injuries. Sam tries to sleep with his arm on her shoulder and tries to stay awake to "keep an eye on my best girl." This has also taken a toll on the family, and no one sleeps through the night for fear that Helen will try to get up and have a serious fall. Sam states that "she seems to have her days and nights mixed up." ADLs continue to require setup and cueing for sequencing.

Four weeks into the 9-week certification period, it became evident that Helen and Sam would not be able to return to their home unless 24-hour caregiver support was available. Today, when you arrive, Peggy is home. When she comes to the door, she steps outside to talk to you and begins to cry. "Mary just gave me her notice. She has to go home to care for her grandchildren during the summer when school is out because her daughter just found a job and will not be home during the day. She will only be able to work for 2 more weeks! I don't know what we're going to do. I cannot quit my job. Do you think that Mother and Daddy will ever be able to return home and live on their

Continues

CASE
1

Helen *Continued*

own again? I really thought that when mother got to my house that she would be okay, that her mind would clear. Last night, my father said that he didn't think that he and mother would ever get back to their home. He thinks that they should go to a nursing home! He said that he wouldn't mind going if Mother were with him. It broke my heart—I feel like I've let them down, and I don't know what to do."

This case study illustrates many aspects of aging that people don't like to think about. Everyone dreads putting a loved one in a nursing home; however, coping capacities are finite, as evident in this case. In this situation the ideal resolution would be to find a high-quality nursing home facility close to Peggy and her family where Helen and her husband can live together in an apartment-like arrangement. Helen would then get the care she needs, and family members would be free to provide love and support rather than being physically and financially drained.

Speaking of

Health and the "Old Codger"
COLLEEN CRONIN
74-YEAR-OLD RETIRED NUTRITIONIST

Today, when I was talking to my daughter, I learned a new word: "senescence." When my doctor told me that I had dementia, I didn't know I had a medical condition . . . I figured all older people had dementia. I have had a lot going on in the last few years. I've had trouble sleeping, had blurry vision, couldn't keep my eyes on a line of print, had trouble getting to the bathroom fast enough, and have had trouble with my balance.

My doctor tested everything. I had my eyes tested, my brain scanned, and my balance evaluated. No one found anything. So I quit talking about it—it was just old age. I tried to hide my growing difficulties from my kids, and from my friends. But it kept getting worse.

After two serious falls, I was getting scared. I talked to the doctor again, and she sent me for an MRI. This test showed that I had adult-onset hydrocephalus.

I was lucky. I had a cerebroperitoneal shunt (a "brain drain," according to my son) put in 2 weeks ago, and my dementia has begun to resolve. I am still forgetful, I still lose things, but, according to my daughter, this is "senescence" rather than dementia. She says that senescence is normal in a 74-year-old, while dementia is not. So, I guess what I'm left with is normal old-age forgetfulness, called *senescence,* and the disease of dementia was treated by the shunt.

This experience has taught me many things. I know first-hand how confusing it is when you are scared and worried but keep hearing from others how good you are looking. There is so much that people cannot see. I also learned how hard it is to sort out the "physical symptoms" from the emotional ones, like grief at the loss of my husband of 50 years, loneliness, and stress.

I had many health-care workers who listened and worked with me. That really helped—knowing that they would not just write me off as a crazy old codger. I learned that aging and senescence cause many changes, but even when you are 74 years old, not every problem is inevitable with aging.

Speaking of

The Simple Things

BARBARA HAASE, MHS, OTH, BCN
OCCUPATIONAL THERAPIST

RICHARD HAASE, MA
REHABILITATION COUNSELOR

She was dying. She, her husband of 39 years, and her family all knew it; yet they at times denied it. She had been well taken care of at the hospital, by many of the same nurses she had trained there. Now she was home, for her final days, to die.

Her caregivers through Hospice were good at their jobs. They came every day to give her a bed bath, to provide supplementary feedings, to adjust the morphine, and to provide support to her and her family. There were good days and bad—those days when she reminisced through pictures of happier times and those when she lived for the next push on her morphine drip. There were quiet times, storytelling, and many tears.

It is the simple things, at times like this, that mean so much. What do you do for a person who is dying, especially when it is your mother? My mother lived a full and active life. She raised three kids and was beginning to enjoy grandchildren. She was a registered nurse professionally. Her life was beautiful, and she handled dying with grace and without fear. The greatest gift I gave her during these last days, in addition to just being with her, was arranging for Hospice to bring in a shower seat so she had a shower. What a joy this was for her.

As an occupational therapist, I have met and worked with people of all ages, from all walks of life, and at different stages of their lives. The study of aging and cognition were part of my master's specialization. I have gained considerable experience with the clinical aspects of aging. Sometimes, as a therapist, it feels better to be using a new technology, because this may be what the consumer wants, or a sophisticated research protocol, because it reflects my own clinical talents. But, as my mother reminded me, it is not high tech or research that are important. In reality, the simple things, the daily life activities, are the most important.

REFERENCES

Ahmed, I., & Takeshita, J. (1996). Late-life depression, *Generations, 20*(4), 17–22.

Albert, M. S., Savage, C. R., Jones, K., Berkman, L., Seeman, T., Blazer, D., & Rowe, J. W. (1995). Predictors of cognitive change in older persons: MacArthur studies of successful aging. *Psychology and Aging, 10*, 578–589.

American College of Sports Medicine. (2000). *ACSM's guidelines for exercise testing and prescription* (6th ed.). Philadelphia: Lippincott, Williams and Wilkins.

American Occupational Therapy Association. (2002). Occupational Therapy Practice Framework: Domain and process. *American Journal of Occupational Therapy, 56,* 609–639.

Bahr, S., & Peterson, E. (Eds.) (1989). *Aging and the family.* Lexington, MA: D. C. Heath.

Barrett-Connor, E., & Palinkas, L. (1994). Low blood pressure and depression in older men: A population-based study. *British Medical Journal, 308*(6926), 446–450.

Binstock, R. H., & George, L. K. (1996). *Handbook of aging and social sciences* (4th ed.). San Diego, CA: Academic Press.

Blair, S. N. (1993). 1993 C. H. McCoy research lecture: Physical activity, physical fitness, and health. *Research Quarterly for Exercise and Sports, 64*(4), 365–376.

Blair, S. N., Kohl, H. W., Barlow, C. E., Paffenbarger, R. S., Gibbons, L. W., & Macera, C. A. (1995). Changes in physical fitness and all-cause mortality: A prospective study of healthy and unhealthy men. *Journal of the American Medical Association, 273*(14), 1093–1098.

Blair, S. N, & Wei, M. (2000). Sedentary habits, health, and function in older women and men. *American Journal of Health Promotion, 15*(1), pp. 1–8.

Bottomley, J. M., & Lewis, C. B. (2002a). Comparing and contrasting age-related changes in biology, physiology, anatomy, and function. In *Geriatric rehabilitation: A clinical approach* (pp. 50–75). Upper Saddle River, NJ: Prentice Hall.

Bottomley, J. M., & Lewis, C. B. (2002b). Describing psychosocial aspects of aging. In *Geriatric physical therapy* (pp. 76–100). Norwalk, CN: Appleton and Lange.

Bottomley, J. M., & Lewis, C. B. (2002c). Integumentary treatment considerations. In *Geriatric physical therapy* (pp. 484–527). Norwalk, CN: Appleton and Lange.

Bundy, A. C. (2001). Leisure. In B. R. Bonder & M. B. Wagner (Eds.), *Functional performance in older adults* (2nd ed.) (pp. 196–217). Philadelphia: F. A. Davis.

Castor, T., & Carter, T. (1995). Low vision: Physician screening helps to improve patient function. *Geriatrics, 50(12)*, 51–58.

Cerny, F. J., & Burton, H. W. (2001). Aging. In *Exercise physiology for health care professionals* (pp. 257–271). Champaign, IL: Human Kinetics.

Cohen, M. (1999a). Cardiac considerations in the older adult. In T. L. Kauffman (Ed.), *Geriatric rehabilitation manual* (pp. 24–29). Philadelphia: Churchill Livingston.

Cohen, M. (1999b). Pulmonary considerations in the older adult. In T. L. Kauffman (Ed.), *Geriatric rehabilitation manual* (pp. 29–34). Philadelphia: Churchill Livingston.

Cole, K., Rotella, D., & Harper, J. (1999). Mechanisms for age-related changes of fingertip forces during precision gripping and lifting in adults. *Journal of Neuroscience, 19*, 3228–3247.

Cook, N. R., Evans, D. A., Scherr, P. A., Speizer, F. E., Vedal, S., Branch, L. G., Huntley, J. C., Hennekens, C. H., & Taylor, J. O. (1989). Peak expiratory flow rate and 5–6 year mortality in an elderly population. *American Journal of Epidemiology, 160*, 66–78.

DeCarlo, T. J. (1974). Recreation participation patterns and successful aging. *Journal of Gerontology, 29*, 416–422.

Fiatarone, M. A., O'Niell, E. F., Ryan, N. D., Clements, K. M., Solares, G. R., Nelson, M. E., Roberts, S. B., Kehayias, J. J., Lipsitz, L. A., & Evans, W. J. (1994). Exercise training and nutritional supplementation for physical frailty in very elderly people. *New England Journal of Medicine, 330(25)*, 1769–1775.

Finch, C. E., & Tanzi, R. E. (1997). *Science, 278*, 401–411.

Fries, J. F. (1980). Aging, natural death, and the compression of morbidity. *New England Journal of Medicine, 303*, 130–136.

Frontera, W. R., Meredith, C. N., O'Reilly, K. P., Knuttgen, H. G., & Evans, W. J. (1988). Strength conditioning in older men: Skeletal muscle hypertrophy and improved function. *Journal of Applied Physiology, 64*, 1038–1044.

Guccione, A. A. (2000). Implications of aging population for rehabilitation: Demography, mortality, and morbidity. In A. A. Guccione (Ed.), *Geriatric physical therapy* (2nd ed.) (pp. 3–16). Philadelphia: Mosby.

Gutmann, E., & Hanzlikova, V. (1976). Fast and slow motor units in aging. *Gerontologist, 22*, 280–300.

Hagberg, J. M. (1987). Effect of aging on decline of VO_{2max} with aging. *Federal Proceedings, 46*, 1830–1833.

Herzog, A. R., Kahn, R. L., Morgan, J. N., Jackson, J. S., & Antonucci, T. C. (1989). Age differences in productive activities. *Journal of Gerontology: SOCIAL SCIENCES, 44*, S129–S138.

Herzog, A. R., & Morgan, J. N. (1992). Age and gender differences in the value of productive activities. *Research on Aging, 14(2)*, 169–198.

Hills, G. A. (2002). The changing realm of the senses. In C. B. Lewis (Ed.), *Aging: The health care challenge* (4th ed.) (pp. 83–103). Philadelphia: F. A. Davis.

Hogstel, M. (2001). *Gerontology: Nursing care of the older adult.* Albany, NY: Delmar Thomson Learning.

Katzel, L. I., Bleeker, E. R., Colman, E. G., Rogus, E. M., Sorkin, J. D., & Goldberg, A. P. (1995). Effects of weight loss vs. aerobic exercise training on risk factors for coronary disease in healthy obese, middle-aged and older men. *Journal of the American Medical Association, 74(24)*, 1915–1921.

Kaufman, S. R. (1986). The ageless self: Sources of meaning in late life. Madison, WI: University of Wisconsin Press.

Kausler, D. (1991). *Experimental psychology and human aging* (2nd ed.). New York: Springer-Verlag.

Kee, C. (1990). Sensory impairment: Factor X in providing nursing care to the older adult. *Journal of Community Health Nursing, 71(1)*, 45–52.

Kimmel, D. C., Price, K. F., & Walker, J. W. (1978). Retirement choice and retirement satisfaction. *Journal of Gerontology, 33(4)*, 575–585.

Kline, D., & Scialfa, C. (1997) Sensory and perceptual functioning: Basic research and human factors implications. In A. D. Fisk & W. A. Rogers (Eds.), *Handbook of human factors and the older adult* (pp. 27–54). New York: Academic Press.

Larsson, L. (1982). Physical training effects on muscle morphology in sedentary males at different ages. *Medicine and Science in Sports and Exercise, 14*, 203–206.

Legters, K. (2002). Fear of falling. *Physical Therapy, 82(3)*, 264–272.

Lewis, C. B., & Kellems, S. (2002). Musculoskeletal changes with age: Clinical implications. In C. B. Lewis (Ed.), *Aging: The health care challenge* (4th ed.) (pp. 104–126). Philadelphia: F. A. Davis.

McArdle, W. D., Katch, F. I., & Katch, V. L. (1996). *Exercise physiology* (4th ed.). Baltimore: Williams and Wilkins.

McAuley, E., Katula, J., Mihalko, S. L., Blissmer, B., Duncan, T. E., Pena, M., & Dunn, E. (1999). Mode of physical activity and self-efficacy in older adults: A latent growth curve analysis. *Journal of Gerontology, B, 54*, P283–292.

Moncur, C. (2000). Posture in the older adult. In A. A. Guccione (Ed.), *Geriatric physical therapy* (2nd ed.) (pp. 265–279). Philadelphia: Mosby.

Mutchler, J. E., Burr, J. A., Massagli, M. P., & Pienta, A. M. (1999). Work transitions and health in later life. *Journal of Gerontology, B, 54*, S252–S261.

Mutchler, J. E., Burr, J. A., Pienta, A. M., & Massagli, M. P. (1997). Pathways to labor force exit: Work transitions and instability. *Journal of Gerontology, B, 64*, S4–12.

National Council on the Aging, Inc. (2002). *American perceptions of aging in the 21st century.* Washington, DC: National Council on the Aging, Inc.

Orlander, J., Kiessling, K.-H., Larsson, L., & Karlsson, J. (1978). Skeletal muscle metabolism and ultrastructure in relation to age in sedentary men. *ACTA Physiology Scandinavia, 104*, 249–261.

Papalia, D. E., Camp, C. J., & Feldman, R. D. (1996). *Adult development and aging.* New York: McGraw-Hill.

Patten, C., & Craik, R. L. (2000). In A. A. Guccione (Ed.), *Geriatric physical therapy* (2nd ed.) (pp. 78–109). Philadelphia: Mosby.

Payne, V. G., & Isaacs, L. D. (2001). *Human motor development: A lifespan approach* (5th ed.). Boston: McGraw-Hill.

Peel, C. (1996). The cardiopulmonary system and movement dysfunction. *Physical therapy, 76*, 448–455.

Pohl, P., Winstein, C., & Fisher, B. (1996). The locus of age-related slowing: Sensory processing in continuous goal-directed aiming. *Journal of Gerontology*, 51, 94–102.

Ragheb, M., & Griffith, C. (1982). The contribution of leisure participation and leisure satisfaction to life satisfaction of older persons. *Journal of Leisure Research, 14*, 295–306.

Reynolds, P. (1991). Characteristics of aging skeletal muscles. *Physiotherapy Theory and Practice, 7(3)*, 157–162.

Riley, K. P. (2001). Cognitive development. In B. R. Bonder & M. B. Wagner (Eds.), *Functional performance in older adults* (2nd ed.) (pp. 138–152). Philadelphia: F. A. Davis.

Rowe, J. W., & Kahn, R. L. (1987). Human aging: Usual and successful. *Science, 237*, 143–149.

Rowe, J. W., & Kahn, R. L. (1997). Successful aging. *The Gerontologist, 37(4)*, 433–440.

Royal College of Psychiatrists. (2003). Bereavement. Retrieved August 14, 2003, from http://www.rcpsych.ac.uk/info/help/bereav/.

Russell, R. (1987). The relative contribution of recreation satisfaction and activity participation to the life satisfaction of retirees. *Journal of Leisure Research, 19*, 273–283.

Saltin, B., Blomquist, G., Mitchell, J. H., et al. (1968). Responses to exercise after bedrest and after training. *Circulation, 38 (Suppl. VII)*, 1–78.

Schunk, C. (2001). Cognitive impairment. In A. A. Guccione (Ed.), *Geriatric physical therapy* (2nd ed.) (pp. 150–160). Philadelphia: Mosby.

Searle, M. S. (1991). Leisure, aging, and mental health: A review of the clinical evidence. *Topics in Geriatric Rehabilitation, 7(2)*, 1–12.

Settersten, R., & Hagestad, G. (1996a). What is the latest? Cultural age deadlines for family transitions. *Gerontologist, 36*, 178–188.

Settersten, R., & Hagestad, G. (1996b). What is the latest II? Cultural age deadlines for educational and work transitions. *Gerontologist, 36*, 602–613.

Shumway-Cook, A., & Woollacott, M. (2001). *Motor control: Theory and practical applications* (2nd ed.). Philadelphia: Lippincott, Williams and Wilkins.

Sinaki, M., Itio, E., Wahner, H. W., Wollan, P., Gelzcer, R., Mullan, B. P., Collins, D. A., & Hodgson, S. F. (2002). Stronger back muscles reduce the incidences of vertebral fracture: A prospective 10-year follow-up of post-menopausal women. *Bone, 30(6)*, 826–841.

Sinaki, M., & Mikkelsen, B. A. (1984). Postmenopausal spinal osteoporosis: Flexion versus extension exercises. *Archives of Physical Rehabilitation, 65*, 593–596.

Singleton, J. F. (1985). Retirement: Its effects on the individual. *Adaptation and Aging, 6(4)*, 1–6.

Smith, E. L., & Gilligan, C. (1983). Physical activity prescription for the older adult. *The Physician and Sports Medicine, 11(8)*, 91–101.

Spirduso, W. W., & Cronin, D. L. (2001). Exercise dose-response effects on quality of life and independent living in older adults. *Medicine and Science in Sports and Exercise, 33(6), Suppl.*, S598–608.

Spirduso, W. W. (1980). Physical fitness, aging, and psychomotor speed: A review. *Journal of Gerontology, 35(6)*, 850–865.

Sterns, H. L., Junkins, M. P., & Bayer, J. G. (2001). Work and retirement. In B. R. Bonder and M. B. Wagner (Eds.), *Functional performance in older adults* (2nd ed.) (pp. 179–195). Philadelphia: F. A. Davis.

Stevens-Long, J., & Commons, M. (1992). *Adult life* (4th ed.). Mountainview, CA: Mayfield.

Swank, A. M., Funk, D. C., Durham, M. P., & Robers, S. (2003). Adding weights to stretching exercises increases passive range of motion for healthy elderly. *Journal of Strength and Conditioning Research, 17(2)*, 374–378.

Thompson, L. V. (2000). Physiologic changes associated with aging. In A. A. Guccione (Ed.), *Geriatric physical therapy* (2nd ed.) (pp. 28–55). Philadelphia: Mosby.

Turrell, G., Lynch, J. W., Kaplan, G. S., Everson, S. A., Helkala, E-L., Kauhanen, J., & Salonen, J. (2002). Socioeconomic position across the lifecourse and cognitive function in late middle age. *Journal of Gerontology B, 57*, S43–51.

Unger, J. B., McAvay, G., Bruce, M. L., Berkman, L., & Seeman, T. (1999). Variations in the impact of social network characteristics on physical functioning in elderly persons: MacArthur studies of successful aging. *Journal of Gerontology, B, 54*, S245–251.

U. S. Census Bureau (2001). Population Profile of the United States: 2000 Internet Release. Washington, DC: U. S. Census Bureau [producer and distributor]. Retrieved August, 2002. *http://www.census.gov/population/pop-profile/2000/profile2000.pdf.*

Vita, A. J., Terry, R. B., Hubert, H. B., & Fries, J. F. (1998). Aging, health risks, and cumulative disability. *New England Journal of Medicine, 338(15)*, 1035–1041.

Williams, H. (1990). Aging and the development of eye-hand coordination. In C. Bard, M. Fleury, & L. Hay (Eds.), *Development of eye-hand coordination across the lifespan* (pp. 327–357). Columbia, SC: University of South Carolina Press.

World Health Organization. (2002). *ICF: International Classification of Functioning and Disability.* Geneva, Switzerland: World Health Organization.

Zimmer, Z., Hickey, T., & Searle, M. S. (1997). The pattern of change in leisure activity behavior among older adults with arthritis. *Gerontologist, 37(3)*, 384–392.

Family and Disablement in Adulthood

Christine L. Raber, MS, OTR/L
Assistant Professor
Department of Occupational
Therapy
Shawnee State University
Portsmouth, Ohio

Objectives

Upon completion of this chapter, the reader will be able to

▓ Discuss the impact of illness and disease on adults.

▓ Describe the process of disablement during adulthood.

▓ Identify the influence of illness and disability on adult developmental life tasks.

▓ Discuss the issues related to living with a family member who is disabled.

▓ Explain the ways in which disability impacts participation in major life activities.

▓ Define self-advocacy and discuss its role in adaptation to disability for individuals with disabilities, and for their families.

Key Terms

acquired limitations	chronology	prognosis
acute	congenital	self-advocacy
attitude	malingering	sick role
barrier-free design	normalization	support and relationships
chronic	occupation	

THE EXPERIENCE OF ILLNESS AND DISEASE IN ADULTHOOD

An *illness* encompasses the particular ways in which a pathology or impairment interferes with everyday function (Beer, 2003). Illness and diseases that affect a person's health status have a significant impact on both the innate domains of human performance (affective, cognitive, and psychomotor) and on the domains of physical, psychological, and social function in daily life. While a change in health may appear to primarily affect function in one performance domain, the other domains are often affected by this disruption in the usual state of balance and well-being for a person. For example, consider a common occurrence: contracting the flu during the winter months. A person typically experiences the common physiologic symptoms of nausea, vomiting, fever, and muscle aches that impact on the psychomotor domain and make even simple physical tasks, like getting out of bed, difficult. While the flu typically does not create symptoms that interfere with the affective or cognitive domains of performance, these areas may be affected as a result of the short-term physical changes brought on by the virus. For example, missing work or school may create anxiety about completing assignments, and decision-making skills may be decreased as a result of a fever. Through this simple example, you can see that changes in one's body function or structure tend to have an interactive effect on all areas of function.

Throughout this chapter we will explore the disablement process in adults and its impact on the person and her family or support system. As you recall from Chapter 1, the ICF provides a model for understanding human function and impairment. The relationships between health conditions and activity limitation are multifaceted and nonlinear, and these complex relationships represent a dynamic interaction between the individual and his environment (World Health Organization, 2002). Being able to identify the factors that contribute to disablement is an essential task for rehabilitation professionals if they are to be successful in providing the services that maximize function and independence for persons with disabilities. By the end of this chapter, you should be better able to identify how multiple factors, particularly family and significant others, interact to create a person's experience with disability.

Two distinguishing features related to illness and the perception of disease are the chronology and severity of a disease. **Chronology** refers to the timing of the onset of the condition (for example, at what point in the lifespan the condition occurs), as well as the length of time that the condition persists. Medical terminology often uses the terms *acute* and *chronic* to characterize the length of time the person has been experiencing a particular condition. For example, an **acute** condition, such as a bone fracture due to an accident, is typically time-limited and presents a different set of needs from a **chronic** condition, such as rheumatoid arthritis, which is expected to continue indefinitely after diagnosis. Severity of the condition may relate to the magnitude and frequency of symptoms experienced that interfere with daily functioning. Many chronic conditions, such as multiple sclerosis, exhibit exacerbating and remitting symptom patterns, while progressive decline is the hallmark of chronic conditions such as amyotrophic lateral sclerosis (ALS). Some conditions are marked by a major event in which significant declines in function occur, as in a cerebrovascular accident or traumatic brain injury.

Together with chronologic issues, these variations in prognosis both within and across conditions create some of the challenges that affect function, recovery, and disability status. **Prognosis** is "the prospect of survival and recovery from a disease as anticipated from the usual course of that disease or indicated by special features of the case" (Merriam-Webster, 2002, retrieved July, 20, 2003, from http://dictionary.reference.com/search?q=prognosis). In time-limited conditions, expectations for recovery without further impairment are typical and are experienced by individuals and their families differently from conditions in which uncertainty exists about the amount of recovery to previous levels of function that will occur.

In many chronic conditions, such as Alzheimer's disease, continued decline is expected as part of the disease's progression. Prognosis and amount of resulting impairment may also be influenced by lifestyle choices associated with management of the disorder, as is the case in conditions such as diabetes and hypertension. Differences in illness experiences also exist between **acquired limitations,** such as traumatic brain injury or spinal cord injury, and **congenital** limitations, such as cerebral palsy. In any case, it is important for rehabilitation professionals to take these variable condition-related factors into account when providing services to individuals with disabilities.

Adulthood is the longest phase of human life and is seen as a period of health for the majority of individuals. In young adulthood most health-related concerns develop as a result of accidents and/or engagement in risky health behaviors, including sexually transmitted diseases (Merluzzi & Nairn, 1999). As individuals approach middle age, health concerns may begin to develop, particularly related to lifestyle behaviors that create increased risk for medical conditions, such as a sedentary lifestyle, obesity, smoking, and work habits that contribute to injury (Merluzzi & Nairn, 1999). When adults enter the later years, there is an increased incidence of chronic conditions, but these often do not affect individuals at the level of disability, and the majority of older adults manage at least one chronic health condition (such as hypertension or arthritis) without significant changes in normal daily functioning (National Center for Health Statistics, 1995). This being said, the overall incidence of disability in older adults does increase (Verbrugge, 1994).

Throughout adulthood, psychiatric conditions, such as substance abuse and schizophrenia, as well as mood, anxiety, and personality disorders, may occur and contribute to changes in health and level of disability (Kaplan & Sadock, 1998). In fact, during adulthood, one in five adults experiences a mental illness, and recent research indicates that even when compared with other diagnoses, mental illness is a major contributor to disability (U.S. Department of Health and Human Services [USDHHS], 1999).

The impact of disease or disorders of any type on function in adulthood is related to *contextual factors.* Personal Factors are the ICF contextual influences within the person, and may include motivation, coping skills, habits, lifestyle, and demographic characteristics such as gender and social background. An example of a Personal Factor could be the amount of education a person has, which influences her ability to manage health behaviors effectively. Environmental Factors include two levels: individual and services or systems. Both levels relate to the physical and social environment and include the home, workplace, community services, and relationships with family, friends, and others. Beginning to understand the disablement process for any individual requires an assessment of the ways in which these contextual factors affect the person's experience and abilities.

THE DISABLEMENT PROCESS IN ADULTHOOD

Disablement refers to the experience of change in functional ability that results in a different way of being in the world. Understanding the process of disablement has received increased attention in the past quarter-century, and it has been framed in both medical and social perspectives (Bickenbach et al., 1999). The ICF represents an attempt to create a biopsychosocial model—that is, one that synthesizes the biologic, individual, and social perspectives of ability and disability (World Health Organization, 2002). Several models of disablement were described in Chapter 1, and you will note that the delineation of what constitutes "disability" varies, both with regard to a person's experience and in the accepted definitions of disability.

In adulthood, the level of impairment that constitutes disability is influenced by several factors: degree of interference with daily activities as experienced by the person, chronologic age, level of intrinsic and extrinsic resources, attitudes, and societal barriers (World Health Organization, 2002). There is an important distinction between an adult's view of himself as disabled and society's view of the person as disabled. While the person may function well in his own home, he often needs help to access community activities and public transportation. The drawing in Figure 17–1 shows the use of a commercial bus lift. These lifts cannot be operated by the person getting on the bus, and are available only on some public buses. While the individuals using them do not view themselves as disabled, they are viewed by society as disabled (Nagi, 1991).

Disability frequently is created not by the person's level of functional impairment or her abilities to manage a disability, but by societal barriers such as the attitudes of others, discrimination in employment, and lack of access to services, spaces, and places in the community (World Health Organization, 2002). Alternately, individuals may view themselves as disabled and have challenges due to Personal Factors that may affect or limit their ability to use or develop effective coping skills. Emotional responses to disability are varied and deeply entwined with the person's overall function (Versluys, 1996).

STRUCTURE AND FUNCTION IMPAIRMENT

Disability status is influenced by the nature of the condition creating impairments in the ICF category of

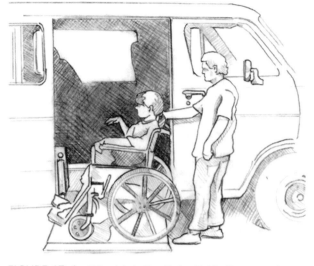

FIGURE 17–1   Wheelchair User Trying Public Transportation

Body Structure or Function. Activity limitations acquired by the sudden onset of an event, such as cerebrovascular accidents or traumatic brain injuries, typically involve a period of instability that may improve as a result of medical management and rehabilitation, and then the condition becomes stable after this period of recuperation.

Finally, coexisting conditions, such as diabetes and a recent myocardial infarction, affect impairment levels and functioning. While it is helpful to understand how these condition-related variations affect a person's body structure and/or function, ultimately rehabilitation professionals need to bring their primary focus to a person's functional abilities, since impairments do not exhibit a linear relationship to disability status.

ACTIVITIES AND PARTICIPATION IMPAIRMENTS

Across various theories, the predominant developmental life tasks of adults include separation and individuation from family of origin, development of one's own family, financial/career independence, and successful navigation of life events throughout adulthood. As has been noted in the preceding chapters, many different theorists have outlined the developmental tasks of adulthood, each with his or her own focus on the outcomes and behaviors that constitute "successful" negotiation of life tasks. One overarching similarity across theories relates to a person's ability to successfully manage life roles in a manner that is acceptable to both the individual and the standards of his cultural group. Examples of some common life roles that adults in the United States engage in are worker, home maintainer, family member, friend, student, and group or organization member. Differences in culture, values, family and

societal expectations, and so forth create a range of tasks and activities that are expected and associated with each role (Christiansen & Baum, 1997).

The ICF classifies the range of *life tasks* under Activities and Participation, which includes the areas of learning and applying knowledge, general tasks and demands, communication, mobility, self-care, domestic life, interpersonal interactions and relationships, major life areas (involving education and employment), and community, social, and civic life (World Health Organization, 2002). The Occupational Therapy Practice Framework (American Occupational Therapy Association, 2002) identifies *life tasks* as areas of occupation, which include *activities of daily living* (ADLs), *instrumental activities of daily living* (IADLs), work/school, play, leisure, and social participation. Specific descriptions of the broad life tasks discussed by adult developmental theorists, such as Erikson's task of generativity for middle adulthood or Maslow's hierarchy of needs, are presented in Chapter 2 of this text.

PERSONAL CONTEXTS

Support and relationships are considered ICF *contextual factors* that influence a person's disability status. Immediate (spouses, siblings, children, parents) and extended (aunts, uncles, cousins) family members assume many roles and responsibilities in response to their family member's impairments or disability. These responses may serve as facilitators or barriers for adults experiencing impairments that create changes in function. For example, a spouse may provide opportunities to resume household chores and responsibilities as part of the recovery process, and this may facilitate the person's resumption of previous roles (i.e., home maintainer) and minimize disability. On the other hand, barriers to function and magnifying of a disability may take the form of a spouse responding to the person with behaviors that are overly protective and that maintain the person in a dependent or helpless role. Families are complex, dynamic systems that are a significant influence on the individual's functional abilities. Understanding the role of family in a person's recovery and experience of disability is therefore an essential contextual factor to be evaluated by rehabilitation professionals.

Finally, age and life stage will impact the disablement process as well. While chronologic age is not the best indicator of life stage or developmental tasks being undertaken in adulthood, it can provide a general indicator. In early adulthood (ages 18–34 years), the major life-stage emphasis is on affirming one's identity and establishing one's independence, while middle adulthood (ages 35–64 years) is marked by attainment of meaning and balance in one's life goals (such as family and careers), and development of the ability to adapt to life's many changes (Merluzzi & Nairn, 1999; Schuster, 1992b).

Consolidation of life experiences, adjustment to changes in life roles, and the validation of the meaning of one's life characterize later adulthood (age 65 and older) (Merluzzi & Nairn, 1999; Schuster, 1992b).

Specific developmental life tasks may be further assessed and explained through the use of theories of adult development, and these theories and associated practice frames of reference are useful to assist professionals in identifying major life tasks as a means of further understanding a person's life context when facing disability. For example, a young mother with a spinal cord injury may identify her major concerns as being unsure of her physical capabilities for her role as a parent of an infant, whereas a middle-aged divorced father with multiple sclerosis may identify his major concerns as being worried about difficulties with work performance and maintaining his ability to sustain an income. Understanding life stages and the roles associated with these stages is essential for rehabilitation professionals to develop interventions that accurately address the needs of the person and assist in maximizing function and minimizing disability.

ENVIRONMENTAL CONTEXTS

Impairments in body functions or structures create challenges to the successful engagement in life tasks, and disability can result from this gap between abilities and task demands. The rehabilitation process is designed to assist individuals with learning the skills that will enable them to cope with their disability, whether this occurs through remediation of abilities or compensation for lost abilities (Moyers, 1999). However, for this process to be successful, rehabilitation professionals must understand the contextual factors that are the backdrop for a person's functioning in daily life. ICF classifies environmental contextual factors as products and technology, the natural environment and human-made changes to the environment, support and relationships, attitudes, and services, systems, and policies. Each of these factors relates to the physical and/or social environment in which people carry out their daily lives, and these contexts must be considered when determining the impact of disability on adult developmental life tasks. One obvious environmental concern for the adult with limited mobility is the ability to use public buildings and recreational sites. **Barrier-free design** is a strategy recommended to all builders to make industrial design and technology accessible to the broadest possible spectrum of society. A goal of this approach is to have not two sets of technology/design for society, but rather one universal standard that remains accessible to all. Table 17–1 presents some Internet-based examples of resources for barrier-free design.

Understanding the demands of activities that affect a person's participation in life tasks is required in order to make the connection between a person's abilities

and his challenges in participation. Further discussion of the personal contextual factors of motivation, values and self-advocacy, and the major life tasks of work and leisure for adults follows. Environmental contextual factors are discussed at greater length later in this text.

LIVING WITH A DISABLED FAMILY MEMBER

Family members are often a primary source of support for individuals as they navigate the world with a disability. In Chapter 9 you learned about family systems and the family life cycle theory. Chapter 13 presents examples of how relationships with family members are affected by developmental changes and increasing social demand. With aging, all parties in the relationship find themselves facing new and often unexpected challenges in relating to each other. The context of the social environment is a critical factor in understanding a person's experience and response to living with a disability.

As we consider families as an environmental context of "support and relationship," it is important to remember that the ICF classification of family as a contextual factor focuses on the physical and emotional support a family member provides for a person. The ICF classification system does not incorporate the attitudes of family members providing the support (World Health Organization, 2002).

Attitudes by family, others, and society are a contextual factor defined as "general or specific opinions and beliefs . . . . about the person or about other matters (e.g., social, political, and economic issues) that influence individual behaviour and actions" (World Health Organization, 2002, p. 143). Chapter 4 introduced issues of culture and cultural sensitivity to the student of development. Family culture plays a primary role in caregiving and in empowering individuals who have activity limitations. For example, it has been proposed that Euro-American philosophies of social Darwinism have contributed to social intolerance and stigmatization of children with chronic conditions (Starn, 1996). To illustrate the differences between the ICF category of "support and relationships" and the category of "attitude," consider the following case:

Mark is a 16-year-old with systemic juvenile rheumatoid arthritis. He was diagnosed at age 5 when he began having high, daily fevers and a rash on the trunk and extremities. He is able to walk for short distances but has a significant leg-length difference and a secondary scoliosis. Mark's family has been aggressive in seeking medical management and therapy for Mark. They have been active in local parent support groups, and have served on a consumer board for the local parks to increase accessibility in the community recreation programs.

TABLE 17–1	Barrier-Free Design Resources

Center for Inclusive Design and Environmental Access   http://www.ap.buffalo.edu/~idea/
Dedicated to improving the design of environments and products by making them more usable, safer, and appealing to people with a wide range of abilities, throughout their lifespans.

The Center for Universal Design, North Carolina University, Raleigh, North Carolina   http://www.design.ncsu.edu/cud/
A national research, information, and technical assistance center that evaluates, develops, and promotes accessible and universal design in buildings and related products. They are using a combination of text and multimedia modes for presentation of their information to ensure access to all users.

Dynamic Living   http://www.dynamic-living.com/DLHome.htm
Offers information on kitchen appliances, unique daily living products, and home automation products that promote a convenient, comfortable, and safe home environment for people of all ages. Useful information for seniors and people with mobility challenges.

The Home Modification Action Project   http://www.usc.edu/go/hmap/
Provides information on home modifications so that frail older and disabled persons have the choice to age in place, and the provision of care can take place in a supportive environment. Site is designed for builders, homeowners, and those who have a loved one with access needs.

Liberty Resources' Link to World Wide Web Resources on Accessibility and Housing   http://www.libertyresources.org /housing/ph-index.html
Liberty Resource Inc. is a nonprofit, consumer-driven organization that advocates and promotes independent living for persons with disabilities.

Missouri AgrAbility Project   http://www.fse.missouri.edu/agrability/
This state program provides appropriate education and assistance designed to promote independence in production agricultural and rural living. The Missouri AgrAbility Program provides professional training, on-the-farm assessment, technical assistance, information dissemination, and referral to other service providers.

National Institute on Disability & Rehabilitation Research   http://www.ed.gov/offices/OSERS/NIDRR/
Promotes the coordination of research about individuals with disabilities through the federal government and ensures that the general public, services, and agencies have access to research results.

National Resource Center on Supportive Housing   http://www.homemods.org
The center's mission is to make supportive housing and home modification a more integral component of successful aging, long-term care, preventive health, and the development of elder-friendly communities.

Trace Research and Development Center   http://trace.wisc.edu/world/
Gives basic info about concepts like universal and flexible design and also about many related guidelines, standards, tools, and ideas.

U.S. Department of Housing and Urban Development (HUD)—Accessible Housing Designs   http://www.hud.gov /access.html
Links to information about accessibility that is required by different federal laws, about accessibility that is voluntary, and about innovative accessible designs for multifamily and single-family housing.

Mark's father was an avid basketball player in high school and currently coaches the high school basketball team. Although both Mark and his father have been aware for some time that Mark would not be able to participate in competitive sports, fitness and sports are very much a part of the family culture. Mark's father proclaims a "use it or lose it" philosophy and has rejected the adaptive devices offered by the occupational and physical therapist to assist Mark in school activities. The teachers pressure Mark to use the adaptive devices, but Mark sees these as evidence of his inadequacies. Mark had been looking forward to taking driver's education in school this year, only to find that his physical limitations make it impossible to drive without adaptations to the vehicle. Mark did not explain this to his parents; rather, he told them that he did not want to drive. He has been spending more time alone at school, is often withdrawn, and is rude to his teachers and classmates. He now refuses to participate in many classroom activities or at home.

In Mark's case, the family provides excellent physical support, but the family sports culture marginalizes

Mark and his accomplishments. By refusing to accept adaptive equipment for Mark, the family has demonstrated an attitude of intolerance for Mark's activity limitations. This attitude is disabling for Mark, both in the school setting and in his consideration of new tasks like driving. Because driving is such a significant social milestone in the United States, Mark is likely to be further stigmatized by his decision throughout his adolescence.

This case may help those outside of the family better appreciate the contradictions that often are brought to the forefront when disability occurs within the family. For example, in one study that explored the cultural issues of mothers caring for a family member with AIDS, it was found that fears of stigma affected caregivers' level of disclosure, despite possessing competing values about truthfulness (Boyle, Bunting, Hodnicki, & Ferrell, 2001). In Mark's case, the family stigma associated with devices to accommodate his activity limitations has created a barrier to function when none need exist.

FAMILY CAREGIVERS

A huge body of research and literature defines caregiving for a range of disabilities and discusses the issues families face when they assume a caregiving role for their family member with a disability. The challenges faced by family members involve managing not only the day-to-day physical and emotional needs of their family member with a disability, but managing their own stress levels and emotional responses to providing this level and type of care. The research on caregiving and mental health consistently indicates that caregiving results in some level of burden, and that the risk for mental health problems, particularly depression, is high (Pruchno, 2000). Mobility and access remain one of the most difficult issues for the adult with activity limitations. Even with good resources, the demands of equipment and ADL care require the support of other persons. While children can attempt to lend support, as illustrated in Figure 17–2, the physical, emotional, and social barriers to participation may be difficult to overcome.

With aging, the needs of family members change over time, and as described in Chapter 13, roles and responsibilities need to be renegotiated (Zarit, Johansson, & Jarrott, 1998). Meeting the day-to-day needs of the family creates anxiety and changes in the relationships, and this anxiety differs according to caregiving contexts (e.g., spouses caring for partners versus children caring for parents) (Cavanaugh, 1998). Cavanaugh (1998) also notes that for spousal caregiving, loss of companionship

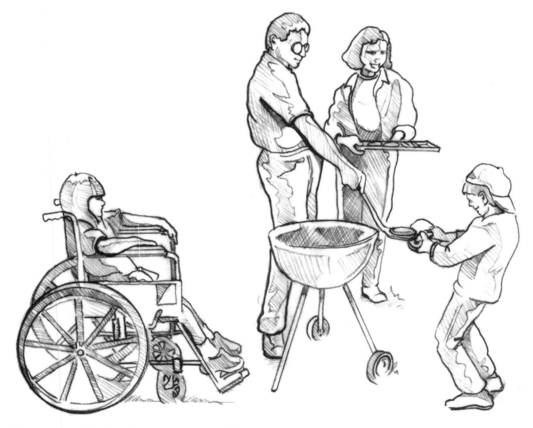

FIGURE 17–2 Fatigue and mobility limitation can interfere socially.

and intimacy is often a negative outcome, whereas caring for a parent can infringe on other life roles and daily routines.

It is important to note that the dynamics of caring for an adult with a disability do not equate to the caregiving dynamics associated with caring for children with disabilities. Despite the physical and emotional dependencies that may occur in adults with various disabilities, it is crucial to identify the developmental levels and life stages achieved both prior to, and during, the onset and aftermath of disability. This awareness for caregivers can help with fostering maximal independence and preventing excess dependency in their family members.

AREAS OF OCCUPATION

First introduced in Chapter 1, **occupation** is a meaningful action in the context of a person's life. Occupation contributes to personal competence and feelings of mastery in the individual (Larsen, Wood, & Clark, 2003). Activity limitations can impair the person's ability to be successful in the areas of ADLs, IADLs, work, social participation, play, leisure, education, and communication. While many of these areas of occupation have been discussed in earlier chapters, there are some additional impacts on adults and adult roles that need elaboration.

To aid this discussion, review the ICF model from Chapter 1, here called Figure 17–3. You can see the ICF categories of Body Structures and Functions, and under these categories the components described in the *Guide to Physical Therapy Practice* (American Physical Therapy Association, 2001) and the *Occupational Therapy Practice Standards* (American Occupational Therapy Association, 2002). In these models, the terms *illness* and *sickness* are not used. In fact, only the *Guide to Physical Therapy Practice* (American Physical Therapy Association, 2001) retains the use of the word *disability*. Dr. Brundtland, director general of the World Health Organization, describes the

ICF	Health Condition											Contextual Factors									
	Body Structures and Functions			Activities and Participation								Personal Factors			Environmental Factors						
OT Practice Framework	Body Structures	Body Functions	Motor Skills	Process Skills	ADL	IADL	Work	Social Participation	Play	Leisure	Education	Communication Skills	Routines	Habits	Roles	Spiritual	Cultural	Social	Physical	Temporal	Virtual
	Client Factors		Performance Skills (*with communication skills)		Areas of Occupation							*	Performance Patterns			Context					
PT Guide to Practice (Negative Aspects from ICF)	Pathology and Impairment			Functional Limitation																	
				Disability																	

FIGURE 17–3 In the ICF, disabilities are viewed as interactions between health conditions and contextual factors. The shaded area exemplifies environments that are optimally inclusive.

rationale for this revised terminology: "More than any-thing, the ICF is based on the value of inclusion, and on a universal model of disability. It rejects the view that disability is a defining feature of a separate minority group of people" (2002, retrieved July 23, 2003, from http://www.who.int/director-general/speeches/2002 /english/20020418_disabilitytrieste.html).

The field of medical sociology has long recognized *disability* as socially constructed, illustrated by the large body of literature on "the sick role." Talcott Parsons, in 1951, noted that (p. 431) "illness is a state of distur-bance in the 'normal' functioning of the total human individual, including both the state of the organism as a biological system and of his personal and social ad-justments. It is thus partly biologically and partly so-cially defined. Participation in the social system is al-ways potentially relevant to the state of illness, to its etiology and to the conditions of successful therapy, as well as to other things." It was Parsons who first coined the phrase, the "sick role."

ILLNESS AND THE SICK ROLE

Illness is the particular way a pathology or impairment interferes with everyday function (Beer, 2003). Parsons takes this conception further, stating that in our society there are predictable ways for an ill person to behave, to receive social support for her illness. As Parsons de-scribed it, for a person to assume the **"sick role"** and therefore be free from blame for her condition, these four conditions must be met:

- The individual is exempt from normal social role responsibilities, like going to work.
- The sick person cannot be expected, by "pulling herself together," to get well by an act of will. Because she cannot will herself well, she will be "taken care of."
- The person must be active in expression of and in behaviors supporting her desire to "get well."
- The person must seek and comply with the expectations of technically competent help (adapted from Parsons, 1951, p. 437).

If you are limited to bed, wear your pajamas all day, and look pitiful, you are afforded special care and priv-ileges. If you cannot perform your daily occupations because of some pathology, and you behave in a man-ner that suggests that you are trying to return to your occupational roles, society will release you from per-formance expectations for the duration of the illness.

Parsons also notes that "the privileges and exemp-tions of the sick role may become objects of a 'secondary gain,' that the patient is positively motivated, usually un-consciously, to secure or to retain" (Parsons, 1951,

p. 439). This is what we currently call **"malingering."** A person who malingers enjoys exemption from work and social demands, and either exaggerates his disability or fails to follow through on intervention strategies aimed at returning him to the workforce.

The societal response to illness as a form of de-viance requiring expert assistance is the fundamental premise of the *medical model*. This model also establishes physicians as the gatekeepers to the label of *disability* and empowers them to certify who is eligible for social support services like workers' compensation (Albrecht, 1992). The medicalization of illness and disability is a cultural phenomenon and is strongly challenged by persons with longstanding activity limitations who see themselves as "differently abled" rather than disabled.

NORMALIZATION

In our society there is a negative stigma associated with the label *disabled*. For adults acquiring a condition that results in chronic activity limitations, and for the par-ents accepting a developmental difference in their child, it has been documented that the persons in-volved begin to see the lifestyle changes caused by a medical condition as "ordinary." This process is **normalization** and is a positive adaptation in parenting a child with special needs (Deatrick, Knafl, & Walsh 1988). Normalization reflects an internalization of the specialized habits and routines associated with activity limitations to such a degree that they are integrated as ordinary personal and family occupations (Cronin, 2003). The normalization process represents the suc-cessful integration of activity limitations into daily occu-pations in a manner that enhances function.

THE WORLD OF WORK: ISSUES FOR PERSONS WITH DISABILITIES

Productivity relates to a range of activities including paid employment, volunteering, skills in obtaining and keeping a job, and home maintenance. These activities represent participation in a highly valued aspect of Western society. For individuals with acquired activity limitations, the loss of income represents not only a fi-nancial loss but a loss of identity as well. The vast major-ity of individuals with disabilities indicate that a primary goal is paid employment. However, significant system barriers exist that prevent a substantial portion of these individuals from maintaining gainful employment. In fact, it is estimated that nearly two thirds of all working-age adults with disabilities are not in the workforce, and it is hypothesized that policy disincentives and lack of physical access are among the major types of barriers that prevent employment for such individuals (National Institute on Disability and Rehabilitation Research [NIDRR], 1999). Examples of these barriers include eligibility requirements for federal disability income benefits, limited knowledge and/or skills of employers to implement job accommodations, attitudinal barriers of employers, and lack of skills in self-advocacy by individuals with disabilities.

While a "sick" person is excused from paid labor, the person with persistent activity limitations who does not "work" will be labeled as *disabled,* and in some cases as a "malingerer." Financial losses are often associated with being disabled for both the person with a disability and his family. Young adults who sustain injuries that result in disability, such as spinal cord injuries and traumatic brain injury, face different challenges than adults in middle and older age. In the case of young adults, determining a career path is a normative life task that is often significantly disrupted by the onset of disability. Adults who have already established a career face the need to readjust their career focus due to limitations created by the disability, and they may need to change career areas entirely.

Type and severity of disability will also influence the amount of change in the life task of work that is experienced by an individual, regardless of age. Family members often support their loved ones financially, and this situation may become a source of increased conflict, for both the person with a disability and the family member. Additionally, family members may have difficulty empowering the person with a disability to take on productive life roles, both inside and outside the home, due to changes in the quality or quantity of activity the person with a disability may be able to successfully complete. Caregivers often unwittingly create excess disability through these actions.

CHANGES IN LEISURE PARTICIPATION

Participation in leisure for adults is not clearly addressed in the ICF. The Occupational Therapy Practice Framework (American Occupational Therapy Organization, 2002) defines **leisure** as an occupation that is intrinsically motivating and nonobligatory. Participating in leisure activities has the power to meet many human needs, such as relaxation, emotional expression, self-development, socialization, and experiencing pleasure in life (Olson & Roarty-O'Herron, 2000). Disability presents multiple barriers to leisure participation and often results in the total cessation of previously treasured leisure occupations. Barriers to participation may include decreased capability to perform the activity at necessary or desired levels of satisfaction, a myriad of environmental barriers, and discrimination resulting in

lack of access to leisure options, particularly travel and social activities. Loss of the opportunity and means to travel was noted as major loss for individuals and their spouses following the onset of a stroke (Mumma, 1986/2000).

Decreased community participation may be due to environmental and transportation barriers as well as stigma or discrimination. The energy and amount of effort required by the individual and/or their caregivers may also result in decreased leisure participation. Regardless of the type of barriers to leisure participation, the loss of previously enjoyed activities represents a loss of an important source of identity and coping for individuals with disabilities. Increasingly, communities are including public recreational sites that use principles of barrier-free design, allowing access to playgrounds, hiking paths, parks and golf courses (Figure 17–4). These accessible leisure sites are limited and not available to all persons.

While many rehabilitation professionals address leisure participation and community reintegration in formal rehabilitation settings, carryover is often limited, and resources for community involvement are sorely lacking. Consumers with disabilities are demanding equal access and are creating, often with their family members, resources for leisure participation. The Internet has become a growing source of these resources and permits a new level of engagement for many with disabilities. As individuals progress through the recovery process, it is the responsibility of rehabilitation professionals to be aware of options and resources for addressing the major life task of leisure participation. By attending to leisure needs, individuals with disabilities and their families may experience the opportunity to reduce stress, increase self-confidence and self-esteem, integrate the development of new skills, increase coping skills, affirm their identity, and experience pleasure in their lives.

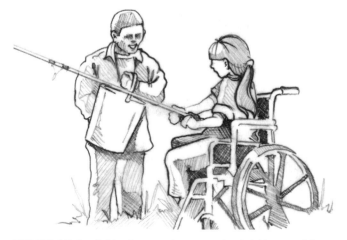

FIGURE 17–4 Fishing is an outdoor sport that is fairly accessible to the motivated wheelchair user.

SELF-ADVOCACY: AN EMPOWERMENT TOOL

Self-advocacy can be defined as advocating for one's needs and rights, and the disability rights movement has championed the development of this skill for individuals with disabilities. In response to the pervasive discrimination and stigma experienced by individuals with disabilities, many different groups in the disability community have organized, advocated for, and won fundamental changes in public policy that ensure the rights of individuals with disabilities. The most recent major legislative change was the enactment of the Americans with Disabilities Act (ADA) in 1990 (Fleischer & Zames, 2001). The ADA contains statutes that ensure access to public spaces and employment protections, among other provisions for the nearly 54 million individuals whose conditions qualify under the ADA definition of disability (Fleischer & Zames, 2001).

Many support networks are available for individuals with disabilities, and their services range from local support groups for individuals and their families to major resource catalogs, referral sources, and services regionally, nationally, and on-line. Given the complicated network of federal, state, and private resources available to individuals with disabilities, these support and advocacy organizations are essential for education and assistance in accessing the services.

SUMMARY

This chapter has provided an overview of the role of family in the disablement process for adults. Probably the most important take-away message is to understand how context, particularly family context, contributes to the experience of disability for adults.

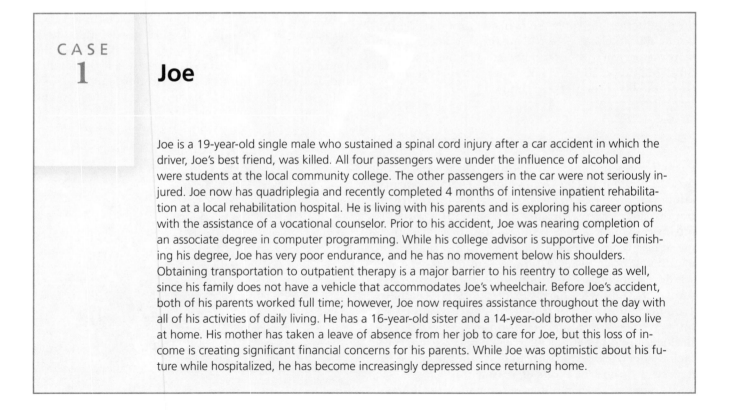

CASE

1

Joe

Joe is a 19-year-old single male who sustained a spinal cord injury after a car accident in which the driver, Joe's best friend, was killed. All four passengers were under the influence of alcohol and were students at the local community college. The other passengers in the car were not seriously injured. Joe now has quadriplegia and recently completed 4 months of intensive inpatient rehabilitation at a local rehabilitation hospital. He is living with his parents and is exploring his career options with the assistance of a vocational counselor. Prior to his accident, Joe was nearing completion of an associate degree in computer programming. While his college advisor is supportive of Joe finishing his degree, Joe has very poor endurance, and he has no movement below his shoulders. Obtaining transportation to outpatient therapy is a major barrier to his reentry to college as well, since his family does not have a vehicle that accommodates Joe's wheelchair. Before Joe's accident, both of his parents worked full time; however, Joe now requires assistance throughout the day with all of his activities of daily living. He has a 16-year-old sister and a 14-year-old brother who also live at home. His mother has taken a leave of absence from her job to care for Joe, but this loss of income is creating significant financial concerns for his parents. While Joe was optimistic about his future while hospitalized, he has become increasingly depressed since returning home.

CASE
2

Mary

Mary is a 45-year-old married female with three children, ages 5, 8, and 10. She was diagnosed with multiple sclerosis 3 years ago. Until recently she had been managing her symptoms well and continued to work part-time at a local library and care for her children with increased assistance from her husband. However, after a recent exacerbation of her illness, she has lost more function and now is unable to work or drive. Mary is experiencing increased difficulty with meal preparation and child-care responsibilities, and her mother-in-law has been assisting her on a daily basis. While Mary appreciates the help from her mother-in-law, their relationship has always been turbulent and conflicted due to personality differences. Mary's husband tends to be caught in the middle in these conflicts, and he typically avoids confrontation by working on household projects. Mary's doctor has recommended therapy services from the home health agency, and while Mary is reluctant, she agrees. Mary has never received any rehabilitation services since being diagnosed, and she tends to feel she can handle her disease and does not want to be seen as "handicapped."

CASE
3

Ed

Ed is a 74-year-old widowed male who currently lives alone in a two-story home. His wife died 9 months ago, and since that time Ed's functional abilities have declined markedly. His two adult children, a son and a daughter, both live over 2 hours away from him, but each child and their families see him at least once a month. Ed's daughter, Sarah, is a registered nurse and has noticed several concerns in the last two months. She observed that Ed has lost at least 20 pounds and that he frequently has spoiled food in his refrigerator. Ed has also stopped his daily habit of going to the local coffee shop for breakfast with his group of friends. Sarah suspects that Ed is not taking his medications correctly and that he has had several falls, though Ed denies both of these concerns, stating, "I'm fine, really." Ed's son, Sam, has noticed that his father is not attending to the yard work or household chores with his usual interest and skill level. In fact, Ed recently said he should just hire someone to mow for him, a task he previously took great pride in and enjoyed immensely. Ed has moderate osteoarthritis, hypertension, low back pain, and a history of a heart attack 6 years ago. When Ed's wife was living, she motivated him to take care of himself, but now Ed states, "What's the difference?" when prodded by his children to take better care of his health. It has become apparent to Sarah and Sam that Ed is not doing well, and Sarah suggests to her father that he come and live with her. After making this suggestion, Sarah and Sam bring their father to the gerontology clinic for a full assessment and recommendations for assistance with caregiving.

Hanging on to Loved Ones and Home

CORRIE A. MANCINELLI, PT, PhD
CONSULTANT PHYSICAL THERAPIST TO THE WEST VIRGINIA UNIVERSITY 65+ CLINIC

It is hard to tell a patient that he can no longer safely provide care for his chronically ill wife. This is a true, yet not unique, experience I have had as a therapist.

Mr. A. is an 80-year-old gentleman with severe ankylosing spondylitis who sustained a fracture around a total hip replacement. His wife has Parkinson's disease. Mr. A. provided care for Mrs. A. until the fracture. This acute event interfered with Mr. A.'s abilities to function in his own home. He was no longer able to care for himself, let alone Mrs. A. They lived in a first-floor apartment with barriers such as thick carpet and a very small bathroom. She spent most of her time in a wheelchair and had a history of falling. He was ambulatory with a rolling walker, but his mobility was markedly limited. He certainly was not able to help her with transfers, bathing, dressing, or meal preparation.

After 4 months of admissions to acute-care hospitals and rehabilitation facilities followed by extensive home health and outpatient rehabilitation, Mr. A. recovered enough to provide care for himself, but not for his wife. Mrs. A. was no longer a candidate for home health services covered under Medicare because of limited potential to improve. Neither Mr. nor Mrs. A. was eligible for daily aid services provided by the local senior center. The only option for care that remained for her was an extended-care nursing facility. Mrs. A. was willing to accept that she was no longer able to remain at home. She did not want to burden her husband. He, on the other hand, was distraught about not being able to provide for her. He did not want to accept the fact that it was unsafe for both of them to remain in their apartment. He felt as though he was "letting down the love of his life." His core family values were also being disrupted because he was taught from a very young age to take care of all family, no matter how large the task. Mr. A. was losing his sense of purpose. He had to rely on his only daughter to visit daily, bathe his wife, cook their meals, and put her to bed. His daughter did this in addition to working full-time and being a mother of two busy teenage boys. She became worn from providing the intensity of care that was needed. In a very short time, Mr. A. became aware that the circumstance was emotionally and physically draining for his daughter and unsafe for his wife. He recognized that it was time for Mrs. A. to become a resident in an extended-care nursing facility. He said, "It is selfish of me to want my wife at home now."

Mr. and Mrs. A. celebrated their last evening of being together at home as a couple for 50-plus years. They did so with a mutual respect and a deep love for each other. Mrs. A. went to the nursing home the next day. Now Mr. A. calls and visits Mrs. A. daily. He reports that he feels lonely at times without her but recognizes that she is safer in the nursing home.

Sometimes people are not able to see dangerous home situations because they are not willing to accept disability for themselves or their loved ones. Mr. A. was unrealistic about his disablement and ability to provide care for his wife. For healthcare providers, it is important not only to respect family values and traditions as much as possible, but to also see the dangers that prevail in life circumstances that are unstable because of injury or disease. Mr. A. once again has a sense of purpose because he knows that his wife looks forward to his phone calls and visits. He also has learned that he still can provide for her emotional needs, even though he cannot provide for her physical needs. During a recent follow-up phone call, he said to me that his "love for her exceeds his need for her." He didn't realize that he contributed to my understanding of care and support of family just through that statement. I will carry that with me throughout my remaining professional years.

REFERENCES

Albrecht, G. (1992). *The disability business: Rehabilitation in America*, Sage Library of Social Research 190. Newbury Park, CA: Sage.

American Occupational Therapy Association. (2002). Occupational Therapy Practice Framework: Domain and process. *American Journal of Occupational Therapy, 56(6)*, 609–639.

American Physical Therapy Association. (2001). *Guide to physical therapist practice* (2nd ed.). Alexandria, VA: American Physical Therapy Association.

Bickenbach, J. E., Chatterji, S., Badley, E. M., & Ustun, T. B. (1999). Models of disablement, universalism and the international classification of impairments, disabilities, and handicaps. *Social Science and Medicine, 48*, 1173–1187.

Boyle, J. S., Bunting, S. M., Hodnicki, D. R., & Ferrell, J. A. (2001). Critical thinking in African-American mothers who care for adult children with HIV: A cultural analysis. *Journal of Transcultural Nursing, 12(3)*, 193–202.

Brundtland, G. (2002). Director-general's speech to the WHO Conference on Health and Disability. Retrieved July 23, 2003, from http://www.who.int/director-general/speeches/2002/english/20020418_disabilitytrieste.html.

Cavanaugh, J. C. (1998). Caregiving to adults: A life event challenge. In I. H. Nordhus, G. R. VandenBos, S. Berg, & P. Fromholt (Eds.), *Clinical geropsychology* (pp. 131–135). Washington, DC: American Psychological Association.

Christiansen, C., & Baum, C. (1997). *Occupational therapy: Enabling function and well-being* (2nd ed.). Thorofare, NJ: Slack.

Cronin, A. (2003). Mothering a child with hidden impairments. *American Journal of Occupational Therapy* (in press).

Deatrick, J. A., Knafl, K. A., & Walsh, M. (1988). The process of parenting a child with a disability: Normalization through accommodations. *Journal of Advanced Nursing, 13*, 15–21.

Fleischer, D. Z., & Zames, F. (2001). *The disability rights movement: From charity to confrontation*. Philadelphia: Temple University Press.

Kaplan, H., & Sadock, B. (1998). *Synopsis of psychiatry, behavioral sciences/clinical psychiatry* (8th ed.). Baltimore: Williams and Wilkins.

Larson, E., Wood, W., & Clark, F. (2003). Occupational science: Building the science and practice of occupation through academic discipline. In E. Crepeau, E. Cohn, & B. Schell (Eds.), *Willard and Spackman's occupational therapy* (10th ed.) (pp. 15–26). Philadelphia: Lippincott.

Merluzzi T. V., & Nairn, R. C. (1999). Adulthood and aging: Transitions in health and health cognition. In T. L. Whitman, T. V. Merluzzu, & R. D. White (Eds.), *Life-span perspectives on health and illness* (pp. 189–206). Mahwah, NJ: Lawrence Erlbaum Associates.

Moyers, P. A. (1999). The guide to occupational therapy practice. *American Journal of Occupational Therapy, 53*, 247–298.

Mumma, C. M. (1986/2000). Perceived losses following stroke. *Rehabilitation Nursing, 25(5)*, 192–196.

Nagi, S. (1991). Disability concepts revisited: Implications for prevention. In A. M. Pope & A. Tarlov (Eds.), *Disability in America: Toward a national agenda for prevention* (pp. 309–339). Washington, DC: National Academy Press.

National Center for Health Statistics. (1995). *Trends in the health of older Americans, 1994.* (DHHS Pub. No. [PHS 95]–1414). Washington, DC: U.S. Government Printing Office.

National Institute on Disability and Rehabilitation Research. (1999). NIDRR's long-range plan. Retrieved December 10, 2001, from the National Center for the Dissemination of Disability Research Web site: http://www.nidrr.org/new/announcements/nidrr_lrp/index.html.

Olson, L. J., & Roarty-O'Herron, E. A. (2000). Range of human activity: Leisure. In J. Hinojosa and M. Blount (Eds.), *The texture of life: Purposeful activities in occupational therapy.* (pp. 258–288). Bethesda, MD: American Occupational Therapy Association.

Parsons, T. (1951). *The social system.* England: RKP.

Pruchno, R. A. (2000). Caregiving research: Looking backward, looking forward. In R. L. Rubinstein, M. Moss, & M. H. Kleban (Eds.), *The many dimensions of aging.* New York: Springer.

Schuster, C. S. (1992a). Developmental frameworks of selected stage theorists. In C. S. Schuster & S. S. Ashburn (Eds.), *The process of human development: A holistic life-span approach* (3rd ed.) (pp. 893–896). Philadelphia: J.B. Lippincott Company.

Schuster, C. S. (1992b). Developmental tasks of life phases. In C. S. Schuster & S. S. Ashburn (Eds.), *The process of human development: A holistic life-span approach* (3rd ed.) (pp. 881–882). Philadelphia: J.B. Lippincott.

Verbrugge, L. M. (1994). Disability in later life. In R. P. Abeles, H. C. Gift, & M. G. Ory (Eds.), *Aging and quality of life* (pp. 30–95). New York: Springer.

Versluys, H. P. (1996). Evaluation of emotional adjustment to disabilities. In C. A. Trombly (Ed.), *Occupational therapy for physical dysfunction* (4th ed.) (pp. 225–234). Baltimore: Williams and Wilkins.

U.S. Department of Health and Human Services. (1999). *Mental health: A report of the surgeon general.* Rockville, MD: U.S. Department of Health and Human Services, Substance Abuse and Mental Health Services Administration, Center for Mental Health Services, National Institutes of Health, National Institute of Mental Health.

World Health Organization. (2002). ICF: International Classification of Functioning and Disability. Geneva, Switzerland: World Health Organization.

Zarit, S. H., Johansson, L., & Jarrott, S. E. (1998). In I. H. Nordhus, G. R. VandenBos, S. Berg, & P. Fromholt (Eds.), *Clinical geropsychology* (pp. 345–360). Washington, DC: American Psychological Association.

Special Topics in Human Performance

Environmental Contexts

Diana Middleton-Davis, OTR/L
Assistant Professor
Division of Occupational Therapy
West Virginia University
Morgantown, West Virginia

and

Anne Cronin, PhD, OTR/L, BCP
Associate Professor
Division of Occupational Therapy
West Virginia University
Morgantown, West Virginia

Objectives

Upon completion of this chapter, the reader should be able to

▓ Understand the complex relationship between environmental contextual factors and function for individuals of all ages.

▓ Define the three environmental contexts as identified by the ICF.

▓ Differentiate accessibility, universal design, and negotiability in the environment.

▓ Understand the distinctions between traditional health care and client-centered care.

▓ Describe the relationships among attitudes, roles, and habits.

▓ Discuss the implications of assistive technology for expanding environmental access.

Key Terms

accessibility
assets
assistive technology (AT)
attitudinal environment

client-centered care
natural environment
negotiability
physical environment

Products and Technology
universal design
virtual environment

INTRODUCTION

The ICF presents a radical redefinition of health. It is based on the premise that international stability and economic growth are grounded in the health of the population. Dr. Gro Harlem Brundtland, director-general of the World Health Organization, states, "Only healthy people with the support of a functioning health sector can ensure sustainable development of their societies. A loss of health is a loss not only to the person but also to the person's family and society as a whole" (retrieved August 14, 2003, from http://www.who.int /director-general/speeches/2002/english/20020418 _disabilitytrieste.html).

Throughout this textbook there have been multiple references to the *contextual factors* in the ICF (World Health Organization, 2002). With the ICF document, the international community has made a strong statement that function and participation are not simply based on features intrinsic to the individual, but that complex external factors are integral to determining functional capacity. Within the ICF, *environment* refers to the complex contexts that individuals encounter in their daily activities and participation. Thus, *environment* as defined by the ICF includes the "physical, social and attitudinal environment in which people live and conduct their lives" (World Health Organization, 2002, p. 22). The ICF goes on to state, "The factors are external to individuals and can have a positive or negative influence on the individual's participation as a member of society, on performance of activities of the individual or on the individual's body function or structure" (World Health Organization, 2002, p. 22). Environments can have a facilitating or an inhibiting effect on development and aging based on the unique qualities of the individuals and the environments within which they carry out their daily tasks (Corcoran & Gitlin, 1997). This chapter will review each of the three aspects of an individual's environmental context.

The ICF classifies three types of environmental factors: *Products and Technology, Natural Environment* and Human-Made Changes to the Environment, and *Support and Relationships,* Attitudes, Services, Systems, and Policies (World Health Organization, 2002). Each of

these types will be covered briefly in terms of the needs and practice guidelines of occupation and physical therapists.

PHYSICAL ENVIRONMENT

The **physical environment** includes both the natural and man-made features of the space the person occupies. The **natural environment** includes physical features of the outdoor environment such as land forms, distances between resources, terrain, plants, animals, and bodies of water. Climate also impacts human function. Climatic features such as seasonal variations and unexpected natural events (hurricanes, earthquakes, etc.) are part of the natural environment. Because the ICF is focused on human function, the human population who share the same pattern of environmental adaptation are considered part of the natural environment. Humans impact the natural environment in many ways. Human-caused changes to the natural environment can include large-scale disruption to people's day-to-day lives. Examples of this include war, environmental disasters, and land, water, or air pollution (World Health Organization, 2002). The physical environment has a pervasive influence on all human activities and participation. For example, features of the physical environment can influence such diverse things as the rate of child development (Maleta et al., 2003), mother-child dynamics (Olson & Esdaile, 2000), the ability to engage in productive paid work (Bootes & Chapparo, 2002), and the possibility of becoming independently mobile (Jones, McEwen, & Hansen, 2003).

PRODUCTS AND TECHNOLOGY

The ICF category of **Products and Technology** refers to the physical items that people come in contact with while completing their daily activities. These items can include fundamental needs like food and medications or complex items such as regional land-use policies, including the design, planning, and development of space. Although integrally involved with people in clinical situations, rehabilitation professionals must be skilled in both using and adapting products and technologies of all types. Some selected subtypes of products and technologies are presented in Table 18–1 with a discussion of limitations in clinical application.

As rehabilitation specialists, we tend to think of specialized adaptations, but products and technology also relate to ordinary everyday items. For example, the ability to don and doff items of clothing is an important developmental milestone for children. As children gain control over their lives, this is often expressed by their ability to shed their clothing on their own. As their motor, visuospatial, and cognitive skills develop, they master the ability to choose and don their own clothing. The skills developed and necessary for this major landmark can vary widely between cultures. The skills necessary to don the typical American clothing items of jeans, shirt, socks, and shoes are very different from the skills needed by a female youth from India donning a sari independently for the first time.

As individuals age and experience motor and visual changes associated with natural aging, the experience of dressing oneself can once again gain significance in determining the ability of the older individual to continue living independently. The buttons, snaps, and zippers that challenged the 4-year-old with poor motor skills can once again become challenging as difficulties with vision and motor changes brought about by arthritis or Parkinson's disease change the function of the older individual. Oftentimes the older person alters his wardrobe choices to increase his independence. These changes can include the use of elastic-waist skirts and pants, pullover tops versus button-down, and loafers or slip-on shoes versus tennis shoes. The older individual from a different culture might find the changes associated with aging uniquely challenging.

TABLE 18–1	Selected Subtypes of ICF Products and Technologies	
Product	**ICF Definition (World Health Organization, 2002)**	**Example of Limitation**
Products or substances for personal consumption	Any object or substance gathered, processed, or manufactured for ingestion, including food and medicines	Limitations affect social function. An adolescent who has cerebral palsy and limited abilities to chew and swallow will not be able to participate in class pizza parties.
Products and technology for personal use in daily living	Equipment, products, and technologies used by people in daily activities	Limitations may be culturally influenced. A child who cannot manage eating utensils may be socially limited in a Western culture, where this is not accepted; however, in a Pakistani culture, this would be acceptable.
Products and technology for personal indoor and outdoor mobility and transportation	Equipment, products, and technologies used by people in activities of moving inside and outside buildings	Limitations may be environmentally determined. Many shopping malls now offer rental of motorized scooters for persons with limited mobility. These devices would not be equally useful in a street market with curbs, uneven pavement, and gravel paths.
Products and technology for communication	Equipment, products, and technologies used by people in activities of sending and receiving information	Limitations influence ability to communicate. Telephone access to emergency rescue systems is widely available. Persons with speech or hearing impairments will not be able to use this safety program.
Products and technology for employment	Equipment, products, and technology used for employment to facilitate work activities	Limitations may impact ability to perform employment tasks. Traditional storage and filing cabinets are not accessible to persons who cannot stand.

ASSETS

The role that **assets,** or "products or objects of economic exchange such as money, goods, property and other valuables which an individual owns or to which he or she has rights of use" (WHO, 2002, p. 98), play is highly variable based upon culture, personal values, and services available. Children are often raised within the asset boundaries set by their parents or caretakers. The amount of assets possessed by parents can either facilitate or inhibit development of children. Those raised in poverty oftentimes have decreased opportunities in childhood compared with children raised in affluent environments. The true impact this has on the development of children, though, is a complicated equation in which the society's values, supports, and political environment must be included. The effect of assets on development and aging is often tempered or worsened by the effects of other environmental factors such as support and relationships, attitudes, and services, systems, and policies. Decreased socioeconomic status has been related to increased occurrences of mental illness in all ages. Franks, Gold, and Fiscella (2003) report "lower socioeconomic status (SES) and being black are associated with lower reported health status and higher mortality" (p. 2505). The effects of the physical environment on health and social participation are generally underestimated by therapists. Physical environments that provide access and opportunity for participation were found to be conducive to fostering occupational performance (Rebeiro, 2001).

As individuals age, assets continue to affect aging and the experience of the older individual. In most societies aging is associated with a decrease in income as the individual passes from worker to retired person, or as changes in motor, visual, and cognitive systems dictate a change in employment. This loss of monetary assets has a direct effect on health and wellness in the aged population. Seniors who have collected greater assets during their life have more flexibility to pick and choose where and how they want to live during retirement than seniors who were unable to accumulate financial assets as working individuals. Frail, disabled, and widowed elders who live alone are more likely to have limited assets and report more depression, loneliness, and sleep problems. Hays and George (2002) report that these same widowed elders "use more formal home-care services; have less access to help in emergencies; and are at greater risk of unstable living arrangements and of institutionalization compared to similar elders living with others" (p. 284).

In American society the transition from worker to retiree is often marked by the transition from health insurance with prescription-drug coverage to health insurance without prescription coverage. Medical advances have increased the average life expectancy of most Americans; however, these medical advances are often achieved by the use of expensive medications.

The older person with limited financial assets is likely to cut corners, choosing to sacrifice her quality of living by reducing her household expenses or by choosing to compromise her health by taking less medication than what is recommended by her physician. The Medicare Prescription Drug Improvement and Modernization Act, signed into law in December 2003, attempts to address this problem by providing discount cards for seniors, providing low-income seniors with additional benefits, and initiating a Medicare Prescription Drug Benefit beginning in 2006 (American Association of Retired Persons, 2004).

PRODUCTS OF ARCHITECTURE, BUILDING, AND CONSTRUCTION

Most architecture and buildings are designed for average-sized adults with normal motor, cognitive, and sensory perceptual function. The fixtures and architectural details of most settings are not intended for use by those of small stature or those with motor, visual, and/or cognitive deficits. When we discuss the impact of architectural or building products and their effects of development, we need to think in terms of the people using them and the activities for which they are used. Providing **accessibility** in an environment means removing barriers that prevent people with activity limitations from the use of services, products, and information available in that environment. Many access-related technologies have become prevalent because they assist all persons, not just those with limitations. Some of these common access features are curb-cut ramps along the sidewalks, the bell that chimes when an elevator is about to arrive, and the door that opens automatically on your approach. Table 18–2 lists the government laws mandating accessibility in several countries.

When considering the impact of the environment on function, accessibility is not an end point but a beginning. Accessibility is a subcategory of **negotiability,** which is the ability to access a feature of the environment and use it for its intended purpose in a manner acceptable to the person (Guccione, 2000). Negotiability is more than the ability to move around objects within the environment; it is also the ability to operate switches, doors, sinks, and so forth. An example of a negotiability limitation is illustrated in Figure 18–1. Even a highly motivated younger sibling will not be able to access and use the older child's toys when his mobility is dependent on a supportive walker.

Another challenge faced by preschool children attempting to gain independence in their environment can be found in the bathroom. Early attempts to use the toilet are complicated by the height and size of the toilet. Children often use potty chairs so that they do not have to climb up onto the toilet and do not have to worry

TABLE 18–2	Examples of Government Laws Mandating Accessibility
Australia	Australia passed the Disability Discrimination Act of 1992 with specific provisions to accommodate people with disabilities.
Canada	The Policy on the Provision of Accommodation for Employees with Disabilities became effective July 1, 1999, and outlines responsibilities regarding the employment accommodation of employees with disabilities.
United Kingdom	The Disability Discrimination Act 1995 refers to accessibility in employment issues and the provision of goods, facilities, and services. Another act, the Special Educational Needs and Disability Act 2001, extends this act to schools.
United States	Legislation relating to accessibility in the United States involves several laws. Those discussed in this text are Section 508 of the Federal Rehabilitation Act, the Individuals with Disabilities Education Act (IDEA), and the Americans with Disabilities Act (ADA). These are all discussed in detail in Chapter 21.

Adapted from World Health Organization, 2002.

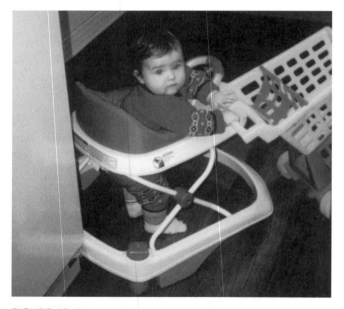

FIGURE 18–1   This little boy is frustrated in his attempts to access the toy cart. He has a limitation in negotiability.

about falling through the seat. Conversely, as people age, the toilet again poses a challenge in that it becomes too low to sit on comfortably or to rise from easily. In these situations raised toilet seats and grab bars are necessary.

For users with impairments, barriers to accessibility are myriad. Table 18–3 presents some of the typical barriers encountered by persons using a wheelchair. Examples are given for entering a building, for kitchen areas, and for school. There are as many other possible barriers as there are occupational environments.

The concept of **universal design** is gaining popularity in American home design as a result of a rapidly aging population. "Universal design is the design of products and environments to be usable by all people, to the greatest extent possible, without the need for adaptation or specialized design. . . . The intent of universal design is to simplify life for everyone by making products, communications, and the built environment more usable by as many people as possible at little or no extra cost. Universal design benefits people of all ages and abilities" (Center for Universal Design, 1997, retrieved August 26, 2003, from www.design.ncsu.edu/cud/univ_design/ud.htm).

Universal design refers to designing homes that are accessible to people of all ages and multiple levels of physical abilities. It can be used to create homes that allow people to "age in place." Families can conceivably move into a home with small children and remain in the same home comfortably through retirement without requiring major structural redesign as normal aging and disabling illness occur. Some universal-design concepts include doors that are wide enough for wheelchairs throughout the house, a bedroom and accessible bathroom on the main floor of the house, one-level construction, low and high counters in kitchens, lever-type door handles and faucet controls, and easy-to-maneuver floor coverings.

NATURAL ENVIRONMENT AND HUMAN-MADE CHANGES TO ENVIRONMENT

The ICF category of Natural Environment and Human-Made Changes to Environment refers to features of physical geography and population. Shumway-Cook et al. (2003) reports that mobility disability results, in part, from avoidance of physically challenging features within the environment. For example, persons living in a mountainous terrain will have different mobility

TABLE 18–3	Typical Barriers Encountered by Persons Using a Wheelchair

Entering a Building

Parking	Space too narrow to permit transfer to a wheelchair.
	Space not level.
	Curb or step to be negotiated.
	Parking meter out of reach.
Approach	Street between parking space and building entrance.
	No curb-cut or traffic light at crossing.
	No snow removal.
	Step between sidewalk and entrance to be negotiated.
Entrance	Doors too narrow for wheelchair.
	Distance between outer and inner door too short to negotiate in wheelchair.
	Excessive force needed to operate doors.

Household Kitchens

Room Layout	Small "alley" style layout does not allow for wheelchair negotiability.
	Appliances poorly located for negotiability.
	Appliance doors open downward and block access to interior of appliance.
	Sinks too high for wheelchair users.
	Appliance and light switches high on wall, requiring one to reach across countertop or cooking surface.
	Storage areas too high.
	Cabinets and cooking areas reached only by parking wheelchair parallel to area.

Schools

Lecture areas	No level station for wheelchair.
	No writing surface to accommodate person in a wheelchair.
	Aisles too steep or too narrow.
	Internet hookups and electric outlets placed in fixed station where wheelchair user cannot work.
Campus	Storage lockers with combination locks above eye level.
	Travel between buildings involves steps, steep ramps, and delayed snow removal.
	Accessible transportation and parking limited.
	Crowded hallways difficult to negotiate in allotted time.
	Water fountains and pay phones out of reach.

challenges than do persons living on an open plain. Issues of terrain are common in the authors' home state of West Virginia. The beautiful and rugged environment is much admired for adventure sports, and for the adventurous child, as illustrated in Figure 18–2, but it is very limiting for the wheelchair user.

While there are adventurous persons who try mountain climbing, sailing, and sky diving in spite of their wheelchairs, people more typically feel discouraged by obstacles rather than challenged by them (Shumway-Cook et al., 2003). On a less dramatic scale, persons living in rural areas may be unable to use motorized scooters or power wheelchairs safely, although their urban counterpart will find these tools invaluable. Population density can influence the availability of services and the perception of security. For example, an elderly person in a rural area may have no close neighbor and feel isolated.

Climate is another physical feature that can greatly impact function. Persons living in cold climates will have the health and mobility challenges posed by extreme weather, ice, and snow. Retired persons with the financial means to relocate during the winter months are called "snow birds" as they annually migrate to warmer climates. Temperature extremes can be a health risk for persons with cardiovascular and respiratory limitations.

Earthquakes, floods, and volcanoes are listed as aspects of the natural environment by the ICF model. For therapists this seems far beyond our scope of consideration, but in fact it can easily become a variable in intervention planning. For example, along the Mississippi River there are occasional severe floods. These floods cause obvious immediate problems but also cause lasting problems in the form of contaminated wells, damaged structures, increased insect populations, and

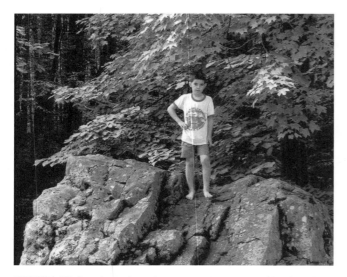

FIGURE 18–2 Physical terrain can pose insurmountable obstacles for persons with mobility impairments.

mildew inside living structures. This type of natural event can leave a person who has managed independently for years suddenly needing support for ordinary ADLs and IADLs. The frail elderly person who has been managing marginally may be forced out of his home if accommodation cannot be made.

Likewise, human disruptions of the natural environment can disrupt people's day-to-day lives. Examples of this are the self-imposed and government limitations on community access following terrorist threats and toxic pollution. The ICF document includes many more types of constraints imposed by natural environments and human-made changes to the environment. These concerns, while important, are similar in scope to the flood example earlier. While not typically a focus of rehabilitation professionals, environmental challenges impact people in myriad ways, and it is important to recognize and address these challenges as you consider the needs of the person.

An increasingly important environment for function is the **virtual environment,** defined as an "environment in which communication occurs by means of airways or computers and an absence of physical content" (American Occupational Therapy Association, 2002, p. 623, Table 4). Virtual play, leisure, and work are emerging trends in society. Concepts of universal design accessibility and negotiability are equally applicable to the virtual environment and to the physical environment.

SUPPORT AND RELATIONSHIPS

Support and Relationships in the ICF document refers to "people or animals that provide practical physical or emotional support, nurturing, protection, assistance and relationships to other persons, in their home, place of work, school or at play or in other aspects of their daily activities" (World Health Organization, 2002, p. 12). *Relationships* include immediate family, extended family, friends, acquaintances, peers, colleagues, neighborhood and community members, people in positions of authority, and people in subordinate positions. The effect these relationships have on the development and aging of individuals differs according to the varieties of possible relationships that may exist. As discussed in Chapter 9, children who have healthy relationships with parents or caregivers have a better chance of developing normally in areas of motor, cognitive, and psychological aspects than children who do not. Additionally, older women who are childless are more likely to end up living in a nursing home than are women who have been mothers (Aykan, 2003).

FAMILIES

In contemporary American culture, increasing geographic mobility has led to the emergence of small immediate family groups living separately from their extended family. Children are often raised in a home with just their parents and siblings, with only occasional contact with grandparents, aunts and uncles, and cousins. This change to the smaller family unit has increased the importance of the relationships maintained with parents and siblings. It also increases the importance of relationships with friends, neighbors, and other community members. Families have an extensive impact on daily function. Ingoldsby, Shaw, and Garcia (2001) found that boys who were exposed to high levels of family conflict were likely to have performance problems at school. Similarly, Slomkowski et al. (2001) found parallel patterns of delinquency among siblings of both sexes.

On the positive side, having a partner has a protective effect on the physical declines associated with normal aging (Bisschop et al., 2003). These authors also reported that an expanded social network could have a positive impact on physical functioning in the presence of chronic conditions. As individuals age, a lack of stability in relationships and access to children, grandchildren, and spouses can have a negative effect (Unger et al., 1999). Older individuals are more likely to experience isolation and its associated problems. Isolation has been shown to increase incidence of depression and chronic medical conditions (Unger et al., 1999). Older individuals may also experience a loss of supportive relationships due to attrition. They may experience the slow loss of friends and family through death and illness and experience changes in relationships as friends move away. A lack of centralized extended family impacts the support experienced by the older citizen dealing with issues of poor health, acute or chronic disability, and financial insecurity. The decreased proximity of family and other close relationships can increase the likelihood of facility placement versus discharge home following acute or chronic illnesses (Jette, Tennstedt, & Crawford, 1995). Lack of physical family support can also increase the financial burden of disease by increasing the necessity of third-party paid caregivers in the home.

PEOPLE IN POSITIONS OF AUTHORITY

The ICF category of "People in Positions of Authority" is a broad one that includes teachers, employers, supervisors, health professionals, and caregivers. These people are defined as individuals who have decision-making responsibilities for others and who have socially defined influence (World Health Organization, 2003). The environmental influence of people in positions of authority is difficult to isolate or represent based on a few research studies. The concept of **client-centered care** that is accepted as a positive practice standard in the rehabilitation fields reflects recognition and concern for the influence of power in relationships. **Client-centered** means "a collaborative relationship with individuals in the client's environment to assist the client to obtain the skills and make modifications to remove barriers" (Christensen & Baum, 1997, p. 593). As therapists we have a privileged relationship and a responsibility to recognize the potential influence we may have in the individual's pursuit of functional performance. Townsend (2003) reflects on the social and ethical responsibilities of therapists in their role as authority figures. In the many decisions we as therapists guide, we have a responsibility to weigh our expectations and responsibilities as we offer advice. In the case of the aging father newly confined to a wheelchair for mobility, therapists will feel pressure to be cost-effective, but a standard type wheelchair may be difficult for the client with poor upper-body strength or an active lifestyle to manage. Our responsibility in client-centered practice is to learn about people's lifestyle and expectations for independent mobility as they consider types of wheelchairs and other such equipment.

ATTITUDES

Attitudes as an environmental consideration—that is, **attitudinal environment**—relates to observable consequences of customs, practices, ideologies, values, norms, factual beliefs, and religious beliefs (World Health Organization, 2001). Attitudes influence individual behavior and social life at all levels, including some unconscious levels. As students in the health professions, you probably consider yourself to have an

open and positive attitude toward persons with activity limitations. Yet the popular culture of magazines, movies, and the Internet provide many not-so-subtle messages about persons who function differently. In searching for photos for this text, the authors were surprised to find many Internet images of persons with Down syndrome in the preschool years but few images of adult or aging persons with Down syndrome. Why? This difference in availability in images is not the case for typically developing children. Do people with Down syndrome lose their appeal or become embarrassing as they age? This is an example of a societal attitude that is not evident to the casual observer.

Auslander and Gold (2000) analyzed the portrayal of persons with disabilities in popular press materials in both Canada and Israel. These authors found that persons with physical disabilities received the most, and the most positive, media attention in both countries. Interestingly, mental health disabilities were second on the list, with persons with developmental disabilities coming in last in terms of both the frequency and tone of media attention. These authors emphasize, "The press has an important role in reflecting and shaping public attitudes. In many ways media coverage reinforces negative attitudes towards people with disabilities, particularly those with psychiatric and developmental disabilities" (Auslander & Gold, 2000, p. 430).

ROLES

The "sick role" described earlier in this text provides an example of societal-level opinions and beliefs that are reflected in family, teachers, roommates, employers, and other community members about how a person should behave if she is to be given respite from performing her expected roles. People with emotional distress or cognitive impairment are less likely to be afforded the sick role because they don't look or act sick.

Another widely held societal attitude is the value of a strong "work ethic." Work, especially paid work, is highly valued in American culture. Persons who engage in unpaid work, like housework and child-care, may be less valued even though they are equally productive. Because of this, persons who leave paid-work positions because of activity limitation or to provide caregiving support may feel devalued and perceive a loss of status.

A final example of a socially prescribed role is the role of mother. Mothers as portrayed in the media and in the literature purporting "family values" are vital to the physical, emotional, behavioral, and moral performance of their children. Mothering is put on a pedestal as a core building block of society, yet mothers are often isolated and have limited fiscal resources. Mothers of children who have activity limitations, especially activity limitations like attention deficits that do not conform to the "sick role," are openly criticized and marginalized. Cronin (2003) found a consistent pattern of discord and lack of support from both school and health-care providers reported by mothers of children with attention deficit disorder.

HABITS

Within the ICF model, *attitudes* include "customs, practices, rules and abstract systems of values and normative beliefs that arise within social contexts and that affect or create societal and individual practices and behaviours, such as social norms of moral and religious behaviour or etiquette; religious doctrine and resulting norms and practices; norms governing rituals or social gatherings" (World Health Organization, 2002, p. 192). Chapter 4 of this text deals extensively with culture and cultural issues. What remains to be covered are customs in the form of habits or routines that impact function on a societal level. Fitzgerald (1997) reports, "Science, bureaucracy and organized religion have played an important role in shaping the construction of disability—as the broken, incomplete and imperfect self, as the case requiring management, and as the object of pity and charity" (p. 407). When students select careers in health professions, they often comment that they "really want to help people." This is a positive, socially endorsed value. The desire to help people can be generous and adaptable, but it also can be based in the belief that people who are different are in some way unfortunate, and worthy of charity. Echoing the stance of the national disability rights movement, Fitzgerald notes that "concepts such as the medical model of disability and the evolving genetic model of disability have shaped the way in which we construct disability and, consequently, the way in which we treat people with disability—through isolation, segregation, and elimination" (p. 407). The client-centered approach to intervention is a movement away from this traditional "helping" ideal and should help the person new to these professions challenge her own thinking in her approaches to persons in her professional practice.

Habits are behaviors that are performed automatically and with thought (Christiansen & Baum, 1997). Habits include talking louder to older persons, talking to attending adults rather than to the person in the wheelchair, and assuming that the medical community understands the day-to-day needs of an individual on the basis of his medical label. In this sense, habits are a reflection of societal and personal attitudes. Habits can be beneficial, in that they allow us to focus our thoughts elsewhere while performing routine tasks, but they must be identified and considered carefully as they relate to our interactions with other people.

SERVICES, SYSTEMS, AND POLICIES

The ICF addresses many services, systems, and policies that affect function. Before moving forward in the discussion of how these things affect development and aging, it is important to differentiate the terms. The ICF defines *services* as "services that provide benefits, structured programs and operations, in various sectors of society, designed to meet the needs of individuals" (World Health Organization, p. 192). *Systems* are "administrative control and organizational mechanisms, and are established by governments at the local, regional, national, and international levels" (World Health Organization, p. 192). *Policies* are "constituted by rules, regulations, conventions, and standards established by governments at the local, regional, national and international levels, or by other recognized authorities" (World Health Organization, p. 192).

Within the American government structure, policies are the legislative actions taken by the federal, state, or local governments to meet perceived needs. Medicare and Medicaid provide examples of this. These programs were established by federal legislation to establish insurance for the elderly, disabled, and impoverished. The influence on development and aging of services, systems, and policies cannot be overstated. This topic will not be covered in detail here, because the following chapter presents an overview of policy and legislation. The presence of services can compensate for multiple other negative environmental factors including poverty, lack of supportive relationships, and physical barriers (Franks, Gold, & Fiscella, 2003).

ASSISTIVE TECHNOLOGY

Assistive technology (AT) refers to "equipment or devices designed to help persons with disabilities increase functional capacities or meet the requirements of daily living" (Christiansen & Baum, 1997, p. 592). There have been a series of policies and legislation providing some support for the use of assistive technologies as an educational and a rehabilitation tool. These will be briefly outlined and then discussed in terms of their scope as services, systems, and policy.

As early as the 1980s it was evident that the growing potential and scope of AT could provide opportunities for increased independence and participation in all of life's activities (OSERS, 1989). The Technology Related Assistance for Individuals with Disabilities Act of 1988 (Tech Act) (P.L. 100-407) was the first legislation to provide federal funds to states to develop training and delivery systems for assistive technology devices and services. To receive these funds, states were required to develop technology-related services for individuals with disabilities of all ages. Table 18–4 illustrates how the Tech Act mandate separates into aspects of policy, systems, and services.

DRIVER'S LICENSE LAWS

Another example of policy, systems, and services that is a little closer to home are the driver's license laws (see Table 18–5). A rite of passage of adolescence is gaining independence by obtaining a driver's license. The minimum driving age is set by individual states but overall is 16 years of age. As the development of adolescent motor, perceptual, and cognitive skills have become better understood, states have begun to introduce graduated licensing laws. Under these laws there are benchmarks set before adolescents are allowed to do certain things. Most graduated laws institute a curfew for driving for the first 2 years. Limits are also set on the number of passengers that can be in the car. Under graduated licensing the state also establishes more severe penalties for moving violations and may suspend the license until the adolescent is 18 years old. Graduated licensing is intended to restrict driving in highly challenging situations such as late at night or with maximal distractions in the car until the driver has developed the skills to handle these situations.

In this case legislation carefully controls who gets a driver's license, but for health-care providers, the concern often becomes whether an individual can drive safely enough to keep a license. Current studies indicate that by 2030, elderly drivers will account for 18.9 percent of all vehicle miles driven, and the number of elderly traffic fatalities will more than triple by the year 2030 (Arizona Governor's Office on Highway Safety, 2001). This number of fatalities will be 35 percent greater than the total number of alcohol-related traffic fatalities in 1995 (Arizona Governor's Office on Highway Safety, 2001).

Currently, few elders lose their licenses before being involved in a serious accident. Many states have considered enacting a policy to place some sort of retesting or other restriction on older drivers. One suggestion offered by the National Motorists Association recommends establishing a system to evaluate the driving competency of motorists who, through objective screening criteria, come to the attention of the licensing authority. They suggest that there should be a process by which the licensing agency could be petitioned to do an evaluation of a given license holder based on first-hand knowledge of family members, a law enforcement agency, or the courts. In fairness, there should also be an appeal process for the person who loses his license (National Motorists Association, 2003).

TABLE 18–4	Technology-Related Assistance for Individuals with Disabilities Act of 1988 (Tech Act)
Policy	P.L. 100-407
Systems	TITLE I—STATE GRANT PROGRAMS
	Sec. 101. Continuity grants for states that received funding for a limited period for technology-related assistance.
	Sec. 102. State grants for protection and advocacy related to assistive technology.
	Sec. 103. Administrative provisions.
	Sec. 104. Technical assistance program.
	Sec. 105. Authorization of appropriations.
Services	Statewide, consumer-responsive programs of technology-related services for individuals with disabilities of all ages.

TABLE 18–5	Driving Laws within the ICF Categories of Services, Systems, and Policies
ICF Category	**Driving**
Policy	State laws for obtaining license
Systems	Department of Motor Vehicles
Services	Testing; different-colored licenses; licenses that are oriented differently

SUMMARY

Although recognition of the many aspects and influences of environmental factors on human function predated the ICF model, these factors have never before received sufficient focus by either health-care providers or policymakers. Aspects of the environment are also addressed in the discussions of culture and policy.

Although it is more comfortable to look within the scope of your professional experience to define roles and prescriptive strategies for interacting with clients and families, an effective clinician will consider the context and perspective of his consumer and be adaptable to best serve the needs of that person and the family.

Speaking of

Barriers

MARYBETH MANDICH, PT, PhD
PEDIATRIC PHYSICAL THERAPIST

There is a song about West Virginia that refers to the majestic and grand West Virginia hills. Well, majestic and grand they may be to some, but to others with disabilities, they are real barriers. Some years ago, I was asked by the mother of a teenage girl with spina bifida to serve as an outside expert on a case involving the local school system. The situation was that this young lady was fairly independent in mobility, especially using her manual wheelchair. However, when the girl entered high school, she was confronted with a new physical barrier. The high school was built as a campus arrangement, with different buildings for different activities and classes. Unfortunately, the cafeteria was a great distance from the classroom. The walkway between buildings was paved, but not covered, and the terrain was very hilly, typical of West Virginia. This created a natural physical barrier. Initially, the young woman valiantly tried to propel her wheelchair to the cafeteria. However, she was always late for lunch and consequently late in returning to her classroom. The school imposed a solution to this problem. They said the girl had to stay in the classroom each day, and someone would bring her a lunch tray.

Congratulations . . . the physical barrier was conquered! However, another barrier was created—a social one. Any of us who have lived through high school know how important lunchtime is. It's a time to visit with friends who may not share your classes. It's a time to gossip and flirt and cram for quizzes. In the long run, it was the social, not the physical, barrier that presented a bigger obstacle to this young woman.

It was at this point that the concept of reasonable accommodation came in. I believe it was a reasonable accommodation to allow this young lady to leave for the cafeteria early, get her lunch before the crowds came, and still be able to fully participate in lunchtime with her classmates and peers. In bad weather, the option to remain in the classroom could be presented to the girl. That was my "expert" (or commonsense) recommendation. But the school resisted—now presenting an attitudinal barrier. Eventually, by threatening to take the case to the courts, the mother was able to get the school system to agree to the reasonable accommodation. But it was quite a battle for all of us, not least for the young lady.

Barriers encountered by people with disabilities are sometimes obvious and sometimes subtle. Even in this simple story of one person, multiple barriers are present. Some of the barriers are not created by people, but some of them are. I think it's our job to be social activists, to be conscious of barriers of all types, and to be vigilant in eliminating or minimizing their impact on quality of life for our clients.

REFERENCES

American Association of Retired Persons (AARP). (2004). Medicare changes that could affect you. Retrieved June 3, 2004, from http://assets.aarp.org_/articles/legislative /prescriptiondrugs/medicare_changesTEMP.pdf.

American Occupational Therapy Association. (2002). Occupational Therapy Practice Framework: Domain and process. *The American Journal of Occupational Therapy, 56(6),* 609–639.

American Physical Therapy Association. (2001). *Guide to physical therapist practice* (2nd ed.). Alexandria, VA: American Physical Therapy Association.

Arizona Governor's Office on Highway Safety. (2001). Elderly drivers. Retrieved August 26, 2003, from http://www .azgohs.state.az.us/elderly_drivers.html.

Auslander, G., & Gold, N. (2000). Media reports on disability: A binational comparison of types and causes of disability as reported in major newspapers. *Disability and Rehabilitation, 21,* 420–431.

Aykan, H. (2003). Effect of childlessness on nursing home and home health care use. *Journal of Aging & Social Policy, 15 (1),* 33–54.

Bisschop, M., Kriegsman, D., van Tilburg, T., Penninx, B., van Eijk, J., & Deeg, D. (2003). The influence of differing social ties on decline in physical functioning among older people with and without chronic diseases: The Longitudinal Aging Study Amsterdam. *Aging Clinics Experimental Research, 15(2),* 164–173.

Bootes, K., & Chapparo, C. (2002). Cognitive and behavioural assessment of people with traumatic brain injury in the work place: Occupational therapists' perceptions. *Work, 19(3),* 255–268.

Brundtland, G. (2002). Retrieved August 14, 2003, from http://www.who.int/director-general/ speeches/2002/ english/20020418_disabilitytrieste.html.

Center for Universal Design. (1997). What is universal design? Retrieved August 26, 2003, from http://www .design.ncsu.edu/cud/univ_design/ud.htm.

Corcoran, M., & Gitlin, L. (1997). The role of the physical environment in occupational performance. In C. Christiansen & C. Baum (Eds.), *Occupational therapy: Enabling function and well-being* (2nd ed.) (pp. 337–360). Thorofare, NJ: Slack.

Cronin, A. (2000). Mothering a child with a hidden disability. *American Journal of Occupational Therapy, 58(1),* 83–92.

Fitzgerald, J. (1997). Reclaiming the whole: Self, spirit and society. *Disability and Rehabilitation, 19,* 407–413.

Franks, P., Gold, M., & Fiscella, F. (2003). Sociodemographics, self-rated health, and mortality in the U.S. *Social Science & Medicine, (56) 12,* 2505–2515.

Guccione, A. (Ed.) (2000). *Geriatric physical therapy* (2nd ed.). Philadelphia: Mosby.

Hays, J., & George, L. (2002). The life-course trajectory toward living alone: Racial differences. *Research on Aging, 24(3),* 283–307.

Ingoldsby, E., Shaw, D., & Garcia, M. (2001). Intrafamily conflict in relation to boys' adjustment at school. *Developmental Psychopathology, 13(1),* 35–52.

Jette, A. M., Tennstedt, S., & Crawford, S. (1995). How does formal and informal community care affect nursing home use? *Journal of Gerontology Series-B Psychological Sciences and Social Sciences, 50(1),* S4–S12.

Jones, M., McEwen, I., & Hansen, L. (2003). Use of power mobility for a young child with spinal muscular atrophy. *Physical Therapy, 83(3),* 253–262.

Law, M. (2002). Participation in the occupations of everyday life. *American Journal of Occupational Therapy, 56(6),* 640–649.

Maleta, K., Virtanen, S. M., Espo, M., Kulmala, T., & Ashorn, P. (2003). Seasonality of growth and the relationship between weight and height gain in children under three years of age in rural Malawi. *Acta Paediatrics 92(4),* 491–497.

National Motorists Association. (2003). NMA's position on elderly driving. Retrieved August 26, 2003, from http://www.motorists.org/issues/elderly/elderly.htm.

Olson, J., & Esdaile, S. (2000). Mothering young children with disabilities in a challenging urban environment. *American Journal of Occupational Therapy, 54(3),* 307–314.

Rebeiro, K. L. (2001). Enabling occupation: the importance of an affirming environment. *Canadian Journal of Occupational Therapy, 68(2),* 80–89.

Shumway-Cook, A, Patla, A. E., Stewart, A., Ferrucci, L., Ciol, M. A., & Guralnik, J. M. (2002). Environmental demands associated with community mobility in older adults with and without mobility disabilities. *Physical Therapy, 82(7),* 670–681.

Slomkowski, C., Rende, R., Conger, K., Simons, R., & Conger, R. (2001). Sisters, brothers, and delinquency: Evaluating social influence during early and middle adolescence. *Child Development, 72 (1),* 271–283.

Townsend, E. (2003). Reflections on power and justice in enabling occupation. *Canadian Journal of Occupational Therapy, 70(2),* 74–87.

Tryssenaar, J., Jones, E. J., & Lee, D. (1999). Occupational performance needs of a shelter population. *Canadian Journal of Occupational Therapy, 66(4),* 188–196.

Unger, J., McAvay, G., Bruce, M., Berkman, L., & Seeman, T. (1999). Variation in the impact of social network characteristics on physical functioning in elderly persons: MacArthur studies of successful aging. *Journal of Gerontology Series-B Psychological Sciences and Social Sciences, 54(5),* S245–251.

World Health Organization. (2002). *ICF: International classification of functioning and disability.* Geneva, Switzerland: World Health Organization.

CHAPTER 19

Wellness and Health Promotion

Ralph Utzman, PT, MPH
Assistant Professor
Division of Physical Therapy
West Virginia University
Morgantown, West Virginia

and

Bernadette Hattjar, MEd, OTR
Occupational Therapy
Florida A & M University
Tallahassee, Florida

Objectives

Upon completion of this chapter, the reader should be able to

■ Discuss and define wellness, substance abuse, and safe sex.

■ Identify several health indicators.

■ Differentiate morbidity and mortality in population studies.

■ Outline the functional impact of personal behavior on wellness, including use of tobacco and tobacco products.

■ Describe addiction and the impact of addictive behaviors on function.

■ Delineate the fastest growing health threats in contemporary society.

■ Discuss the differences in mental health concerns at differing points in the lifespan.

■ Differentiate overweight and obesity, and the impact of these on wellness.

■ Argue the relationship between access to health care and wellness in populations.

Key Terms

addiction	leading health indicators	physical activity
dementia	mental health	safe sex
determinants of health	morbidity	sexuality
gateway drugs	mortality	substance abuse
gender identity	obese	wellness
Healthy People 2010	overweight	

INTRODUCTION

Wellness not only is the absence of illness but includes the motivation to be involved in life, to have a sense of control over one's actions, and to desire interaction and connection with other individuals, and, perhaps most prominently, wellness enhances our sense of self-esteem and self-worth. The *American Heritage Dictionary* (2000c) defines wellness as "the condition of good physical and mental health, especially when maintained by proper diet, exercise, and habits" (http://dictionary .reference.com/search?q=wellness). In this context, wellness may be viewed as the ingredient that enhances our life. Wellness may also be viewed as a blending of the physical, psychosocial, and spiritual realms. Wellness is a triangulated concept where, if all components work in concert, a positive outcome is achieved.

Chapter 1 introduced readers to the ICF model of Function, Disability, and Health. The ICF model does not specifically discuss wellness, but rather describes how people live with their health condition. This chapter will discuss the ICF model as it relates to wellness and health promotion and introduce readers to the *Healthy People 2010* initiative. Using the leading health indicators provided by the *Healthy People 2010* document (U.S. Department of Health and Human Services, 2000) as a guideline, this chapter presents an overview of major health concerns in the United States. **Leading health indicators** are health concerns selected to represent the trends in population health in the United States at the beginning of the twenty-first century.

Individuals often engage in social or seemingly innocent activities that detract from concepts of wellness and end up paying a high personal price for that involvement. Personal or environmental factors, such as smoking, substance abuse, irresponsible sexual behavior, emotional distress/stress, and lack of access and/or utilization of health care are considered *risk factors*. Risk factors are associated with increased susceptibility to injury, disease, impairment, or death.

ICF MODEL FOR HEALTH AND WELLNESS

The ICF model provides an updated framework for the discussion of disability, health, and wellness. While previous models of disability and health focused primarily on constructs such as disease, limitations, and risk factors, the ICF model emphasizes function, activities, and participation (World Health Organization, 2001). In the ICF model, health influences, and is influenced by, function and disability, implying an interaction between the ICF categories of Body Structure and Function, Activities, and Participation. In review, the ICF model defines *body structures* as anatomic parts of the body and *body functions* as physiologic functions of those parts. *Activities* are tasks or actions performed by an individual, such as getting out of bed, sleeping, drinking, or walking. *Participation* represents involvement in life situations in a social context, such as fulfilling occupational or family roles (World Health Organization, 2002).

Function and disability are impacted by contextual factors. Environmental Factors are factors that are external to the person, whereas Personal Factors represent a person's demographic, behavioral, and psychosocial characteristics. Environmental Factors are discussed at length in Chapter 18. Also related are policy factors as discussed in Chapter 20.

Both individual health care and public health interventions seek to improve health and wellness. To select the most appropriate interventions, health-care and public health professionals must partner with clients to identify the modifiable contextual factors that are contributing to function and disability, and determine how function and disability are impacting health and wellness.

HEALTHY PEOPLE 2010

In 1979 the first *Healthy People* report was published. In the report, the U.S. surgeon general set forth national goals for reducing morbidity and mortality. This

TABLE 19-1	*Healthy People 2010* Leading Health Indicators

- Physical activity
- Overweight and obesity
- Tobacco use
- Substance abuse
- Responsible sexual behavior
- Mental health
- Injury and violence
- Environmental quality
- Immunization
- Access to health care

document was developed by consensus among several hundred national organizations and state, federal, and local health agencies. *Healthy People 2010* serves as a mechanism to identify the health of the U.S. population, set goals for the nation's health, and provide mechanisms to measure progress (U.S. Department of Health and Human Services, 2000). In addition, each state has produced a companion document that provides specific goals for that state's population. The national and state companion documents are useful tools for directing health-promotion activities at many levels, including policymakers, government agencies, educational institutions, health systems, community groups, and individual health-care providers.

Healthy People 2010 is based on **determinants of health,** or factors that influence overall health and well-being. According to this model, health is determined by biologic factors, behaviors, social and physical environments, and public policies and interventions. Readers should note the similarity between these determinants and the ICF model's construct of *contextual factors.*

Healthy People 2010 outlines 10 *leading health indicators,* or key concerns for public health (Table 19–1). The remainder of this chapter will discuss each of these health indicators, except environmental quality, which is addressed in Chapter 18. Interested readers should also study *Healthy People 2010: Understanding and Improving Health,* available for download from http://www.healthypeople.gov/.

PHYSICAL ACTIVITY

The human body was designed for physical activity. In all stages of life, movement and activity can have a profound effect on health. **Physical activity** is any activity that requires physical exertion that the individual participates in to develop or maintain fitness. Physical activity places stresses on the neurologic, musculoskeletal, and cardiopulmonary systems that are necessary for growth, development, and function. Despite the many benefits of regular physical activity, Americans are not getting enough exercise to promote optimum health. It is estimated that 300,000 people died in the United States in 1990 due to inactivity and poor diet habits (McGinnis & Foege, 1993).

Regular physical activity is related to decreased morbidity and mortality for people of all ages. **Morbidity** is "the rate of incidence of a disease" (American Heritage Dictionary, 2000b). **Mortality,** in contrast, reflects the death rate in a given population. People who exercise regularly benefit from increased strength, increased bone density, and lower body fat. Physical activity decreases the risk of heart disease, stroke, high blood pressure, diabetes, and certain types of cancer. Evidence also suggests that exercise is good for mental health (U.S. Department of Health and Human Services, 2000; Singh, Clements, & Fiatarone, 1997). People can benefit from regular physical activity regardless of age or disability.

The Centers for Disease Control and Prevention (CDC) and the American College of Sports Medicine recommend that adults accumulate at least 30 minutes of moderate physical activity per day at least 5 days per week (Pate et al., 1995). Moderate physical activity produces a feeling of exertion while allowing a person to converse normally (Figure 19–1). Studies have shown that people who exercise regularly have lower risk of overall mortality (Blair et al., 1995; Lee, Hsieh, & Paffenbarger, Jr., 1995). However, about 30 percent of adults do not participate in any leisure-time physical activity (Centers for Disease Control and Prevention, 2001b).

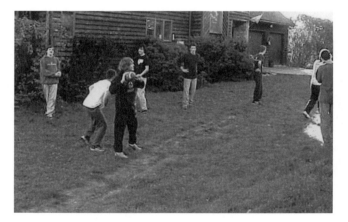

FIGURE 19–1 Physical activity is necessary for good health throughout the lifespan. Even for adults, physical activity can be fun.

Children are also not getting enough exercise. The CDC recommends that adolescents be physically active in sports, physical education, or other activities on a daily basis, and participate in at least three 20-minute sessions of aerobic exercise per week (National Center for Chronic Disease Prevention and Health Promotion, 2003). For elementary school children, the CDC recommends a minimum of 30–60 minutes of developmentally appropriate physical activity every day (National Center for Chronic Disease Prevention and Health Promotion, 2003) (Figure 19–2). While research shows that youth are generally more active than adults, almost one third don't get the recommended amount of moderate to vigorous activity (Centers for Disease Control and Prevention, 2002c). Physical activity and grade level in school are inversely related (Centers for Disease Control and Prevention, 2002c).

Similar trends are apparent in older adults. As adults age, they tend to get less exercise (National Center for Chronic Disease Prevention and Health Promotion, 2003a). The CDC recommends that older adults perform at least 30 minutes of aerobic activity three to five times a week, as well as participate in flexibility and strength-building exercises. As many as 44 percent of adults aged 75 or older get no physical activity at all (National Center for Chronic Disease Prevention and Health Promotion, 2003b). The benefits of exercise for the elderly are numerous. One study found that the average medical costs for women 75 and older who exercise are 38 percent less than costs for those who do not exercise (Pratt, Macera, & Wang, 2000). Exercise can improve balance and strength, and has been shown to reduce risk of falls in elderly women (Campbell et al., 1997) (Figure 19–3). In one study, older women with osteoarthritis of the knee who began an exercise program had less pain and better function than those who did not exercise (Kovar et al., 1992). Regular exercise has been shown to reduce depression in older adults (Singh et al., 1997), as well as maintain cognitive function (Barnes, Yaffe, Satariano, & Tager,

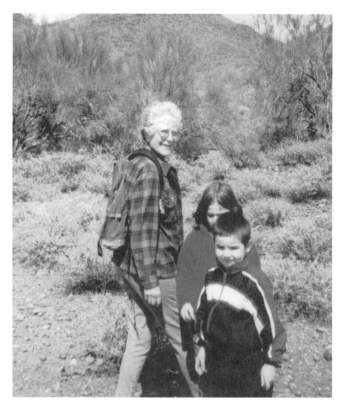

FIGURE 19–3   Exercise has many physical, cognitive, and emotional benefits for older adults.

2003; Yaffe, Barnes, Nevitt, Lui, & Covinsky, 2001; Kramer et al., 1999).

People with disabilities can also benefit greatly from regular physical activity. In fact, the benefits of physical activity for those with disabilities are similar to the benefits for everyone else. In addition, exercise can help people with disabilities improve functional abilities and participation through improved strength, flexibility, dexterity, balance, and endurance. People with disabilities are highly susceptible to developing further health problems (Rimmer, 1999). This susceptibility is often due to barriers to regular physical activity as much as it is due to disability itself (Rimmer, 1999).

Interventions to increase physical activity range from those targeted at individuals, to those targeted at communities, to those targeted at changing public policy. An example of individual intervention is the PACE+ approach described by Prochaska (Prochaska, Zabinski, Calfas, Sallis, & Patrick, 2000). The Patient-Centered Assessment and Counseling for Exercise Plus Nutrition tool can be administered by paper or computer in the health-care provider's waiting room. The results provide a framework for review and counseling regarding the client's exercise and eating habits (Prochaska et al., 2000).

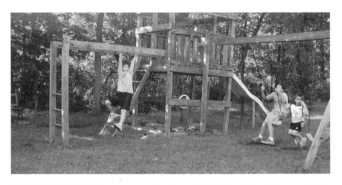

FIGURE 19–2   Elementary school–aged children should accumulate at least 30–60 minutes of age-appropriate activity every day.

These types of provider-based interventions are important. In a study of older adults, nearly half stated that their health-care providers did not ask them about their exercise habits (Centers for Disease Control and Prevention, 2002b). Those who did not receive counseling regarding physical activity were less likely to exercise than those who did (Centers for Disease Control and Prevention, 2002b). Developing home-based exercise programs is also an effective strategy to encourage physical activity in the elderly (Campbell et al., 1997).

Work-based fitness programs serve as an example of interventions aimed at populations. Because of the potential cost savings of a healthier workforce, many large employers have begun providing fitness programs for their employees. In fact, the growth in employer-based exercise programs exceeded targets set by *Healthy People 2000* (National Center for Health Statistics, 1997).

Unfortunately, there is an opposite trend among public schools requiring physical education classes. Since 1991 the number of high school students participating in physical education classes has declined, with less than a third of students participating daily (Centers for Disease Control and Prevention, 2002c). Considering the decreasing levels of exercise among youth, changes in public policy aimed at increasing the amount of physical education in schools represent a much needed intervention.

Finally, interventions are needed to address barriers to physical activity for those with disabilities. James Rimmer (1999) suggests that physical and occupational therapists are uniquely qualified to act as consultants to communities and fitness centers in developing exercise programs and facilities for people with disabilities.

OVERWEIGHT AND OBESITY

As stated in the previous discussion, more than a quarter of a million Americans died in 1990 due to poor exercise and dietary habits. Obviously, those who are sedentary are more likely to be overweight or obese. Other factors, such as diet, genetics, and social/environmental influences, play a role as well. Due to the high health, monetary, and social costs of overweight and obesity, it is important that habits to maintain a healthy weight begin in childhood and continue across the lifespan.

The terms *overweight* and *obesity* are often used interchangeably, but they represent different degrees of the problem. People with a **body mass index (BMI)** of 25–29.9 kg/m² are considered **overweight,** while those with a BMI of 30 kg/m² or higher are considered **obese** (National Heart Lung and Blood Institute, 1998). BMI is calculated by dividing weight (in kilograms) by the square of height in meters. According to the Behavioral Risk Factor Survey System, the number of adults who

are obese has risen each year since 1991, from 12 percent to 21 percent in 2001 (Mokdad et al., 1999; Mokdad et al., 2000; Mokdad et al., 2001; Mokdad et al., 2003). The numbers for children are just as staggering. Over 10 percent of all children under 18 were overweight or obese in 2001 (Centers for Disease Control and Prevention, 2002c).

The health impact of being overweight or obese is serious. Besides being at higher risk for heart disease, osteoarthritis, high blood pressure, and certain cancers, those who are overweight are seven times more likely to develop diabetes (Mokdad et al., 2003). Besides being the fifth deadliest disease in the United States, diabetes causes high levels of morbidity. It damages circulation in the heart, eyes, kidneys, and the extremities. Diabetes causes more than 60 percent of the amputations not caused by trauma (Centers for Disease Control and Prevention, 2002a). In 1999 nearly 115,000 Americans underwent renal dialysis or transplant due to diabetes (Centers for Disease Control and Prevention, 2002a).

The longer a person lives with diabetes, the more likely it is that the person will develop serious complications. Over the past two decades people have been developing the disease at increasingly younger ages. In fact, children are now developing Type II diabetes mellitus, which was previously known as *adult-onset diabetes* (Rosenbloom, Joe, Young, & Winter, 1999). Eight out of ten children who develop Type II diabetes are overweight (American Diabetes Association, 2003). The increased prevalence of diabetes in adults and children, as well as the increase in overweight and obesity, has been attributed to an increasingly sedentary lifestyle that includes foods high in fats and sugars.

Interventions aimed at increasing physical activity can be helpful in reducing or maintaining body weight. In addition, alterations in dietary habits are important. Eating a diet low in fat and sugar and high in dietary fiber can help maintain healthy body weight and reduce the risks of developing diseases related to obesity. The CDC has developed the "5 a Day" campaign, which encourages people to eat at least five servings per day of fruits and vegetables. Besides helping maintain a healthy weight, diet and activity modifications have been shown to cut the risk of developing Type II diabetes in half (Centers for Disease Control and Prevention, 2002a).

For clinicians in rehabilitation fields, obesity is a persistent problem. In both community and institutional settings, persons need help in learning and in supporting healthy lifestyle choices. In addition to addressing problems of diet and exercise, there are many ADLs and IADLs (defined in Chapter 1) that are impacted by obesity. The clinician will often be involved in home and equipment modifications for the obese client.

SMOKING AND TOBACCO-PRODUCT USE

Once viewed as an indicator of adulthood or social savvy, smoking is now regarded as one of the most detrimental and easily accessible contributors to ill health. Each day more than 6,000 persons under the age of 18 begin smoking, and more than 3,000 become daily smokers (Giovino, 1999). A 1998 CDC surveillance summary focusing on youth risk behaviors in alternative high schools reports that male students in grade 12 (93.0 percent) were more likely than female students in grade 12 (86.8 percent) to have tried cigarette smoking. White students (94.9 percent) were significantly more likely than black and Hispanic students (82.3 percent and and 90.1 percent, respectively) to have tried cigarette smoking, use smokeless tobacco (12.6 percent versus 3.9 percent and 4.2 percent, respectively), or smoke cigars (42.9 percent versus 35.3 percent and 33.3 percent, respectively).

Throughout the lifespan, the negative effects of tobacco use increase. In younger people, smoking can cause fertility problems. Smoking during pregnancy severely increases health risks to the unborn child. Smokers are generally at risk for poorer health at all ages. Smokers have a higher risk of high blood pressure or hypertension (contributors to stroke and heart attacks), cancer (lung, especially), and adverse respiratory conditions (bronchitis, emphysema, chronic obstructive pulmonary disease). Smokers also tend to have thicker, rougher skin and show the appearance of aging earlier. Smoking constricts blood vessels and reduces the amount of blood flowing to the skin, thereby depleting oxygen and essential nutrients (Health 50+, 2002). Tobacco product use is an example of an environmental feature that may impact the ICF domains of Body Structure and Function as well as Activities and Participation.

Tobacco contains the drug *nicotine,* a powerful and naturally occurring nerve stimulant. It is extremely toxic and has been classified as the most addictive drug in existence. **Addiction** is defined as "compulsive physiological and psychological need for a habit-forming substance" (American Heritage Dictionary On-line, 2003). Once ingrained as an addiction, the automatic response of smoking or using a tobacco product is difficult to extinguish. Even in cases of illness, tobacco use is difficult to eliminate. Bak et al. (2002) studied smoking-cessation patterns in individuals who experienced their first *cerebrovascular accident (CVA)*. The cessation of smoking after a CVA is widely recommended to reduce the risk of myocardial infarction and recurrent stroke. A total of 551 patients (81 percent) participated in an admission and post-hospitalization follow-up study. Of these individuals, 198 (38.7 percent) were smokers upon admission for treatment of CVA. Six

months after a CVA, only 43 of these individuals (21.7 percent) had given up smoking.

Most smokers have unsuccessfully attempted to quit. A concept widely used in the field of smoking cessation research is the *stage of change* concept, which views four different variables: current behavior, the number of "quit" attempts, the intention to change, and the amount of time elapsed since quitting smoking (Etter & Sutton, 2002). When using the stage of change to assess smoking cessation or the true intent to quit smoking, one must consider how these four variables are combined, measured, and tracked. Etter and Sutton (2002) indicate that it may be preferable to assess each element independently to ensure a complete and accurate picture of the cessation success or failure level.

Currently, various over-the-counter smoking cessation products, such as chewing gum, inhalers, and nicotine patches, are readily available. Although the mechanisms of delivery are different, nicotine is present in all these products. The idea behind these products is to deliver a dose of nicotine in a less "noxious" format than a cigarette, and to decrease the nicotine dose over time. A recent follow-up study conducted by Yudkin, Hey, Roberts, Welch, Murphy, and Walton (2003) found that 5 percent of all trial participants ($n = 1686$) in a 1991 study of the effectiveness of using a nicotine patch to stop smoking remained smoke-free. Nine percent of the subjects stopped smoking for one year afterward but relapsed. Since the impact of smoking is so great, and has proved to be so difficult to reverse, it is prudent to reinforce the notion that not beginning to smoke is the best prevention method. If one is a smoker, quitting is the best line of physical defense.

Smoking has been linked to many physical problems, including osteoporosis (Blum et al., 2000; Harris et al., 2002), cardiopulmonary problems, lung cancer, circulatory problems, stroke, myocardial infarction (Centers for Disease Control and Prevention, 1994), and chronic obstructive pulmonary disease. As with obesity, the secondary impacts of tobacco use are widespread and are seen by both physical and occupational therapists in community and institutional settings.

ANECDOTAL REPORT

After a long, hard battle with lung cancer, Mr. S. has come home from the hospital under the care of a local hospice agency. Mr. S. began smoking at the age of 14 and had smoked a pack or two of cigarettes per day up until a partial lung resection last year. Despite repeated bouts of radiation and chemotherapy, the tumor grew and spread. After discussing his situation with his daughter and his physicians, he has decided to spend his remaining time at home with his family.

As part of his hospice care, physical and occupational therapy consults have been requested. After several hospitalizations and surgeries, Mr. S. is very weak and debilitated. He needs help to walk short distances and he becomes short of breath with basic activities such as dressing. During their first visit, the therapists learn that his daughter, Diane, has quit her job at a local factory to care for her father. They teach Mr. S. and Diane strategies for safe mobility, comfortable positioning, and energy conservation.

After the therapy session, Diane follows the therapist out to the front porch. She expresses concern about her ability to care for her father without neglecting her own husband and teenage daughters. As she lights a cigarette, she states that she knows she should quit. She has tried several times but finds the cravings for cigarettes in times of stress too difficult to resist.

SUBSTANCE ABUSE

The use of legal and illegal substances and the detrimental effects of the use of these substances are widely documented. **Substance abuse** is the overindulgence in and dependence on an addictive substance, especially alcohol or a narcotic drug (American Heritage Dictionary Online, 2003). According to the American Council for Drug Education, alcohol is the oldest and most widely used drug in the world. Alcohol is legal and readily accessible.

The American Academy of Pediatrics (AAP) cites alcohol and tobacco as leading **gateway drugs** (2002). Gateway drugs are substances that seem to open the entrance into harder-drug use (Figure 19–4). The AAP points out that

- Alcohol and tobacco are usually the first drugs that young people try.
- High school seniors who smoke every day are 10 times more likely to use cocaine regularly than are seniors who don't smoke on a regular basis.
- Adolescents who drink heavily or who "binge drink" are more likely to use other drugs than are nondrinkers or moderate drinkers (AAP, 2002).

The use and abuse of alcohol can affect an individual from the prenatal period to old age. *Fetal alcohol syndrome (FAS)* results from prenatal exposure to alcohol. Babies and children with FAS are subject to a variety of developmental, learning, and behavioral problems throughout the lifespan due to in utero ingestion of alcohol. FAS results in brain damage in various regions (Kodituwakku, Kalberg, & May, 2002) and thwarted brain development (Andrew, 2000). Prenatal exposure to alcohol may also affect *executive functioning*, the ability to plan and guide behavior to achieve a goal in an efficient manner (Kodituwakku, Kalberg, & May, 2002). Physiologically, infants born to mothers who drink alcohol during pregnancy have an increased risk of

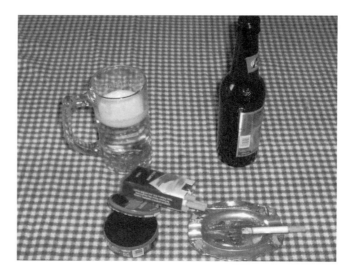

FIGURE 19–4   Use of tobacco and alcohol by teens and young adults may pave the way for use of other, "harder" drugs.

prematurity, lower birthweight, irritability, and poor skills for attachment (Wooster, Grey, & Gifford, 2001).

Adolescents who engage in drinking have a higher likelihood of transitioning to heavier alcohol use and the use of drugs (Blow, 1997). Adolescents who engage in the use of illegal drugs like cocaine, marijuana, and inhalants may experience significant adjustment problems in regard to education (truancy, more frequent absences, poor grades), have difficulty in adjusting to adult roles and responsibilities, and are more likely to become involved in deviant behaviors (Bonder, 1998).

Throughout the adult decades of life, alcohol abuse impacts all occupational performance areas. This impact is magnified in later adult years. Adults over the age of 65 are more likely to be affected by at least one chronic illness that can make them more vulnerable to the negative effects of alcohol. Substance abuse, particularly of alcohol and prescription drugs among adults age 60 and over, is one of the fastest growing heath problems facing the country. It is estimated that 17 percent of older adults abuse alcohol and misuse prescription drugs (Brennan & Moos, 1996). Older adults may attempt to self-medicate with alcohol or prescription drugs. These individuals also may identify themselves as being lonely and as having "lower life satisfaction" (Blow, 1997).

Alcohol consumption is the major contributor for *alcohol-induced liver disease (ALD)*. Approximately 10–35 percent of heavy drinkers develop alcoholic hepatitis, and 10–20 percent develop cirrhosis (Maher, 1997). In the United States cirrhosis is the seventh leading cause of death among young and middle-aged adults. Approximately 10,000–24,000 deaths from cirrhosis may be attributable to alcohol consumption each year (DeBakey, Stinson, Grant, & Dufour, 1996).

Alcohol impacts health professionals in a variety of ways. Occupational therapists work in programs to help persons who abuse alcohol and other substances (Ward, 2003). Both physical and occupational therapists work with people with dementia, amnesic disorders, and movement dysfunction that may be caused by prolonged use of alcohol.

RESPONSIBLE SEXUAL BEHAVIOR

Sexuality is defined by Encarta (2000) as "the state of being sexual," "involvement in sexual activity," and "sexual appeal." Thus, sexuality includes not only the act of having sex, but the more complicated elements of emotion, physiologic drive, pregnancy, birth control, and sexually transmitted diseases. Prior to the introduction of the birth control pill in 1960, sex was something performed for procreation and only rarely and, in certain circles, for entertainment or pleasure. The pill changed how we think and practice sex as a society. The ultimate outcome of sex potentially changed because the consequence was no longer the conception of a baby but the completion of a pleasurable act. This changed consequence in turn impacted emotional and psychosocial issues related to commitment, marriage, and the connection with another person. These changed attitudes were, and remain, the keystone of the "sexual revolution."

Throughout the lifespan, sexuality is incorporated into our persona with varying degrees of intensity. Sexuality may be affected by factors such as infertility, pregnancy, and aging (Read, 1999). **Gender identity,** defined as "the sense of identification with either the male or female sex, as manifested in appearance, behavior and other aspects of a person's life" (Gale Encyclopedia of Childhood and Adolescence, 1995), defines an individual's approach to and the manifestation of sexuality.

Children learn about sexuality by watching and listening to both children and adults around them and from their own exploration (Windham, 1998). The groundwork for future sexuality is sometimes laid in childhood games and in mutual sexual exploration with siblings or peers of a similar age. Boys and girls are mature enough in the early periods of childhood (age 6–12 years) to intuitively know that boys and girls are "different," and that "I am a boy (girl)." This is one of the foremost developmental tasks, and it is frequently accomplished by being accepted by same-sex peers (Carter, 1999).

The postpuberty years are aligned with the development of a sense of autonomy, the development of a personal identity, a refinement of values, the development of future life directions, the onset of dating, and, most likely, the initial sexual experience. The World Health Organization (WHO) identifies the *transitional stages of adolescence* as periods when the individual progresses from the initial appearance of secondary sexual characteristics to full sexual maturity; the stage when the psychological processes and modes of identification for the individual evolve from those of a child to those that characterize an adult; and a period in which the individual passes from a state of total social and economic dependence to one of relative independence.

On the average, the first sexual experience occurs somewhere between the ages of 16 and 18 (BBC News, 1999; WHO, 1998). Recent reports substantiate that regular sexual activity that is enjoyable continues well into the seventh decade of life (Read, 1999). The onset of having sex brings with it the issues of safe sex and the use of birth control. **Safe sex** is defined as "sexual activity in which safeguards, such as the use of a condom and the avoidance of high-risk acts, are employed to reduce the chance of acquiring or spreading a sexually transmitted disease" (American Heritage Dictionary, 2000).

Sexually transmitted diseases (STDs), once called *venereal diseases,* are among the most common infectious diseases in the United States today. In the year 2000 more than 65 million people in the United States were living with an incurable sexually transmitted disease (Centers for Disease Control and Prevention, 2000c). In spite of this, STDs are one of the most underrecognized health problems in the country today. Although as individuals we tend to consider STDs a private problem, outside the scope of our career as healthcare providers, this is not true.

The Occupational Therapy Standard of practice lists sexuality and sexual behaviors as ADLs. Our tendency to omit sexuality and sexual behavior from our consideration is of concern, because this hesitancy can "reinforce the societal myth that people with an illness or disability are asexual" (McKenna, 2003, p. 542). Physical and occupational therapists can play key roles in supporting the renewal of sexual function following serious injury or illness, and are often involved in providing school-based therapy to adolescents considering, or currently engaged in, sexual behaviors.

MENTAL HEALTH AND EMOTIONAL ISSUES

Mental health is "a state of emotional and psychological well-being in which an individual is able to use his or her cognitive and emotional capabilities, function in society, and meet the ordinary demands of everyday life" (American Heritage Dictionary On-line, 2003). The phrase *mental health* is used interchangeably with the phrase *emotional wellness.* Mental health is an invisible barrier that separates functional and productive individuals from those deemed to be dysfunctional or disturbed. The ICF included a detailed description of mental functions, discussed in Chapter 3 of this text, that relate to specific aspects of mental health. Mental health is a dynamic process that is greatly influenced by the individual's developmental and contextual factors.

CHILDHOOD AND ADOLESCENCE

In childhood and adolescence, mental health is defined as the achievement of expected developmental, cognitive, social, and emotional milestones. This identification is further highlighted by the individual's ability to cope effectively, initiate and maintain secure attachments with others, and develop satisfying social relationships. Mentally healthy children and adolescents are able to enjoy a positive quality of life; function well at home, at school, and in their community; and are free from disabling symptoms of psychopathology (Hoagwood et al., 1996).

ADULTHOOD

In adulthood, the longest phase of human life, mental health is demonstrated by the successful performance of the mental functions related to work, education, and personal relationships. In adulthood there are ongoing developmental tasks and periods of special vulnerability that need to be navigated (Kaplan & Sadock, 1997). The adult period of life is characterized by the presence of both predictable and unexpected stressors that can create havoc in the day-to-day world. Commonly identified adult stressors are listed in Table 19–2.

LATE ADULTHOOD

The mental health problem most commonly associated with late adulthood is dementia. **Dementia** is the "deterioration of intellectual faculties, such as memory, concentration, and judgment, resulting from an organic disease or a disorder of the brain. It is sometimes accompanied by emotional disturbance and personality changes" (American Heritage Dictionary, 2000a). Estimates are that 5 percent of people over age 65 have severe dementia, and an additional 15 percent have milder versions of the condition (Kaplan & Sadock, 1997). While dementia can lead to significant disablement, it remains a condition impacting 20 percent or less of the elderly population.

Older people are faced with a series of losses. Depression associated with grief and bereavement is a common, often untreated mental health issue in the aged population. In this population, depression "is

often accompanied by physical symptoms or cognitive changes that mimic dementia" (Kaplan & Sadock, 1997, p. 65). Somatic complaints and subclinical symptoms of anxiety or depression are commonly overlooked in primary care settings. Failure to detect individuals who have truly treatable mental disorders represents a serious public health problem (NIH Consensus Development Panel on Depression in Later Life, 1992).

A longitudinal study by Jonsson, Josephesson, and Kielhofner (2000) reflected that "how persons achieve meaning in their occupations, maintain a balance in occupational life, and reorganize occupational behavior patterns all are potentially illuminated in the retirement process" (p. 463). In this study the greatest proportion of those persons who were negative and expected retirement to be a negative change found this to be true for them. Subjects with the negative expectations reported that there was not enough to do to occupy their time. One subject described rationing available activities so that she would have one task for each day of the week. Another kept herself busy with her house and with sorting papers but saw these activities as having little value. Individuals who feel isolated and feel that their daily occupations have no value are at risk for depression and other mental health conditions.

In contrast, subjects who had previously seen work as positive and saw retirement as positive were more likely to take responsibility for their retirement situations. Some continued to work in an unpaid status, and others found productive ways to spend their time. For about one third of the subject group, the retirement outcome was different from their preretirement expectation. For some of these people, the difference was because they acted decisively to avoid potentially negative outcomes. Others had unexpected experiences that altered their expected outcome. These results suggest that through planning and active participation in meaningful daily occupations, individuals can positively influence the outcome of their own retirement transition.

INJURY AND VIOLENCE

Many health problems such as diabetes, heart disease, and cancer are chronic diseases that result from the cumulative effects of years of health behaviors and environmental exposures. In contrast, injuries from accidents and violence affect people of all ages and represent a leading cause of death for children and young adults.

Rehabilitation specialists are frequently involved in the care of persons recovering from injuries. Serious injuries, like head injuries, can lead to physical, emotional,

TABLE 19–2	Commonly Identified Adult Stressors
Divorce or break-up of romantic relationship	Approximately one-half of all marriages end up in divorce; 30–40 percent undergoing a divorce report a significant increase in symptoms of depression and anxiety; divorce may include the addition of economic stressors and single or shared parenting stressors.
Death of child or spouse	Although strong emotional distress is common and usual, the conventional approach for diagnosis is to *not* diagnose depression or emotional distress during the arbitrary period of bereavement, usually considered to be 2 months.
Chronic strain	This category takes into account poor physical health, relationship problems, conflicts with parents, siblings, and children, work and coworkers' problems, and problems with friends and neighbors.
Past trauma	Trauma experienced in childhood may resurface during the adult years. This may include but is not limited to the following: sexual abuse; neglect; the death of a significant person, including a parent, sibling, or friend; substance abuse; parental divorce; and psychopathology.
Domestic violence	Domestic violence affects victims who are overwhelmingly female and children who witness the violence. These victims are at a much higher risk for mental health problems as well as physical injury and death. Children who witness the violence are at a higher risk for acute and long-term emotional disturbances, including nightmares, depression, learning difficulties, and aggressive behavior. The observance of violence may place children at risk for the use of violence as they mature.
Life-threatening assault or accident	Life-threatening experiences may relate to, more commonly, urban violence or assault, but may also figure within the context of "act of God" occurrences like hurricanes, floods, or tornados, or the horror of the 9-11 event in New York City.
Racism and discrimination	Prejudice and discrimination based on the color of one's skin, sex, nationality, or family of origin can create ongoing and indefinable emotional distress. This may be directed toward, for example, the lack of a promotion because of one's sex, the ineligibility to join an organization because of the color of one's skin, or the lack of opportunity provided because of one's physical limitations.
Economic hardships	Economic hardships may relate to employment problems or the lack of employment, divorce or the absence of financial support, spending tendencies of the individual, or educational or motivational deficits.

and social problems for individuals and their families (Cronin, 2001). In this section we will discuss some of the more common sources of injury for children and adults.

ACCIDENTS AND VIOLENCE IN CHILDHOOD

In 2001 unintentional injury was the number one cause of death among American children and teens (Arias & Smith, 2003). A majority of accidental deaths are due to motor vehicle accidents; even more children are injured in auto accidents and survive with temporary or permanent disabilities. Nearly half the accidental deaths in the United States involve motor vehicles (Arias et al., 2003). The costs of motor vehicle accidents, including medical costs, lost productivity, and other direct and indirect

costs, are estimated at $150 billion per year. Thirty-eight percent of all motor vehicle accidents are related to alcohol. Use of seat belts and child safety seats (Figure 19–5) and reductions in drunk driving could prevent many deaths and injuries for people of all ages (Centers for Disease Control and Prevention, 2001a).

However, 15 percent of parents admit that their children do not always wear appropriate restraints or use safety seats (Behavior Risk Factor Survey System [BRFSS], 1995–2001). Fourteen percent of youth in grades 9 through 12 stated that they rarely, if ever, use safety belts when riding in a car driven by someone else (Youth Behavior Risk Factor Survey [YBRFS], 2001). Thirteen percent of teenagers admitted driving under the influence during the previous month, and 31 percent admitted riding with someone else who had been drinking (YBRFS, 2001).

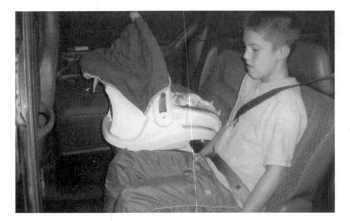

FIGURE 19–5   Proper use of child restraints and safety belts can prevent death and serious injury from car crashes.

Intentional injury is also an important health problem in children. Violence (i.e., assault or homicide) was the fourth leading cause of death for ages 1 through 14, and the second leading cause for ages 15 through 24 (Arias et al., 2003). It is estimated that more than 900,000 children were victims of abuse or neglect in 2001; but 1,300 of these children died. Over one fourth of those abused were 3 years old or younger. Of children who died of abuse, 40 percent were less than 1 year old (U.S. Department of Health and Human Services, Administration on Children, Youth, and Families, 2003). Health-care providers need to familiarize themselves with the signs and symptoms of child abuse, state laws regarding mandatory reporting of suspected abuse, institutional policies and procedures, and community support services for abused children and their families.

Parents or other caretakers do not inflict all intentional injuries. Twenty percent of female high school students report having been physically or sexually abused in the context of dating (Centers for Disease Control and Prevention, 2001c). The U.S. homicide rate among children 15 years old and younger is higher than the combined rates of 25 other industrialized countries (Centers for Disease Control and Prevention, 2001c). The CDC has called on schools to work with communities to develop programs to reduce violence, homicide, and suicide among youth. The American Occupational Therapy Association has identified such programs as an emerging area of importance for occupational therapists.

ACCIDENTS AND VIOLENCE IN ADULTHOOD

As stated earlier, motor vehicle accidents account for an overwhelming number of injuries and deaths among people of all ages, and violence is a leading cause of death in young adults. Other sources of injury

in adults include work-related accidents and, for older adults, falls in the home. Although fatal work-related injuries have declined over the past two decades, nearly 17 workers died each day in 1997 due to work-related injury (National Institute for Occupational Safety and Health [NIOSH], 2002a). Leading causes of these occupational injuries were motor vehicle accidents and homicide. Fatalities were most common in the construction, transportation, public utilities, agriculture, forestry, and fishing industries (NIOSH, 2002a).

Still, many injuries occur on the job each day that are not fatal. According to the National Institute for Occupational Safety and Health, nearly 6 million occupational injuries occurred in 1997 (2002b). Nonfatal injuries are most common in the agriculture, construction, manufacturing, and transportation and utilities industries. Many work-related injuries involve sprains and strains; nearly half of such injuries involve the spine (National Institute for Occupational Safety and Health, 2002b). Physical and occupational therapists are uniquely qualified to provide consultation and perform research regarding worksite/task modification and fitness programs that prevent worker injuries.

As adults age, they become more susceptible to accidental falls. Injuries sustained in falls are the leading cause of injury, death, and disability in people over 65 years of age (Centers for Disease Control and Prevention, 2000b). Use of certain medications, environmental factors, and decline in muscle strength, balance, vision, or proprioception can contribute to falls. Older adults who fall may fracture a hip; nearly half who do never regain their previous level of function (Centers for Disease Control and Prevention, 2000b). Caring for a person with a hip fracture, including medical care and care provided by the family, can cost as much as $18,000 for the first year after the injury (Centers for Disease Control and Prevention, 2000b). The majority of hip fractures occur in women. Other risk factors include osteoporosis, low BMI, and decreased physical activity. Interventions for reducing risk of falls and fall-related hip fractures include individualized exercise programs, medication review, counseling, and environmental modifications. Community-based programs that incorporate these elements have shown promise in reducing the rate of falls in older adults; more research in this area is needed (Centers for Disease Control and Prevention, 2000b).

IMMUNIZATION

Immunizations, or vaccinations, are given for protection from infectious diseases. The first vaccine was developed in the 1700s for smallpox. Vaccines are often made from materials extracted from infectious organisms or from organisms that are closely related to the infectious organism. When a vaccine is introduced into the body, antibodies are formed that provide immunity from the disease in question. Vaccines are typically harmless, although allergic reactions or minor side effects occur in a very small percentage of people.

Immunizations have been credited with greatly reducing death and disability due to infectious diseases during the twentieth century. Incidence of smallpox, diphtheria, polio, measles, mumps, and rubella have declined by more than 99 percent (Campbell & Bryant, 2001). In order to maintain reductions in these diseases, efforts to maintain and improve vaccinations for children and adults in the United States continue.

Vaccinations are necessary for school-age children, adolescents, and adults as well. Children who do not receive the appropriate immunizations as infants should receive them before starting school. Children and young adults who spend time in classrooms or dormitories have a greater chance of being exposed to infectious diseases. Also, immunity provided by some vaccinations fades over time, making boosters necessary. This is the case with tetanus and diphtheria; it is recommended that adults have a booster at least once every 10 years (Centers for Disease Control and Prevention, 2003). Older adults and adults with certain chronic conditions should have immunizations for the flu and pneumonia. Currently the CDC recommends an annual influenza shot for adults over 50 (Centers for Disease Control and Prevention, 2000a). Pneumococcal vaccine is recommended for those over 65 (Peter & Gardner, 2001).

Despite the successes of vaccination programs in the United States during the past century, concerns about infectious diseases still exist. An outbreak of measles occurred in 1989 and 1990. Nearly half of the cases occurred in unvaccinated preschool children, many of whom were nonwhite. The cause of the outbreak was identified as failure to properly vaccinate children at the appropriate age (1991). As a result, changes in immunization policies and practices have been proposed and initiated. These changes include improved availability of vaccines, improved recognition by providers of those in need of immunizations, and delivery of promotional campaigns for providers and the public (1991; Peter et al., 2001). It is recommended that all health-care workers and students maintain proper immunizations to limit risks to themselves and their patients (Peter et al., 2001).

ENVIRONMENTAL QUALITY

As noted in Chapter 1 of this text, a unique aspect of the ICF classification system is the inclusion of environmental factors as part of the classification. Increasingly, social scientists and other professionals are recognizing the importance of the role of environmental factors in either facilitating functioning or creating barriers for people with disabilities (World Health Organization, 2002). The inclusion of environmental quality as a health threat in *Healthy People 2010*, consistent with the ICF, refers to the natural environment consisting of both the physical environment and the social environment. The physical environment "includes the air, water, and soil through which exposure to chemical, biological, and physical agents may occur" (Healthy People 2010, http://www.healthypeople.gov/document/html/uih/uih_4.htm#environqual). The social environment includes features such as housing, transportation, urban development, land use, industry, and agriculture (*Healthy People 2010*).

HEALTH-CARE ACCESS ISSUES

The number and percentage of Americans without health insurance continue to increase. Census Bureau figures released in September 2003 showed that 43.6 million Americans (15.2 percent) of the population now lack health insurance (U.S. Census, 2003). There is a great deal of variation in the degree of lack of health-care insurance from state to state, with states in the Southwest and Southeast having the highest percentage of uninsured people. There is also a great disparity in the degree of underinsurance by ethnic group. Twelve percent of non-Hispanic whites are uninsured, compared with 21.5 percent of blacks and 34 percent of Hispanics.

The figures about access to health insurance provide only part of the picture. Many persons with basic health insurance do not have coverage for mental health conditions. In 1999, in the surgeon general's report (U.S. Department of Health and Human Services), Dr. David Satcher shared these findings:

- Mental health disorders were as common in minorities as in nonminorities.
- Members of minority groups were less likely to receive treatment.
- Mental health care may be inferior and/or the patient may be misdiagnosed.
- Minority groups are overrepresented in populations at risk for mental illness, i.e., homelessness, incarceration, poverty.
- Reduced health-care access may be due to language barriers, financial costs, lack of health insurance, and the stigma of being labeled mentally ill.

The United States spends far more on health care than does any other country. In 2000 the United States spent $4,719 per person, or over 13.5 percent of the gross national product, on health-care costs (Hatcher Agency, 2003). Rural health-care providers are in a different position than their urban counterparts in regard to serving the uninsured. Urban health-care providers are able to provide unreimbursed services to the extent that other health-care revenues generated cover fixed costs (salaries, benefits, utilities, rent, licensing, etc.) and provide enough of a profit margin to absorb the cost of caring for nonpaying patients. When managed-care plans reduce payments to providers, the cushion used to provide care to the uninsured and underinsured disappears. The rural health-care setting is commonly composed of fewer health-care providers. Many rural regions of the country do not have "safety net" providers eligible for public grant dollars to help underwrite the costs of caring for the uninsured or underinsured (National Rural Healthcare Association, 1999).

SUMMARY

Occupational and physical therapists typically provide clinical services in response to specific functional needs; however, there is an increasing role for community-based programs aimed at wellness and prevention. Many existing wellness programs are multidisciplinary and address the key health indicators presented in this chapter. In addition to providing education and advocacy in wellness programs, rehabilitation specialists can serve as program development consultants in home health and in industry. Increasingly, occupational therapists have been providing mental health interventions in nontraditional settings like soup kitchens and with the homeless (Hodges & Segal, 2002; Shordike & Howell, 2001).

Speaking of

Wellness

ANNE CRONIN, PhD, OTR/L, BCP
PEDIATRIC PHYSICAL THERAPIST

I remember being an occupational therapy student, and being sure that much of what we learned was useless and not related to what I would really do. And later, as an experienced teacher of occupational therapy, I remember being taken aback when asked to teach a course for OT students on wellness. "We work with people who have impairments," I said. "I wouldn't begin to know how to approach wellness as an OT." Beware of limiting your vision.

I did end up teaching the wellness class, and I came to realize that a very large part of my clinical practice was about wellness and prevention, within a population of children with impairments. Later, I was asked to consult in an inpatient rehabilitation program for children with clinically severe obesity. By now I recognized that (1) you never know when knowledge will be helpful, and (2) OTs excel in wellness and prevention—but obesity?

Persons with clinically severe obesity (100 lbs or 100 percent over their healthy weight) can have many problems participating in their daily occupations. The teens I saw could not fit into a shower or get up from a tub. They had many personal hygiene problems, including cleaning up after toileting. In the supported environment of the rehabilitation center I saw these children blossom, but I also recognized that they would be returning to their homes and communities soon—back to the homes and communities where they had originally acquired all of that weight. In searching for community connections, I learned about the lack of low-cost noncompetitive fitness programs in most communities. In our school district the middle school students rotate through gym class for one 6-week period during the entire school year, and there are no school-supported gym programs during the summer.

As health professionals, we need to understand and integrate current trends in health care and community health problems and advocate for low-cost community-based fitness programs for our clients. Don't limit your vision, or your potential to build successful clinical interventions in nontraditional "wellness" settings. People with and without activity limitations benefit from health and are best able to perform to the top of their ability in an environment that supports their health.

REFERENCES

Adams, R. D., Victor, M., & Ropper, A. H. (1997). *Principles of neurology* (6th ed.), New York: McGraw-Hill.

American Academy of Pediatrics. (2002). *Tobacco and alcohol: Gateway drugs?* Retrieved October 7, 2003, from http://www.aap.org/advocacy/chm99tobacfact.htm.

American College of Obstetricians and Gynecologists. (1999). *How to prevent sexually transmitted diseases.* Retrieved October 7, 2003, from http://www.medem.com/search/article_display.cfm?path=n:andmstr=/ZZZZQP7DD27C.html.

American Diabetes Association. (2003). *Children and diabetes.* Retrieved April 12, 2003, from http://www.diabetes.org/main/application/commercewf?origin=*.jspandevent=link(B4_3).

American Heritage® dictionary of the English language (4th ed.). (2000a). Houghton Mifflin Company. *Dementia.* Retrieved October 7, 2003, from http://dictionary.reference.com/search?q=dementia.

American Heritage® dictionary of the English language (4th ed.). (2000b). Houghton Mifflin Company. *Morbidity.* Retrieved October 7, 2003, from http://dictionary.reference.com/search?q=morbidity).

American Heritage® dictionary of the English language (4th ed.). (2000c). Houghton Mifflin Company. *Wellness.* Retrieved October 7, 2003, from http://dictionary.reference.com/search?q=wellness.

Andrew, G. (2000). *FAS setting up for success.* Retrieved October 7, 2003, from http://www.albertadoctors.org/publications/digest/2000/mar-apr-2000/fas/html.

Arias, E., & Smith, B. L. (2003). Deaths: Preliminary data for 2001. *National vital statistics report 5[51],* 1–45. Hyattsville, MD: National Center for Health Statistics, Centers for Disease Control and Prevention.

Bak, S., Sindrup, S., Alslev, T., Kristensen, O., & Gaist, D. (2000). Cessation of smoking after first-ever stroke: A follow-up study. *Stroke, 33 (9),* 2263–2269.

Bancroft, J. (1989) *Human sexuality and its problems* (2nd ed.) (pp. 282–285). Edinburgh: Churchill Livingstone.

Barnes, D. E., Yaffe, K., Satariano, W. A., & Tager, I. B. (2003). A longitudinal study of cardiorespiratory fitness and cognitive function in healthy older adults. *Journal of the American Geriatrics Society, 51,* 459–465.

Batshaw, M. L., & Conlon, C. J. (1997). Substance abuse: A preventable threat to development. In M. L. Batshaw (Ed.), *Children with disabilities* (4th ed) (pp. 143–162). Baltimore: Brookes.

BBC News. (1998). *UK youth tops global sex league.* Retrieved October 7, 2003, from http://news.bbc.co.uk/1/hi/health/454760.stm.

Blair, S. N., Kohl, H. W., III, Barlow, C. E., Paffenbarger, R. S., Jr., Gibbons, L. W., & Macera, C. A. (1995). Changes in physical fitness and all-cause mortality. A prospective study of healthy and unhealthy men. *Journal of American Medical Association, 273,* 1093–1098.

Blow, F. (1997). Substance abuse among older adults: Treatment improvement protocol. *U.S. Department of Health and Human Services and SAMHSA National Clearinghouse for Alcohol and Drug Information.* Series 26. Retrieved October 7, 2003, from http://www.health.org/govpubs/BDK250/default.aspx.

Blum, R., Beuhring, T., Shew, M., Bearinger, L., Sieving, R., & Resnick, M. (2000). The effects of race/ethnicity, income, and family structure on adolescent risk behaviors. *American Journal of Public Health, 90(12),* 1879–1884.

Bonder, B. (1995). *Psychopathology and function.* Thorofare, NJ: Slack.

Brennan, P., & Moos, R. (1996). Late-life drinking behavior: The influence of personal characteristics, life context, and treatment. *Alcohol Health and Research World, 20(3),* 197–221.

Campbell, A. J., Robertson, M. C., Gardner, M. M., Norton, R. N., Tilyard, M. W., & Buchner, D. M. (1997). Randomised controlled trial of a general practice programme of home-based exercise to prevent falls in elderly women. *British Medical Journal, 315,* 1065.

Campbell, A. L., & Bryant, K. A. (2001). Routine childhood immunizations. *Primary Care, 28,* 713–738, vi.

Carter, D. (1999). Sexual development in childhood—News/reference. *PENpages.* Retrieved October 7, 2003, from http://www.penpages.psu.edu/penpages_reference/28507/28507315.html.

Centers for Disease Control and Prevention. (1999). *CDC surveillance summaries,* October 29, *48(SS07),* 1–44.

Centers for Disease Control and Prevention. (2000a). Prevention and control of influenza: Recommendations of the advisory committee on immunization practices. *Morbidity and Mortality Weekly Report, 49(RR03),* 1–38.

Centers for Disease Control and Prevention. (2000b). Reducing falls and resulting hip fractures among older women. *Morbidity and Mortality Weekly Report, 49(RR02),* 1–12.

Centers for Disease Control and Prevention. (2000c). *Tracking the hidden epidemics: STDs in the United States.* Centers for Disease Control and Prevention.

Centers for Disease Control and Prevention. (2001a). Motor-vehicle occupant injury: Strategies for increasing use of child safety seats, increasing use of safety belts, and reducing alcohol-impaired driving. *Morbidity and Mortality Weekly Report, 50(RR07),* 1–13.

Centers for Disease Control and Prevention. (2001b). Physical activity trends—United States, 1990–1998. *Morbidity and Mortality Weekly Report, 50(9),* 166–169.

Centers for Disease Control and Prevention. (2001c). School health guidelines to prevent unintentional injuries and violence. *Morbidity and Mortality Weekly Report, 50(RR22),* 1–46.

Centers for Disease Control and Prevention. (2002a). *National diabetes fact sheet: General information and national estimates on diabetes in the United States* (Rep. No. NIH 02-

3892). Atlanta, GA: U.S. Department of Health and Human Services.

Centers for Disease Control and Prevention. (2002b). Prevalence of health-care providers asking older adults about their physical activity levels—United States, 1998. *Morbidity and Mortality Weekly Report, 51(19),* 412–414.

Centers for Disease Control and Prevention. (2002c). Youth risk behavior surveillance—United States, 2001. *Morbidity and Mortality Weekly Report, 51(SS04),* 1–64.

Centers for Disease Control and Prevention. (2003). Recommended childhood and adolescent immunization schedule. *Morbidity and Mortality Weekly Report, 52(04),* Q1–Q4.

Cronin, A. F. (2001). Traumatic brain injury in children. *American Journal of Occupational Therapy, 55 (4),* 377–384.

DeBakey, S. F., Stinson, F. S., Grant, B. F., & Dufour, M. C. (1996). Surveillance report #41. *Liver cirrhosis mortality in the United States, 1970–93.* Bethesda, MD: National Institute on Alcohol Abuse and Alcoholism.

Encarta. (2002). *Sexuality.* Retrieved October 7, 2003, from http://encarta.msn.com/encnet/features/dictionary/DictionaryResults.aspx?search=sexuality.

Etter, J., & Sutton, S. (2002). Assessing "stage of change" in current and former smokers. *Addiction, 97(9),* 1171–1182.

Gale Encyclopedia of Medicine. (1995). *Gender identity.* Retrieved October 7, 2003, from http://www.findarticles.com/cf_dls/PI/search.jhtml?isp=FAandcat=refandcat=healthand key-%2.

Giovino, G. (1999). Epidemiology of tobacco use among U.S. adolescents. *Nicotine and Tobacco Research 1 (Supp. 1),* S31–S40.

Global Birth Control Usage. (2003). *What women want: International survey of birth control methods.* Retrieved October 7, 2003, from http://www.birthcontrolresources.com/results/htm.

Grunbaum, J., Kann, L., Kichen, S., Ross, J., Gowda, V., Collins, J., & Kolbe, L. (1999). Youth risk behavior surveillance—National alternative high school youth risk behavior survey, United States, 1998. *Morbidity and Mortality Weekly Report, 48* No. SS-7.

Hatcher Agency. (2003). *Healthcare statistics.* Retrieved April 6, 2004, from http://www.hatcheragency.com.

Health 50+. (2003). Smoking health risks. *Health Topics.* Retrieved October 7, 2003, from http://www.50plushealth.co.uk/index.cfm?articleid=903.

Health Matters. (1999). *An introduction to sexually transmitted diseases.* National Institute of Allergy and Infectious Diseases or the National Institute of Health, July 1999. Retrieved October 7, 2003, from http://www.niaid.nih.gov/factsheets/stdinfo.htm.

Hoagwood, K., Jenson, P., Petti, T., & Burns, B. (1996). Outcomes of mental health care for children and adolescents: I. A comprehensive conceptual model. *Journal of the American Academy of Child and Adolescent Psychiatry, 35(8),* 1055–1063.

Hodges, J., & Segal, S. (2002). Goal advancement among mental health self-help agency members. *Psychiatric Rehabilitation Journal, 26(1),* 78–85.

International Longevity Center—USA. (2000). Nearly half of older Americans say "these are the best years of my life" new survey shows. Retrieved October 7, 2003, from http://www.ilcusa.org.

Jonsson, H., Staffan, J., & Kielhofner, G. (2000). Evolving narratives in the course of retirement: A longitudinal study. *American Journal of Occupational Therapy, 54(5),* 463–470.

Kaplan, H., & Sadock, B. (1997). *Kaplan and Sadock's synopsis of psychiatry* (8th ed.). Philadelphia: Williams and Wilkins.

Kodituwakku, P., Kalberg, W., & May, P. (2003). The effects of prenatal alcohol exposure on executive functioning, *National Institute on Alcohol Abuse and Alcoholism Publications.* Retrieved October 7, 2003, from http://www.niaaa.nih.gov/publications/arh25-3/192-198.htm.

Kovar, P. A., Allegrante, J. P., MacKenzie, C. R., Peterson, M. G., Gutin, B., & Charlson, M. E. (1992). Supervised fitness walking in patients with osteoarthritis of the knee. A randomized, controlled trial. *Annals of Internal Medicine, 116,* 529–534.

Kramer, A. F., Hahn, S., Cohen, N. J., Banich, M. T., McAuley, E., Harrison, C. R., Chason, J., Vakil, E., Bardell, L., Boileau, R. A., & Colcombe, A. (1999). Aging, fitness and neurocognitive function. *Nature, 400,* 418–419.

Lee, I. M., Hsieh, C. C., & Paffenbarger, R. S., Jr. (1995). Exercise intensity and longevity in men. Harvard Alumni Health Study. *Journal of the American Medical Association, 273,* 1179–1184.

London, K. (1982). The history of birth control, *Yale-New Haven Teachers Institute.* Retrieved October 7, 2003, from http://www.yale.edu/ynhti/curriculum/units/1982/6/82.06.03x.html.

Maher, J. (1997). Exploring alcohol's effects on liver function. Retrieved April 6, 2004, from http://www.niaaa.nih.gov/publications/arh21-1/05.pdf, in National Institute on Alcohol Abuse and Alcoholism's *Alcohol's Effect on Organ Function,* 21(1).

McGinnis, J. M., & Foege, W. H. (1993). Actual causes of death in the United States. *Journal of the American Medical Association, 270,* 2207–2212.

McKenna, K. (2003). Sexuality and disability. In E. Crepeau, E. Cohn & B. Schell (Eds.), *Willard and Spackman's occupational therapy (10th ed.).* Philadelphia: Lippincott, Williams and Wilkins.

Mokdad, A. H., Bowman, B. A., Ford, E. S., Vinicor, F., Marks, J. S., & Koplan, J. P. (2001). The continuing epidemics of obesity and diabetes in the United States. *Journal of the American Medical Association, 286,* 1195–1200.

Mokdad, A. H., Ford, E. S., Bowman, B. A., Dietz, W. H., Vinicor, F., Bales, & Marks, J. S. (2003). Prevalence of obesity, diabetes, and obesity-related health risk factors, 2001. *Journal of the American Medical Association, 289,* 76–79.

Mokdad, A. H., Serdula, M. K., Dietz, W. H., Bowman, B. A., Marks, J. S., & Koplan, J. P. (1999). The spread of the obesity epidemic in the United States, 1991–1998. *Journal of the American Medical Association, 282,* 1519–1522.

Mokdad, A. H., Serdula, M. K., Dietz, W. H., Bowman, B. A., Marks, J. S., & Koplan, J. P. (2000). The continuing epidemic of obesity in the United States. *Journal of the American Medical Association, 284,* 1650–1651.

National Center for Chronic Disease Prevention and Health Promotion. (2003a, March 3). *Can inactivity hurt my health?* Retrieved April 14, 2003, from http://www.cdc.gov/nccdphp/dnpa/physical/importance/inactivity.htm.

National Center for Chronic Disease Prevention and Health Promotion. (2003b, January 15). *Promoting active lifestyles among older adults.* Retrieved April 8, 2003, from http://www.cdc.gov/nccdphp/dnpa/physical/lifestyles.htm.

National Center for Chronic Disease Prevention and Health Promotion. (2003, April 1). *Are there special recommendations for young people?* Retrieved April 8, 2003, from http://www.cdc.gov/nccdphp/dnpa/physical/recommendations/young.htm.

National Center for Health Statistics. (1997). *Healthy People 2000 Review 1997* (Rep. No. 97-1256). Hyattsville, MD: U.S. Department of Health and Human Services.

National Heart Lung and Blood Institute. (1998). Treatment guidelines. In *Clinical guidelines on the identification, evaluation, and treatment of overweight and obesity in adults: Evidence report* (pp. 56–93). Bethesda, MD: National Institutes of Health.

National Institute of Health Consensus Development Panel on Depression in Late Life. (1992). *Mental health: A report of the surgeon general.* Retrieved October 7, 2003, from http://www.surgeongeneral.gov/library/mentalhealth/chapter5/sec/2.html.

National Institute for Occupational Safety and Health. (2002a). *Worker health chartbook 2000: Fatal injury* (Rep. No. 2002-117). Cincinnati, OH: U.S. Department of Health and Human Services, Centers for Disease Control and Prevention, National Institute for Occupational Safety and Health.

National Institute for Occupational Safety and Health. (2002b). *Worker health chartbook 2000: Nonfatal injury* (Rep. No. 2002-119). Cincinnati, OH: U.S. Department of Health and Human Services, Centers for Disease Control and Prevention, National Institute for Occupational Safety and Health.

National Rural Health Association. (1998). Access to health care of the uninsured in rural and frontier America. Retrieved October 7, 2003, from http://www.nrharural.org/dc/issuepapers/ipapers15.html.

National Vaccine Advisory Committee. (1991). The measles epidemic: The problems, barriers, and recommendations. *Journal of the American Medical Association, 266,* 1547–1552.

Pate, R. R., Pratt, M., Blair, S. N., Haskell, W. L., Macera, C. A., Bouchard, C., et al. (1995). Physical activity and public health. A recommendation from the Centers for Disease Control and Prevention and the American College of Sports Medicine. *Journal of the American Medical Association, 273,* 402–407.

Peter, G., & Gardner, P. (2001). Standards for immunization practice for vaccines in children and adults. *Infectious Disease Clinics of North America, 15,* 9–19.

Pratt, M., Macera, C. A., & Wang, G. (2000). Higher direct medical costs associated with physical inactivity. *The Physician and Sportsmedicine, 28,* 63–70.

Prochaska, J. J., Zabinski, M. F., Calfas, K. J., Sallis, J. F., & Patrick, K. (2000). PACE+: Interactive communication technology for behavior change in clinical settings. *American Journal of Preventive Medicine, 19,* 127–131.

Read, J. (1999). ABC of sexual health: Sexual problems associated with infertility, pregnancy, and ageing. *British Medical Journal, 313(7183),* pp. 587–589.

Rimmer, J. H. (1999). Health promotion for people with disabilities: The emerging paradigm shift from disability prevention to prevention of secondary conditions. *Physical Therapy, 79,* 495–502.

Rosenbloom, A. L., Joe, J. R., Young, R. S., & Winter, W. E. (1999). Emerging epidemic of type 2 diabetes in youth. *Diabetes Care, 22,* 345–354.

Rouya, A. (2001). Breaking barriers to healthcare: Does race determine one's accessibility to healthcare? *Berkeley Medical Journal,* Spring 2001. Retrieved October 7, 2003, from http://www.ocf.berkeley.edu/~issues/spring01/barrier/html.

Shordike, A., & Howell, D. (2001) The reindeer of hope: An occupational therapy program in a homeless shelter. *Occupational Therapy in Health Care 5(1/2),* 57–68.

Singh, N. A., Clements, K. M., & Fiatarone, M. A. (1997). A randomized controlled trial of progressive resistance training in depressed elders. *Journals of Gerontology. Series A, Biological Sciences and Medical Sciences, 52,* M27–M35.

U.S. Census Bureau. (2003). Health Insurance Coverage: 2002. Retrieved April 6, 2004, from http://www.census.gov/prod/2003pubs/p60-223.pdf.

U.S. Department of Health and Human Services. (1999). *Mental health: A report of the surgeon general—Executive summary.* Rockville, MD: U.S. Department of Health and Human Services, Substance Abuse and Mental Health Services Administration, Center for Mental Health Services, National Institutes of Health, National Institute of Mental Health.

U.S. Department of Health and Human Services. (2000). *Healthy people 2010: Understanding and improving health* (2nd ed.). Washington, DC: U.S. Government Printing Office.

U.S. Department of Health and Human Services. (2001). *Mental health: A report of the surgeon general—Chapter 4, Stressful life events.* Rockville, MD: U.S. Department of Health & Human Services, Substance Abuse and Mental Health Services Administration, Center for Mental Health Services, National Institutes of Health, National Institutes of Mental Health.

U.S. Department of Health and Human Services, Administration on Children, Youth, and Families. (2003). *Child Maltreatment 2001.* Washington, DC: U.S. Government Printing Office.

Ward, J. (2003). Adults with mental illness. In E. Crepeau, E. Cohn, & B. Schell (Eds.), *Willard and Spackman's occupational therapy* (10th ed.) (pp. 835–866). Philadelphia: Lippincott, Williams and Wilkins.

Webster's Revised Unabridged Dictionary. (1998). *Sexual.* Retrieved October 7, 2003, from http://dictionary.reference.com/search?q=Sexual%20.

Windham, A. (1999). Children and sexual development. Retrieved October 7, 2003, from http://www.effect.net.au/scallywags/may99/childandsd.htm.

World Health Organization. (2003). *Situationer.* Retrieved October 7, 2003, from http://www.doh.gov.ph/ayhd/htm/situationer.htm.

World Health Organization. (2002). ICF: Introduction. In *ICF: International Classification of Functioning, Disability, and Health.* Geneva, Switzerland: World Health Organization.

Yaffe, K., Barnes, D., Nevitt, M., Lui, L. Y., & Covinsky, K. (2001). A prospective study of physical activity and cognitive decline in elderly women: Women who walk. *Archives of Internal Medicine, 161,* 1703–1708.

Yudkin, P., Hey, K., Roberts, S., Welch, S., Murphy, M., & Walton, B. (2003). Abstinence from smoking eight years after participation in randomized controlled trial of nicotine patch. *British Medical Journal, 327(7405),* 28–29.

CHAPTER 20

Public Policy and Health Care

Barbara L. Kornblau, JD, OT/L,
FAOTA, DAAPM, CCM, CDMS
Professor
Occupational Therapy and Law
Nova Southeastern University
Fort Lauderdale, Florida

and

Sandee Dunbar, DPA, OTR/L
Associate Professor
Nova Southeastern University
Fort Lauderdale, Florida

Objectives

Upon completion of this chapter, the reader should be able to

■ Describe the process of public policymaking.

■ Identify key public policy issues related to health care.

■ Identify the role of the health professional in public policy advocacy.

■ Explain three ways in which public policy can have an impact on clinical practice.

■ Explain how the ADA, IDEA, Fair Housing Act, Medicare, and Medicaid affect clinical practice and the lives of those we serve.

■ Explain how public policy relates to the Environmental Factors context described by the ICF document.

Key Terms

Americans with Disabilities Act
  (ADA)
Balanced Budget Act of 1997 (BBA)
co-insurance
deductible

Fair Housing Act Amendments of
  1988 (FHAA)
Individuals with Disabilities
  Education Act (IDEA)
Medicaid

Medicare
prospective payment system (PPS)
Rehabilitation Act of 1973
TriAlliance of Health and
  Rehabilitation Professions

INTRODUCTION

Why is public policy important to health-care professionals? The ICF (World Health Organization, 2002) reflects the importance of public policy at local, national, and international levels in their discussion of environmental contexts. Much of what has been presented earlier in this text is influenced by public policy decisions. Requirements for immunizations, school lunches, and wheelchair accessibility are all aspects of public policy. This chapter briefly introduces some of the major policy features of the contemporary health-care environment.

While many health-care practitioners chose their craft because of a desire to help people or make a difference in people's lives, one cannot ignore the impact of public policy on one's practice or potential practice. When politicians, regulatory bodies, courts, and others struggle to make changes in public policy, health-care professionals must keep a close watch on those changes and the impact the changes have on the work they do or can do. With the stroke of a governmental pen, health-care professionals can find an area of practice severely curtailed or expanded by budgetary constraints, new systems of reimbursement, regulatory reform, appellate court decisions, and other policy changes.

For example, when Congress passed the **Balanced Budget Act of 1997 (BBA),** a new system of reimbursement was initiated in long-term-care facilities under Medicare called the **prospective pay system (PPS)** (Balanced Budget Act of 1997, 1997). Under the PPS, the amount of reimbursement for a particular service is predetermined, irrespective of actual cost. This differs from *retrospective payment,* where actual costs are reimbursed (Shi & Singh, 2001). As a result of this shift in the reimbursement system, the amount of therapy provided to residents of long-term-care facilities plummeted, and thousands of occupational and physical therapists and assistants were laid off. Therapy companies that acted as middlemen, employing occupational and physical therapists and assistants and providing services to such facilities, found there was no longer a market for these services. All of a sudden,

unemployed therapists flooded the employment market, causing a sharp drop in salaries and a severe decline in enrollment for occupational and physical therapy educational programs. Further, older adults served in long-term-care facilities saw services severely curtailed as their access to occupational therapy and physical therapy practitioners decreased. Thankfully, in many cases, that situation has corrected itself, and therapists and assistants are again providing care to clients in these facilities.

Another example of how public policy affects health care is the $1,500[1] cap on outpatient occupational therapy services, physical therapy, and speech services. With the passage of the BBA, Congress assigned a dollar-amount limit of $1,500 to certain outpatient occupational therapy services, physical therapy, and speech pathology services combined. For the first time under Medicare, Congress cut services by placing an arbitrary dollar-amount limit on a covered service. The **TriAlliance of Health and Rehabilitation Professions,** comprising the American Occupational Therapy Association, the American Physical Therapy Association, and the American Speech and Hearing Association, successfully lobbied for a moratorium on the $1,500 cap, delaying the effects of the cap by two years. This lobbying continued in response to the proposed lifting of the moratorium on the cap in 2003 with an extension of the moratorium and the hope of eliminating the cap on a permanent basis.

THE MAKING OF PUBLIC POLICY

State and federal governments play a primary role in the development of public policy, which they express through laws and funding mechanisms. For example, in response to a noticeable increase in the needs of children with autism, the Florida legislature passed a law funding regional centers for autism and related disorders. Among

---

[1]This amount as of this writing is now equal to $1,590.

other services provided, these centers included a mandate to educate parents and providers about treatment and other needs of children with autism. Occupational and physical therapy practitioners benefited from the services provided under this law.

Sometimes the government expresses public policy through implementing regulations or guidelines. For example, in the area of ergonomics the Department of Labor has gone back and forth over whether or not it should institute mandatory workplace design, or *ergonomic,* regulations. After much debate and discussion, the ergonomic regulations—which if mandatory would have broadly expanded a practice area for occupational and physical therapy practitioners—became merely recommended guidelines.

Public policy is sometimes made by the judicial branch of government—that is, the courts. The U.S. Supreme Court makes policy when it rules on cases brought before it. For example, in *Olmstead v. LC* (1999) the Court ruled that states could not force segregation of individuals with disabilities into state institutions in order to receive services. According to the Court, states must provide a range of services in the community so society does not prevent individuals with disabilities from participating in community life—an opportunity afforded to individuals without disabilities. This policy opened opportunities for occupational and physical therapy practitioners to serve more individuals with disabilities in community-based programs as the states scrambled to put together Olmstead-compliance plans.

Laws do not change by themselves. Occupational and physical therapy practitioners can play a key role in advocacy for public policies that help those they serve. As professionals, readers must endeavor to familiarize themselves with the key public policy initiatives that will affect their practice and the people they serve and stay current with these issues on an ongoing basis. This chapter examines some of those public policies with which rehabilitation professionals regularly work: Medicare and Medicaid, the Fair Housing Act, the Individuals with Disabilities Education Act (IDEA), and the Americans with Disabilities Act (ADA). While this chapter provides readers with background information, readers must keep in mind that, as the previous examples showed, these policies often change based upon the passage of new laws and regulations and appellate court decisions.

PUBLIC POLICY AND DISABILITY

Since the 1960s and the initiatives of President Lyndon B. Johnson, there has been a large amount of legislation directed at policy areas such as health care and civil rights for individuals with disabilities. Every piece of legislation impacts not only the individuals directly affected, but also those professionals who provide services in the field of disability. A few landmark pieces of legislation are presented in the following paragraphs. Each piece of legislation mentioned has a significant day-to-day impact on the practice of rehabilitation.

MEDICARE

Medicare, created in 1965 as Title 18 of the Social Security Act, is a health insurance program run by the federal government. Originally intended for individuals over age 65, in 1972 Medicare coverage was extended to younger individuals with permanent disabilities and individuals with permanent kidney failure requiring dialysis or transplant (end-stage renal disease, or ESRD). The Centers for Medicare and Medicaid Services (CMS)[2] oversee the Medicare program, which provides services to 39 million Americans (Booth, 2002). By 2030 CMS estimates that Medicare will serve 77 million Americans (Booth, 2002).

When the Medicare program started in 1966, more than 19 million individuals enrolled. By 1970 there were 20 million Americans enrolled (Booth, 2002), and by 1980, more than 28 million individuals were enrolled. As the numbers grew, so did expenses. Hospitals initially received reimbursement using a cost-based system. They received payment of a fee for their services plus additional funds for certain other allowable costs. However, because of rising costs, the government changed its payment system for hospitals from a cost-based system to a PPS, under which, as explained earlier, a set amount of money is received by the facility based upon the patient's diagnosis. This situation shifted costs to long-term-care facilities and home-health-care programs as patients found themselves quickly discharged to these alternatives to hospitalization. With the passage of the Balanced Budget Act of 1997, Congress sought to decrease long-term-care costs by instituting a PPS in long-term-care facilities (Balanced Budget Act of 1997, 1997). It also sought to control outpatient costs by putting a dollar-amount cap on certain outpatient therapy services (Balanced Budget Act of 1997, 1997). Additional laws and regulations will soon put similar controls on occupational and physical therapy in other Medicare-covered settings.

Though CMS oversees the Medicare program, it contracts with *fiscal intermediaries* to handle the actual claims for benefits. Such intermediaries are usually insurance companies under contract with the government to review the claims for services such as

---

[2]This agency was formally known as the Health Care Financing Administration (HCFA).

occupational and physical therapy and decide whether to pay them.

Medicare plays a key role in the provision of occupational and physical therapy services as a major source of health-care reimbursement for older adults and individuals with disabilities. Occupational and physical therapy practitioners will find themselves working under Medicare programs if they work in long-term-care facilities, home-health-care programs, inpatient or outpatient hospital programs, free-standing clinics, rehabilitation centers, private practices, and other settings. Providing services under Medicare means therapists must write thorough documentation to justify treatment so it can withstand any audits the fiscal intermediaries may undertake.

As a significant source of reimbursement, occupational and physical therapy practitioners should familiarize themselves with the basics of how Medicare works and stay current with the changes that happen in public policy regarding Medicare. For example, as discussed in Chapter 18, in 2003 Congress mandated several different ways to cover prescription drugs under the Medicare program, a service not presently covered. Changes that affect therapy practice can occur, and therapists must make themselves aware of the changes as they happen and proactively look at proposed changes.

Medicare consists of two types of insurance: *Part A,* which covers hospital insurance, and *Part B,* which covers medical benefits. Part A covers some of the cost of hospital stays, skilled-nursing-facility stays, home-health-care services, hospice care, and blood received in a hospital or skilled nursing facility. Part B covers some of the cost of medical and other services, including occupational and physical therapy, clinical laboratory services, home health care, and outpatient hospital services, including blood received as an outpatient (Centers for Medicare & Medicaid Services, 2003).

Most people over age 65 and eligible for Part A receive it without the need to pay a premium because the individual, or his spouse, paid a Medicare tax through his employer for a period of 10 years or more. An individual (or her spouse) over 65 who did not pay Medicare taxes may purchase Part A coverage if she is a U.S. citizen or permanent resident (Unknown, no date given).

Individuals under 65 may receive Part A coverage without paying a premium if they have received disability benefits under Social Security or the Railroad Retirement Board for a period of 24 months. Individuals with Lou Gehrig's disease need not wait 24 months but are eligible for premium-free Part A coverage the first month they receive social security disability benefits. Individuals with end-stage renal disease are also entitled to premium-free Part A (Unknown, no date given). While Part A is premium-free for most Medicare beneficiaries, everyone pays a fee for Part B coverage (Centers for Medicare & Medicaid Services, 2003).

When Congress passed the Medicare law, it did not include coverage for occupational therapy services. Over time, the American Occupational Therapy Association (AOTA) lobbied members of Congress to include occupational therapy services in Medicare. Gradually, occupational therapy coverage found its way into the services provided, with some exceptions. For example, occupational therapy services were not covered in home health care. After extensive lobbying campaigns, occupational therapy services were accepted as a covered service in home health care with some limitations. While physical therapy and speech and language pathology services are considered primary services, occupational therapy is not. In order for an occupational therapist to see a home-care patient, someone else on the team—physical therapist, speech and language pathologist, or nurse—must open the case and "recommend" or refer the patient to occupational therapy. The American Occupational Therapy Association continues to lobby to fix this quirk in the system.

Under Medicare today, covered occupational and physical therapy services are reimbursed under both Part A and Part B. Part A covers certain services provided in skilled nursing facilities and home-health-care settings. Part B covers outpatient occupational and physical therapy services provided in hospitals and outpatient clinics, and outpatient therapy services provided by home-care agencies (Centers for Medicare & Medicaid Services, 2003).

Some services provided under Medicare require that patients pay co-insurance or deductibles before becoming eligible for Medicare reimbursement. **Co-insurance** is health (or prescription) insurance in which the insured is obligated to accept payment on a claim at some predetermined value (Merriam-Webster, 1996). A **deductible** is "a clause in an insurance policy that exempts the insurer from paying an initial specified amount in the event that the insured sustains a loss" (American Heritage Dictionary, 2000, http://dictionary.reference.com/search?r=2&q=deductible). For example, Part B Medicare patients must pay 20 percent for all outpatient occupational and physical therapy services. Under Part A, patients pay a significant deductible and/or co-insurance for their hospital stay, and only a certain number of days are covered. Under Part A, patients pay nothing for their first 20 days in a skilled nursing facility but must pay an amount just over $100 per day for days 21 through 100 (Centers for Medicare & Medicaid Services, 2003).

To avoid some of these charges, or lessen the amount of them, some Medicare beneficiaries join *Medicare Managed Care Plans.* These plans must offer, at a minimum, the benefits offered by Part A and Part B; however, they often offer a broader range of coverage of services, such as drug coverage and lower co-insurance and deductibles. This is in exchange for limiting the choices of health-care providers to primary-care providers and other restrictions. The Medicare Managed Care Plans usually limit the amount of occupational and physical therapy services.

Another policy-related issue under Medicare is that only the durable medical equipment it views as "medically necessary," such as wheelchair rental, are covered. It will not pay for shower/tub benches, raised toilet seats, or grab bars, which are often necessary following an accident or illness. Also, some fiscal intermediaries pay for certain interventions that others do not. These concerns point to the need for occupational and physical therapy professionals to know the provisions of Medicare, advocate for changes to the program that benefit those we serve, and keep up with changes as they occur.

MEDICAID

Enacted into law in 1965 as Title 19 of the Social Security Act, **Medicaid**[3] is a joint federal/state program that provides basic medical care to approximately 36 million medically indigent individuals. Such individuals qualify for Medicaid based on their low income or their qualifications for public assistance programs such as *Supplemental Security Income (SSI)*. Unlike the case with Medicare, Medicaid recipients do not pay premiums for the health-care benefits they receive, since the Medicaid program provides services to the poor. However, under certain limited circumstances, states may impose nominal deductibles or co-payments on certain recipients (Social Security Administration, 2001). Also unlike Medicare, the type, amount, scope, and type of benefits offered vary by state. The state determines its own eligibility standards, sets the rates for payment for services to providers, and administers its own program (Wilmer, 2002). For example, some states, such as New York, cover occupational therapy benefits for adults, while other states, such as Florida, do not necessarily provide coverage for occupational therapy services in the adult population.

States must cover "categorically needy individuals." Categorically needy individuals usually include

- Low-income families with children.
- Individuals receiving SSI.
- Pregnant women, infants, and children with incomes less than a specified percent of the federal poverty level.
- Qualified Medicare beneficiaries (Social Security Administration, 2001).

In addition to the required coverage for the categorically needy, states may optionally choose to cover the cost of medical care for persons considered "medically needy." These individuals include those who would qualify for Medicaid on the basis of their need for services but their income, while not enough to pay for the medical services they need, exceeds the program's limits. Since "medically needy" programs are optional, not all states have them. States can elect coverage for other optional groups, such as

- The medically needy aged, blind, or disabled individuals.
- Members of families with dependent children who have too much income and/or resources to be eligible for cash assistance but not enough for medical care.
- Aged and disabled persons with incomes less than 100 percent of the poverty level.
- Institutionalized persons with incomes no greater than 300 percent of the SSI federal benefit rate (Social Security Administration, 2001).

Though states are not required to provide services to the medically needy, if they do elect to cover them, they must provide, at a minimum, the following:

- Prenatal care and delivery services for pregnant women
- Ambulatory services to individuals under age 18 and individuals entitled to institutional services
- Home health care to individuals entitled to nursing facility services
- If the state plan includes services either in institutions for mental diseases or in intermediate care facilities for the mentally retarded (ICF/MRs), it must offer either of the following to each of the medically needy groups: (1) the services contained in 42 CFR sections 440.10 through 440.50 and 440.165 (to the extent that nurse-midwives are authorized to practice under state law or regulations); or (2) the services contained in any seven of the sections in 42 CFR 440.10 through 440.165 (Dulany, 2002c)

In order to receive federal funds for Medicaid, the state must provide categorically needy individuals with at least the following minimal services:

- Inpatient hospital services
- Outpatient hospital services
- Rural health clinic services
- Laboratory and X-ray services
- Nursing facility services
- Home health care for individuals age 21 or older
- Family planning services and supplies
- Early and periodic screening, diagnosis, and treatment for individuals under age 21

---

[3]In California, the Medicaid program is called *Medi-cal.*

- Certified midwife services and physician services
- Certified pediatric and family nurse practitioner services
- Federally qualified ambulatory and health center services

In addition to these required services, states can choose to provide other services, such as prescription drug, occupational therapy, and physical therapy services.

Though all states are required to provide some basic services, there are some exceptions to these rules. Under the law, states can request a *waiver* of the Medicaid rules from the Secretary of Health and Human Services to try innovative or experimental programs to enhance the provision of benefits in a cost-effective manner (Dulany, 2002a). For example, the state of "Chaos" may place its Medicaid recipients into *health maintenance organizations (HMOs)* as a method of expanding coverage and keeping costs in check. However, just because "Chaos" does this, it does not mean that the state of "Grace" will have all of its Medicaid recipients in HMOs, because each state is different.

Occupational and physical therapists will find that coverage for therapy services varies by state as well. Some states may cover therapy services for children but not adults, for example. Others may cover therapy services only for individuals with disabilities. Some may limit the number of visits allotted for therapy services. As states experience budget deficits and competition for limited funds, therapists may find currently existing coverage for occupational and physical therapy in jeopardy. Occupational and physical therapists should familiarize themselves with the benefits available in their own states and advocate for coverage for the clients they serve. Each state maintains a Web site with up-to-date information on its own Medicaid program. Readers can reach their own state's Medicaid program Web site from links located at http://cms.hhs.gov/medicaid/stwebsites.asp.

As the government changes its policy emphases, new programs may come and go. For example, various grant-funded demonstration projects currently exist under Medicaid to promote increased employment of individuals with disabilities (Dulany, 2002b). As with all public policy, Medicaid provisions change, and those changes can affect occupational and physical therapy practice as well as the individuals we serve. Therefore, therapists should keep up with the latest changes in Medicaid and anticipate changes before they become law.

REHABILITATION ACT

The **Rehabilitation Act of 1973** (also called the *Rehab Act*) was one of the first significant pieces of civil rights legislation for individuals with disabilities (Lunnen,

1999). *Section 504* of the Rehabilitation Act is often cited because it contains language indicating that individuals with disabilities cannot be discriminated against in any program (including public education) that receives federal sources of funding. This law obviously paved the way for more comprehensive legislation relating to the right to education for individuals with disabilities (Lunnen, 1999).

INDIVIDUALS WITH DISABILITIES EDUCATION ACT (IDEA)

In 1975 Congress passed the Education for All Handicapped Children Act of 1975. The intent of this act was to provide adequate education for "handicapped children," assist states in providing these services, and evaluate the effectiveness of implemented programs in the United States (Mills, 1996). It was created to address the problem of 8 million disabled children with unmet educational needs in the public school system, and another 1 million children with special needs who did not even attend school due to their disabilities (Mills, 1996). Legislative changes that led to the Education for All Handicapped Children Act were a result of parent advocacy groups that increased awareness of disabled students' needs (Rosenbaum, 1998). The key ethical issue of ensuring equal educational opportunities for all children was a critical factor in establishing this law. This law was considered the most important legislation related to children's services at the time. The congressional commitment to furthering educational standards for children with disabilities was exemplified at the time by congressional authorization to pay 40 percent of the cost of educating children with disabilities, increasing to 66 percent through Part B state grants by 2001 (Mills, 1996). The government provides federal funds to state and local educational agencies for the sole purpose of providing special education and related services to children with disabilities.

The implementation of the Education for All Handicapped Children Act allowed numerous therapists to have a role in the public education sector as related service providers. This increased the number of job opportunities and resulted in a new awareness of what therapists can contribute outside the medical model. Many students have benefited from the provision of educationally relevant services within the school environment. Parental and professional advocacy was shown to have made a difference for children with special needs.

IDEA TODAY

In 1990, Congress amended the Education for All Handicapped Children Act, changing the name to the

Individuals with Disabilities Education Act, which is commonly represented by the acronym **IDEA.** Additions included the expansion of services for younger children and more parental involvement in program planning and decision making.

In June of 1997 the IDEA was amended and reauthorized and is now known as *Public Law 105-17* (Individuals with Disabilities Education Act of 1997, 1997). The IDEA (1997) continues to ensure that special education is provided for students with disabilities within the public education setting. This legislation requires public school personnel to meet the unique needs of individual students in a "free and appropriate" manner (Osborne, 1999).

In order to understand current issues related to IDEA, it is important to highlight some historical perspectives and purposes of the amendments that included provisions for disciplinary action for children with disabilities and an increased role for general education teachers. Amendments also emphasize increased team involvement, including parents, in the decision-making processes.

The IDEA (Individuals with Disabilities Education Act Amendments of 1997, 1997) was again considered for reauthorization beginning in 2002–3. Key points under discussion include school district management of disciplinary actions; continued federal support for special education and related services; over-identification of minority children; and preventive services. The reauthorization process presents another opportunity for parents and professionals to advocate and become politically involved to ensure improved services for children and families. As of May 2004, the Senate passed a bill to reauthorize IDEA that differed from the House bill passed in 2003. As occurred in 1997, a special joint committee will meet to resolve these differences (Wrightslaw, 2004).

POLITICAL ACTION REGARDING IDEA

A current concern of parents is the ability of the school district to suspend and even expel children with disruptive behaviors, which was not the case before the 1997 amendments. In this regard, the legal standpoint of dismissal has clashed, and will clash, with the parents' views of what is considered ethical for their children.

Proper implementation of IDEA 1997 and full participation of parents can limit dissatisfaction among the family members. The importance of proper notification of meetings and parent participation in decision making is evident in cases such as *Union School District v. Smith* (1994). In this case, the parents of a child with autism sought reimbursement for private clinic services after a dispute with school officials about appropriate placement (Daniel, 2000). The school district claimed that the parents were unwilling to accept appropriate

public school placement. However, the school had not provided information to the parents about alternatives or available resources within the public school setting. The court stated that these aspects of IDEA should be enforced. This case not only illustrates the significance of adhering to the amendments, but it focused on a child in one diagnostic category that then led to mandates to the school district that are common in these types of court cases. It is interesting to note that children with autism quite often have behavioral problems, requiring some type of behavioral plan and disciplinary approach. This provides opportunities for occupational therapists, in particular, to become more involved in psychosocial aspects of participation in daily occupations related to the school environment.

Health professionals can become more involved in advocacy on many levels. Specific examples of involvement related to IDEA include the following actions:

1. Increase awareness of the specific policy and the parameters of service as they relate specifically to occupational and physical therapists.
2. Seek out information from your professional organizations.
3. Read updates on the law through school-based and professional Listservs.
4. Communicate and collaborate with parents regarding children and family rights.
5. Become involved with professional organizations' political action committees.
6. Contact your congressional representatives regarding your support for IDEA.
7. Work collaboratively with special and general education teachers to ensure best practice standards.

Other types of involvement can include advocacy within the school environment. The collaborative language of the changes in IDEA between general education teachers, special education teachers, and related services calls for a greater transdisciplinary emphasis in individual program planning and implementation. One of the concerns, however, is the effectiveness of a general education teacher when confronted with a child who has a pattern of disruptive behavior, such as verbal outbursts or physical aggression.

The expectation that general education teachers can manage these types of challenges is high and perhaps unreasonable. Although involvement of general education teachers is a distinct part of the amendments, there are no specific guidelines as to the proper and adequate training of personnel for these types of experiences. The individual school districts must clarify the intent of the law and independently prepare general educators for these increased challenges. Future strategies should incorporate more training for general educators in behavioral management strategies and in dealing with varying abilities of children with special needs.

With school violence on a significant rise, schools need to take a proactive stance to ensure the full and safe participation in activities for all students. Children with special needs may have patterns of behavior that are disruptive or aggressive. Dayton (2000) considers the initial *Individualized Education Plan (IEP)* meeting to be an optimal time for discussing behavioral management plans before negative incidents occur. The IEP also can provide a framework for positive behavioral support. Sugai and Tindal (1993), among others, advocate for a multilevel approach to managing behaviors, with the lower level consisting of milder strategies and the higher level incorporating structured behavioral plans based on functional behavior assessments.

Preventive strategies that schools could incorporate include the provision of consistent structure, early notification to students when schedules or routines change, the inclusion of the student in the decision-making process when feasible, and encouraging parents to participate more in the classroom setting than is typical. Consistency affords a sense of security for those students who have difficulty with change and transitions to other activities. This consistency can help to minimize behavioral problems. In addition, the consistency of consequences for negative behaviors and reinforcements for positive behaviors can minimize problems. Students who are cognitively able to contribute to their own program plan by stating the factors that precede outbursts or problems should be allowed to do so. A forum should exist that incorporates their participation and input into program planning. At times, this could incorporate their contribution to even the behavioral intervention plan. Parent participation in the classroom might also help to raise the awareness of teacher challenges and empower the parents even more to contribute at the IEP meetings. Parents may also feel that they have an opportunity to try strategies in the classroom themselves before dismissing them, or advocating for another methodology in the IEP meeting. Therapists working in the school environment can assist in facilitating optimal implementation of IDEA through these specific strategies and others.

FAIR HOUSING ACT AMENDMENTS (FHAA)

The **Fair Housing Act Amendments of 1988 (FHAA)** amended Title VIII of the Civil Rights Act of 1968, 42 U.S.C. 3601 et seq., to add "individuals with disabilities"[4] to the list of people protected from housing

discrimination under the existing law that protected individuals based on race, color, religion, sex, national origin, and familial status (Fair Housing Act Amendments, 1988). The definition of "individuals with disabilities" in FHAA is the same as the ADA's definition. The FHAA requires that housing providers must make reasonable accommodations to rules, policies, and practices or services when the accommodation is necessary to allow a person with a disability equal enjoyment of a dwelling or common areas (24 CFR §100.204). The FHAA also makes it unlawful discrimination to refuse to allow a person with disabilities to make reasonable modifications to a dwelling or a public or common area—at that person's own expense—so the person can gain full use and enjoyment of the premises (24 CFR §203).

AMERICANS WITH DISABILITIES ACT (ADA)

Congress passed the **Americans with Disabilities Act (ADA)** in 1990, Pub. L. No. 101-336, (1990) 42 USC 12101 et seq., to promote the civil rights of individuals with disabilities in the mainstream of society in employment, state and local government services, places of public accommodations, transportation and telecommunication (Americans with Disabilities Act, 1990). Prior to the passage of the ADA, the Rehabilitation Act of 1973 (Rehab Act) afforded individuals with disabilities some protection in employment and the provision of other services if provided by federal government agencies or private entities that benefited from, or received, federal funds (Section 504 of the Rehabilitation Act of 1973, 1973). By enacting the ADA, Congress expanded the public policy goals of the Rehab Act, broadening its reach to private entities. Table 20–1 lists the five titles of the ADA.

Title I of the ADA prohibits discrimination against individuals with disabilities in employment by a private, nongovernment employer (*University of Alabama v. Garrett*, 2001). Included in the definition of *discrimination*

TABLE 20–1	Americans with Disabilities Act—Five Titles
Title I	Employment
Title II	State & Local Government Services & Transportation
Title III	Public Accommodations
Title IV	Telecommunications
Title V	Miscellaneous Provisions

---

[4]Though the law uses the term "handicap," this text uses the phrase "individuals with disabilities," since the latter reflects more contemporary terminology known as "people first" language.

is the failure to make reasonable accommodations for qualified individuals with a disability. Rehabilitation professionals often become involved in employment cases where their skills can promote better function in the workplace. The ADA opened the doors to certain practice areas for therapy practitioners. Case study 2, titled "Nancy," at the end of this chapter, illustrates the role of the occupational or physical therapy practitioner under the employment provisions of the ADA.

Some worry that the ADA interferes with business operations and forces employers to do things they do not want to do. However, the ADA does not require that employers hire everyone with a disability who fills out an employment application. Rather, the ADA aims to level the playing field so individuals with disabilities have an opportunity for employment in positions for which they can perform the essential functions and for which they are qualified. Thus, an employer would not have to hire an individual with a disability who could not do the job or was not qualified for the position. Not every employee is entitled to an accommodation in the workplace. There is a three-step inquiry process to determine whether an employee needs or is entitled to an accommodation, shown in Table 20–2.

The first question is whether the worker is an individual with a disability. There are three definitions of *disability*, and the worker must meet one of them. The worker must show that she has a physical or mental impairment that substantially limits one or more major life activities, has a history of such an impairment, or is currently regarded as having such an impairment. If

the worker meets the definition, the next inquiry is whether she is qualified for the job (See Table 20-2). Finally, if the individual is a qualified individual with a disability, the final question is whether the accommodation is reasonable.

Though the ADA sounds like a rosy solution for our clients, the courts have interpreted this law in a very narrow way, and many individuals find they do not qualify as having a disability. However, therapy practitioners can play an advocacy role with their patients and clients who plan to go back to work. Patients and clients need to familiarize themselves with their own workplace limitations and learn about accommodations that can enable their work performance and participation. Educating clients can go a long way toward returning them to the workplace with needed accommodations or alternative ways to perform job tasks.

Therapy practitioners can also help assess the precise limitations that affect a person's performance. In *Williams v. Toyota Motor Mfg.* (Williams v. Toyota Motor Mfg., 2002), the U.S. Supreme Court said that when one claims a limitation in the "major life activity of performing manual tasks, the central inquiry must be whether the claimant is unable to perform the variety of tasks central to most people's lives, not whether the claimant is unable to perform the tasks associated with her specific job." Therapy practitioners can answer this inquiry.

Title II of the ADA applies to services provided by state and local governments. State and local governments must make the programs and services they provide

| TABLE 20–2 | Reasonable Accommodations Decision Progression© |

Step I: Is the Worker an Individual with a Disability?

1. a physical or mental impairment that substantially limits one or more major life activities;
2. a history of having had such an impairment; or
3. Regarded as having such an impairment.

***If the worker is *not* an individual with a disability, the employer does not have to accommodate.

Step 2: Is the Worker a Qualified Individual with a Disability?

1. Individual satisfies the requisite skills, experience, education, and other job-related requirements of the job; and
2. Individual can perform the essential functions of such position with or without reasonable accommodations.

***If the Worker is *not* a qualified individual with a disability, the employer does not have to accommodate.

Step 3: Is the Accommodation Reasonable?

1. How much does the accommodation cost in relationship to the size and budget of the business?
2. Are there tax credits or deductions or outside funding sources to pay for the accommodation?
3. Does the accommodation interfere with the operation of the business or the ability of other employees to perform their duties?

***If it is *not* reasonable, the employer does not have to accommodate.

Used with permission of ADA Consultants, Inc.

accessible to individuals with disabilities. This could include, for example, access to classes provided at public universities, to voting, and to parks and recreational programs. State and local governments may look to therapy practitioners for ideas on ways to provide access to their programs and services to individuals with disabilities.

Title III of the ADA provides that privately owned places of public accommodations must allow access for their customers with disabilities to the goods, services, facilities, and advantages they offer to the public. These places include, for example, theaters, doctors' offices, golf courses, hotels, retail establishments, day-care centers, gas stations, and hospitals. This section of the ADA helps those we serve participate in community life. Places of public accommodations are required to make reasonable accommodations for individuals with disabilities so they may enjoy what these accommodations offer to the public. These privately owned places of public accommodations cannot refuse to serve individuals with disabilities and cannot segregate individuals with disabilities. For example, a day-care center cannot refuse admission to a child simply because the child is

an individual with a disability. A movie theater must offer amplifiers for those with hearing impairments. A doctor's office must allow a service animal to accompany an individual with a disability to a doctor's appointment. Often, places of public accommodations need assistance and consultation to develop reasonable accommodations. Occupational and physical therapy practitioners can provide this assistance. They can also help their clients problem-solve the types of accommodations they will need to function more independently in the community.

Title IV of the ADA sets up a system of telecommunications for individuals with hearing impairments. A relay service is in place to allow communication through Telecommunication Devices for the Deaf (TDD) with those who do not have hearing impairments. These *text telephones* can allow individuals with hearing impairments access to telephone services. Title IV also requires closed-captioning for federally funded public service announcements. This is good information to share with clients as the population ages and occupational and physical therapists find themselves dealing with more individuals with hearing impairments.

SUMMARY

Occupational and physical therapists do not practice in isolation from the politics of policies and laws in the United States. Certain laws protect the rights of those we serve. As professionals, therapists have a professional responsibility to familiarize ourselves with laws

and policies that affect therapy practice and the lives of those we serve. Advocating for these laws promotes independence for our clients and patients and is part of our professional responsibility.

CASE

1

Mrs. Johnson

While recovering from a fractured hip, Mrs. Johnson is diagnosed with multiple sclerosis. Occupational therapy recommends that her family install grab bars in the bathroom of her apartment and a raised toilet seat. Physical therapy recommends a parking space close to her apartment due to her limited endurance. A home program is set up for Mrs. Johnson to perform her exercises in her apartment complex's swimming pool. Since she requires assistance in the pool, a member of her church has volunteered to help her in the pool, and the therapists have trained this person to assist her. Shortly before her discharge, the family reports to the therapists that the landlord refused to allow them to put in a grab bar. He also will not give Mrs. Johnson a parking space close to the building, because no one has "reserved" parking in the complex. The family further reports that the complex's pool rules do not allow guests in the pool after 3:00 in the afternoon weekdays and not at all on weekends. These are

Continues

Case 1   Continued

the only times her church member can help Mrs. Johnson with her home water-exercise program. Everyone is frustrated and angry over all of the plans that were made and are now thwarted.

Not all is lost, however. The FHAA of 1988 considers Mrs. Johnson's landlord's behavior discrimination—discrimination against individuals with disabilities for housing opportunities. Occupational and physical therapy practitioners can help their clients advocate for their rights in situations like this. This advocacy makes a significant difference in people's lives and in some situations can make the difference between living independently and living in a nursing home or other institution.

In this case study, it would be a reasonable accommodation to modify the pool rules for Mrs. Johnson so she could enjoy the pool with the assistance of her fellow church member during normally "non-guest" hours. This could be done by adding grab bars to help Mrs. Johnson get in and out of the pool. It would also be reasonable to assign Mrs. Johnson a parking space close to the building even though no one else has an assigned space. Failure to make these accommodations would be discrimination. Should Mrs. Johnson face this restriction, she can file a complaint for discrimination to the U.S. Department of Housing and Urban Development at http://www.hud.gov /complaints/housediscrim.cfm.

CASE
2

Nancy

Nancy, a nurse with post-polio syndrome and arthritic changes, finds herself tiring easily at work. She requests accommodations from her employer to decrease the amount of energy she expends on the job. She suggests that she use a scooter at work to cut down the number of steps she must take during her workday. Nursing management makes it very clear that it cannot possibly imagine "a nurse in a wheelchair." With her employer unwilling to make this accommodation, Nancy files a complaint for employment discrimination with the Equal Employment Opportunity Commission. The Human Resources Department, alerted to the complaint, calls in an occupational therapist for advice on how to make reasonable accommodations in the workplace. The occupational therapist performs a job analysis and determines that the scooter is a safe accommodation that meets Nancy's needs and does not interfere with her job performance except during emergencies. After some hand-holding with the nurse managers, the hospital administration allows Nancy to perform her nursing job using a scooter during non-emergency job functions. The occupational therapist recommends relocating the charts to a more convenient location. The final recommendation gives Nancy her own key to the supply closet so she need not go back and forth from the patient rooms to the nurse's station repeatedly to get the key. Staff readily accepts the final recommendations, Nancy's complaint is settled, and Nancy continues in her staff nursing position.

Oh! The Politics of Health Care!

HUGH MURRAY, PT, DMDT
PRESIDENT, HUNTINGTON PHYSICAL THERAPY

When I graduated from PT school back in the dark ages I was excited about my future. I possessed a solid base of knowledge. This solid base was a little information on just about everything. The chance to learn more was on the horizon, and coming toward me hourly. I was excited about life, about gaining more knowledge, and about the success I was having with patients in their recovery. I was now flying along, not to be stopped or to even be slowed in my pace toward the goal of learning more and successfully treating *my* patients. I was working in an acute care hospital. The Physical Therapy Department was located between the emergency room and radiology. This was a great location to observe more and enhance my education.

All was going along well until certain events in my life radically changed my rose-colored glasses perception of health care. I was of the opinion that I could evaluate and treat patients as if I were an island. An island of health care! Evaluating and treating patients with the best education I could achieve, some minimal experience, and the most recent research I read the night before was my life's work. That was my professional track.

This happy little freight train quickly derailed from that track. Here are just a few examples:

- A disgruntled patient confronted me early one morning, stating that Workers' Compensation had stopped his benefits because of the "noncompliant" letter I sent to his doctor.
- A doctor was upset with me because I told the patient he had a disk problem. What does a diagnosis mean, anyway? Do I have the right to do this—or is it limited to the doctor?
- The director of the department met with me to provide an "in-service," because Medicare was changing the regulations and now there were certain treatments for which there was no reimbursement. Now I could not provide this service because there was no payment. But I thought I was supposed to provide the best and most appropriate treatment dictated by my professional judgment, not by what would be reimbursed.
- The hospital was unionized, and my fellow employees voted to strike. They walked out and did not return for 28 days. Some employees did not return for 9 months due to scheduling. (I worked 12-hour days for 28 days in Central Supply because the patient census had dwindled.) Administration wants the PT staff to join the union. What does that mean to me personally? Is this professionally ethical?
- The legislature in its great wisdom has decided chiropractors can provide physical therapy—but did not conversely decide that physical therapists could provide chiropractic care. In the meantime, the political action committee (PAC) for PT raised $3,000—while the chiropractic PAC raised $40,000. I wonder if this has anything to do with the legislative initiative.
- Our state practice act is up for "review" in 2009; we could all be unlicensed then.
- Medicare has a $1,500 cap on physical therapy and speech therapy as *one* health-care provider, but a $1,500 cap on OT as a separate provider. How did that happen???

I did not receive any education regarding these politics in PT school.

I still love the profession of physical therapy after gaining more experience over all of these years. But what I know now is, there never was an island for my practice. It was a myth! I am part of a huge political system that impacts my ability to deliver care as well as the scope of care I can legally provide. For that reason, I have worked over the years to become politically informed *and* politically active. I think this is a responsibility we all must accept. I remain in the trenches because I am still excited regarding life, my continuing acquisition of knowledge, and the success I am having with my patients.

But, oh! The politics of health care!

REFERENCES

The American Heritage® Dictionary of the English Language. (2000). (4th ed.). Boston: Houghton Mifflin.

Americans with Disabilities Act. (1990). *42 USC 12101 et seq.*

Balanced Budget Act of 1997. (1997). P. L. 105-33.

Booth, J. G. (March 6, 2002). *Medicare's milestone.* Centers for Medicare & Medicaid Services. Retrieved June 1, 2003, from http://cms.hhs.gov/about/history/ mcaremil.asp.

Centers for Medicare & Medicaid Services. (2003). *Medicare & you 2003.* U.S. Department of Health & Human Services. Retrieved June 1, 2003, from www.medicare .gov/publications/pub/pdf/10050.pdf.

Daniel, P. (2000). Education for students with special needs: The judicially defined role of parents in the process. *Journal of Law and Education, 29(1),* 1–30.

Dulany, J. (2002a, July 24, 2002). *1115 waiver research and demonstration projects.* Centers for Medicare and Medicaid Services. Retrieved May 31, 2003, from http://cms.hhs .gov/medicaid/1115/default.asp.

Dulany, J. (2002b, December 2, 2002). *Demonstration to maintain independence and employment.* Center for Medicare & Medicaid Services. Retrieved May 31, 2003, from http://cms.hhs.gov/twwiia/independ.asp.

Dulany, J. (2002c, September 3, 2002). *Medicaid services.* Center for Medicare & Medicaid Services. Retrieved May 31, 2003, from http://cms.hhs.gov/medicaid/mservice .asp.

Education for All Handicapped Children Act of 1975. (1975). *20 U.S.C. 33 §1401 et. seq.*

Fair Housing Act Amendments Act of 1988. (1988). *42 U.S.C. 3601 et. seq.*

Individuals with Disabilities Education Act. (1990). *20 U.S.C. 33 §1401 et. seq.*

Individuals with Disabilities Education Act Amendments of 1997. (1997). *20 USC 33 §1401 et seq.*

Lunnen, K. (1999) Physical therapy in the public schools. In J. Tecklin (Ed.), *Pediatric physical therapy* (2nd ed.) (pp. 562–578). Philadelphia: Lippincott, Williams & Wilkins.

Mills, D. (1996). Beyond weapons: The case for including a dangerousness exception to the "stay put" provision of the Individuals with Disabilities Education Act (IDEA). *Journal of Juvenile Law, 17,* 94–106.

Olmstead v. L.C. (1999). S. Ct. (Vol. 119, pp. 2176).

Osborne, A. (1999). Students with disabilities. *The Yearbook of Education Law, 139-79.*

Rosenbaum, P., King, S., Law, M., King, G., & Evans, J. (1998). Family-centered service: A conceptual framework and research review. *Physical and Occupational Therapy in Pediatrics, 18(1),* 1–20.

Section 504 of the Rehabilitation Act of 1973. (1973). *29 USC 794.*

Shi, L., & Singh, D. A. (2001). Delivering health care in America: A systems approach. Gaithersburg, MD: Aspen Publications.

Social Security Administration. (March 2001). *Social Security Handbook §2309. Medical assistance.* Social Security Administration. Retrieved May 31, 2003, from http://www.ssa.gov/OP_Home/handbook/handbook.23 /handbook-2309.html.

Union School District c. Smith. (1994). *F.3d* (Vol. 15, pp. 1519): 9th Cir. Ct App.

University of Alabama v. Garrett. (2001). U.S. (Vol. 531, pp. 356).

Unknown. (no date given). *Who is eligible for Medicare?* Centers for Medicare & Medicaid Services. Retrieved June 1, 2003, from http://medicare.custhelp.com/cgi-bin/ medicare.cfg/php/enduser/std_adp.php?p_sid=y_l _cIKg&p_lva=&p_faqid=10&p_created=993576517&p_sp =cF9zcmNoPSZwX2dyaWRzb3J0PSZwX3Jvd19jbnQ9Mjk zJnBfcGFnZT0x&p_li=.

Williams v. Toyota Motor Mfg. (2002). U.S. (Vol. 534, pp. 184).

Wilmer, T. (2002, 9/6/02). *Overview of the Medicaid Program.* Center for Medicare & Medicaid Services. Retrieved May 31, 2003, from http://cms.hhs.gov/medicaid/mover.asp.

World Health Organization. (2002). *ICF: International Classification of Functioning and Disability.* Geneva, Switzerland: World Health Organization.

Wrightslaw. (2004). IDEA alert: Senate passes bill to reauthorize IDEA by 95-3 vote. Retrieved June 4, 2004, from http://www.wrightslaw.com/nltr/04.

CHAPTER 21

Assessment of Human Performance across the Lifespan

Toby Long, PhD, PT
Associate Professor, Department
of Pediatrics
Associate Director for Training,
Center for Child and Human
Development
Director, Division of Physical
Therapy, Center for Child and
Human Development
Georgetown University,
Washington, D.C.

Objectives

Upon completion of this chapter, the reader should be able to

▨ Differentiate the processes of examination, evaluation, assessment, and screening.

▨ Use the results of these processes in clinical decision making.

▨ Describe a wide variety of measurement tools and their theoretical underpinnings.

▨ Describe models used to assess individuals.

Key Terms

arena assessment	ecological approach	routines-based assessment
assessment	evaluation process	screening process
bottom-up assessment	evaluative assessment strategy	standardized test
criterion-referenced	judgment-based assessment	top-down assessment
discriminative index	norm-referenced	

INTRODUCTION

The use of formal measurement strategies by physical therapists and occupational therapists has increased dramatically over the last 30 years. Several factors have influenced this change in practice. First, public policy and legislative initiatives have provoked therapists and other professionals to reassess basic methods of collecting developmental, behavioral, or functional information. The passage of Part B (PL 94-142) of the Individuals with Disabilities Education Act (IDEA) in 1975 required therapists working in educational systems to serve children within an educational framework, work in a multidisciplinary team, and recognize the interrelatedness of motor skills with other areas of development. Since that time, therapists have broadened their systems and strategies of gathering information about a child's performance and provision of service to include collaboration with the family and other team members.

Contemporary evaluation and assessment strategies, in conjunction with intervention, support collaboration among family and team members, integration of findings across domains and environments, as well as reporting of findings in a manner that is family-centered and culturally sensitive. Finally, the Joint Commission on the Accreditation of Healthcare Organizations (JCAHO, 1994) stresses the importance of establishing an effective information-collecting system to

- Quantify the impact of routine caregiving on patients' lives.
- Establish an accurate and reliable system on which to base clinical decisions.
- Evaluate the effectiveness of caregiving.

A second factor is that research over the last 20 years has clearly indicated that the areas of performance typically measured by therapists (behavior, motor, language, cognition, etc.) are interdependent (Greenspan & Meisels, 1993). Biologic, cultural, and environmental variables are recognized to support, facilitate, or impede the development of infants and young children or the performance of mature individuals. For therapy to be meaningful, therapists must not only be knowledgeable in how neuromotor development occurs but also in how it may be affected by sociocultural and environmental parameters. For example, muscle tone in a developing child may be affected if a caregiver does not encourage independent movement or if she holds or positions a child in certain ways (Cintas, 1995). Additionally, cognitive skills are enhanced if a child moves independently within the environment (Bertenthal, Campos, & Barrett, 1984). Measurement tools are required to document domains and relationships of performance.

The third factor that has influenced the measurement process, the development of measurement instruments, and therapeutic intervention is the application of the *systems perspective* of motor development (Case-Smith, 1996; Piper, 1993). Traditional measurement instruments used by therapists are based on the *neuromaturational theory* of motor development advanced by McGraw (1945) and Gesell (1945) or the identification of impairments. The neuromaturational theory is based on the assumption that as the *central nervous system (CNS)* matures, motor development will proceed in a hierarchical fashion. Accordingly, development occurs in a cephalocaudal and proximal-distal direction at a specific rate. As the infant develops, higher centers of the CNS inhibit lower centers, so that voluntary movements can occur when reflexes are integrated. This framework is also applied to adults (Hanson, 1999).

Dynamical systems theory, described in earlier chapters of this text, views the development of motor skills as emerging from the interactions of many subsystems within a specific task (Heriza, 1991). These subsystems include the musculoskeletal system (joint mobility, muscle strength, and static postural alignment), movement patterns (motor milestones, reflexes and reactions, coordination, balance, endurance), functional performance, sensation (visual, vestibular, proprioceptive, auditory, and tactile), and perception. According to Heriza (1991), an assessment following a system paradigm should identify age-appropriate tasks, transition periods, the subsystems influencing movement, and contextual variations. Therapists providing services to individuals throughout the lifespan are mandated legally, regulated through funding sources, and encouraged by research findings and theoretical frameworks to use accurate information-collecting systems.

These interdependent domains are consistent with the perspective of the ICF, although most of the tests discussed in this chapter were developed independently before the ICF framework was adopted. Throughout this chapter, comments will be included to relate the assessment information to the ICF model.

PURPOSE OF COLLECTING INFORMATION

Therapists collect information to describe characteristics of an individual. The process involves a variety of methods to gather information. These include (1) chart reviews; (2) interviewing family members and other primary caregivers, teachers, and health professionals involved in the care of the child, client, or patient; (3) observing the client in natural settings; (4) family reports; and (5) direct testing using standardized, objective measurement tools or clinical observations.

Irrespective of the age of the client, therapists collect information for several purposes:

- To identify risk in an individual or group of individuals
- To contribute to the diagnostic process
- To determine eligibility for service
- To determine change in function over time
- To determine efficacy of intervention
- To conduct research

The procedures, strategies, and types of tests chosen to collect information will be driven by the purpose and by what type of information is needed.

DEFINITIONS

Although the terms *screening, evaluation, assessment,* and *examination* are commonly used interchangeably, various systems or regulatory bodies uniquely define them. The most specific of the definitions is found in the Individuals with Disabilities Education Act (IDEA). IDEA defines evaluation, assessment, and screening as they relate to early intervention and educational programs (IDEA, 1997). The **screening process** is used to detect whether a child's behavior or skill development is at a level that places him at risk for a developmental problem, concern, or delay. The screening process should be brief, and the test used should be easy to administer by a variety of people (physicians, therapists, nurses,

teachers, and, in some cases, parents). Screening instruments should be reliable and accurate. Therapists providing services to adults are mandated by Medicare regulations (CMS, 2001) to screen individuals to determine the need for further assessment or evaluation. According to the *Guide to Physical Therapists Practice, Second Edition* (APTA, 2001), physical therapists conduct screenings to determine the need for prevention services; for further examination, intervention, or consultation with a physical therapist; or for referral to another practitioner. The *Occupational Therapy Standards* (2002) has a similar recommendation for the use of screening tools.

The **evaluation process** is a more complex process. Evaluations are used to help make a diagnosis, identify atypical development, or determine eligibility for services. Instruments used as part of an evaluation process are usually norm-referenced, standardized tools. A **standardized test** is an evaluation instrument that has uniform procedures for administration and scoring (Richardson, 2001). **A norm-referenced** test is a type of standardized test that has been given to a large number of individuals that serve as a normative sample (Richardson, 2001). Therapists using a norm-referenced test can compare the performance of the individual tested to those of other "normative" individuals with similar qualities. For example, a 10-year-old is tested on balance and coordination by comparing hers to the performance of others in her age group. Descriptive scores that are meaningful to laypersons, like age-equivalent scores, can be obtained from norm-referenced tests.

While tests are available that measure discrete aspects of function such as motor performance, many tests are comprehensive developmental scales, covering more than one area of function. Evaluation methods include what Kirshner & Guyatt (1985) refer to as a **discriminative index,** meaning that which distinguishes between individuals or groups on specific dimensions, such as the acquisition of developmental milestones. Discriminative measures determine if a child's behavior is typical for his age and are used to determine eligibility for services. Many of the tools traditionally used by therapists in pediatrics, such as the Bayley Scales of Infant Development-II and the Peabody Developmental Motor Scales-2, fall into this category. The American Physical Therapy Association (2001) defines *evaluation* as a process used to interpret the information collected during the examination process. The American Occupational Therapy Association (1995) defines *evaluation* as a process used to collect and interpret information to plan intervention.

Physical and occupational therapists are often involved in the assessment process. **Assessments** often use comprehensive strategies and tools to delineate strengths and needs, develop appropriate intervention plans and strategies, and determine change in individuals. An assessment is most meaningful when it represents typical performance (Shelton, 1989). Thus, the assessment process should gain information regarding the child's or adult's abilities and behaviors across domains and environments (Cicchetti & Wagner, 1990). Therapists conducting assessments use a variety of methods to gather information. The assessment process also gains valuable information through *ecological* and *performance appraisals* (portfolios). The emphasis in an **ecological approach** to assessment is on documenting the individual's success in participating in activities and routines across domains and environments. Ideally, the assessment is conducted in the environment where the individual (child or adult) is expected to perform the skill so that the skills demonstrated also reflect the context of performance. Judgment-based assessments document the client's, parents', or caregiver's perceptions of the individual's performance. According to Kirshner and Guyatt (1985), an assessment can be "evaluative." An **evaluative assessment strategy** is one that measures the magnitude of change in an individual over time on a specific dimension. The overall purpose of an assessment is to describe an individual's strengths and needs to help design appropriate individualized therapeutic intervention plans.

PLANNING INFORMATION-GATHERING STRATEGIES

Prior to examining, evaluating, or assessing a client, careful planning of the process is imperative to insure that the information is collected efficiently and is meaningful to the client and client family. The following questions guide the therapist in choosing the appropriate strategy and tool.

1. *Why do you need to collect information?* Before collecting any type of information about a client, the therapist must be clear on the purpose. Ask yourself if you are collecting information to help determine a diagnosis, to plan a comprehensive therapeutic program, to determine change over time, to do research, and so on. The process of collecting information and the type of information collected will be done efficiently and targeted to meet the needs of the therapist and the client if the therapist is clear on the purpose.

2. *What information do you need to collect?* Once the purpose of your information-collecting process is determined, the type of information needing to be collected is decided upon. Listed in Table 21–1 are the types of information that the American Physical Therapy Association (2001) indicates that a physical therapist may need to collect. It is probably unnecessary, however, to collect all this information. Given the current care-delivery climate, especially in regard to productivity demands, efficient use of the therapist's time is important. Collecting information that focuses on the purpose will increase efficiency.

3. *How should you collect the information?* Most therapists take an active role in the collection of information. Therapists assume the responsibility of physically examining an individual. However, there are other methods of gathering information, depending on your purpose and the information needing to be collected. Meaningful information can be

TABLE 21–1	Categories of Tests and Measures Based on APTA Guidelines
Aerobic capacity/endurance	Muscle performance: strength, power, endurance
Anthropometric characteristics	Neuromotor development
Arousal, attention, cognition	Sensory processing
Assistive technology	Orthotic, protective, supportive devices
Circulation	Pain
Cranial and peripheral nerve integrity	Posture
Environmental: home, work, school, etc.	Prosthesis
Ergonomics, body mechanics	Range of motion
Gait, locomotion	Reflex integrity
Balance	Self-care
Integument integrity	Home management
Joint integrity	Respiration
Motor function	Play and leisure

American Physical Therapy Association, 2000. Preferred Physical Therapist Practice Pattern is a service mark of the American Physical Therapy Association. All rights reserved.

collected through the following methods. Most often a comprehensive procedure will involve one or more of these methods:

- Chart review
- Parent/family report
- Interviews
- Naturalistic observation
- Clinical observation
- Standardized tools

The purpose of collecting the information and the type of information needing to be collected will guide the therapist on which method would be most appropriate. For example, if the purpose of the exam is to design a therapeutic program to assist the client in walking up and down the stairs to his apartment, the preferred method of determining what may be preventing him from doing this task would be observing him in the natural environment, that is, the stairs in the apartment complex. If the purpose were to help a team determine if the difficulties a school-aged child is demonstrating are consistent with the eligibility for special education and related services categories under IDEA, formal standardized testing would be appropriate.

To determine which methods would be most appropriate and would efficiently answer the specific referral question, a therapist should determine the following: where should the information be collected, when should it be collected, and what strategies and/or tools are available to collect this type of information?

4. *What does it mean?* Once the information is collected, the therapist is in a position to determine the therapy diagnosis, prognosis, and design for a comprehensive plan of care. Interpreting the information collected is the skill that differentiates the professional therapist from the technician. Understanding psychometric qualities of testing instruments, test mechanics, and the relationship that test results have with individuals with disabilities is required to accurately interpret test data.

MODELS USED TO GATHER INFORMATION

This section will discuss five models used to gather information about functional motor performance. Three of the models—top-down, routines-based, and arena—are more applicable for assessment procedures. The bottom-up approach is primarily used for evaluation purposes, and the fifth model, the judgment-based approach, is used for both assessment and evaluation.

Bottom-Up Assessment

Traditionally, therapists have relied on a **bottom-up assessment** to gather information regarding motor performance (Campbell, 1991). The bottom-up model

typically measures body-level structure and function and is *diagnostic-prescriptive*, meaning that deficits or impairments are delineated in specific areas, leading to a program designed to remediate those deficits. This model is most appropriate for (1) evaluation and (2) designing intervention that targets impairments such as decreased joint range of motion or muscle weakness. This model, illustrated in Figure 21–1, is less helpful when designing functionally orientated intervention plans needed to improve outcomes within the daily lives of individuals.

Top-Down Assessment

The **top-down assessment** collects information on the ICF areas of activity and participation and environment. As noted previously, assessment procedures are often used for program planning. Therapeutic programs are functionally orientated and are geared to the accomplishment of outcomes. In the top-down model, illustrated in Figure 21–2, *desired outcomes* guide the assessment process. These are statements that describe what the team (clients, parents, caregivers, and professionals) would like to see happen in the individual. Outcomes can be general ("I'd like to see Anna move around") or specific ("Mr. O'Neill needs to walk from his bed to the bathroom"). A good example of a standardized top-down assessment is the *Assessment of Motor and Process Skill Test* (Fisher, 2001). Assessment

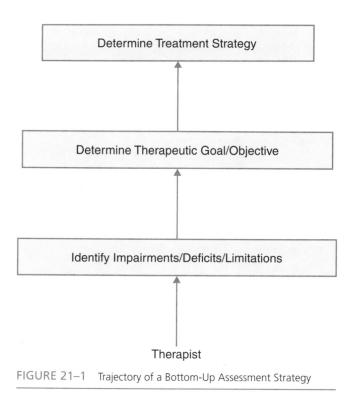

FIGURE 21–1   Trajectory of a Bottom-Up Assessment Strategy

Family/Team

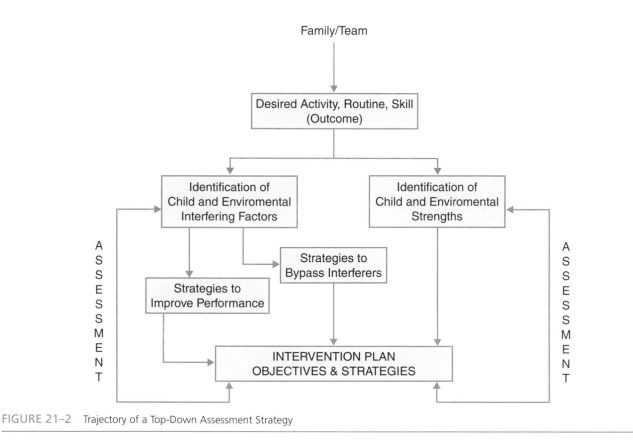

FIGURE 21–2   Trajectory of a Top-Down Assessment Strategy

procedures that operationalize the top-down approach answer the following questions (Campbell, 1995):

- What environmental factors and/or performance components are interfering with or facilitating the performance of the desired outcome?
- Into what specific objectives can the outcome be divided to minimize the immediate and long-term negative effects of identified interferers?
- What intervention approaches, models, and strategies will be used to promote immediate and long-term attainment of the desired outcome?

Routines-Based Assessment

As part of the family-centered intervention planning process, McWilliam (1992) promotes the **routines-based** model of assessment. Consistent with the top-down approach, a routines-based assessment model judges the capabilities of the individual within everyday routines and activities. Like the top-down model, the routines-based model assesses participation and environmental factors. An example of a standardized routines-based assessment is the *transdisciplinary play-based assessment* (Linder, 1993). A routines-based assessment identifies those factors (person-specific and environmental) that interfere with or promote the performance of a specific functional task within a specific routine. For example, a therapist would assess

a client's stair-climbing ability while the client (child or adult) is ascending stairs to go to his bedroom to take a nap, or descending to the basement to obtain a toy or do laundry. The use of routines to assess behaviors is helpful for program planning because

- Routines are meaningful to clients, parents, and caregivers.
- The use of routines promotes the delineation of functional outcomes and intervention strategies.
- Observation of a client across domains, contexts, and environments is most efficiently done in naturally occurring routines.

Although this approach is designed to be used with children, it is easy to see how it could be adapted to be used with adults. Like children, adults participate in ongoing routines and activities. When assessing impairments in isolation, a therapist makes assumptions about the impact these impairments have on function. The routines-based approach allows objective assessment of performance, which is the focus of intervention.

Arena Assessment

The **arena assessment** (Stewart, 2001), primarily used in early intervention, is the simultaneous observation of a child by various disciplines. This process can also be used in an adult rehabilitation setting or geriatric setting where the emphasis is to provide team-based services and reduce duplication of services. The purposes of an arena assessment are to

- Obtain an integrated, holistic view of the client.
- Determine the interrelationship of skills across domains.
- Decrease handling of the individual by multiple professionals.
- Decrease repetitive questioning of the family or client.

The arena assessment can streamline case management and promote integrated service delivery. It can be time-consuming, however. In order for all members of the team to gain the information they need, pre-assessment planning is needed as well as a great deal of collaboration among team members.

Judgment-Based Assessment

The **judgment-based assessment** format enables therapists to obtain task-specific information about an individual from those who see him perform on a regular basis (Haley, Baryza, & Blanchard, 1993). Thus, for young infants, asking parents and caregivers to fill out a form or answer a series of questions regarding the child's behavior would yield information (1) that is meaningful to parents and caregivers and (2) that parents and caregivers

would consider typical behavior for the child. The same can be done for adults, asking either the adult herself or family members and other caregivers.

MEASUREMENT INSTRUMENTS

Literally hundreds of tools are available to therapists for collecting information about an individual's physical status. It is impossible to cover all these tests or tools in one chapter. The following section will discuss a sampling of tools that are specific to a variety of areas of interest to a physical or occupational therapist. Table 21–2 is a list of resources that contain reviews or descriptions of some instruments that therapists may find helpful.

Many tools used by therapists are standardized tools. As explained earlier in this chapter, a standardized measurement instrument is one in which the procedures used to collect the information and score the performance of the individual are the same across examiners. Gathering information in a standardized manner increases the reliability of the method. A standardized tool can be either norm-referenced (discussed earlier) or criterion-referenced. **Criterion-referenced** tests are designed to measure performance on specific tasks (Richardson, 2001). Most academic tests are criterion-referenced. Table 21–3 compares the two types of standardized measurement instruments.

TABLE 21–2	Selected Resources on Testing Instruments

- Asher, I. E. (1996). *Occupational therapy assessment tools: An annotated index* (2nd ed.). Bethesda, MD: American Occupational Therapy Association.
- Aylward, G. P. (1994). *Practitioner's guide to developmental and psychological testing.* New York: Plenum.
- Bagnato, S. J., Neisworth, J. T., & Munson, S. M. (1997). *LINKing assessment and early intervention: An authentic curriculum-based approach.* Baltimore: Brookes.
- Gibbs, E. O., & Teti, D. M. (1990). *Interdisciplinary assessment of infants: A guide for early intervention professionals.* Baltimore: Brookes.
- Guralnick, M. J. (2000). *Interdisciplinary clinical assessment of young children with developmental disabilities.* Baltimore: Brookes.
- Hinojosa, J., & Kramer, P. (1998). *Evaluation: Obtaining and interpreting data.* Bethesda, MD: AOTA Press.
- Lewis, C. B., & McNerney, T. (1994). *The functional outcomes tool box.* Washington, DC: Learn Publications.
- Long, T. M., & Toscano, K. (2002). *Handbook of pediatric physical therapy* (2nd ed.). Philadelphia: Lippincott, Williams & Wilkins.
- Meisels, S. J., & Fenichel, E. (1996). *New visions for the developmental assessment of infants and young children.* Washington, DC: Zero to Three: National Center for Infants, Toddlers and Families.
- Vance, H. B. (1993). *Best practices in assessment for school and clinical settings.* Brandon, VT: Clinical Psychology Publishing.
- Van Deusen, J., & Brunt, D. (1997). *Assessment in occupational therapy and physical therapy.* Philadelphia: W. B. Saunders.

TABLE 21–3	Standardized Measurement Instruments

Norm-Referenced	Criterion-Referenced
1. Standard point score.	Cutoff scores.
2. Evaluates individual performance against group.	Performance against standard.
3. May or may not be related to therapeutic or instructional content.	Content-specific.
4. Normal distribution of scores.	Variability of scores not desired.
5. Maximizes differences among individuals.	Discriminates.
6. Requires diagnostic skills.	Provides information to plan intervention.
7. Not sensitive to effects of therapy.	Sensitive to effects of therapy.
8. Not concerned with task analysis.	Depends on task analysis.
9. Summative.	Formative.

NEUROMOTOR STATUS

Therapists assess the neuromotor status of an individual to determine if neurologic impairments are present. This type of test provides information on the ICF Body Structure and Function level. Typically, therapists assess range of motion, muscle tone, postural responses, and reflex development. Neuromotor assessments are done in a variety of settings. In the neonatal intensive care unit, neuromotor status is used to determine if an infant's behavior is typical for his postconceptual age. Therapists also use neuromotor status to help determine recovery after a stroke or other type of CNS insult.

ASHWORTH SCALE

The *Ashworth scale* (Ashworth, 1964) was the first tool developed to assess the severity of spasticity. The examiner rates the resistance encountered when passively moving specific muscle groups through their range of motion. This scale, presented in Table 21–4, is commonly used in clinical settings and for research purposes for clients throughout the lifespan. Interrater reliability on a modified version of the scale has been shown to be high (Bohannon & Smith, 1987). The validity of the scale decreases with the number of times it is repeated.

FUGL-MEYER (FM) SCALE

The Fugl-Meyer scale of functional return after hemiplegia (FM) (Fugl-Meyer, Jaasko, Leyman, Olsson, & Steglind, 1975) is a quantitative tool based on the stages of motor recovery following stroke as described by

Brunnstrom (1970). Items assessed include muscle tone, state of motor recovery, synergy, speed of movement, and prehension patterns. The items are assessed while the client performs increasingly complex neuromotor activities.

INFANT MOTOR SCREEN (IMS)

The *Infant Motor Screen (IMS)* (Nickel, 1989) is a 25-item, criterion-referenced test used to determine the neuromotor status of infants prematurely born at 4–16 months corrected age. The items on the test were adapted from the *Milani-Comparetti Motor Development Screening Test* (Stuberg, 1992) and the *Movement Assessment of Infants* (Chandler, Swanson & Andrews, 1980) to assess muscle tone, primitive reflexes, automatic responses, and symmetry. A significant asset of this tool is that it takes into consideration the degree of prematurity.

NEONATAL NEUROBEHAVIORAL EXAMINATION (NNE)

The *Neonatal Neurobehavioral Examination (NNE)* (Morgan, Koch, Lee, & Aldag, 1988) is a criterion-referenced exam used to determine the neurobehavioral status of infants at 32–42 weeks postconception. Therapists who serve infants in the neonatal intensive care unit use this test to determine if a child's development is progressing as would be expected for her postconception age. Twenty-seven items are divided into three sections: tone and motor patterns, primitive reflexes, and behavioral responses. The tool was standardized on infants born full-term and those born preterm at risk for neuromotor difficulties.

TABLE 21–4	Modified Ashworth Scale for Grading Spasticity

Grade	Description
0	No increase in muscle tone.
1	Slight increase in tone, manifested by a catch and release or by minimal resistance at the end of the range of motion when the affected part(s) is moved in flexion or extension.
1+	Slight increase in muscle tone, manifested by a catch followed by minimal resistance throughout the remainder (less than half) of the range of motion.
2	More marked increase in muscle tone through most of the range of motion, but affected part(s) easily moved.
3	Considerable increase in muscle tone; passive movement difficult.
4	Affected part(s) rigid in flexion or extension.

Reprinted from Bohannon, R.W., & Smith, M.B. (1987). Interrater reliability of a modified Ashworth scale of muscle spasticity. *Physical Therapy, 67(2)*, 206–207, with permission of the American Physical Therapy Association. This material is copyrighted, and any further reproduction or distribution is prohibited.

AGE-RELATED MOTOR PERFORMANCE

Tools that fall under this category are the most widely used by physical and occupational therapists to determine motor skill acquisition. They are most often norm-referenced and are most effective in determining if a child is meeting developmental expectations. These tools are less helpful once a child is determined to have a developmental disability.

ALBERTA INFANT MOTOR SCALE (AIMS)

The *Alberta Infant Motor Scale (AIMS)* (Piper & Darrah, 1993) was designed to identify gross motor delays in infants up to 18 months of age. It can be used as a screening tool or as part of an assessment to measure gross motor skill maturation over time. The authors of the AIMS clearly indicate that the test is not to be used for older children with known disabilities who are functioning below the 18-month level or to monitor progress of therapy in children with known disabilities.

AIMS is a norm-referenced instrument with strong psychometric characteristics. It can be given by a variety of health-care professionals who have a background in infant motor development. Test administration involves the observation of 58 items, divided among four positions: prone, supine, sitting, and standing. Within each position, three components of movement are evaluated: weight-bearing, posture, and antigravity movements. Minimal handling of the child is required, and the test can be completed in 15–30 minutes.

ASSESSMENT, EVALUATION, AND PROGRAMMING SYSTEM FOR YOUNG CHILDREN (AEPS)

The *Assessment, Evaluation, and Programming System for Young Children (AEPS)* (Bricker, 1993) is an example of the dozens of criterion-referenced tools used by therapists to determine developmental skill acquisition across domains (motor, language, cognition, adaptive, and socioemotional). Like most criterion-referenced tools, the tasks on the AEPS are arranged in a hierarchical fashion, and each skill is further divided into subcomponents. Criterion-referenced tools can be used for programming planning and may contain curricula linked to the tasks on the test. Other commonly used criterion-referenced tools include the *Hawaii Early Learning Profile (HELP)* (Park, 1992) and the *Carolina Curriculum for Infants and Toddlers with Special Needs* (Johnson-Martin, Jens, Attermeier, and Hacker, 1990).

BAYLEY SCALES OF INFANT DEVELOPMENT-II (BSID-II)

The *Bayley Scales of Infant Development–II (BSID-II)* (Bayley, 1993) is the most widely used infant developmental tool available. The tool consists of three scales that can be used independently: the mental scale, motor scale, and behavioral scale. The tool is a reliable and valid measure of developmental skill acquisition in young children from birth to 42 months of age. Items are arranged in a hierarchical fashion. An index score is calculated to judge the degree of delay. An age-equivalent score can also be obtained. The BSID-II is used extensively in follow-up programs for infants prematurely born, for early intervention, and for research purposes. It is recommended that users of the BSID-II have extensive knowledge of infant development and experience in testing and interpreting the results of infant tests.

BRUININKS-OSERETSKY TEST OF MOTOR PROFICIENCY (BOT)

The *Bruininks-Oseretsky Test of Motor Proficiency (BOT)* (Bruininks, 1978) is one of the few norm-referenced tools for children over the age of 5 years. It can be given to children from 4.6 years of age through 14 years of age to provide information on both gross and fine motor skills. The BOT is administered to children with less obvious neuromotor difficulties and is widely used with children suspected of having a *development coordination disorder (DCD)* (Dewey & Wilson, 2001). The test is divided into eight subtests that form a gross motor composite and a fine motor composite. The items assess sophisticated motor skill performance rather than skill acquisition. Movement components assessed include coordination, speed, refinement, dexterity, and balance.

GROSS MOTOR FUNCTION MEASURE (GMFM)

The *Gross Motor Function Measure (GMFM)* (Russell, Rosenbaum, Avery, & Lane, 2002) is a reliable and valid tool for evaluating change in gross motor function for children with cerebral palsy, describing a child's current level of motor function, and helping to determine treatment goals. The tool can be used for a child of any age; however, it has been validated only on children between 5 months and 16 years. It has 88 items of gross motor function divided into five dimensions: lying and rolling, sitting, crawling and kneeling, standing, and walking, running, and jumping. The child is rated on how much of each skill he can complete. Qualitative performance is minimally considered. Scoring yields a percent of accomplishment on each of the dimensions. Change over time is calculated as percent change. The GMFM is a very easy-to-use tool, providing quantitative information on change in performance on basic developmental skills.

PEABODY DEVELOPMENTAL MOTOR SCALE–2 (PDMS-2)

The *Peabody Developmental Motor Scale–2 (PDMS-2)* (Folio & Fewell, 2000) is used to assess developmental motor skill acquisition in children from 1 week of age to 6 years. It consists of two scales—gross motor and fine motor—which can be administered independently.

Each of the scales is subdivided into subtests that assess specific motor skill components such as manual dexterity, balance, reflex development, and so forth. The test is used to determine degree of accomplishment of tasks to determine the skill level of an individual child and her strengths and weaknesses in motor skill acquisition. The tool is norm-referenced, yielding standard scores that are used to compare motor performance with a peer group and calculate an age-equivalent score. Accompanying the PDMS-II test is a book of developmentally appropriate activities that coincide with the test items. These can be used to assist with program planning and intervention.

TODDLER AND INFANT MOTOR EVALUATION (TIME)

The *Toddler and Infant Motor Evaluation (TIME)* (Miller & Roid, 1994) was developed to measure functional movements in an infant's natural environment. It identifies children with mild to severe motor problems, revealing patterns of movements and evaluating motor development over time to assist in intervention planning and treatment efficacy research. TIME is used for children 4–42 months of age to evaluate motor dysfunction. It is divided into eight subtests, five of which have been standardized and norm-referenced.

The child's spontaneous movements in various positions are recorded, as well as her sequence of movements and any abnormal movements. The parents interact with, handle, and position the child with the examiner's instructions and guidance. TIME can be used as a comprehensive motor evaluation or assessment tool. As an evaluation tool, it identifies motor dysfunction. Repeated measures can be taken with this test, making it useful for the assessment of motor development over time as well as for the assessment of treatment efficacy and/or motor maturation.

TIME is a valuable clinical tool. It incorporates dynamic systems theory into the assessment of motor functions and development. It links a child's function, quality of movement, and motor skills. Comprehensive and detailed, this test provides excellent visual descriptors of the motor components being assessed. It uses primarily naturalistic observation to gather data; thus it recognizes the importance of evaluating typical movements as they are impacted by the child's environment.

AGE-RELATED SENSORY PROCESSING

According to the *sensory integration framework* proposed by Ayres, the proximal senses (vestibular, tactile, proprioception) are critical for individuals to interact with the environment (Parham & Mailloux, 2001). These tests measure function in the Activities and Participation domain of the ICF. Although some body function aspects, like assessment of equilibrium reactions and motor planning, are included in some of these tests, the information is interpreted in the context of participation.

SENSORY PROFILE(S)

The original *Sensory Profile* (Dunn, 1999 to 2001) was designed for children 3–10 years of age. Since 1999 two additional profile questionnaires have been published. The *Infant/Toddler Sensory Profile* covers children from birth to 36 months and the *Adolescent/Adult Sensory Profile* covers individuals over the age of 11. All the tools help determine the contribution of sensory processing to the client's daily performance patterns, obtain information about everyday sensory experiences, determine the impact on behavior in different settings, and generate an individualized profile of sensory processing across four quadrants: low registration, sensation seeking, sensory sensitivity, and sensation avoiding.

TEST OF SENSORY FUNCTIONS IN INFANTS

The *Test of Sensory Functions in Infants (TSFI)* (DeGangi & Greenspan, 1989) was developed to screen and quantify sensory processing and reactivity in infants. The test includes five subdomains of sensory processing: reactivity to tactile deep-pressure, adaptive motor responses, visual-tactile integration, ocular-motor control, and reactivity to vestibular stimulation. Infants 4–18 months of age can be screened using the TSFI. The test is most accurate in identifying infants without sensory processing disorders and infants of 10–18 months with sensory dysfunction because definitive sensory processing dysfunction does not emerge until late in the 1st year of life. Because limited normative data are available, total test scores are used to make screening decisions. The individual subtests, however, can be used in conjunction with other standardized developmental and neuromotor tests when making clinical decisions and recommendations (DeGangi & Greenspan, 1988).

TEST OF SENSORY INTEGRATION (TSI)

The *Test of Sensory Integration (TSI)* (DeGangi & Berk, 1987) was the first tool developed to assess sensory processing in preschool-aged children. The test has three components that assess vestibular-based functions: postural control, bilateral motor integration, and reflex development. It is used with children 3–5 years of age. When used with other developmental tools the TSI provides additional information to determine strengths and weakness in basic sensory processing.

The administration of the test requires a great deal of physical handling of the child and subjective interpretation of performance, leading to low interrater reliability. The TSI is best used as part of a comprehensive evaluation of sensory-motor, neuromotor, and motor skill development.

SENSORY INTEGRATION AND PRAXIS TEST (SIPT)

The *Sensory Integration and Praxis Test (SIPT)* (Ayres, 1991) is a battery of tests used to assist in the evaluation of sensory integration in children 4–8 years of age. The SIPT is a lengthy test to administer and score. It consists of a variety of complex tasks assessing tactile and vestibular processing: form and space perception and visuomotor coordination, praxis, and bilateral integration and sequencing. Test administration, scoring, and interpretation are likewise complex. To administer the test a therapist must have advanced training and become certified in the administration of the test.

FUNCTIONAL SKILLS

Another category of tests measures specific aspects of the ICF Activities and Participation domain. *Functional skills* in this context consist of a wide variety of skills, including *activities of daily living (ADLs)* and *instrumental activities of daily living (IADLs)*. The IADLs are complex skills needed across the lifespan to function independently in home, school, employment, and community environments. Contemporary service provision to individuals with activity limitations emphasizes the accomplishment of ADLs, IADLs, and the component skills that interfere with the accomplishment of these tasks (Guccione, 2000).

BARTHEL INDEX

The *Barthel Index* (Mahoney & Barthel, 1965) is one of the oldest measures of self-care and is widely used in rehabilitation settings. The index consists of 10 activities that are rated by a rehabilitation professional from direct observation or client interview. The scoring is an ordinal scale that quantifies level of dependence in these specific activities. Although widely used and clinically respected, little research has been done documenting the psychometric integrity of the measure. There is information that the Barthel index correlates with clinical outcomes and functional status in adults who have had a stroke or other severe disabilities (Granger, Hamilton, & Gresham, 1988; Granger, Albrecht, & Hamilton, 1979).

FUNCTIONAL INDEPENDENCE
MEASURE (FIM)

The *Functional Independence Measure (FIM)* (Granger, 1990) and its pediatric counterpart (WeeFIM) (Granger et al., 1991) assess a person's degree of independence in a variety of ADLs. Items include self-help skills, mobility, communication, social adjustment, and problem solving. The FIM is widely used in rehabilitation settings and is part of a comprehensive outcome database management system. A large literature base describes the FIM's utility. Studies include prediction of the burden of care (Granger, Hamilton, & Gresham, 1988), measure of change in performance following rehabilitation (Heinemann, Linacre, Wright, Hamilton, & Granger, 1994), and prediction of outcome following stroke (Oczkowski & Barreca, 1993). There is less information available on the WeeFIM.

PEDIATRIC EVALUATION OF
DISABILITY INVENTORY (PEDI)

The *Pediatric Evaluation of Disability Inventory (PEDI)* (Haley, Coster, Ludlow, Haltiwanger, & Andrellas, 1992) determines functional capabilities and performance, monitors progress in functional skill performance, and evaluates therapeutic or rehabilitative program outcomes in children with disabilities. It can also be used for children without disabilities from 6 months to 7 years and 6 months of age. PEDI is a norm-referenced test with strong psychometric characteristics. The test is divided into three subtests, focusing on functional skills: self-care, mobility, and social function. In addition, environmental modifications and amount of caregiver assistance are systematically recorded. Information can be obtained through parental report, structured interview, or professional observation of a child's functional behavior. PEDI is a reliable and valid assessment of functional performance in children with significant cognitive and physical disabilities.

SCHOOL FUNCTION ASSESSMENT (SFA)

The *School Function Assessment (SFA)* (Coster, Deeney, Haltiwanger, & Haley, 1998) is used within the educational environment to assess function and to guide program planning for students with disabilities in kindergarten through sixth grade. Nonacademic tasks divided among those areas assessing level of participation, amount of task assistance or modification, and level of performance in cognitive or physical tasks are judged by teachers and other providers of services in the educational environment. The SFA is a criterion-referenced test, using a judgment-based format to gather information on the typical performance of a child from a variety of individuals involved in his education. It yields detailed information across domains and environments that requires collaboration from those that know the student well. The SFA is targeted specifically to an educational environment. Information gathered is directed specifically to the nonacademic components of school functioning and specifically links assessment results to individualized education program (IEP) development.

SCALES OF INDEPENDENT
BEHAVIOR REVISED (SIB-R)

The *Scales of Independent Behavior, Revised (SIB-R)* (Bruninks, Woodcock, Weatherman, & Hill, 1996) is a comprehensive tool assessing adaptive behavior (motor skills, social interaction and communication skills, personal living skills, and community living skills). It also has a screening form and a problem-behavior scale. The tool is norm-referenced and is appropriate for individuals from birth through 99 years. In a judgment-based format the client, parent, or caregiver rates the client's ability and competence on a variety of developmental, functional, or behavioral tasks. The community-living subsection of the tool provides a wealth of information on the client's ability to negotiate around the community and perform expected activities and routines. Items rated include carrying groceries up and down stairs, crossing streets, and planning trips and destinations.

PLAY AND LEISURE

It is becoming more important to clients that therapists assist them in maintaining an active lifestyle along with functional skills. As life expectancy continues to increase, it is becoming more important for older Americans to remain active and retain interest in a wide variety of play and leisure activities.

ACTIVITY INDEX

The *Activity Index* (Nystrom, 1974, Gregory, 1983) consists of two instruments that when used together provide information on the meaning and significance of activity among older adults. One instrument is the *Activity Patterns and Leisure Concepts among the Elderly* (Nystrom); the other is *Occupational Behavior and Life Satisfaction among Retirees* (Gregory). Nystrom's interview rates the degree of participation in 25 activities and preferences for activities. Gregory's self-completed questionnaire rates activities according to degree of enjoyment, internal versus external motivation, and sense of competence. Little research is available for these tools. The psychometric qualities of the tools are poor, so these tools are best used as guides for therapists and to help identify areas of interest.

THE REVISED KNOX PRESCHOOL PLAY SCALE (PPS) (KNOX, 1997)

The most commonly used play scale is the *Knox Preschool Play Scale (PPS)* (Morrison & Metsger, 2001). First developed in 1974, it has undergone two revisions. PPS quantifies the child's play skills to determine a play age and develop a play profile. Although it yields a measure of a child's skills within a play situation, the degree of playfulness should also be addressed. The *Test of Playfulness* (Bundy, 1997) attempts to capture the degree to which a child spontaneously demonstrates play that is intrinsically motivated, internally controlled, and not bound by objective reality (Bundy, 1993).

INDIVIDUALIZED PROGRAM PLANNING

As noted previously, most therapists collect information to help develop an effective therapeutic intervention program. *Individualized program planning* is becoming the norm across the lifespan. The use of tools that help clients identify areas of importance to their own lifestyle will assist with individualizing program plans. Identifying factors that may be interfering with what a client considers significant is most important in operationalizing an individualized program addressing functional outcomes within a natural environment.

CANADIAN OCCUPATIONAL PERFORMANCE MEASURE (COPM)

The *Canadian Occupational Performance Measure (COPM)* (Law, Baptiste, Carswell, McColl, Polatajko, & Pollack, 1994) is appropriate for clients of any age. The purposes of the COPM are to obtain the client's perception of self-care status, productivity, leisure, and change in status over time. Using a semi-structured interview, COPM helps clients and/or family members articulate their difficulties, needs, and goals within naturally occurring activities and routines. The tool has been shown to be responsive to changes noted in performance and personal satisfaction of performance over time in clients receiving therapeutic services (Law, Polatajko, Pollock, McColl, Carswell, & Baptiste, 1994).

FUNCTIONAL OUTCOMES ASSESSMENT GRID (FOAG)

The *Functional Outcomes Assessment Grid (FOAG)* (Campbell, 1993) is used by an interdisciplinary team to develop goals for children with disabilities in direct relation to the functional outcomes determined by the team; monitor change over time; and determine appropriate level of service. It is appropriate for all individuals with disabilities regardless of age. The FOAG is based on the American Occupational Therapy Association's document

Uniform Terminology for Occupational Therapy, 2nd edition (1994). Individualized observation of functional skill performance is done to determine which components (physical, environmental, behavioral, sensory) are impacting positively or negatively on the child's performance of a skill. Each component is scored on a five-point scale from no problems to significant problems that impact on or prevent skill performance. Those factors that impact significantly on performance of team-based outcomes are targeted for intervention. The FOAG operationalizes the top-down model of measurement as well as the routines-based model. It is highly useful for individuals with complex needs whose development is known to be atypical and whose disability affects a broad spectrum of functional skills. It is most helpful when used as a collaborative team decision-making tool, facilitating integrated service provision. The FOAG directly links assessment to program planning and is individualized to meet the unique needs of the client.

ASSESSMENT OF MOTOR AND PROCESS SKILLS (AMPS)

The *Assessment of Motor and Process Skills (AMPS)* (Fisher, 2001) is a qualitative observational assessment used to measure the performance of domestic (instrumental) or basic (personal) ADLs. The quality of a person's ADL performance is assessed by rating the effort, efficiency, safety, and independence. AMPS is unique in that it uses a framework and language consistent with the ICF. This is a top-down test of occupational performance and is not designed to be used to determine the presence of neuromuscular, biomechanical, cognitive, or psychosocial impairments.

MODEL OF HUMAN OCCUPATION (MOHO) ASSESSMENTS

Several top-down assessment instruments have been developed to extend specific understanding of functional aspects of occupation. Several of these assessment instruments address ICF Environmental Factors. This aspect of these tools provides important insight into the context for functional performance. An example is the *Work Environment Impact Scale (WEIS)*. WEIS (Corner, Kielhofner, & Lin, 1997) is a semi-structured interview that evaluates features in the work environment that support or impede occupational performance. It is designed to measure the impact of the work setting on the person's performance, satisfaction, and perception of well-being.

Another MOHO tool is the *Pediatric Volitional Questionnaire (PVQ)* (Kafkes et al., 2001). The PVQ focuses on the ICF Personal (contextual) Factors of volition and motivation in preschool children. A similar tool for adults is the *Volitional Questionnaire* (Gloria de las Heras, Geist, & Kielhofner, 2001).

SUMMARY

The last 20 years have seen significant changes in providing therapeutic intervention to individuals with motor dysfunction. These changes have primarily occurred in methods of gathering information about a client's functional status and delivering appropriate functionally oriented services. Therapists are revising traditional service delivery models to reflect the growing emphasis on providing integrated therapeutic services within inclusive settings. The physical and occupational therapists' expertise in motor development, the effects of sensory motor skills on function and other developmental areas, and their ability to task-analyze is being applied more broadly to the benefit of clients of all ages.

This chapter outlines models of information-gathering used by therapists to evaluate and assess infants, young children, adolescents, and adults. It also reviewed several measurement tools used by physical and occupational therapists. Instruments are used as one component of the measurement process to (1) screen individuals for potential concerns, (2) evaluate individuals to determine diagnosis or eligibility for services, or (3) assess clients to plan therapeutic intervention or to determine effects of intervention. Therapists should be aware of the purpose of each tool and the information they would like to gain before selecting an instrument. They may need to use a variety of tools and strategies to meet their screening, evaluation, or assessment objectives.

In addition to the measurement instrument used to gather information, a comprehensive measurement strategy should encompass principles that recognize that the assessment of individuals of all ages is complex and requires an appreciation of the client's abilities within a functional context. (Greenspan & Meisels with the Zero to Three Work Group on Developmental Assessment, 1996) (Table 21–5).

The therapist needs to appreciate that the assessment or evaluation of neuromotor, sensorimotor, and functional status can be influenced by the interaction of the client with significant others, the environment, and the individual's own neurobehavioral state. This is especially critical with very young infants and when establishing intervention priorities, outcomes, and goals and strategies. Collaborating with family members, other professionals, and caregivers will increase the likelihood that the therapist's findings will reflect the individual's capabilities across environments and current capacities and strengths, as well as identify barriers to optimal development. Individualized assessment of a client's skills should capture movement patterns, components of movement, and the use of movement within a functional activity in addition to sensory processing and developmental skill acquisition.

In creating an information-collection procedure, it is important to determine if your strategies are meeting the guidelines of contemporary service delivery. The checklist for assessment standards in Table 21–6 is a series of questions used to create systems of assessment that are relevant to the client, the family, and other team members and can be used to create meaningful therapeutic programs.

TABLE 21–5	**Principles of Appropriate Assessment**

1. Assessment is a collaborative process involving multiple sources of information and multiple components.
2. An assessment should follow an individualized sequence and procedure.
3. The client's relationship and interactions with his or her most trusted caregiver should form the cornerstone of an assessment. This is especially relevant for very young children.
4. Assessment should emphasize attention to the client's needs, desires, and outcomes.
5. The assessment process should identify the client's current competencies and strengths as well as the deficits, weaknesses, and impairments.
6. The process of assessment is the first step in an intervention process.
7. Assessment of a client's status should occur in the context of naturally occurring activities and routines.

Adapted from Greenspan & Meisels with the Zero to Three Work Group on Developmental Assessment (1996). In S.J. Meisels & E. Fenichel (Eds.), *New visions for the developmental assessment of infants and young children.* Washington, DC: Zero to Three, National Center for Infants, Toddlers, and Families.

TABLE 21–6	Checklist for Assessment Standards

Area of Validity	Questions
Treatment	1. Does the assessment identify feasible goals and objectives? 2. Does assessment information assist in the selection or use of therapeutic methods or approaches? 3. Does assessment contribute to evaluating intervention effects?
Social	1. Does assessment identify goals and objectives that are judged as worthwhile and appropriate? 2. Are assessment methods and materials acceptable to participants? 3. Does the assessment detect significance of change?
Convergent	1. Are several types of assessment materials and approaches used? 2. Is information collected from several settings and sources, especially family members and other caregivers? 3. Are assessments done on more than one occasion?
Consensual	1. Is information pooled and perspectives shared? 2. Do team dynamics favor collaboration and negotiation? 3. Are decisions truly consensual?

CASE

1

Andrew

Andrew was born with a congenital heart defect, which was repaired when he was an infant. He has been healthy and has not had any cardiac-related problems since infancy. He has, however, been diagnosed with severe spastic diplegia and language-processing deficits. He uses a walker and wears ankle-foot orthoses (AFOs). His parents, Ms. King, a dentist, and Mr. Hammer, an architect, are very proud of Andrew's school performance thus far. During preschool and early elementary school he attended a self-contained, noncategorical program in a special education wing in an elementary school. He did extremely well there and subsequently moved to a third-grade class with typically developing peers. Andrew now is on the playground with children in other grades; he goes on field trips, goes outside the classroom for art, gym, and music, and is handling more homework. He has been followed by the same therapist since preschool. While he was in the noncategorical program the therapist saw him twice weekly in the therapy room for 45-minute sessions. He is now receiving therapy using a collaborative-consultation model. A 3-month review of Andrew's *individualized education program (IEP)* is coming up. The therapist is part of the review team.

Andrew's condition has been diagnosed, and it has already been determined that he is eligible for special education and related services. Documenting his degree of delay in the acquisition of motor skills and his neuromotor status is unnecessary to review his IEP. At this point it is important to gather information about Andrew's performance in the classroom and within the school environment. This type of information will allow the team to determine if any additional services and supports are needed to help him meet the expectations of his present environment. *School function assessment* (SFA) is designed to assess this type of information and would provide excellent information to the team to determine his needs. This test will be completed by all members of the team who see Andrew throughout the day. They will indicate from their perspective how well Andrew is meeting expectations placed on him. The team members will indicate what types of supports and modifications he needs to accomplish tasks and whether or not he is participating in all activities within the school. The information gained from SFA will help the team delineate areas of strengths and needs and further refine his IEP.

CASE
2

Allison

Allison is 15 years old. She was born full term, weighing 6 pounds, 5 ounces. Although the pregnancy was without problems, delivery was quite difficult. Ms. Anderson, Allison's mother, was in labor for 22 hours before it was decided to do a cesarean section. Allison was in distress, and she experienced hypoxia in the neonatal period. She was stabilized in the delivery room. She needed to stay in the NICU for only 5 days. She was discharged to home in what was considered "good shape." The pediatric resident noted that her muscle tone was "within normal limits," and "primitive reflexes were present and well developed," while range of motion was "full." The Andersons became concerned about Allison's development at about 6 months of age when she was not rolling over or sitting when placed. The pediatrician referred her to physical therapy at that time.

Initially Allison received therapy through her local early intervention program, then through her preschool program. For the last 10 years Allison has attended her local public school and has been integrated into classrooms with her peers. She has received many special services over the years, including PT, OT, and speech and language therapy. She uses a power-drive wheelchair and a computerized communication system. Over the last 3 years there has been an emphasis on academic skills; thus PT has not been an integral part of her program. However, a physical therapist has been available to consult and collaborate with the other team members as needed.

Allison's parents have noticed that Allison is in her wheelchair just about all the time. They are concerned that she may be developing knee flexion contractures that are preventing her from taking full weight during a standing transfer maneuver. They have called for an IEP meeting, at which time they would like to know if Allison could benefit from PT so she does not lose the ability to transfer independently.

Allison is well known to this school system and to the therapists who provide services. The questions that Allison's parents have are clear and specific. The therapists are responsible for answering the questions of the parents and determining if therapeutic intervention would be of benefit to Allison. The *functional outcome assessment grid* would provide information specific to the question the family has. The grid will delineate which movement components are interfering with Allison's ability to transfer. At this point there is no need to collect information regarding motor skill acquisition. The team is convening to discuss a very specific family concern. Problem solving and meaningful program planning will take place if the therapist brings to the team specific information on what interferes with or promotes Allison's ability to transfer.

CASE
3

Bill

Bill is a 72-year-old father of three children and grandfather to a 2-year old girl. He practices law part-time for the firm he has been a partner in for the last 25 years. He lives in the suburbs of a metropolitan area with his wife, who is a high school principal. The couple have a very active lifestyle. They golf, play tennis (Bill competes nationally in his age group), bike-ride, and socialize with friends and family. When Bill was in his mid-40s he underwent cardiac bypass surgery. Until

Continues

Case 3 Continued

recently he has had no residual problems. Recently he has been diagnosed with congestive heart failure. As an in-patient he was seen by a physical therapist. She did a thorough full-system examination and identified several impairments, including limited endurance and generalized weakness.

Because Bill is an active individual, it is imperative to maintain his activity level. In addition to collecting system-oriented information, it would be helpful to identify areas of interest that Bill would like to participate in, areas of self-care and leisure that are important for him to maintain, and any interferers that may prevent him from participating in his routine activities. A combination of objective measurements such as cardiopulmonary status, manual muscle tests, and self-completed questionnaires to identify outcomes will be necessary to plan a meaningful therapeutic program. As Bill has been an active and robust individual, his needs go well beyond basic ADLs. He may require more intensive intervention to return to his typical activity level.

Speaking of

So Many Tests, So Little Time

JENNY PATTERSON, OTR/L
STAFF OCCUPATIONAL THERAPIST, TERTIARY CARE TRAUMA CENTER

In OT school we learned about a lot of different tests appropriate for a variety of different conditions. As the professors were teaching us about each of the tests, I wondered if I would really need to know them all. During my clinical rotations, I found that therapists often cut corners in regard to assessment in order to save time. After graduation, I was hired as an occupational therapist in a 365-bed acute-care hospital and quickly learned that time spent with patients had to be extremely productive. From the beginning, my caseload included trauma patients, neuro patients of all types, and patients with vision impairments, as well as patients with many other diagnoses. At first, I was overwhelmed with the "nuts and bolts" of being an occupational therapist. It took a while to get comfortable with ordinary practice and to learn about the facility's policies and procedures. Once I had become comfortable in the work setting, I rediscovered many of the assessment tools that I had been exposed to as a student, my favorite of which is the LOTCA (Loewenstein Occupational Therapy Cognitive Assessment). Because the LOTCA consists of several subtests that can be administered all at once or broken down during several sessions, it has been valuable in allowing me to manage time effectively. It also allows me to zero in on cognitive performance deficits that may affect a patient's independent functioning at home and in the community. Most patients in an acute-care setting are most concerned about getting well. However, many fail to plan for accommodations secondary to activity limitations. Assessment helps me anticipate problems and educate my patients about possible limitations and accommodations. In the hospital, patients have a fairly structured environment and schedule. As a result, cognitive problems such as lack of initiation of tasks, disorganized thought patterns, or lack of awareness of safety hazards may not be apparent initially. These cognitive problems could prevent the person from being safe in their own home or community, and/or keep them from performing activities of daily living. With careful testing using a tool like the LOTCA, occupational therapists can provide clients and families with information and strategies to prepare for the future.

REFERENCES

American Occupational Therapy Association. (1994). *Uniform terminology for occupational therapy: Application to practice* (2nd ed.). Rockville, MD: American Occupational Therapy Association.

American Occupational Therapy Association. (1995). Commission on Practice. *OT Week,* July, 10.

American Occupational Therapy Association. (2002). Occupational Therapy Practice Framework: Domain and process. *The American Journal of Occupational Therapy, 56,* 609–639.

American Physical Therapy Association. (2001). *Guide to physical therapist practice* (2nd ed.). Alexandria, VA: American Physical Therapy Association.

Ashworth, B. (1964). Preliminary trial of carisoprodol in multiple sclerosis. *Practitioner, 192,* 540–542.

Ayres, J. (1991). *Sensory integration and praxis test.* Los Angeles: Western Psychological Services.

Bayley, N. (1993). *Bayley scales of infant development-II.* San Antonio: The Psychological Corporation.

Berenthal, B., Campos, J., & Barrett, K. (1984). Self-produced locomotion: An organizer of emotional, cognitive, and social development. In R. Ende & R. Herman (Eds.), *Continuities and discontinuities in development* (pp. 175–209). New York: Plenum.

Bohannon, R. W., & Smith, M. B. (1987). Interrater reliability of a modified Ashworth scale of muscle spasticity. *Physical Therapy, 67,* 206–207.

Bricker, D. (1993). *Assessment, evaluation, and programming system for infants and children.* Baltimore: Brookes.

Bruininks, R. H. (1978). *Bruininks-Oseretsky test of motor proficiency.* Circle Pines, MN: American Guidance Service.

Bruininks, R. H., Woodcock, R. W., Weatherman, R. F., & Hill, B. K. (1996). *Scales of independent behavior—revised.* Chicago: Riverside Publishing.

Brunnstrum, S. (1970). *Movement therapy in hemiplegia.* New York: Harper & Row.

Bundy, A. (1993). Assessment of play and leisure: Delineation of the problem. *American Journal of Occupational Therapy, 47,* 217–222.

Bundy, A. (1997). Play and playfulness: What to look for. In L. D. Parham & L. S. Fazio (Eds.), *Play in occupational therapy for children* (pp. 52–66). St. Louis: Mosby.

Campbell, P. H. (1991). Evaluation and assessment in early intervention for infants and toddlers. *Journal of Early Intervention, 15,* 36–45.

Campbell, P. H. (1995). Medical and physical needs of students in inclusive settings. In N. G. Haring & L. T. Romer (Eds.), *Welcoming students who are deaf-blind into typical classrooms* (pp. 277–306). Baltimore: Brookes.

Case-Smith, J. (1996). Analysis of current motor development theory and recently published infant motor assessments. *Infants and Young Children, 9,* 29–41.

Chandler, L. S., Swanson, M. W., & Andrews, M. S. (1980). *Movement assessment of infants.* Rolling Bay, WI: Infant Movement Research.

Cicchetti, D., & Wagner, S. (1990). Alternative assessment strategies for the evaluation of infants and toddlers: An organizational perspective. In S. J. Meisels & J. P. Shonkoff (Eds.), *Handbook of early childhood intervention.* New York: Cambridge University Press.

Cintas, H. L. (1995). Cross-cultural similarities and differences in development and the impact on parental expectations on motor behavior. *Pediatric Physical Therapy, 7,* 103–111.

CMS. (2001). *Federal Register, 66(152),* August 7.

Corner, R., Kielhofner, G., & Lin, F. L. (1997). Construct validity of a work environment impact scale. *Work, 9(1),* 21–34.

Coster, W., Deeney, T., Haltiwanger, J., & Haley, S. (1998). *School function assessment.* San Antonio: Therapy Skill Builders.

DeGangi, G., & Berk, R. (1987). *Test of sensory integration.* Los Angeles: Western Psychological Services.

DeGangi, G., & Greenspan, S. (1988). The development of sensory functions in infants. *Physical and Occupational Therapy in Pediatrics, 8,* 21–33.

DeGangi, G., & Greenspan, S. (1989). *Test of sensory functions in infants.* Los Angeles: Western Psychological Services.

de las Heras, C. G., Geist, R., & Kielhofner, G. (2001). Volitional Questionnaire. Retrieved April 10, 2004, from http://www.uic.edu/ahp/OT/MOHOC/clinical_instruments.html.

Dewey, D., & Wilson, B. N. (2001). Developmental coordination disorder: What is it? *Physical and Occupational Therapy in Pediatrics, 20,* 5–28.

Dunn, W. (1999). *Sensory profile.* San Antonio: Psychological Corporation.

Dunn, W. (2001). *Adolescent/adult sensory profile.* San Antonio: Psychological Corporation.

Dunn, W. (2001). *Infant/toddler sensory profile.* San Antonio: Psychological Corporation.

Fisher, A. G. (2001). *Assessment of motor and process skills (Vol. 1)* (User manual). Fort Collins, CO: Three Star Press.

Folio, M., & Fewell, R. (2000). *Peabody developmental motor scale—2.* Allen, TX: DLM Teaching Resources.

Fugl-Meyer, A. R., Jaasko, L., Leyman, I., Olsson, S., & Steglind, S. (1975). The post-stroke hemiplegic patient: 1. A method for evaluation of physical performance. *Scandinavian Journal of Rehabilitation Medicine, 7,* 13–31.

Gesell, A. (1945). *The embryology of behavior: The beginnings of the human mind.* Philadelphia: J. B. Lippincott.

Granger, C. (1990). *Functional independence measure.* Buffalo, NY: Uniform Data System for Medical Rehabilitation, State University of New York.

Granger, C., Braun, S., Griswood, K., Heyer, N., McCabe, M., Msau, M., & Hamilton, B. (1991). *Functional independence measure for children.* Buffalo, NY: Uniform Data System for Medical Rehabilitation, State University of New York.

Granger, C. V., Albrecht, G. L., & Hamilton, B. B. (1979). Outcome of comprehensive medical rehabilitation: Measurement by Pulses Profile and the Barthel Index. *Archives of Physical Medicine and Rehabilitation, 60,* 145–154.

Granger, C. V., Hamilton, B. B., & Gresham, G. E. (1988). The stroke rehabilitation outcome study—Part 1: General description. *Archives of Physical Medicine and Rehabilitation, 69,* 505–509.

Greenspan, S. I., & Meisels, S. (1993). *Toward a new vision for the developmental assessment of infants and young children.* Arlington, VA: Zero to Three, National Center for Clinical Infant Programs.

Greenspan, S. I., & Meisels, S. J., with the Zero to Three Work Group on Developmental Assessment. (1996). In S. J. Meisels & E. Fenichel (Eds.), *New visions for the developmental assessment of infants and young children.* Washington, DC: Zero to Three, National Center for Infants, Toddlers, and Families.

Gregory, M. D. (1983). Occupational behavior and life satisfaction among retirees. *American Journal of Occupational Therapy, 37,* 548–553.

Guccione, A. (2000). Functional assessment of the elderly. In A. Guccione (Ed.), *Geriatric physical therapy* (2nd ed.) (pp. 123–133). St. Louis: Mosby.

Haley, S. M., Baryza, M. J., & Blanchard, Y. (1993). Functional and naturalistic frameworks in assessing physical and motor disablement. In I. Wilhelm (Ed.), *Physical therapy assessment in early infancy* (pp. 225–256). New York: Churchill Livingstone.

Haley, S., Coster, W. J., Ludlow, I. H., Haltiwanger, J. T., & Andrellas, P. (1992). *Pediatric evaluation of disability inventory.* Boston: PEDI Research Group, Department of Rehabilitation Medicine, New England Medical Center Hospital.

Hanson, C. (1999). Proprioceptive Neuromuscular Facilitation. In C. M. Hall & L. T. Brody (Eds.), *Therapeutic exercise: Moving toward function* (pp. 233–251). Philadelphia: Lippincott, Williams & Wilkins.

Heinemann, A. W., Linacre, J. M., Wright, B. D., Hamilton, B. B., & Granger, C. V. (1994). Prediction of rehabilitation outcomes with disability measures. *Archives of Physical Medicine and Rehabilitation, 75,* 133–143.

Heriza, C. (1991). Motor development: Traditional and contemporary theories. In M. J. Lester (Ed.), *Contemporary management of motor control problems: Proceedings of the II Step Conference.* Alexandria, VA: Foundation for Physical Therapy.

Individuals with Disabilities Education Act. (1997). PL 105-17. Individuals with Disabilities Education Act Amendments of 1997. 20 U.S.C. 1400 et seq.

Johnson-Martin, N. M., Jens, K. G., Attermeier, S. M., & Hacker, B. J. (1990). *The Carolina Curriculum for Infants and Toddlers with Special Needs.* Baltimore: Brookes.

Joint Commission on the Accreditation of Health Care Organizations. (1994). *A guide to establishing programs for assessing outcomes in clinical settings.* Oak Brook Terrace, IL: Joint Commission on Accreditation of Health Care Organizations.

Kafkes, A., Basu, S., Geist, R., & Kielhofner, G. (2001). Pediatric Volitional Questionnaire (PVQ). Retrieved April 9, 2004, from http://www.uic.edu/ahp/OT/MOHOC/clinical_instruments.html.

Kirshner, B., & Guyatt, G. (1985). A methodological framework for assessing health indices. *Journal of Chronic Diseases, 38,* 27–36.

Knox, S. (1997). Development and current use of the Knox preschool play scale. In L. D. Parham & L. S. Fazio (Eds.), *Play in occupational therapy* (pp. 35–51). St. Louis: Mosby.

Law, M., Baptiste, S., Carswell, A., McColl, M. A., Polatajko, H., & Pollack, N. (1994). *Canadian occupational performance measure.* Toronto, Canada: CAOT Publications.

Law, M., Polatajko, H., Pollack, N., McColl, M. A., Carswell, A., & Baptiste, S. (1994). Pilot testing of the Canadian Occupational Performance Measure: Clinical and measurement issues. *Canadian Journal of Occupational Therapy, 55,* 63–68.

Linder, T. (1993) *Transdisciplinary play-based assessment.* Baltimore: Brookes.

Mahoney, S. I., & Barthel, D. W. (1965). Functional evaluation: The Barthel Index. *Maryland State Medical Journal, 14,* 61–65.

McGraw, M. B. (1945). *The neuromuscular maturation of the human infant.* New York: Hafner Press.

McWilliam, R. A. (1992). *Family-centered intervention planning: A routines-based approach.* San Antonio: Therapy Skill Builders.

Miller, L. J., & Roid, G. H. (1994). *The TIME: Toddler and infant motor evaluation.* Tucson, AZ: Therapy Skill Builders.

Morgan, A., Koch, V., Lee, V., & Aldag, J. (1988). Neonatal neurobehavioral exam: A new instrument for quantitative analysis of neonatal neurological status. *Physical Therapy, 68,* 1352–1358.

Morrison, C. D., & Metsger, P. (2001). Play. In J. Case-Smith (Ed.), *Occupational therapy for children* (4th ed.). St. Louis: Mosby.

Nickel, R. E. (1987). *The infant motor screen.* Eugene, OR: Child Development and Rehabilitation Center, Oregon Health Sciences University.

Nystrom, E. P. (1974). Activity patterns and leisure concepts among the elderly. *American Journal of Occupational Therapy, 28,* 337–345.

Oczkowski, W. J., & Barreca, S. (1993). The functional independence measure: Its use to identify rehabilitation needs in stroke survivors. *Archives of Physical Medicine and Rehabilitation, 74,* 1291–1294.

Parham, L. D., & Mailloux, Z. (2001). Sensory integration. In J. Case-Smith (Ed.), *Occupational therapy for children* (pp. 329–381). St. Louis: Mosby.

Parks, S. (1992). *Inside HELP Administration and Reference Manual.* Palo Alto, CA: VORT.

Piper, M. (1993). Theoretical foundations for physical therapy assessment in early infancy. In I. J. Wilhelm (Ed.),

Physical therapy assessment in early infancy. New York: Churchill Livingstone.

Piper, M., & Darrah, J. (1993). *Motor assessment of the developing infant.* Philadelphia: W. B. Saunders.

Richardson, P. (2001). Use of Standardized Tests in Pediatric Practice. In J. Case-Smith (Ed.), *Occupational therapy for children* (pp. 217–245). St. Louis: Mosby.

Russell, D. J., Rosenbaum, P. L., Avery, L. M., & Lane, M. (2002). *Gross motor function measure. (GMFM-66 and GMFM-88) user's manual.* London: Cambridge University Press.

Shelton, T. (1989). The assessment of cognition/intelligence in infancy. *Infants and young children: An interdisciplinary journal of special care practice, 1,* 10–25.

Stewart, K. B. (2001). Purposes, processes, & methods of evaluation. In J. Case-Smith (Ed.). *Occupational therapy for children* (pp. 190–213). St. Louis: Mosby.

Stuberg, W. (1992). *The Milani-Comparetti motor development screening test* (3rd ed.). Omaha, NB: Meyer Children's Rehabilitation Center, Media Resource Center.

Glossary

abnormal development A pattern or sequence of behavior acquisition that differs from typical patterns in quality and form. Patterns of abnormal development include aspects that are not seen in the typical sequence, including movement sterotypies that are obligatory and cannot be volitionally suppressed.

abstraction Mental function of considering something as a general idea, quality, or characteristic, as distinct from concrete realities, specific objects, or actual instances; allows the individual to consider new or novel solutions to problems.

accessibility The quality of being at hand when needed; also the attribute of being easily approached or entered. Commonly used in terms of barriers to accessibility for persons with activity limitations.

accommodation From Jean Piaget's theory of cognitive development, a change of function in accordance with the environment or modification of the schema.

acquired disability Disability that is not innate and is acquired by the sudden onset of an event; includes stroke and spinal cord and traumatic brain injury.

acquired limitations Limitation of activity secondary to some acute or chronic condition that reduces an individual's usual age-appropriate activities.

active achievement viewpoint The cultural perspective that, through intervention services, an individual's ability to engage in activities can and should change.

Activities and Participation (ICF) Aspects of human behavior that deal with the range of tasks and behavior associated with a person's life situation.

activities of daily living (ADL) Physical functions of the human being that involve the simplest tasks of self-care.

activity level The amount of physical motion during sleep, eating, play, dressing, bathing, and so forth.

activity limitation In the ICF, phrase used to replace disability; refers to restrictions in activities and participation, due to limitations in structure, function, or contextual factors.

acute Describes an injury, such as a bone fracture, that has a sudden onset and a typically time-limited course of recovery.

adaptability The ease or difficulty with which reactions to stimuli can be modified in a desired way.

adaptation skills The ability to anticipate, correct for, and benefit from the consequences of errors that naturally arise during routine task performance.

adaptive cognition Ability to think in a manner less constrained by the need to find a single answer.

adaptive coping An approach to problem solving that aims to master the situation, or expand resources to deal with the situation. It is primarily used as a coping mechanism when individuals feel that they have a realistic chance to effect change.

addiction Compulsive physiologic and psychological need for a habit-forming substance.

adulthood (late) The years 65 and older. In this age group, physical functioning may be a concern as normal age-related changes taking place in the physiology are possibly compounded by chronic illness and disease. In addition, psychosocial issues may become increasingly paramount as the nuclear family may not be intact and individuals must contend with the loss of close friends and loved ones.

adulthood (middle) Typically, the period of 40–65 years of age, when normal age-related changes in physical functioning begin to occur, a more sophisticated level of thinking is adopted, and changes begin to occur within the family system.

adulthood (young) Typically, the period of 20–40 years of age, when optimal physical functioning and intellectual reasoning prevail, major decisions regarding significant relationships and career choices are often contemplated and made, and a keen sense of identity prevails.

aerobic capacity Maximum energy the body can generate through aerobic processes; represents the functional capacity of the cardiovascular system; also defined as VO2-max, or functional work capacity, and relates to physical endurance as an overall index of aerobic physical fitness.

affective domain Involves feelings, including happiness, sadness, anger, etc., which are all part of the human experience.

age-associated memory impairment (AAMI) Modest loss of memory function in healthy persons over age 50; involves complaints of memory impairment with everyday activities.

agonist Muscle considered to be the prime mover of a motion.

Ainsworth, Mary With Bowlby, studied the effect of early social experience on personality; developed the *strange situation* experimental paradigm, and classified modes of attachment behavior.

Americans with Disabilities Act (ADA) Law passed in 1991 that addresses societal limitations through affirmative action and removal of physical barriers.

anencephaly A defect in brain development resulting in small or missing brain hemispheres; a congenital absence of the brain and cranial vault, with the cerebral hemispheres completely missing or greatly reduced in size.

antagonist Muscle that acts against the given motion of an agonist muscle.

anticipatory awareness Ability to analyze a situation or task and identify potential strengths and weakness.

anticipatory control Alteration or adjustment of the motor program even before any interaction with the environment occurs.

anticipatory grief Characteristics of the grieving process, such as sorrow and disengagement, manifested prospectively, that is, before the loss has actually occurred.

apoptosis Apoptosis is the process of cell death and subsequent waste product removal.

approach/withdrawal The nature of initial responses to new stimuli—people, situations, places, foods, toys, procedures.

apraxia Disorder of motor planning and programming.

arena assessment Simultaneous observation of a client by a variety of disciplines; used when emphasis is to provide team-based services with reduction of duplication.

arteriovenous difference Ability of muscles to extract and metabolically utilize oxygen.

assessment Use of comprehensive strategies and tools to delineate strengths and needs, develop appropriate intervention plans and strategies, and determine change in individuals.

assets Products or objects of economic exchange such as money, goods, property, and other valuables that an individual owns and has rights to use.

assimilation Process of changing elements of the environment so they will fit into the current cognitive structure, or schema.

assistive technology (AT) Assistive technology includes any product, instrument, equipment, or technology adapted or specially designed for improving the functioning of a person with disabilities.

associative learning Learning in which the individual learns to predict relationships and draws on long-term memory to make associations; includes classical conditioning, operant conditioning, declarative learning, and procedural learning.

associative play Behavior common in 2-year-old children; the children enjoy the company of other children but do not organize their play.

astasia An inability in the infant to bear body weight on the legs in the period of integration of primitive postural muscle tone patterns and the emergence of voluntary limb control.

asymmetrical tonic neck reflex (ATNR) Mediates a typical postural set, beginning at birth and peaking over the first 2 months of life; stimulated by turning the head to one side, causing the upper and lower limbs on the side toward which the infant is looking (i.e., the face side) to extend while the upper and lower limbs facing the back of the head (the skull side), flex; creates a postural set symbolic of the en guarde position in fencing, so the pattern is sometimes referred to as the *fencing position;* believed to play a role in establishing linkages between the dominant hand and the eyes, since it tends to be stronger to the right in most infants, and it must be integrated to permit more mature behaviors, such as hands-to-midline and hands-to-mouth, to emerge.

asynchronous development Describes a situation in which the normal developmental progression is highly uneven.

atrial chambers of the heart The two chambers affording entrance to the heart.

at-risk infant Infant whose processes of neonatal development and transition to extra-uterine life are complicated beyond the normal circumstances surrounding birth.

attachment The emotional connection or love between the newborn and his caregiver(s).

attention Mental function that begins prenatally and allows the person to focus on something while simultaneously excluding less important information; the key that opens the door to the information-processing system; the process of detecting and orienting to important or desired environmental stimuli.

attention deficit/hyperactivity disorder (ADHD) Disorder characterized by developmentally inappropriate impulsivity, attention, and, in some cases, hyperactivity that affects 3–5 percent of school-age children.

attitude A contextual factor described in the ICF as general or specific opinions and beliefs about the person or about other matters that influence individual behavior and actions.

attitudinal environment The influence of observable beliefs based upon customs, practices, ideologies, values, norms, facts, and religious beliefs.

attractor well In systems theory of motor control, a preferred pattern; the deeper the attractor well, the more obligatory the pattern.

auditory perception Mental functions involved in discriminating sounds, tones, pitches, and other acoustic stimuli; enables a person to isolate an important sound in a noisy environment.

augmentative/alternative communication Means of communication in a form other than expressive speech output.

authoritarianism Preference for obedience to a clearly identified authority, placing less emphasis on individual freedom.

autonomic nervous system (ANS) Tied to parts of the central and peripheral nervous systems; directed by special parts of the brain and peripheral nervous system.

balance The ability to maintain a postural alignment in relation to gravitational forces and physical displacement.

Balanced Budget Act (BBA) Law passed in 1997 that initiated a new system of reimbursement in long-term-care facilities.

Bandura, Albert Social learning theorist of the twentieth century best known for the concept of modeling.

barrier-free design A design strategy recommended to all builders to make industrial design and technology accessible to the broadest possible spectrum of society. A goal of this approach is to have not two sets of technology/design for society, but rather one universal standard that remains accessible to all.

Bayley, Nancy Directed the Berkeley longitudinal studies of human development and was the author of the prominent Bayley Scales of Infant Development, the gold standard in infant assessment.

behavioral state One of the most important aspects of behavior in the newborn infant; may be defined as the infant's level of arousal mediating the responsivity to environmental inputs.

behaviorism Theoretical perspective that ascribes to the notion that all behavior can be described by the principles of conditioning.

benign senescent forgetfulness (BSF) Brief transitory episodes of cognitive decline attributable to inattentiveness and distractions.

bimanual coordination Process of using each hand differently, with one as a lead hand and the other as an assist.

biologic challenge In adolescence, accepting changes in appearance and function associated with a physically mature body.

biologic risk Related to factors in the infant or the mother that are known to have potentially adverse consequences on the infant; may include genetic problems, disease or disability in the mother or infant, maternal age, maternal smoking or drug use during pregnancy, *intrauterine growth retardation* (IUGR), and prematurity.

blastocyst Multicellular product of conception during the first week; embryonic tissue (inner cell mass) is first differentiated from extra-embryonic tissue (fetal membranes and placenta).

body mass index (BMI) Popular measure of amount of body fat.

body-on-body righting (BOB) A transitional movement pattern that persists through life and aids in the control of posture. In this pattern, when one leg is flexed and rotated across the midline of the body, a segmental rotation of the trunk, shoulder, and then head follows the initial movement.

body-on-head righting reaction (BOH) A transitional movement pattern that persists through life and aids in the control of posture. When the individual's postural orientation is not vertical, such as in prone, the individual moves the head out of alignment with the body into a vertical position.

body schema An internalized sense of the space that the body occupies.

bonding The development of a caring relationship on the part of the caregiver to the infant, characterized by behaviors such as kissing, cuddling, and stroking.

bottom-up assessment Perspective in which deficits or impairments are delineated in specific areas, leading to a program model designed to remediate those deficits.

boundaries Within a family system, lines of demarcation between individuals who are inside or outside a subsystem.

Bower, Gordon Psychologist prominent in the area of memory; studied the use of mnemonics, or memory enhancing devices, to improve retention.

Bowlby, John Psychiatrist who studied social development and attachment in children, including ethologic work. Examined the effects of mother-child separation.

bronchopulmonary dysplasia Progressive scarring of the lungs, creating a emphysematous-like function that is caused by many factors but is probably most closely related to prolonged ventilation of immature lungs, therefore placing infants who do not wean well from the ventilator at risk for this condition.

calibration Judgment of force, speed, and directional control necessary to accomplish a task.

cardiopulmonary system A key physiologic system in mediating behavior, particularly motor behavior; supports characteristics of motor performance such as endurance.

career An organized path of work pursued over some length of time.

career literacy An understanding of the nature of a given career through observation, media, part-time employment, or volunteer work.

caregiver Any individual—including a physician, nurse, social worker, parent, child, or other family member—who assists in the identification, prevention, or treatment of an illness or disability and attends to the needs of a child or dependent adult.

caregiver-child interactions Interactions between caregiver and infant, optimally showing characteristics such as reciprocity and synchrony; goodness of fit is desirable.

Case, Robbie Developmental psychologist who elaborated upon Piaget's theory of cognitive development, emphasizing innate abilities with social and cultural influences.

cataracts Opacity of the lens of the eye due to developmental or degenerative processes.

central nervous system (CNS) The brain and spinal cord; the parts of the nervous system that do not leave the protective covering of the skull and vertebral column.

cephalocaudal Relating to a head-to-tail direction along the long axis of the body.

cephalocaudal folding of the embryo Occurs as the neural plate continues its rapid expansion during the 3rd week and continues through the 4th week postconceptual age; the embryo gradually loses its flattened shape, adopting the curled, or flexed, posture it will maintain until birth.

cerebral hemispheres The two halves of the brain cerebrum; they make up the largest part of the brain.

cerebral palsy Most common congenital disorder, affecting primarily the motor system with secondary impact on multiple functions, including sensory, intellectual, self-care, and language. It is due to a nonprogressive defect or lesion of the brain in early life.

Chess, Stella Theorist who, with Alexander Thomas, developed a classic system for describing and categorizing temperament.

Chomsky, Noam Prominent twentieth-century theorist in the area of language development; known for nativist approach, or the belief that the ability for language acquisition is innate.

chondroskeleton The well-formed cartilaginous skeleton identified at the lowest portion of the skull, the spine, ribcage, scapulas, and extremities by the 10th–11th week postconceptual age.

choreoathetoid Type of cerebral palsy resulting from kernicterus.

chronic Describes conditions such as diabetes, osteoarthritis, and Parkinson's disease that involve gradual, progressive declines over time.

chronic sorrow Recurrent sorrow that occurs when parents encounter repetitively the limitations from their child's enduring impairments.

chronology Chronology refers to the timing of the onset of the condition (for example, at what point in the lifespan the condition occurs), as well as the length of time that the condition persists. Medical terminology often uses the terms "acute" and "chronic" to characterize the length of time a person has been experiencing a particular condition.

classical conditioning Process that enables learning to occur from repeatedly pairing some neutral stimulus with a stimulus that evokes a response.

client-centered care A dynamic strategy in which both professionals and clients work together in a collaborative manner to meet the needs of the client.

cocaine-exposed infants Infants who were exposed through the placental circulation to cocaine; infants are irritable and have difficulty feeding.

cognition How and what we think; the function of the brain that enables interaction with the environment.

cognitive appraisal theory Cognitive appraisal theory was introduced by Lazarus and Folkman (1984) to define psychological stress as a cognitive problem-solving process.

cognitive competencies Mastery of cognitive skills that permit effective and appropriate environmental interactions.

cognitive development Difficult to definitively characterize in the neonate; may include the abilities of discrimination and recognition, as well as a response to both classical and operant conditioning.

cognitive domain Involves thought; includes the ability to express one's self through written and spoken language, the ability to read, think, and perform tasks from planning through completion.

cognitive flexibility The ability to consider alternatives and change strategies or approaches to a problem.

cognitive map Mental manipulations of remembered sensory experiences superimposed on a desired task.

cohesion The tendency to stick together. Cohesion in a family group is the tendency to support one another in a positive way.

coincidence-anticipation timing The ability to initiate and complete a motor pattern with the arrival of a moving object at a previously set interception point.

co-insurance Situation in which an individual has two or more insurance policies, such as Medicare plus private insurance; agreement must be made as to primary and secondary coverage.

collectivistic cultural characteristics The principles or system of ownership and control of the means of production and distribution by the people collectively, usually under the supervision of a government.

colostrum Nutritive substance produced by the mother for the first 48–72 hours after birth that is viscous, clear, and full of antibodies that are passed from mother to infant during breast-feeding.

communication Term that encompasses the ability of humans to interact in ways that enable them to share such functions as basic needs, wants, desires, and ideas.

comparator In motor control theories, used to refer to a neural body, such as the cerebellum, that has access to both expected or programmed and actual or received sensory input about the motor program.

conceptional age Common terminology associated with dating the age of the preterm infant. Also called *postconceptual age.*

concrete operations In Piaget's theory of cognitive development, the third stage, typically roughly equivalent to that displayed by the school-age child. In this stage, the child performs manipulations on the envi-

ronment using organized cognitive structures. Key characteristics displayed by children in this phase are reversibility of actions and mastery of conservation tasks.

conditioned response Learned reaction to a neutral stimulus.

conductive hearing loss Hearing loss caused by a problem with the outer or middle ear.

congenital Condition or trait that exists or dates from birth, such as cerebral palsy.

consciousness A global mental function; involves a level of arousal that permits responsiveness to the environment.

consolidation stage The fifth of Super's (1985) eight stages of career exploration and development. Here the individual is responding to actual work experiences; a vocational path is selected that offers the best chance to obtain satisfaction.

constructive play Play that involves the making or building of things; develops at age 3–4 years and closely parallels the development of manipulation and fine motor skills and executive functions like planning, sequencing, and error detection.

contextual factors In the ICF, those factors that influence how a person is able to respond to a given condition; these factors are intrinsic (personal) or extrinsic (environmental).

control parameters Conditions in existence at the time the task is to be executed.

cooperative play Behavior typical of middle childhood, as in team games where there is social interaction in a group setting, with a sense of group identity.

co-payment In insurance, the percentage of any given product or service for which the individual is responsible for payment.

coping styles The way families "contend with difficulties and act to overcome them"; two styles include *adaptive,* or attempting to manage the situation or solve the problem, and *emotional,* or attempting to manage the emotional response to the situation.

cranial nerves Composed of 12 pairs of nerves that emanate from the nervous tissue of the brain. In order to reach their targets they must ultimately exit/enter the cranium through openings in the skull.

criterion-referenced Type of formative assessment that examines the number of items or criteria an individual can successfully complete as compared with a standard completed by a normative group; is sensitive to intervention and can help guide therapy.

cruising An infant mobility pattern that involves moving the hands along furniture or other environmental features while taking steps sideways to move in a desired direction.

crystallized intelligence Intelligence that reflects the acquired and accumulated education, knowledge, and skills of an individual.

crystallization (stage of career choice) In Super's theory, the stage characteristic of early adolescence where only general ideas regarding a career are formulated.

crystallization of vocational choice Ginzberg's theory of occupational choice in which a single occupation is selected from within a career category, as in selecting nursing from health-related careers.

cultural issues with the newborn The typical parental and interpersonal behaviors that have been passed on as part of a family's culture and affect not only the birth process but the immediate postpartum period as well

cultural practices The actions and occupations that reflect the generally accepted values, beliefs, and behaviors of particular cultural groups.

cultural schemas Divided into four areas: person, self, role, and event; these schemas allow a therapist to systematically view the influence of culture on specific behaviors and characteristics.

culture The characteristic features of a civilization, including its beliefs, spiritual practices, and social institutions.

cycle of violence Concept that a childhood history of physical abuse predisposes a person to violence in later years.

deceleration stage The seventh of Super's (1985) eight stages of career exploration and development. This includes the preretirement phase, during which the individual's attention is on continuing to meet the minimum requirements of the job rather than on enhancing their position. It culminates in leaving the workforce.

decision making Process of evaluating and assimilating all available information in order to arrive at conclusions about problems, goals, and interventions.

declarative learning Learning that the individual is conscious of and makes a conscious effort to support; predominates as the individual attempts to learn a new skill at any age and requires both awareness of and attention to the task.

deductible In insurance, the amount an individual must pay out of his own pocket before the insurance begins to pay; typically calculated on an annual policy year basis.

degrees of freedom In any system, the number of factors that are free to vary.

dementia Deterioration of intellectual faculties such as judgment, concentration, and especially memory, usually due to an identified organic problem. Emotional disturbance and personality changes sometimes occur.

denervation The act of depriving an organ or body part of a nerve supply.

determinants of health Factors that influence overall health and well-being, including biologic factors, behaviors, social and physical environments, and public policies and interventions.

development The changes in performance that are heavily influenced by maturational processes.

developmental coordination disorder (DCD) Problems with cognition, sensory, and motor functions that cause difficulty integrating and coordinating the information from these three areas; roughly 6 percent of school-age children have DCD, which may appear in conjunction with other learning disorders.

developmental crises Crises experienced by families that influence structure and identity of the family unit; they are typically represented across many families and are therefore somewhat predictable.

developmental delay Describes failure of child to acquire normative age-related behaviors; implies the ability to "catch up."

developmental disorder Pervasive and chronic developmental delay, often with scatter in the acquisition patterns of developmental milestones.

developmental life tasks Activities that an individual takes part in that may, for an adult, include separation and individuation from family of origin, development of one's own family, financial/career independence, and successful navigation of life events throughout adulthood.

developmental milestones Skills typical within a culture to a specific age group; useful for screening children, but do not give adequate information to determine whether a delay is based on neuromotor or environmental causes.

developmental theory Theory that attempts to describe change as a function of time.

Dewey, John Theorist who believed in the biologic and social bases to learning and emphasized the school as an instrument of social progress; a major influence on American education systems.

diagnosis The label applied to describe the patterns of signs and symptoms displayed by an individual with a medical complaint.

differentiation Allows cells to become specialized; is at its peak in younger individuals, but begins to decline in the aging adult.

disability Inability to pursue life tasks and roles because of physical or mental impairment.

disablement Sociologic concept commonly used to describe the impact of a disease or disability on human function, recognizing that functional states associated with health conditions are not identical to the conditions themselves.

disablement model A theoretical attempt to categorize activity limitation in terms of an individual's social and cultural environment.

discriminative index Method of distinguishing between individuals or groups on specific dimensions to determine if observed performance is typical, such as in acquisition of developmental milestones.

discriminative touch Aspects of touch that we think consciously about, like how hard, smooth, or curved an object is.

disease Biologically based problem or condition in which a person's functional abilities have been disrupted.

distal transverse palmar arch Flexible arch that balances stability and mobility in the hand; maintained by activity in the hand's intrinsic muscles.

distractibility Refers to the effectiveness of extraneous environmental stimuli in interfering with ongoing behaviors.

dorsal sensory neuron Nerve cell that conducts impulses from a sense organ to the central nervous system.

Down syndrome Fairly common genetically based developmental disorder caused by an extra twenty-first chromosome; physical characteristics and mental retardation are commonly associated with this syndrome.

ductus arteriosus Passageway between the pulmonary trunk and the aorta that normally closes within the first few hours after birth.

dynamic mobility Ability to time, anticipate, and change motions while actively moving.

dynamic postural stability Type of active, adaptive control that allows an individual to change movements without stopping or losing balance; begins around 5 years of age.

dynamical systems theory Has its roots in a theory of human physics, which refers to self-organization of complex particles; states that behavior at any given point in time is the result of variable interactions of a number of complex systems and that behavior is emergent.

dysarthris Paresis, paralysis, or weakness of the oral musculature.

dysmorphism Refers to physical characteristics that are abnormal; often associated with genetic conditions.

Early Intervention (EI) Federally funded incentive program under IDEA, Part C, which provides preventive and ameliorative services for parents of children with developmental delay from birth through 2 years.

ecological approach In assessment, documents the individual's success in participating in activities and routines in the environment where the individual is expected to perform the skill, thereby giving a contextual reference.

ectoderm Among the three primary embryonic cell layers, the one that results in the surface layer of cells forming the skin.

educational participation Adolescent engagement in academics, non-academics (such as hall and lunch time) and school sponsored extracurricular activities.

effector system of motor control Musculoskeletal system; key in executing motor behavior.

efficacy The personal sense that you are competent and effective in your life roles.

egalitarianism Preference for affirmation of the individual allowing for negotiation in authority relationships.

egocentric thinking Thought processes in which one does not understand or consider the possibility that the view may be different for persons on another side of a three-dimensional array; lack of understanding of the feelings or viewpoints of others.

electronic play An intrinsically motivated activity chosen by the child as a form of leisure that involves use of an electronic apparatus such as television.

embryo The developing human from conception to 8 weeks.

embryonic period Period extending to the end of the 8th week after conception, at which point all major body structures have been formed.

emergent awareness Ability to analyze a situation or task and identify potential strengths and weakness.

emergent behavior Alteration of a task in countless ways in order to meet the current conditions.

emergent control In motor-control theories, the ability to alter how a task is performed in accordance with current environmental circumstances.

emotional functions Functions that include specific mental functions related to the feeling and affective reactions of individuals, as well as mental regulation of the appropriateness and degree of emotion within the individual's social and environmental context.

empiricist school Based on belief that the formation of associations between various sensations is the foundation of perception.

endoderm Germ layer from which are formed the digestive system, many glands, and part of the respiratory system.

energy functions Functions that include the physiologic and psychological mechanisms that result in the individual's energy level, motivation, appetite, craving (including craving for substances that can be abused), and impulse control.

engrossment The sense of absorption, preoccupation, and interest that fathers have in their newborn child.

entrainment Rudimentary variation of a linked behavioral and social exchange present at birth.

entrance process In *Theory of Transformed Parenting* by Seidemen & Kleine, occurs when parents receive and respond to the diagnosis of their child's condition.

environmental constraints Prevailing environmental conditions that help shape the movement to be executed.

environmental factors Features that make up the physical, social, and attitudinal environment in which people live and conduct their lives.

environmental fit The concept that an appropriate level of stimulation and support is available to support functional performance of an individual at any age.

environmental risk Related to factors in the infant's environment that may have a potentially adverse effect on the infant, such as low socioeconomic status (SES), inadequate parental caregiving, neglect or abuse, poor nutrition, etc.

epiblasts Outer layer of a blastula that gives rise to the ectoderm.

equilibrium Process of maintaining, through postural adjustments, the center of mass over the base of support.

equilibrium reactions Complex patterns involving rotational movements along the body axis in order to maintain balance that are considered neurologically mature because their presence indicates the integration of earlier primitive and transitional motor patterns.

ergonomics The science of workplace design to promote optimal physical function and to prevent common workplace injuries.

Erikson, Erik One of the few true lifespan theorists; his psychosocial theory related developmental stages to a series of life tasks, or crises that need to be resolved.

error detection Ability to look at one's own work or the work of others and find any errors in the work.

establishment stage The fourth of Super's (1985) eight stages of career exploration and development. In this stage the individual is in actual work situations, experiencing some that fit and others that do not.

ethnicity Generally refers to the influence of both race and culture on behavior and may also refer to shared traits, customs, language, religion, and ancestry.

evaluation process According to IDEA, the process used to help make a diagnosis, identify atypical development, or determine eligibility for services; typically involves both collecting and interpreting information.

evaluative assessment strategy A strategy that measures the magnitude of change in an individual over time on a specific dimension. The overall purpose of an assessment is to describe individuals' strengths and needs to help design appropriate individualized therapeutic intervention plans.

event schemas The manner in which familiar situations are organized, such as the sequence of events on a child's first day of school.

examination Objective means of data collection.

executive functions Control or oversight functions of thought; the mental processes that organize our thoughts for action, including the processes of initiating, abstraction, problem solving, cognitive flexibility, and judgment.

exercise Purposeful physical activity that promotes physiologic and emotional well-being.

experimentation period In Ginzberg's theory of occupational choice, the period involving selection of career category and investigation of options.

explicit memory Also known as declarative memory, it is a type of memory containing knowledge about the world, facts, and figures, much of which can be verbally represented.

expressive language Act of speaking, writing, or signing; precedes receptive language development.

eye-hand coordination Skillful use of the hand under visual guidance; precedes the development of fine hand and eye control.

Fair Housing Act Amendments (FHAA) Fair Housing Act Amendments of 1988 (FHAA) amended Title VIII of the Civil Rights Act of 1968 to add individuals with disabilities to the list of people protected from housing discrimination.

family-centered intervention Interventions in which families play a key role in decision-making, including assigning resources and interpreting needs.

family functions Tasks that families perform to meet the individual and collective needs of the members.

family issues with the newborn Associated with an often challenging transition accompanied by stress and uncertainty that, in most cases, occurs successfully as the infant is integrated into the rhythms of the family life.

family life cycle theory Theory of how families change over time and go through predictable stages, such as coupling, childbearing, having school-age children, having adolescents, launching, postparental, and aging.

family member An immediate or distant relative who may assume many roles and responsibilities in response to their family member's impairments or disability.

family structure Refers to the variety of characteristics that make the family unique, such as membership characteristics, cultural style, and ideological style.

family subsystems Functioning subsystems within the family, such as the marital, parental, or sibling systems; they describe who participates in interaction.

family systems theory Derivative of systems theory, in which the family is seen as a group of individuals with interrelated occupations; the family system is greater than the sum of its parts.

family transitions Interim phases between stages of family life cycles; they require adaptation on the part of the family members.

fantasy period Period of childhood lasting until about age 11 or 12 in which the person expresses a desire to become a teacher, doctor, athlete, superhero, etc.

fantasy play Play that allows children to mentally experiment with new sensations or roles and try out new behaviors for themselves in imagined forms while in a safe environment.

fear of falling (FOF) Multifactorial problem with high incidence in the older adult; associated with poorer health status and functional decline.

feedback In any system, information returned to the source for processing; in motor control, sensory information that is available as a result of movement.

fetal alcohol syndrome (FAS) Syndrome caused by excessive maternal consumption of alcohol during pregnancy; typically includes microcephaly, developmental delay, and dysmorphism in the child.

fetal period The longest period of prenatal development, extending from approximately the 9th week after conception until the moment of birth. This period involves extensive growth as well as complex structural and physiologic refinement of the tissues, organs, and systems that were formed during the embryonic period.

fetal viability Exists when a fetus is sufficiently developed to live outside the uterus.

fetus The developing human after the 8th week; the fetus has rudimentary eyes and eyebrows, ears, arm buds with hands, fingers, leg buds with feet, and toes. (From birth to the 8th week, the developing human is called an *embryo*.)

Fick equation The relationship between cardiopulmonary function and an individual's maximum performance level or functional capacity is expressed by the Fick equation: $VO_{2MAX} = CO \times$ a-vO_2 difference. VO_{2MAX} is the maximum volume of oxygen the body can utilize; CO is cardiac output or the product of heart rate and stroke volume; and a-vO_2 difference is the arteriovenous difference or the measure of the body's ability to extract and utilize oxygen.

figure-ground perception Ability to separate an object of regard from its surroundings.

fine motor control Includes the volitional, coordinated use of the eyes, hands, and muscles of the mouth.

fiscal intermediary Typically, an insurance company under contract with the government to review claims for services.

flow Term used to describe the smoothness and fluidity of movement.

fluid intelligence Capacity to use unique kinds of thinking to solve unfamiliar problems by utilizing short-term memory, creating concepts, perceiving complex relationships, and engaging in abstract reasoning.

foramen ovale Opening between the two atrial chambers of the heart that normally closes within the first 2 weeks after birth.

forebrain The most anterior of the three primary regions of the embryonic brain, from which the telencephalon and diencephalon develop.

formal operations In Piaget's theory of cognitive development, the last and highest phase; the ability to manipulate problems mentally using logic and rules; roughly equivalent to the early adolescent in age.

Fragile X syndrome Sex-linked genetic abnormality that results in intellectual impairment, including mental retardation.

frame of reference Theoretical perspective or viewpoint that organizes the approach to client management.

Freud, Sigmund Father of psychoanalysis; developed familiar concepts such as id, ego, and superego; one of the originators of psychological interventions.

function Action or ability for which a person or thing is specially fitted, used, or responsible for.

functional communication Effective sending and receiving of information.

functional goal The end toward which effort is directed to contribute to the development or maintenance of a larger whole.

functional performance Describes the ability of an individual to participate in activities, tasks, and roles during daily occupations. The four primary forms of occupation in adulthood are work, play, leisure, and self-care.

functional work capacity Maximum energy the body can generate through aerobic processes; represents the functional capacity of the cardiovascular system; also defined as VO2-max or aerobic capacity and relates to physical endurance as an overall index of aerobic physical fitness.

gag reflex Elicited by touch of the posterior half to third of the tongue or the soft palate/uvula region; plays an important role in feeding development in preterm infants.

games with rules Play activities that have explicit rules that are agreed upon by all parties and involve the cooperative play of at least two persons.

gastroesophageal reflux A heartburn-like condition created by stomach content refluxing into the esophagus that is extremely common in premature infants; can produce behaviors such as incoordination in swallowing, feeding aversion, and arching.

gateway drugs Drugs, such as alcohol, that seem to open entrance into harder drug use.

gender identity The sense of identification with either the male or female sex, as manifested in appearance, behavior, and other aspects of a person's life.

gender issues with the newborn Difficult to isolate specifically to the neonatal period and often illustrates cultural practices; in some cultures the birth of a male infant is much more highly prized than the birth of a female infant, and in Western cultures, traditional parents (defined as parents where the father is the primary breadwinner and the mother primary caregiver) tend to interact more with sons than with daughters.

germinal period Period that lasts approximately 2 weeks from conception and ends when the unicellular zygote has implanted in the uterus and has become an embryo, a complex multicellular organism capable of producing all of the organs and tissues of the body.

Gesell, Arnold Director of Yale center for child development; published extensively from his work with developmental norms, and was a strong supporter of the maturationist or "nature" school.

gestalt school Characterized by belief that perception is not a perfect, photographic representation of the world, nor is it a sum of sensations, but that it has a psychological form that represents the world without being identical to it.

gestational age Direct estimate of the duration of the pregnancy, dated from the mother's last menstrual period.

Gibson, Eleanor Perceptual theorist who studied perceptual development and believed that perception is a function of learning to attend to salient features of a stimulus.

Ginzberg, Eli Theorist who proposed that the process of occupational choice follows a developmental progression that begins in childhood and spans into early adulthood, including a fantasy period, a tentative period, and a realistic period.

glaucoma Increased intraocular pressure causing damage and visual loss; one of the leading causes of blindness in individuals over the age of 35.

global mental functions Functions that underlie the other mental activities, including consciousness, energy, and drive, and are crucial to all human activity; they also are important predictive factors in rehabilitation outcomes.

goodness of fit Occurs when the individual's temperament supports the demands and expectations of the environment.

graphomotor skills The collections of conceptual and perceptual motor skills involved in drawing and writing.

grasp reflexes Highly predictable in the newborn; include the plantar grasp reflex and the palmar grasp reflex.

growth Quantitative changes that occur over time in the human (height, weight, physical characteristics, etc.) and underlie human development.

gustatory perception Mental function involved in distinguishing the differences in tastes, such as sweet, sour, salt, and bitter stimuli, detected by the tongue; has functional implications in aging, when diet may be compromised by changes in this perceptual function.

habits Ingrained behaviors that can be performed without conscious thought.

hand preference Consistent choice of the same hand for complex skilled tasks; usually developed by the age of 4.

haptic awareness Involved in distinguishing the differences (without the use of vision) in texture, shape, size, weight, and temperature.

haptic perception Active memory of touch, texture, shape, temperature, and weight that allows an individual to tell you that she has, for example, a penny in her hand even in the absence of sight.

Hayflick limit In humans, the ability of cells to divide and replicate is limited to some genetically predetermined amount referred to as the Hayflick limit (Hayflick, 1974). The ability of cells to reproduce is decreased as one begins to age.

health Refers to the absence of illness and is often culturally mediated with expected behaviors to be demonstrated before an individual can claim to be healthy.

health management A specific self-care skill, as described in the AOTA practice framework. This task includes developing, managing, and maintaining routines for health and wellness promotion.

Healthy People 2010 Document developed by consensus of several hundred national organizations and government agencies to serve as a mechanism to identify the health of the U.S. population, set goals for the nation's health, and provide ways to measure progress.

heart septum Membranous structure between the two heart atria or between the two heart ventricles.

hierarchical models of development Theory tying the acquisition of developmental milestones to the level of brain maturation; models explain human motor behavior, with the cerebral cortex ultimately determining the form and function of human movement.

hindbrain The most posterior of the three primary divisions of the brain in the embryo; develops into the cerebellum, pons, and medulla oblongata.

hippotherapy Use of horseback riding to accomplish therapeutic goals such as improved strength, balance, and posture.

HIV-exposed Infants who contract the HIV virus from their mother.

Holland, John His theory of career selection emphasizes the notion of fit between personality type and career selection.

hyperopia Farsightedness.

hypogeuia Decreased sensitivity to taste in the gustatory system.

hyposmia Decreased sensitivity to smell in the olfactory system.

hypotonia Hypotonia involves decreased resting tension in the muscles (muscle tone). Hypotonia may suggest the presence of central nervous system dysfunction, genetic disorders, or muscle disorders.

hypoxic ischemic encephalopathy (HIE) Lack of oxygen due to asphyxia that can cause insult to the nervous system of a preterm infant.

illness Refers to the negative changes in a person's well-being and social position within a cultural group; is not merely the presence of disease but also reflects the social and cultural interpretation of well-being.

ideologic style Family's beliefs, values, and coping behaviors.

immediate memory Also called *sensory memory;* recall of stimuli within seconds of the event; the ability to remember and act on information immediately preceding the present need for the information.

immunization Injection of small amounts of material from infectious organisms administered to allow the individual to produce antibodies against that organism.

implementation (stage of career choice) In Super's theory, the stage in which young adults begin to explore career possibilities through entry-level jobs and/or professional training.

implicit memory Implicit memory, also known as procedural memory, incorporates skills that are practiced and autonomic and that primarily involve cognitive or motor components.

inclusion Philosophy that all students in school, regardless of strengths/weaknesses, are part of the school community.

independent cultural groups Western cultures that encourage independence and attributes such as inquisitiveness.

Individual Family Support Plan (IFSP) Intervention document mandated by IDEA, Part C, Early Intervention, which includes the goals of the intervention and the expectation of the family.

individualistic cultural characteristics Typical of a culture that values assertiveness in reaching goals, with emphasis on individual over collective welfare.

Individualized Education Plan (IEP) Intervention document mandated by IDEA, Part B, School Programs, which sets the current level of functioning, goals, measurement strategies, and time estimate to achieve the goals.

Individuals with Disabilities Education Act (IDEA) Federal legislation first passed in 1975 as the Education of the Handicapped Act; renamed and reauthorized in 1990 and several times subsequently; guarantees adequate access to and provision of education for children with disabilities, including provisions for related services such as therapies.

infancy Time in the human life cycle from birth through 12 months of age.

inferior pincer grasp Developmental grasp pattern using the distal pads of the thumb and forefinger, with the ulnar fingers inhibited and the thumb in opposition.

in-hand manipulation The process of using one hand to adjust an object for more effective placement or for release; the object remains in that hand and usually does not come in contact with a surface during in-hand manipulation.

initiation Ability to begin something.

instrumental activities of daily living (IADL) Activities of daily living that typically involve cognitive sequencing of chains of behavior; examples include complex tasks, often involving some tool or instrument, such as setting the table, picking up toys, washing vegetables, and folding washcloths.

integration In development, the notion that certain patterns (frequently called reflexes) are no longer characteristic in motor behavior, but may become dominant in the case of stress or injury.

intellectual awareness Capacity to perceive "self" in relatively "objective" terms; includes knowledge about the strategies we employ in our own thinking and the individual's knowledge about personal thoughts and feelings as they impact performance and impact others; may be considered insight into self.

intellectual functions Skills required for the individual to understand and constructively integrate information from all types of mental function; functions that develop and change over the lifespan and are influenced by experience, environmental contexts, and learning.

intelligence Refers to the capacity to acquire and supply knowledge. *Fluid intelligence* refers primarily to novel situations, whereas *crystallized intelligence* refers to the ability to apply strategies consistently and effectively.

intelligence quotient Number held to express the relative intelligence of an individual; determined by dividing mental age by chronological age and then multiplying by 100.

intensity Energy level of responses, regardless of quality or direction.

interactive behaviors All active behaviors that are directed at gaining the attention of others.

interdependent cultural group Mutually dependent group; relying on others but also being responsible for their behavior as well as one's own.

International Classification of Functioning and Disability (ICF) Classification system published by the World Health Organization to provide a scientific basis for understanding and studying functional states associated with health conditions.

interuterine growth retardation Describes infants who are born with low birthweight (less than 2,500 g) and are also *small for gestational age (SGA)*, reflecting poor fetal nutrition during pregnancy, commonly caused by maternal smoking, which deprives the fetus of oxygenation; may cause attentional and activity

disorders, but the outcome appears to interact with the support in the postnatal environment, and a supportive environment may help minimize the consequences.

intimacy Ability to trust, to be autonomous, to have initiative and industry, and to have established personal identity.

intraventricular hemorrhage (IVH) Fragile blood vessels near the ventricles of the brain that can rupture, causing insult to the nervous system of a preterm infant.

isolation Inability to have genuine physical exchanges with others who could offer empathy, understanding, support, encouragement, and insight.

jaundice An increase in bilirubin that causes an infant's skin to have a yellowish cast.

judgment The mental function involved in making a choice, as is involved in making a decision or forming an opinion.

judgment-based assessment Assessment strategy to obtain task-specific information about an individual from those who routinely watch the task performance, as in the case of a schoolteacher reporting on handwriting.

kangaroo care In care of the premature infant, the concept of providing warmth from the temperature of the parents' skin, by placing the baby inside the parents' clothing and against the skin; replaces the warming incubator or isolette.

kernicterus Caused by excessive bilirubin levels that may lead to damage to certain parts of the brain.

kinesthetic awareness Information about movement within the body and changes in limb position.

kinesthetic perception Interpretation of information regarding relative position of body parts, body in space, and awareness of position and movement.

Knowledge of Performance (KP) In motor learning/control theory, the knowledge of qualities of the movement.

Knowledge of Results (KR) In motor learning/control theory, the knowledge of the outcome of the movement; essential for motor learning.

Kohlberg, Lawrence Student of Piaget, who is known for his theory of moral development.

kyphosis Kyphosis is a curving of the spine that causes a bowing of the back, which leads to a forward-bending or slouching posture.

labyrinthine righting reactions Mediate antigravity behaviors that include a number of upper brainstem–mediated responses that either align the body with respect to gravity and/or the support surface or rotate the body parts into alignment with each other, thereby permitting the individual to change positions, as in rolling.

language A learned code, or system, of rules that make it possible for us to communicate ideas and express wants and needs.

language acquisition device (LAD) Innate mechanism that is activated through linguistic input and performs mental operations essential to learning language.

language development Typically defined as a representation of cognitive structure that appears to be present in newborns on a receptive language level.

language disorder Problem with the comprehension and/or production of the language components morphology, syntax, semantics, and pragmatics.

language impairment Any problem in the comprehension and/or production of the language code.

lanugo Coat of delicate, downy hairs that covers the human fetus and newborn infant.

lateral folding of the embryo Occurs by around day 19 or 20, when the embryo begins to fold lengthwise. Lateral folding is the result of expansion of the paraxial mesoderm and the emerging somites.

lateral prehension (also called **lateral pincer** or **key grasp**) Lateral prehension generally describes a grip pattern with the thumb pressing laterally against an object or the base of the first digit. This can be a power grip if the thumb is adducted; a precision grip if the thumb is abducted.

leading health indicators Ten key concerns for public health identified by *Healthy People 2010,* including physical activity, smoking cessation, and reduction of sexually transmitted disease.

learned helplessness Disabling type of social learning in which a person learns that there is no way to succeed after repeatedly experiencing failure, resulting in a passive failure to attempt unfamiliar tasks.

learning Acquisition of new behavior, heavily influenced by environmental exposure as well as feedback and practice.

leisure Time that is not relegated to specific work or purpose but is used for enjoyment; leisure time has varying characteristics at different ages across the lifespan.

level of fixity Refers to how quickly a skill is lost after the child stops performing it for a given amount of time.

limbic system Part of the brain that controls needs, drives, and innate behaviors; very old and buried deep within the cerebral cortex.

lipofuscin Pigmented lipid substance that accumulates in the cytoplasm of all aging cells, including the brain; it is a biologic marker that occurs through peroxidation of lipids and proteins.

literacy Ability to read written language.

locomotor pattern Type of mobility pattern in which the body as a whole is moved, or translated, through space.

long-term memory Memory for an indefinite period of time; storage is widely distributed in the brain.

longitudinal palmar arch Flexible arch that balances stability and mobility in the hand; maintained by activity in the hand's intrinsic muscles.

lordosis Lordosis is an increased curvature of the normally curved lumbar spine.

low vision Very limited sight that can interfere with a person's daily routine activities.

macular degeneration Small hemorrhages in the macular area that lead to gray shadows in center of visual field, making reading, watching television, and fine motor activities difficult.

maintained abilities Abilities that are typically maintained and do not diminish with age, including cultural and academic knowledge, verbal comprehension, vocabulary, number facility, and fluency of retrieval from long-term memory.

maintenance stage The sixth of Super's (1985) eight stages of career exploration and development. The maintenance stage generally begins in the mid-40s and is distinguished by the maintenance of prestige, authority, and responsibility.

malingering The act of intentionally feigning or exaggerating physical or psychological symptoms for personal gain.

Maslow, Abraham Theorist who developed a theory of hierarchy of needs, from the most basic physiologic needs to self-actualization.

mastery motivation Innate drive to find solutions, evolving from playfulness and motivating an individual to learn; helps with the development of a sense of personal value.

maturation Qualitative changes related to organizational and process changes that underlie human development.

mature rotary neck righting (NOB) A transitional movement pattern that persists through life and aids in the control of posture. In this pattern, when the head and neck are rotated across the midline of the body, a segmental rotation of the shoulder, trunk, and then pelvis follows the initial movement.

maximum oxygen consumption (VO2 Max) Maximum energy the body can generate through aerobic processes; represents the functional capacity of the cardiovascular system; also defined as *aerobic* or *functional work capacity* and relates to physical endurance as an overall index of aerobic physical fitness.

McGraw, Myrtle Theorist known for her study of motor development, including the Johnny & Jimmy twin studies, designed to assess the relative impact of nature versus nurture.

meconium Thick, tarry substance that is usually voided in utero as well as for the first few days postnatally.

Medicaid Enacted into law in 1965 as Title 19 of the Social Security Act, a joint federal/state program that provides basic medical care for approximately 36 million medically indigent individuals. Medically indigent individuals qualify for Medicaid based on their low income or their qualifications for public assistance programs such as Supplemental Security Income (SSI).

medical model Emphasizes the person, and that person's impairments, as a cause of disability; it is the traditional approach presented in rehabilitation literature.

medically necessary In insurance, products or services deemed appropriate for coverage, such as wheelchair rental; however, it may eliminate reimbursement for functional aids such as shower/tub benches, raised toilet seats, and grab bars, which are often necessary following an accident or illness.

Medicare A federal health insurance program for individuals over the age of 65, created in 1965 as Title 18 of the Social Security Act; Part A covers hospital insurance and Part B medical benefits, such as outpatient services.

memory The registering and storing of information and retrieving it as needed.

memory functions Functions that include immediate, recent, and remote memory spans, as well as the skills used in recalling and learning, like retrieval of information and remembering.

memory trace In Adam's theory of motor learning, the stored sensory motor plan of a movement.

mental functions Functions of the brain and central nervous system that underlie human learning; they are innate to humans and include both global functions like consciousness, and specific functions like self-control.

mental health Status of emotional and psychological well-being in which an individual is able to use her cognitive and emotional capabilities, function in society, and meet the ordinary demands of everyday life.

mental retardation Description of cognitive function that describes limitations in both intelligence and adaptive functions.

mesenchymal Cells of mesodermal origin that are capable of developing into connective tissues, blood, and lymphatic and blood vessels.

mesoderm Germ layer that forms many muscles, the circulatory and excretory systems, and the dermis, skeleton, and other supportive and connective tissue. It also gives rise to the notochord.

metabolic equivalent unit (MET) A measure of functional capacity. One MET is equal approximately to the body's utilization of 3.5 ml O_2 per kilogram of body weight per minute (ml O_2/kg/min).

metacognition Refers to the use of cognitive skills that provide the basis for transfer and generalization of learned skills to daily functioning; includes monitoring functions and executive functions that help us plan, organize, execute, and evaluate our day-to-day activities.

metalinguistic awareness Ability to engage in introspective tasks that reflect one's use of language.

midbrain The middle of the three primary divisions of the brain in the embryo.

minimal-stimulation protocol In care of the premature infant, the notion that any stimulation is physically stressful; attempts are made to package caregiving procedures and minimize unnecessary episodes of care.

mobility Capability of moving or being moved.

modeling Part of Bandura's social learning theory that proposes that children do not need to be directly reinforced to learn certain social skills; rather, they can learn by watching and receiving vicarious reinforcement.

model of function and disability Model intended to help one visualize components of the current understanding of the implications and consequences of disease or disability for the ability of an individual to function in any or all domains.

model of optimal development Wagner's model of adolescent development encompassing six domains of function: biologic, cognitive, emotional, social, moral, and vocational.

models of disablement Models that include definitions for the terms *disease, impairment, disability,* and *handicap,* in order to permit international communication for the purpose of acquiring data banks used for epidemiology and outcome studies on a large scale.

monitoring function Mental activities that let us think about what we are doing before, during, and after we do it, including intellectual awareness of personal skills, the ability to anticipate task demands or outcomes, the ability to detect errors in one's work, and the ability to organize one's actions to complete a desired task.

mood Refers to the amount of pleasant and friendly or unpleasant and unfriendly behavior in various situations.

mood disorder Disorders in affect, most typically depression and bipolar disorder.

morbidity Rate of incidence of a disease.

Moro reflex Key pattern used in all neonatal assessment to determine neurologic integrity; the infant's head is dropped backward, stimulating the vestibular system of the inner ear, and causing abduction of the arms, followed by adduction of the arms across the chest.

morphology Study of word structure, including alterations in word structure to change word meaning.

mortality Death rate in a given population.

motion hypothesis Notion that self-produced movement is important in the development of depth perception and spatial judgment.

motor behavior Any performance of movement that can be observed or documented.

motor control Study of the neurobiologic processes underlying human movement.

motor development Acquisition of motor behavior that is heavily maturational in origin.

motor learning Both a specific type of learning and an approach to therapeutic intervention following injury that is directed toward searching for a motor solution that emerges from an interaction of the individual with the task and the environment.

motor planning The ability of the brain to conceive, organize, and carry out a sequence of unfamiliar actions. Also known as motor praxis.

motor praxis Ability of the brain to conceive, organize, and carry out a sequence of unfamiliar actions. Also known as motor planning.

motor program Message sent from the CNS to the spinal cord and out to the muscles containing a code of the specific parameters of how the muscular system is supposed to act.

multiple intelligences Intelligences that cannot presently be measured psychometrically, like intrapsychic capacity, in addition to those that can.

multiple role lifestyle Lifestyle involving management of competing career and family roles.

musculoskeletal system Key system in executing motor behavior; considered the effector system of motor control.

myelin Fatty or lipid-based substance that encases nerves and aids nerve conduction velocity.

myelination Developmental process of building a myelin sheath on the nerves to insulate the fibers and ensure that messages sent by nerve fibers are not lost en route.

myopia Nearsightedness.

nativist school Perspective that genetic predisposition and innate ability largely explain the development of perception.

natural environment Animate and inanimate elements of the natural or physical environment, including physical geography, flora and fauna, climate, light, and natural events.

negative reinforcement Process that removes a persistent undesirable stimulus—that is, removes a negative.

negativism Expression of autonomy that includes verbal repetitions of the word "no" and physical resistance in the form of hitting, biting, kicking, and tantrums.

negotiability Ability to access a feature of the environment and use it for its intended purpose in a manner acceptable to the person.

neonatal intensive care unit (NICU) A specialized nursery prepared to take care of infants who require resuscitation and mechanical ventilation.

neonatal motor behavior Reflexive pattern of behavior that dominates the newborn's motor behavior and is emergent, depending on the interaction of a number of systems both intrinsic and extrinsic to the organism; may be best explained by a systems theory of motor control and can be classified as having a very deep attractor well.

neonatal neck-righting reaction First of the rotary righting reactions to develop that allow the infant to transfer from one postural set to another, i.e., prone to supine.

neonatal period Period of the first 4 weeks after birth.

neonate Name given to a baby for the first 4 weeks after birth.

neural plate Region of embryonic ectodermal cells that lie directly above the notochord.

neurogenesis Process by which new nerve cells are generated.

neuromotor behavior The most prescriptive of the neonatal characteristics; includes the behavior of the newborn that is a direct reflection of the parts of the central nervous system.

nonassociative learning Learning in which the individual does not rely on memory or prior experiences to associate with the sensory experience; important in the learning of physical and motor skills, resulting in both transient and long-term modulation at the synaptic level; important in rehabilitation of movement disorders.

nonvolitional behaviors Behaviors that occur with thought or planning.

normalization Normalization reflects an internalization of the specialized habits and routines associated with activity limitations to such a degree that they are integrated as ordinary personal and family occupations. The normalization process represents the successful integration of activity limitations into daily occupations in a manner that enhances function.

norm-referenced Summative assessment in which individual performance is evaluated against the standard deviation of scores obtained from a normative group or population; scores are typically presented as standard scores, z scores, or stanines, referenced to the bell-shaped curve; useful for diagnosis but not sensitive to intervention effects.

notochord Hollow chord at the embryo's midline formed when mesenchymal cells migrate upward between the ectodermal and endodermal layers. The vertebral column will form around this rodlike structure. The notochord provides some stability to the embryo and also serves as "the primary inductor" of early embryonic development.

obesity Indicated by a body mass index (BMI) of $30kg/m^2$.

object play Manipulation of objects in an intrinsically motivated activity that is not focused on some externally imposed goal.

occupation An occupation is a meaningful action in the context of a person's life.

occupational model Theoretical model that focuses on competence in performance of desired human occupations.

Occupational Therapy Practice Framework A classification scheme by the American Occupational Therapy Association that organizes client factors, performance skills, areas of occupation, performance patterns, and context.

older adolescents As defined in Chapter 12, young people ages 16–18.

olfactory perception Mental function involved in distinguishing differences in smells; sometimes used as a tool to help stimulate persons in a coma state; often results in very strong, lasting memories that are usually emotional in nature.

oligohydramnios Insufficient amount of amniotic fluid, sometimes associated with kidney problems in the fetus.

onlooker play Behavior that occurs when children watch other children play without engaging in the play activity themselves.

operant conditioning Type of behavioral conditioning in which the behavioral response is strengthened in the presence of reinforcers.

operating processes In the theory of transformed parenting, the processes of creating a mindset, guarding hope, experiencing chronic sorrow, and adaptation by actions.

optical righting reaction (ORR) A vision-dependent transitional movement pattern that persists throughout life. When the visual field appears tilted, the individual uses visual information to seek a vertical orientation for the body. This response can conflict with the vestibular/gravity-mediated righting responses in some environments, causing disorientation.

oral motor reflexes Reflexes specific to the muscle actions of the mouth and oral area.

organogenesis The development of major organs and organ systems, such as the heart and lungs; occurs during the embryonic period.

orientation An awareness of who you are, where you are, and what time it is.

ossification Formation of bone.

osteopenia Osteopenia refers to decreased calcification or density of bone. Having osteopenia places a person at risk for developing osteoporosis, a more serious condition that causes bones to become brittle and possibly break.

osteoporosis Disease with high incidence and prevalence, especially in women, in which imbalance between bone resorption and bone formation leads to susceptibility to fracture.

overweight For a child, indicated by BMI above the 95th percentile for his age; for an adult, indicated by BMI of 25–29.9 kg/m^2.

palliative coping An emotion-focused form of coping in which the main objective is to feel better through the management of the emotional response to a stressful situation in order to relinquish oneself of the psychological or physical impact.

palmar grasp Pattern that occurs in response to pressure in the palm, causing an infant's fingers to curl around the examiner's finger, appearing to be a grasp.

parallel play Developmentally typical play pattern at 2–4 years, when children are not mature enough to sustain interaction with others. Children bring toys or establish play space near others, yet play independently.

parasympathetic nervous system Mediates basic physiologic behaviors such as digestion, elimination, and sexual function.

passive acceptance viewpoint Cultural perspective that endorses a stance of living in harmony with nature;

one implication is greater acceptance of alterations in structure and function.

patent ductus arteriosus Failure of the ductus arteriosus to close; often seen in premature infants.

Pavlov, Ivan Russian psychologist responsible for description of the classical conditioning paradigm (Pavlov's dogs).

perception Sensation-based complex mental function that allows the brain to recognize and interpret sensory information; requires both attentional and memory functions to be efficient and is influenced by the perceiver's experience and previous knowledge.

perceptual functions Functions that include the mental processes of matching sensations with meaning by using information from the individual's sensory environment.

perceptual learning Complex form of nonassociative learning that does not require prior experience but does require memory; allows an individual to store information to be recalled at some later date after viewing performance of a new skill.

perceptual motor skills Controlled, volitional motor acts that respond in a dynamic way to sensory perceptions.

perceptual trace In Adam's theory of motor learning, a working sensory motor plan that can be modified by experience or feedback.

performance processes In the theory of transformed parenting, reality-construing processes, contextual processes, and operating processes.

performance skills Skills that involve the ability to physically perform within the environment and that can be measured by attributes such as goal achievement, accuracy, and speed.

peripheral nervous system Consists primarily of nerves and nerve roots that connect the control centers of the CNS to external sites, such as muscles, glands, or skin.

periventricular leukomalacia (PVL) Characterized by necrosis and cavitation of the white matter of the brain and may develop following a vascular insult, such as intraventricular hemorrhage, or in isolation, presumably due to some insult to the neural tissue.

persistence The length of time particular activities are pursued by an individual, with or without obstacles.

persistent fetal circulation Occurs when the shunting of blood persists beyond the perinatal period and is treated by aggressive oxygenation through special ventilators or through *extracorporeal membrane oxygenation (ECMO)*.

personal factors Contextual influences on function and activity limitation that are intrinsic, such as gender, age, temperament, and personality.

personality Enduring emotional and behavioral characteristics of an individual.

personality type (A & B) Categories used to describe predominant personality classifications. Type A is more aggressive, ambitious, and typically masculine in traits; Type B is more relaxed, easygoing, and not highly ambitious.

personality type (C & D) Categories used to describe predominant personality types. Type C personalities are described as cooperative and compliant; Type D personalities are described as distressed and negative.

personality type (Holland) One of six personality types associated with fitting certain vocation types.

pervasive developmental disorder (PDD) Name given to spectrum of disorders that have four characteristics in common: impairments in both verbal and nonverbal communication; stereotypical interests, activities, or behaviors; impairments in social interaction; and a history of developmental delay before age 3.

phasic bite reflex Elicited by pressure on the gums, with a normative response being an up-and-down motion of the jaw, that often accompanies feeding behavior.

phonology Rules governing combinations of phonemes to produce words that have meaning.

physical activity Any activity that requires physical exertion that the individual participates in to develop or maintain fitness.

physical environment The natural and man-made features of the space a person occupies.

physical functions Ability to react to and act upon the environment using the existing behavioral repertoire.

physiologic age Ability to adapt to the environment in normal life situations or life crises.

physiologic immaturity Present in preterm infants; adversely affects the development of the lungs, since their development in the last postnatal trimester in utero is in large part what enables the successful transition to extrauterine life at term birth.

Piaget, Jean Twentieth-century psychologist who presented one of the most comprehensive and accepted theories of cognitive development for its time; his theories have influenced numerous subsequent psychological and educational systems.

placing reaction Reaction present in both hands and feet that is facilitated by stroking the back of the hand or top of the foot against a tabletop, causing the infant to lift the limb in flexion, then extend the limb as if to place it on the table.

plantar grasp Pattern representing primitive attempt at balance that occurs in response to pressure across the metatarsal heads, just under the toes, causing grasping by the toes.

plasticity The ability to modify behavioral or neural systems in response to changes in the internal or external environment.

play Human activity voluntarily engaged in for pleasure that reflects individual differences and preferences and becomes more complex as one matures.

playfulness Characteristic pattern of interaction that includes the tendency to seek opportunities for play, to suspend reality, and to behave with spontaneity.

pluripotent cells Primordial cells that may still differentiate into various specialized types of tissue elements.

polyhydramnios An excess of amniotic fluid; may be associated with leakage of fluid from the fetus into the amniotic sac.

positive reinforcement Process that results in increasing the probability that a positive reward will be offered.

positive support reactions One of the key patterns seen in standing, where extension through the lower limbs is mediated when the infant is held in vertical suspension and the feet are placed on the surface; occurs without true weight bearing and must be integrated to permit true weight bearing and walking to occur.

postconceptional age Common terminology associated with dating the age of the preterm infant.

postural control Ability to control your body's position in space, to remain erect in spite of changes in the surface you are walking on.

postural control reflexes Associated with development of postural control, especially as the neonate works against gravity.

postural set Alignment of body parts at any given point in time.

postural stability Ability to keep the body balanced and aligned.

posture Alignment of the body at any given point in time, including both biomechanical and neuromotor elements.

poverty Has been described in terms of absolute and relative levels: *Absolute poverty* refers to severe conditions of inadequate shelter, poor nutrition, and an increased risk for delays or disability. *Relative poverty* describes the condition of those who can afford some basic necessities but are unable to maintain an average standard of living.

power grasp Used for managing large or heavy objects; includes cylindrical grip, spherical grip, hook grip, and lateral prehension.

pragmatics Mental function of understanding the communicative uses of language.

precision grasp Develops after power grasp patterns and emerges in the preschool years; includes palmar prehension and lateral prehension.

prehension Using the hands for grasping, holding, and manipulation of objects.

prelinguistic period Period from birth to 12 months in which developmental changes in cognitive motor and social domains occur; when the period ends, the child can use words to refer to things.

preoperational stage Typically period of 3–6 years; intelligence is demonstrated through the use of symbols, language use matures, and memory and imagination are developed; learning continues to be greatly influenced by experience, and children are egocentric in this period.

presbyastasis Balance and dizziness resulting in disequilibrium in the absence of overt pathology.

presbycusis Age-related inner ear dysfunction that diminishes auditory acuity and is the most common cause of hearing loss in adults.

presbyopia Most common visual problem in older adults; loss of accommodation or ability to focus on near objects.

preterm infant Infant born at less than 37 weeks' gestation.

preterm infant environment Preterm infants are cared for in a very special environment known as the *Neonatal Intensive Care Unit (NICU)* that is typically considered a Level III nursery, meaning it has the technology and staff necessary to resuscitate infants; the nurse-to-infant ratio in a typical NICU is very low, and the necessities of medical caregiving in these nurseries create an abnormal environment for the preterm infant, who normatively should be in a totally flexed position in a dark, aquatic environment.

primitive stepping Spontaneous and reciprocal flexion of one leg and extension of the other in alternating patterns in response to the infant being tipped slightly forward; occurs without true weight bearing and must be integrated to permit true weight bearing and walking to occur.

problem solving Ability to interpret information from the monitoring functions, like error detection, and act on that information to self-correct, leading to effective performance and the ability to appropriately end (or terminate) activities.

procedural learning Learning of tasks that are performed automatically, such as the development of skill in areas like sports and playing musical instruments; occurs after declarative learning is complete.

process skills Skills that allow the transfer and adaptation of previously learned tasks to novel or altered situations.

productivity Those activities and tasks that are done to enable the person to provide support to the self, family, and society through the production of goods and services.

products and technology Natural or human-made products, equipment, and technology in an individual's immediate environment that are gathered, created, produced, or manufactured. It is recognized that any product or technology can be used to improve the function of an individual with an activity limitation and thus be considered "assistive technology."

prognosis The prospect of survival and recovery from a disease as anticipated from the usual course of that disease or indicated by special features of the case.

proprioceptors Sensory receptors located in muscles, tendons, joints, and ligaments that provide information about position and movement of the body in space.

prospective payment system (PPS) A reimbursement system in which the health or long-term-care facility receives a flat-fee reimbursement related to individual diagnosis; designed to control costs and motivate facilities to provide high-quality care with short length of stay.

protective factor Opposite of risk factor. Protective factors are personal or environmental factors that insulate or counteract the potential negative impact of risk factors.

protective reactions Protective reactions, in postural control, are localized reactions to displacement or unexpected postural change. These reactions vary in degree from limb-specific to whole-body reactions based on the degree of displacement. Protective reactions involve a pattern of abduction and extension.

proximal transverse palmar arch Rigid arch that balances stability and mobility in the hand.

proximodistal From the center, or midline, moving outward.

psychological challenges In adolescence, the emotional and cognitive changes associated with the ability to think abstractly.

psychological functions Exemplified by the individual's ability to complete tasks associated with his life roles, as well as gaining the affective behaviors necessary to master the environment.

psychometric approaches to intelligence Define intelligence as the ability to assimilate factual knowledge, to recall either recent or remote events, to reason logically, to manipulate concepts (either numbers or words), to translate the abstract to the literal and the

literal to the abstract, to analyze and synthesize forms, and to deal meaningfully and accurately with problems and priorities deemed important in a particular setting.

psychomotor domain Involves movement and includes all the activities that give an individual mastery over the environment; encompasses both cognitive and affective behavioral domains through cognitive ability, motivation, and affect.

psychomotor functions Mental functions of control over physical and motor skills; include the ability to originate (plan) and initiate (begin) movements, monitor and adjust motions in progress, perform learned tasks automatically without conscious direction, and pace, limit, or end movement based on activity demands.

psychosocial approaches to intelligence State that not all aspects of human learning can be quantified and that there are many types of intelligence, rather than a single intelligence factor.

public policy Standards of administrative control and organizational mechanisms established by governments at the local, regional, national, and international levels and typically expressed through legislation that reflects the values of a society.

pulmonary hypertension Caused by diminished blood flow through the lungs associated with vascular resistance in the lung capillary beds staying extremely high.

punishment Addition of a negative or aversive stimulus to a negative reinforcement situation.

race Distinct biologic attributes possessed by a group of people, including skin color, hair type, and bone structure.

raking A developmental grasp pattern that involves using all of the fingers in a raking motion to slide small objects into the palm to pick them up. This grasp does not persist in typically developing children beyond one year.

rapport talk Use of language in conversation as a way to connect and negotiate relationships, characteristic of young females.

reaction time Time delay between presentation of a stimulus and motor response to that stimulus.

readiness State of being prepared for use or action after sufficient growth and maturation have occurred, irrespective of the amount of exposure provided.

realistic career exploration Ginzberg's theory of occupational choice corresponds to late adolescence, as the young adult develops a chosen career category, taking into account personal abilities and realistic evaluation of constraints.

recall Ability to organize information into usable form, thereby affecting retrieval of information.

recent memory Also called *short-term memory;* recall of stimuli that occurred more than five minutes ago; the most vulnerable in brain injury or disease.

receptive language The understanding of what is said, written, or signed; develops earlier than expressive language.

reflex Stereotypic obligatory response to a given stimulus.

reflex integration Reflexive pattern that is no longer a highly predictable or preferred one, promoting the development of more variable patterns of neuromotor behavior that underlie functional accomplishments.

Rehabilitation Act of 1973 One of the first significant pieces of civil rights legislation for individuals with disabilities; Section 504 is often mentioned because it said that any program that received federal funding, such as public education and transportation, could not discriminate against people with disabilities. This act has been revised and amended several times since its 1973 passage.

reinforcement Consequence to an action that modifies the likelihood of the action being repeated.

report talk Use of language as a way to give information and directives.

respiratory distress syndrome Condition caused by immaturity of the lungs, which results from an infant being born too soon; present in nearly all preterm infants; attributable to a lack of surfactant.

respite care Formal programs providing trained individuals who can care for an individual with a disability, giving regular caregivers short-term relief from daily tasks of caregiving.

response specifications From Schmidt's theory of motor learning, the rules for directing a movement.

restrained formal communication Form of communication characterized by governing one's emotions or passions and adhering to traditional standards of correctness without emotion content.

retinopathy of prematurity (ROP) Condition caused by abnormal vascularization of the eye and related to levels of oxygenation; can range from mild to severe, and in the most severe cases, the infant with ROP is blind.

rhythmicity Refers to the regularity of physiologic functions such as hunger, sleep, and elimination.

righting reaction A category of transitional movement patterns that help the individual maintain a vertical alignment with respect to gravity during movement and position change.

risk factor Personal or environmental factor, as defined in the ICF (World Health Organization, 2002), that leaves the individual at risk or susceptible to injury, disease, impairment, or death.

role schemas A person's social position within a culture and the expected behaviors of a person in that position.

rooting reflex Elicited by peri-oral touch; is the vestige of early patterns allowing newborns of other species born with their eyes closed to seek out the maternal teat.

rotation Involves movements at or near the pads of the fingers that move an object around one or more of its axes.

routine-based assessment Consistent with a top-down model, judges the capabilities of the individual within everyday routines and activities.

safe sex Refers to taking precautions that decrease the potential for transmitting or acquiring sexually transmitted diseases.

sandwich generation Term used to describe the role of middle-aged adults who are "sandwiched" between older and younger cohorts in the population. Additionally, this term serves to describe the middle-aged adult who is concurrently serving in a role of both parent to her own children and adult child of a parent.

sarcopenia An age-related decline in muscle mass and thereby muscle strength.

Schmidt, Richard Originator of the open-loop theory of motor learning, including concept of a motor response schema.

school function assessment (SFA) Judgment-based assessment developed for use with children from kindergarten through sixth grade to help elementary students with disabilities succeed by identifying their strengths and needs in nonacademic functional tasks.

school readiness Mastering of prerequisite developmental criteria for success in the school environment; there are no agreed-upon criteria, but in general a child must be healthy both physically and emotionally.

screening process Process used to detect problems that identify an individual as falling outside age-related norms of function.

Sears, Robert Social learning theorist who combined a number of perspectives, including psychoanalytic and behavioral; he theorized that a child imitates the mother because this is reinforcing.

Section 504 of Rehabilitation Act of 1973 Declares that a person cannot be excluded on the basis of disability alone from any program or activity receiving federal funds.

selective attention A type of attention that involves focusing on a specific aspect of an experience while ignoring other aspects.

self-actualization Highest level in Maslow's hierarchy, defined as the need to become all one can be.

self-advocacy Advocating for one's needs and rights.

self-definition How an individual views himself or herself, including his or her various roles.

self-efficacy Belief in one's personal power to change things, to organize and implement effective strategies to deal with potential situations that may be novel, unpredictable, or stressful.

self-management skills Skill in the general self-care tasks and the more specific skills of organizing time, space, and materials for a specific task.

self-organizing behavior Behavior from a systems perspective; implies an extremely complex interaction between systems, which act together in infinite ways to produce a behavioral result.

self schemas The characteristics and traits a person assigns to self.

semantics Meaning parameter of language.

sensorimotor stage Typically ages 0–2 years; intelligence is demonstrated through motor activity without the use of symbols like written or spoken language, and knowledge of the world is based on the child's physical interactions and experiences.

sensorineural hearing loss Hearing loss due to problems with the inner ear or end organ of hearing.

sensory function in the newborn Refers to the stage at which all senses are functioning, though some may be relied on more than others, with the senses of smell, taste, and touch being highly developed, and hearing and vision being somewhat less developed.

sensory integration Term widely used in the neuroscience literature to describe the brain's ability to automatically combine sensory information from a variety of different senses to permit accurate categorization of perceptual information.

sensory integration theory Describes the senses (auditory, vestibular, proprioceptive, tactile, and visual) as contributing to learning and the development of important functional skills like regulation of activity level and attention span, eye-hand coordination, visual perception, and many metacognitive functions; also states that both the global and specific mental functions that allow us to interact and respond in purposeful ways depend on adequate organization of sensory information.

sensory threshold Refers to the amount of stimulation, such as sounds or light, necessary to evoke discernable responses in an individual.

sentence embedding Process wherein phrases and clauses are combined with other clauses or phrases to create more complex utterances.

separation anxiety Refers to insecurity and emotional distress that occurs when individual is removed from someone or something familiar; tends to lessen over time.

services From the ICF, services that provide benefits, structured programs, and operations, in various sectors of society, designed to meet the needs of individuals.

sexuality The state of being sexual, including not only the physical act but also the more complicated elements of emotion, physiologic drive, pregnancy, birth control, and sexually transmitted disease.

shaping Strategy used with operant conditioning that involves a deliberate and gradual plan to change behavior.

shift movements Movements that occur at the finger and thumb pads with the alternation of thumb and finger movement.

short-term memory Memory that lasts for seconds or minutes; processed in a specific part of the temporal lobe of the brain and is therefore susceptible in diseases such as Alzheimer's.

sibling subsystems Interactions between siblings in a family system.

sick role A social role described by Talcott Parsons in 1959 in which the sick individual is exempt from normal social role responsibilities, such as going to work.

skeletal maturity The attainment of maximal or peak bone mass, usually occurring between the ages of 25 and 35.

Skinner, B. F. The best-known of the behaviorists; developed principles of reinforcement as ways to study and control behavior.

sleep functions Periods of reversible mental disengagement from one's immediate environment accompanied by characteristic physiologic changes.

small for gestational age (SGA) Used to describe infants born at less than the 10th percentile for weight based on gestational age.

social competence Smooth sequence of social skills applied in a dynamic way across various social contexts.

social effects of preterm birth Refers to the result of a preterm birth, in which the infant is typically resuscitated if necessary, shown to the mother, and whisked away to the NICU—which is frequently in a different hospital—leaving the postpartum woman behind and therefore resulting in maternal-infant separation almost immediately.

social environment Those aspects of the environment that include support and relationships that provide physical or emotional support and assistance.

social functions Functions that encompass motor, cognitive, and affective behavioral domains; the ability to participate in a social environment, filling social roles and expectations.

social knowledge The understanding of appropriate social behavior, including decoding and interpreting social cues, searching and selecting an optimal response, and undertaking the correct action.

social learning Acquisition of behaviors within a social context.

social model Model that sees society rather than the individual as the problem, viewing disability as a society-created problem.

social referencing Comparison of self to peers; often begins in the school-age child.

societal-level risk factors Risk factors such as teenage pregnancy and maternal drug and alcohol abuse.

societal limitation An individual's ability to participate in societal functions; some, such as work, may be related to many factors, such as alterations in structure and function, intrinsic factors, and extrinsic factors. Extrinsic factors may be physical, such as barriers, or social, such as attitudes.

sociocultural challenges In adolescence, finding appropriate societal roles that are suitable physically and psychologically.

solitary play Independent play characteristically acquired between 18 months and 4 years of age.

somatic awareness Information about the state of the body (touch, pressure, temperature, pain, etc.).

somatosensory General sensory input to the central nervous system from the body, typically touch and pressure.

spatial awareness Understanding of both near and far space around an individual; assessed by the accuracy of locating items in that space.

Special Olympics International program dedicated to empowering children and adults with disabilities to become more physically fit, respected, and productive through sports training and competition.

special senses Those senses that are unique and supplied by cranial nerves, such as vision, hearing, and taste.

Specific Mental Functions Functions of memory, language, and calculation; more easily quantified than the global functions and more often a focus of intervention following brain injury.

specification (stage of career choice) In Super's theory, a focused development of career ideas characteristic of late adolescence and young adulthood.

speech Oral form of language.

speech disorders Speech sound disorders (phonology), voice disorders (voice generation), and fluency disorders (stuttering).

sports Physical activity engaged in for pleasure or fulfillment, often in competition against self or others; three types of sports focus include competitive, family, and social.

stability limit The farthest that an individual can shift his mass off center without altering his base of support.

stability of temperament Established aspect of personality that can change as the individual gains experience and skills but has been found to be fairly constant within an individual beyond infancy.

standardized tests Measurement instruments in which the procedures used to collect the information and score performance are the same across examiners.

static postural stability Ability to maintain the preferred posture when the body is still; includes the ability to remain upright while sitting in a chair or to stand quietly when waiting in line without leaning against support or sitting.

static visual acuity Refers to the ability to discern details when both the person and the target are static; useful for reaching and grasping objects and the basic hand skills required in infancy and early in the preschool years; permits the development of eye-hand coordination.

stereotypy Intrinsic nonpurposeful movement pattern that repeats itself.

stimulus discrimination Differentiation of stimuli causing a conditioned response to a certain stimuli but not to others.

stimulus generalization Extension of a conditioned response to additional neutral stimuli.

stranger anxiety An innate mistrust or wariness of new or unfamiliar people.

stress Emotional state, generally considered to be unpleasant, that occurs when a person is facing a demanding situation that is appraised by the person as taxing or exceeding her resources and endangering her well-being.

substance abuse Overindulgence in and dependence on an addictive substance, especially alcohol or a narcotic drug; in pregnancy, the use of drugs and alcohol that can result in negative long-term effects for the infant.

successful aging Refers to normal age-related changes that are present without modification of risk and without significant functional change.

suck-swallow reflex The most basic of the neonatal motor behaviors that is associated with the intake of nourishment.

sucking Early oral motor behavior of the neonate that is differentiated from the more mature patterns developed by the end of the 1st postnatal trimester.

suckling Process of pressing the nipple or teat to the hard palate and using a process of positive pressure, or expression, to obtain milk.

Super, Donald Theorist who addressed development of vocation; postulated that through developmental stages, vocational decision making becomes clearer and more realistic as self-concept is refined.

superior pincer grasp Developmental grasp pattern using the distal tips of the thumb and forefinger for precision, with the ulnar fingers inhibited and the thumb in opposition.

support and relationships Contextual factors that influence a person's disability status. Immediate (spouses, siblings, children, parents) and extended (aunts, uncles, cousins) family members assume many roles and responsibilities in response to their family member's impairments or disability. These responses may serve as facilitators or barriers for adults experiencing impairments that create changes in function.

symmetrical tonic neck reflex (STNR) The STNR is a tonic reflex initiated by the infant's head position. When the head and neck are in extension, extensor tone increases in the upper trunk and limbs, with an increase in flexion in the lower limbs. Conversely, when the head and neck are in flexion, flexor tone increases in the upper trunk and limbs, with an increase in extension in the lower limbs.

sympathetic nervous system A division of the nervous system that controls "fight or flight" reactions and is associated with a high level of arousal.

synapse Junction across which a nerve impulse passes from an axon terminal to a neuron, muscle cell, or gland cell.

synaptogenesis The building of specialized junctions at which a nerve cell communicates with a target cell.

syntax Rules governing word order in a language.

systems From the ICF, administrative control and organizational mechanisms established by governments at the local, regional, national, and international levels.

tactile defensiveness Perception of ordinary, nonthreatening touch as aversive.

tactile perception Perception of touch that is important in the processing of somatic, kinesthetic, and haptic awareness.

temperament Collection of inborn differences among individuals that is closely associated with personality; the constitutional disposition of an individual to react in a particular way to situations.

temporal awareness Perception of time as it relates to the planning, sequencing, and altering of movement.

temporal organization Orderly and logically sequencing of steps in task.

tentative period Ginzberg's theory of occupational choice corresponding to ages 13–14 until late adolescence; individual begins to meet realities of career he is suited for, considering economic reality and potential barriers.

teratogen Agent that causes the production of physical defects in the developing embryo.

theory Set of propositions describing operations and causes of natural phenomena.

thermal regulation Refers to the fetus's ability to maintain body temperature outside the womb environment.

Thomas, Alexander Theorist who, with Stella Chess, developed a classic system for describing and categorizing temperament.

thought functions Specific functions related to the presence and development of ideas that emphasize the control of thought in terms of pace, content, and form.

toddling Immature walking pattern characterized by rapidity, wide base of support, and limited rotary movement between shoulder and pelvis.

tonic labyrinthine reflex Reflex that plays a role in mediating the gravity dependency of a human newborn based on the position of the head (body) in space; when the infant is prone, systemic flexion is facilitated, and when she is supine, systemic extension is facilitated, pulling her into gravity.

top-down assessment Assessment in which desired outcomes guide strategy.

transfer pattern Type of mobility pattern that allows individuals to transfer from one postural set to another, as from lying down to sitting.

transformed parenting, theory of Theory developed by Seideman and Kleine in 1995, based on interviews of parents of children with developmental delays; describes processes whereby parents change their envisioned role in order to deal with a child who has impairments or disabilities.

transitions The change from one characteristic life stage to another; for example, the transition from being a childless married couple to becoming parents.

translation Linear movement of the object in the hand from the finger surface to the palm or the palm to the fingers.

TriAlliance of Health and Rehabilitation Professions The largest constituency of health and rehabilitation professionals representing the professions of occupational therapy, physical therapy, audiology, and speech-language pathology; consists of the American Occupational Therapy Association (AOTA), the American Physical Therapy Association (APTA), and the American Speech-Language-Hearing Association (ASHA); represents a joint venture on the part of the three organizations to address issues of mutual concern and to initiate, as appropriate, collective action to enhance their individual responses to major societal problems.

trimester system System in which the human gestational period is divided into periods of 3 months, each being one third of the length of a pregnancy.

trophoblast In the first week of pregnancy, the outer layer of the blastocyst that will give rise to the placenta and other tissues.

Type A personality Originally described by Friedman and Rosenman (1959), this personality type is characterized by intense sustained drive for achievement, competition, and recognition.

Type C personality Type C personalities are described by Denollet (1998) as "cooperative and compliant" with authorities, but unexpressive and unassertive of their own negative emotions. In this case the belief is that unexpressed negative emotions weaken their immune system.

Type D personality Type D personalities are described by Denollet (2000) as a "distressed" personality type—one that has a tendency to experience negative emotions and to inhibit self-expression.

universal design Designing the physical environment, as in the personal home, in such a manner as to be accessible to people of all ages and various levels of physical abilities.

usual aging Refers to normal age-related alteration in physical and cognitive functions, such as increases in blood pressure and blood glucose and modest memory impairment; implies no major pathology, but disease risk factors are present.

vascularization Growth of blood vessels into a tissue or organ, with the result that the oxygen and nutrient supply is improved.

ventral motor neurons Neurons that activate muscle cells.

ventricular chambers of the heart The two chambers that form the lower portion of the heart.

verbal rehearsal In motor learning, characteristic of early stages, where individuals recite key points verbally.

vernix caseosa The fatty matter, consisting chiefly of dead epidermal cells and sebaceous secretions, covering the skin of a fetus and newborn.

very-low-birthweight infants Infants weighing 1,500 g or less.

vestibular perception Awareness of movement in terms of speed and direction; provides information for balance, movement, and personal protection, allowing an individual to walk on uneven surfaces or down darkened stairways without relying on vision.

Vgotsky, Lev Russian theorist who studied cognitive development with an emphasis on sociocultural influence.

vigilance The ability to maintain attention on important aspects of a task for a sustained period.

virtual (electronic) play Intrinsically motivated activity using an electronic device such as television, videogame, or computer for the purpose of enjoyment.

virtual environment Computer or other technology-driven social network of real and virtual human interaction at a communal or larger group level that operates for reasons of tradition, culture, business, pleasure, information exchange, institutional organization, legal procedure, governance, human betterment, social progress, spiritual enlightenment, among other reasons.

visual acuity Ability to focus the eyes in order to distinguish detail in the visual display.

visual discrimination Ability to discriminate visual details, the perception of depth, spatial relations, and directional orientation.

visual identification The matching, categorizing, and recognition of shape, size, color, and other ocular stimuli.

visual perception Most studied type of perception; includes both visual identification and visual discrimination; a key aspect of reading written language.

visual pursuit Slow, smooth eye movements, also known as tracking.

visual scanning Short, rapid changes of fixation from one point in the visual field to another, also known as saccadic eye movement.

visual skills Ability of the individual to use extraocular muscles to direct the eye.

visuospatial perception Perception based on a complex interaction of attention, visual perception, and analysis of speed and trajectory of movement; provides information on the relative position and motion of objects in the environment and interacts with tactile perception to help determine speed of movement needed for a given activity, to adjust the alignment of the body, and to develop the projected action sequences needed to be skilled in sports.

vocational development Typically, vocation is used to describe a "calling," or "life's work"; the term is typically used in describing the affective attachment one has to a career.

vocational self-concept Self-concept as it relates to participation in a particular occupation.

volitional behaviors Behaviors that occur with thought and cognitive planning.

vulnerable abilities Abilities most likely to decrease or diminish with advancing age, including reasoning, perceptual speed, short-term memory, visual processing, and processing speed.

Watson, John First American behaviorist; he viewed the stimulus-response relationship as the essential one between organism and environment.

weight training A planned regimen of exercise using resistance, which is typically in the form of free weights or a weight machine.

wellness Triangulated concept including physical, psychosocial, and spiritual health and well-being.

work Meaningful activity that helps us define our position in society, is an outlet for creativity, is a source of social stimulation, and provides fulfillment.

working memory The type of human memory in which past events are associated with present events.

younger adolescents As defined in Chapter 12, young people from 12 to 15 years of age.

zone of proximal development (ZPD) From Vgotsky's theory, refers to the child's preparedness to learn such that minimal support from the environment will result in learning.

zygote Single diploid cell resulting from the fusion of male and female gametes at fertilization.

Index

Note: Numbers followed by the letter "t" indicate tables; numbers in bold indicate figures.

Finger dexterity, 207
Fiscal intermediaries, 379–380
Fixity, level of, 7
FLAS (Fair Labor Standards Act), 233
Flexibility, 219, 313–314
Flexor postural control, 149
Flow, 179, 220
FLSA (Fair Labor Standards Act), 233
Fluency disorders, 82
Fluid intelligence, 291
FOAG (functional outcomes assessment grid), 402
FOF (fear of falling), 317
Foramen ovale, 116
Force, muscle, 287–288
Formal operations stage, 23, 24, 222
Fragile X disorder, 250
Frames of reference, 12–13, 16. *See also* Theory(-ies)
Free morphemes, 74
Free movement, zone of, 25
Freud, Sigmund, 17–18
   comparison of Erikson's and Piaget's stages with, 24t
   comparison of Erikson's theories and, 19t
Friendships:
   in adolescence, 226, 234
   during middle childhood, 210–211
FSN (Family Support Networks), 256
Fugl-Meyer scale, 397
Full-term infants, *see* Newborns
Function(s), 8–12
   body, 5
   of cognitive domain, 5–6
   defined, 5, 8
   and disablement, 10–11
   emotional, 6
   models of, 9–12
   neuromusculoskeletal and movement-related, 6
   physical, 8–9
   psychological, 9
   psychomotor, 6
   social, 9
Functional asymmetry, 29
Functional capacity, 312
Functional communication:
   in middle childhood, 207
   in preschoolers, 190
Functional independence measure (FIM), 401
Functional limitation:
   in Nagi's disablement model, 10
   in NCMRR model, 11
Functional outcomes assessment grid (FOAG), 402
Functional performance, 292
Functional skills, 400–401

Gag reflex, 119
Game devices, 211
Gardner, H., 44–45
Gastric system, 132
Gastroesophageal reflux (GER), 132
Gateway drugs, 366
Gender:
   and development of moral behavior, 21

   issues with newborns, 130
   and likelihood of poverty, 66
   middle childhood and physical differences in, 200
   and middle childhood peer relationships, 210
Gender differences:
   in dealing with disabled child, 253
   and functional communication in middle childhood, 207
   in strength, 220
Gender identity, 367
Gender identity disorder, 276
General pediatricians, 247
Geneticists, 247
Genital stage, 18
GER (gastroesophageal reflux), 132
Germinal period, 93, 98–100
Gesell, Arnold, 28–30
Gesell Schedules, 28
Gestalt school, 26, **27**
Gestational age, 93, 96, 132
Gestures, 65, 72, 236
Gibson, Eleanor, 26, 27
Gibson, James, 26, 27, 31
Giftedness:
   asynchronous development in, 193
   and loneliness during middle childhood, 205
Gilligan, Carol, 21
Ginzberg's developmental theory, 272, 274t
Glaucoma, 316–317
Global mental functions, 6, 38–39, 43–47
   Energy and Drive Functions, 46
   intellectual, 43–45
   Sleep Functions, 46
   temperament and personality, 45–57
GMFM (gross motor function measure), 399
Goal(s):
   in adolescence, 28
   preestablished, adulthood and lack of, 265
   quality of life as, 13–14
   self-care as, 320
   setting/attaining, 8
Goodness of fit, 45, 171
Grandparents, 166, **168**
   and care of disabled children, 255
   child-care by, 321
Graphomotor skills, 188–189
Grasp:
   in adolescence, 219–220
   in early infancy, 144, 145, **146**
   in late infancy, 152, 154
   in middle childhood, 207
   in middle infancy, 151
   in preschoolers, 181, 182
   in transitional infancy, 157, 158
Grasp reflex, 124
Grief, anticipatory, 134
Grip, 199, 200
Grooming (in adolescence), 227
Gross motor development:
   in early infancy (birth to 3 months), 143–144
   late infancy (7-9 months), 152–154
   in middle infancy (4-6 months), 147–151